Diagnosis and Management of Primary Bone Tumors

Won-Jong Bahk

Diagnosis and Management of Primary Bone Tumors

Volume 2

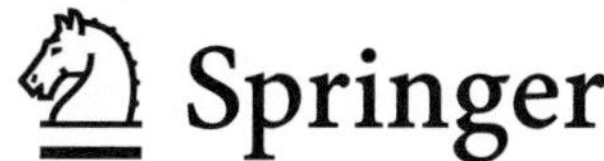

Won-Jong Bahk
Department of Orthopaedic Surgery
The Catholic University of Korea, Uijeongbu St. Mary's Hospital
Uijeongbu-si, Korea (Republic of)

ISBN 978-981-99-5500-8 ISBN 978-981-99-5498-8 (eBook)
https://doi.org/10.1007/978-981-99-5498-8

This Springer imprint is published by the registered company Springer Nature Singapore Pte Ltd.
The registered company address is: 152 Beach Road, #21-01/04 Gateway East, Singapore 189721, Singapore

Contents

Part I

Osteoclastic Giant Cell-Rich Tumors

1 Giant Cell Tumor

1.1 Definition

Conventional giant cell tumor (GCT) of bone is a benign but locally aggressive bone tumor composed of neoplastic component of mononuclear stromal cells and non-neoplastic component of numerous multinucleated osteoclast-like giant cells. Rarely, a frank malignancy can be found in association with conventional GCT as either primary de novo or secondary form of malignant transformation in a recurrent GCT or following radiation therapy for GCT.

1.2 Synonym

Osteoclastoma, but no more recommended to use.

1.3 Incidence

GCT is relatively common, accounting for about 4–7% of all primary bone tumors and about 20% of benign bone tumor [1–5].

1.4 Age

Most patients are between 20 and 40 years of age after epiphyseal closure, while chondroblastoma (CB) typically occurs in patients between 10 and 20 years of age before epiphyseal closure. A peak incidence is in their third decades. It is very rarely seen in patients younger than 15 years with open growth plate (Fig. 1.1e) and older than 60 years (Fig. 1.2a). However, "*fibrous histiocytoma variant*" of GCT typically occurs between 40 and 70 years of age that is older on average by some 10 years than conventional GCT [4].

W.-J. Bahk, *Diagnosis and Management of Primary Bone Tumors*,
https://doi.org/10.1007/978-981-99-5498-8_1

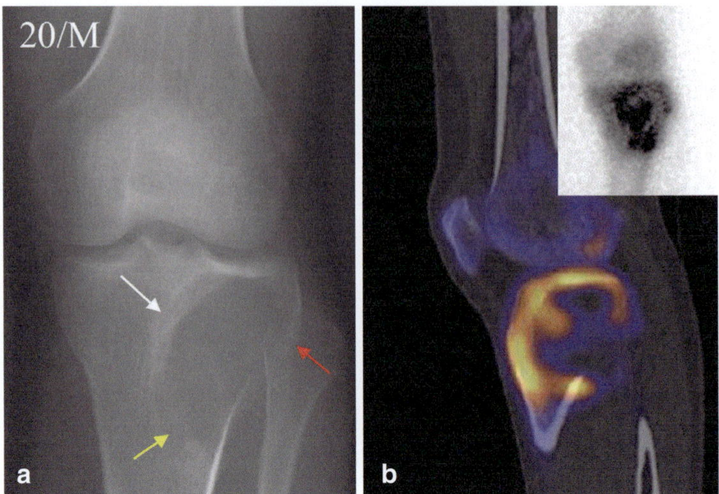

Fig. 1.1 (**a**) Radiograph taken for left knee of 3-month duration in 20-year-old young man shows an eccentric geographic osteolytic lesion having an incomplete rim of sclerosis proximally (white arrow) as well as ill-defined broad zone of transition distally (yellow arrow) in the epi-metaphysis of proximal tibia. Note cortical destruction with a naked soft tissue mass with no reactive bone formation, simulating malignant tumor (red arrow). (**b**) SPECT/CT image reveals an inhomogeneous uptake in left proximal tibia and adjacent soft tissue. Bone scan notes also a heterogenous strong uptake (inset). (**c**) MR images demonstrate an eccentric intramedullary large mass-like lesion with a cortical destruction and naked soft tissue mass formation (red arrows). The SI is intermediate on T1-weighted image and heterogeneously intermediate and high with multiple fluid-fluid levels on T2-weighted image, suggesting underlying solid tumor with secondary ABC. There are peri-tumoral bone marrow and soft tissue edema (asterisks). Post contrast image shows peripheral and septal enhancement of the bone (red arrow) and soft tissue (yellow arrow) lesion. Bone marrow (black asterisk) and soft tissue edema (red asterisk) are also enhanced. (**d**) Follow-up radiograph at 3 years after extended curettage, cementing, and plating under a histologic diagnosis of GCT with secondary ABC demonstrates no evidence of local recurrence. (**e**) Radiograph taken for left knee painful swelling of 4-month duration in 14-year-old girl shows a well-defined, eccentric, geographic destruction with a thin internal rind of reactive sclerosis (yellow arrow) and mild expansion surrounded by outer reactive new bone formation (red arrow), highly suggesting benignancy, in the epi-metaphysis of proximal tibia. Note the growth plate is still opened (black arrows), which would make a presumptive diagnosis of CB more likely than GCT. (**f**) Bone scan typically reveals a strongly increased uptake in the periphery of the lesion (arrow) with central photon defect (asterisk), so-called "*doughnut appearance*." (**g**) MR images demonstrate an eccentric medullary mass-like lesion showing a well-defined, eccentric, lobular lesion with a focal expansion of lateral cortex. The SI is low to intermediate on T1-weighted image and heterogeneous intermediate and high SI on T2-weighted image. Note dark signal of inner thin rim of sclerosis (yellow arrow) and outer rind of new bone formation (red arrow) on both sequences, highly indicating benignancy. The lesion is well enhanced (black asterisk). Peri-tumoral bone marrow (white asterisk) as well as soft tissue edema (yellow asterisk) is weakly enhanced. (**h**) Microscopic examination shows a typical pathologic finding of round to oval mononuclear stromal cell proliferation with evenly scattered multinucleated giant cells indicative of GCT

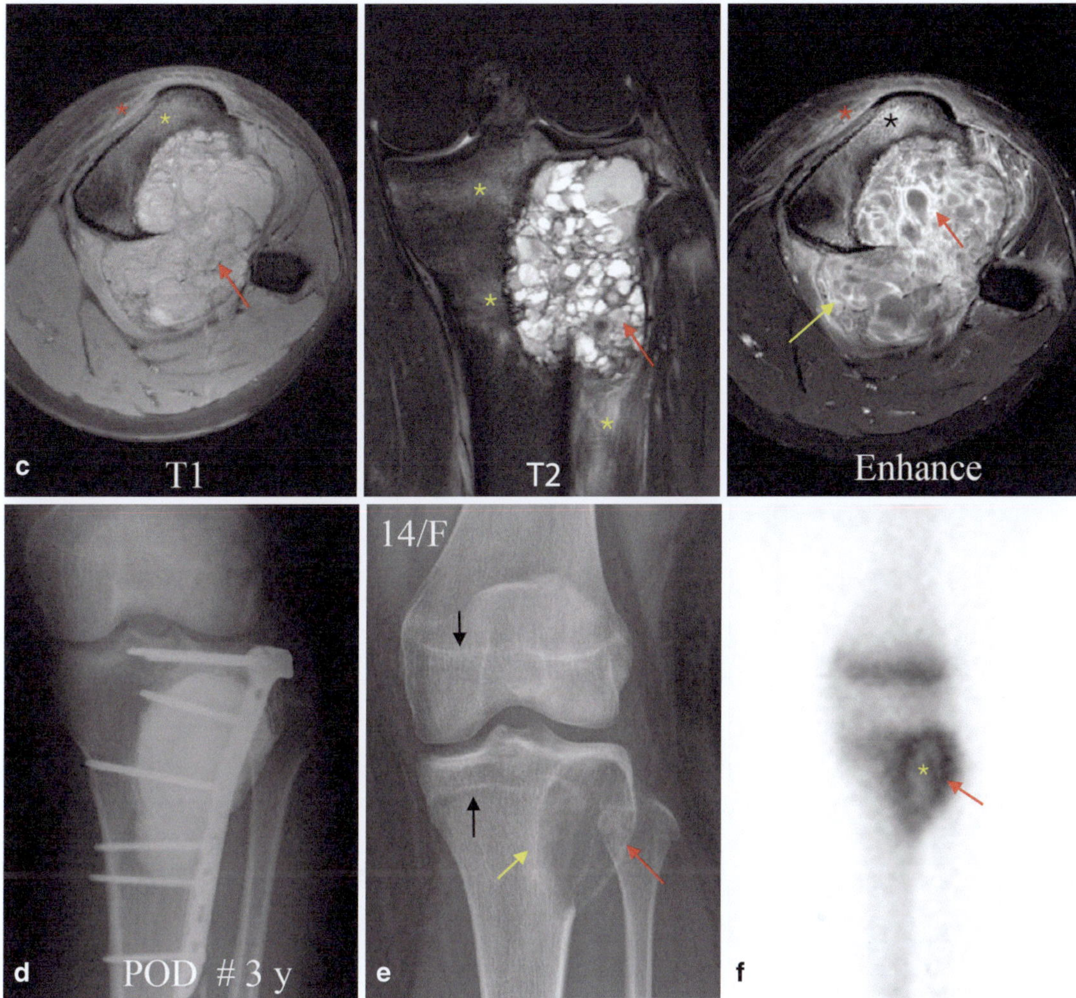

Fig. 1.1 (continued)

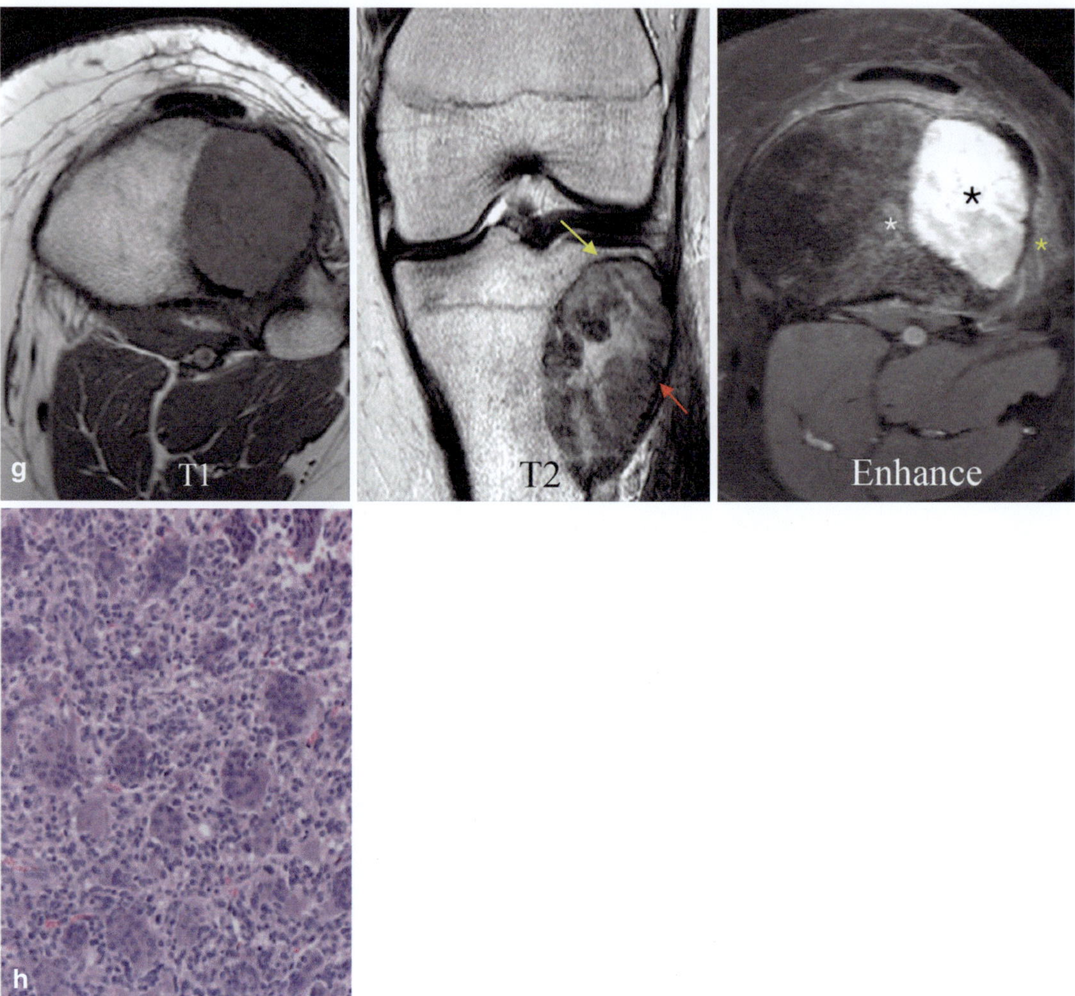

Fig. 1.1 (continued)

Fig. 1.2 (**a**) Radiograph taken for right shoulder pain with motion limitation of 3-month duration after curettage for GCT at another hospital 2 years ago in 64-year-old woman shows a huge expansile multi-lobulated osteolytic lesion with thin rim of surround sclerosis (red arrow) with a part of indiscernible rim (yellow arrow) affecting epimetaphysis of the proximal humerus, suggesting a local recurrence. (**b**) Pinhole bone scan reveals a strong uptake along the periphery (black arrow) with a weak uptake area of intact peripheral rim (blue arrow), which is not clearly seen on radiograph (yellow arrow on (**a**)), suggesting a possible benignancy despite the significant expansion. There is also increase uptake along the septa (red arrow). (**c**) MR images demonstrate a huge intramedullary mass-like lesion with intermediate SI with focal high signals on T1-weighted image and mostly high SI on T2-weighted image. The solid portion of lesion is heterogeneously well enhanced with central non-enhancing area possibly suggesting an extensive necrosis. (**d**) Follow-up radiograph at 3 years after en bloc resection and reconstruction with prosthesis under histologic diagnosis of recurrent conventional GCT notes no evidence of local recurrence

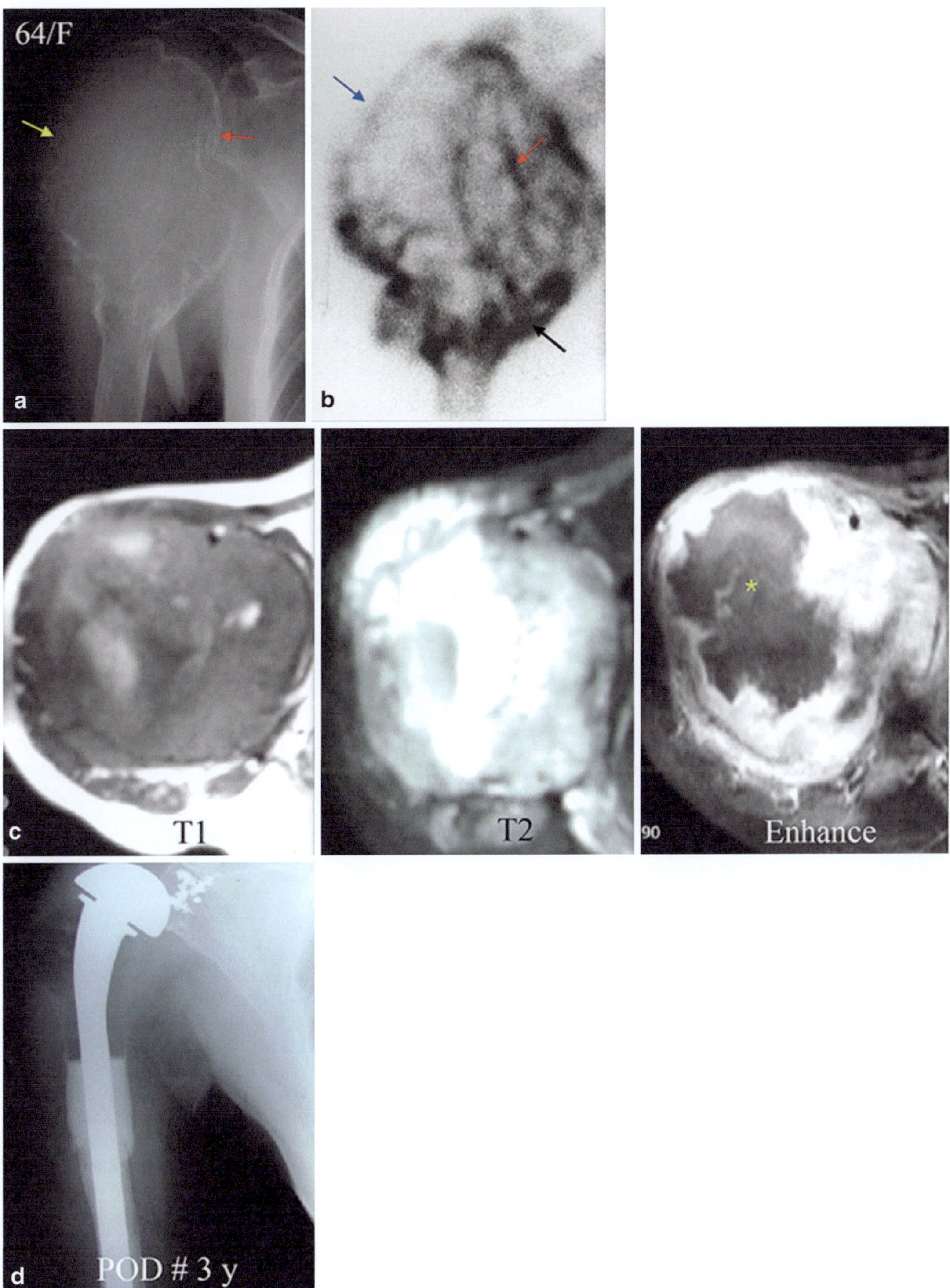
64/F
a
b
c
T1
T2
90
Enhance
d
POD # 3 y

1.5 Location

Vast majority of GCT locate preferentially in the end of the long tubular bones, with the distal femur followed by proximal tibia (knee) occupying over half of the cases, being the most frequent sites. Wrist (distal end of radius), shoulder (proximal end of humerus), and proximal fibular are the next common locations. Majority lesions are originated from the epiphysis and extend to a part of metaphysis (Figs. 1.1, 1.2, 1.3, 1.4, 1.5, 1.6, 1.7, and 1.8). Extremely rare cases may be centered purely in the metaphysis. In a large series of 327 patients managed at the Instituto Rizzoli, only 2 patients have the lesion limited to the metaphysis adjacent to an open growth plate [6]. However, pure diaphyseal location in conventional GCT virtually does not exist. Small number of cases involves patella, craniofacial bones, and small bones of hands and feet (Figs. 1.9, 1.10, and 1.11). When involving the latter small bones, it should be differentiated from GCRG (Figs. 3.1 and 3.2 in Chap. 3). Tarsal bone including calcaneus and talus is also involved in less than 1–2% of all cases [6–8]. Among the axial skeleton, vertebral body and sacrum are the most commonly involved sites. Very rarely, GCT can present as multiple synchronous or metachronous lesions, representing less than 1% of cases [9, 10].

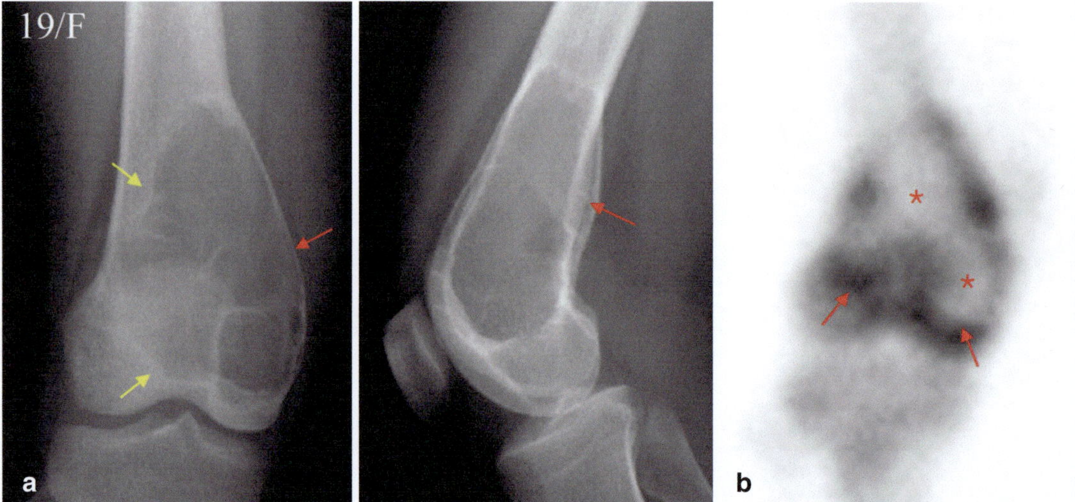

Fig. 1.3 (**a**) Radiograph taken for right knee pain of 5-month duration in 19-year-old young lady shows a well-defined, eccentric, multi-lobulated geographic destruction with moderate expansion affecting epi-metaphysis of right distal femur. Note narrow zone of transition with a thin rim of sclerosis (yellow arrows) and markedly thinned but intact cortex. There is an elevation of the periosteum producing thin periosteal shell of reactive bone (red arrow), which suggest a benignancy despite the large size of destructive lesion with bony expansion. (**b**) Pinhole bone scan reveals a heterogeneously increased uptake along the thin shell and inner septa of the lesion (arrows) with internal central photon defect areas (red asterisks). (**c**) MR images demonstrate a large medullary mass-like lesion with low to intermediate SI on T1-weighted image and heterogeneous low SI mixed with areas of high signal possibly due to hemosiderin, fibrosis, or recent hemorrhage on fat saturated T2-weighted image. Smooth periosteal reaction with cortical thinning is noted medial aspect of lesion, but cortical breakage is not seen (yellow arrows). The lesion is heterogeneously enhanced with non-enhanced areas (asterisks). (**d**) However, a several cortical tiny breaches were found in the cortex (yellow circles) neighboring to the window for curettage on operating field (yellow arrow). Frozen biopsy during surgery confirmed a diagnosis of a conventional GCT. (**e**) Extended curettage was performed using high-speed bur, followed by adjuvant cryosurgery using liquid nitrogen. (**f**) Immediate postoperative surgery shows cement filling and plate fixation for prevention of postoperative fracture. (**g**) However, radiograph taken for a severe knee pain after slip at 4 months after initial surgery notes fracture of medial condyle (red arrow). (**h**) Follow-up radiograph at 5 years after open reduction and additional plate fixation for fracture demonstrates good maintenance with no evidence of local recurrence. (**i**) She has hypertrophied scars (red arrows) but is doing well with a full range of knee motion. The scars become less prominent by scar revision by plastic surgeon (inset)

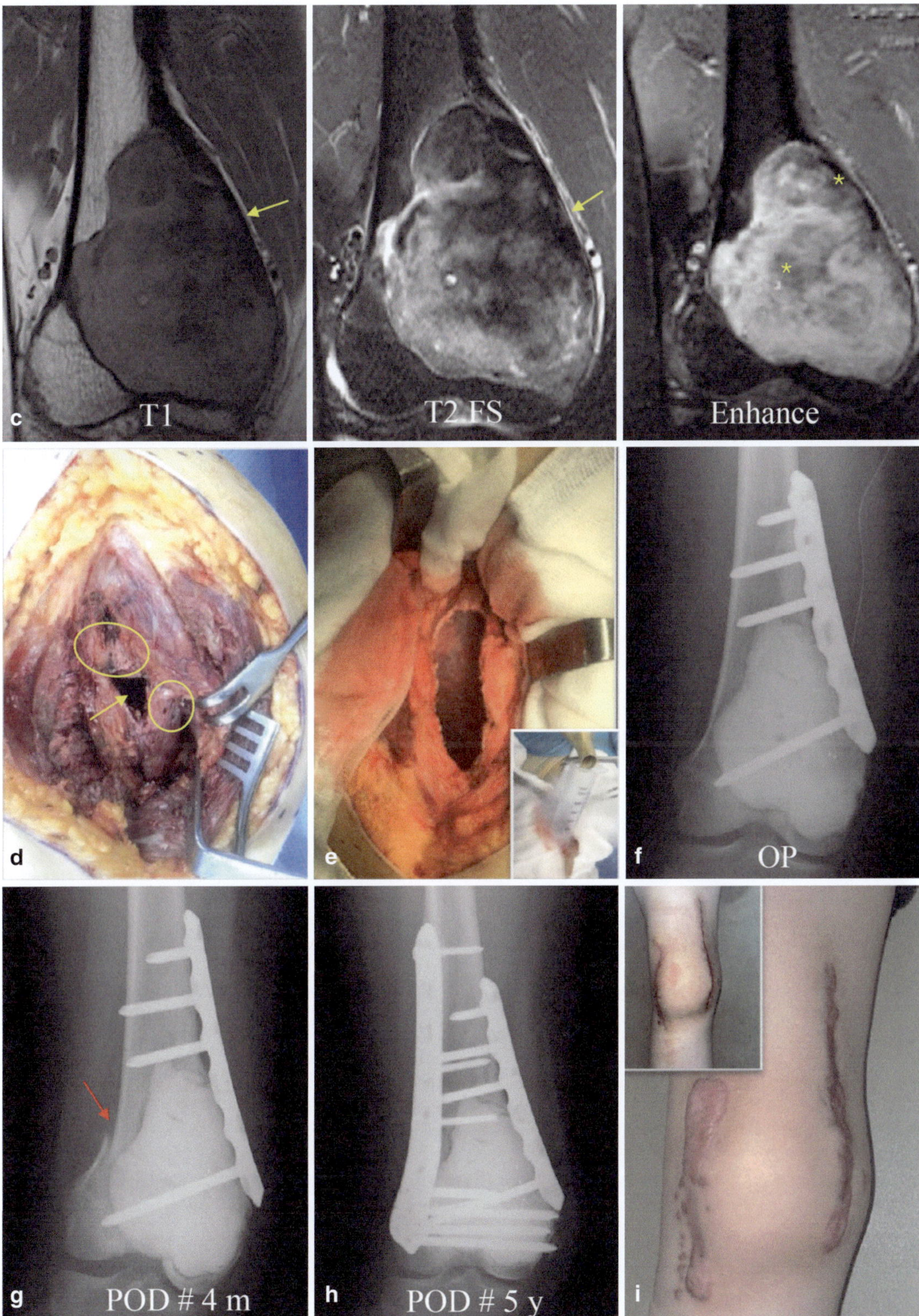

Fig. 1.3 (continued)

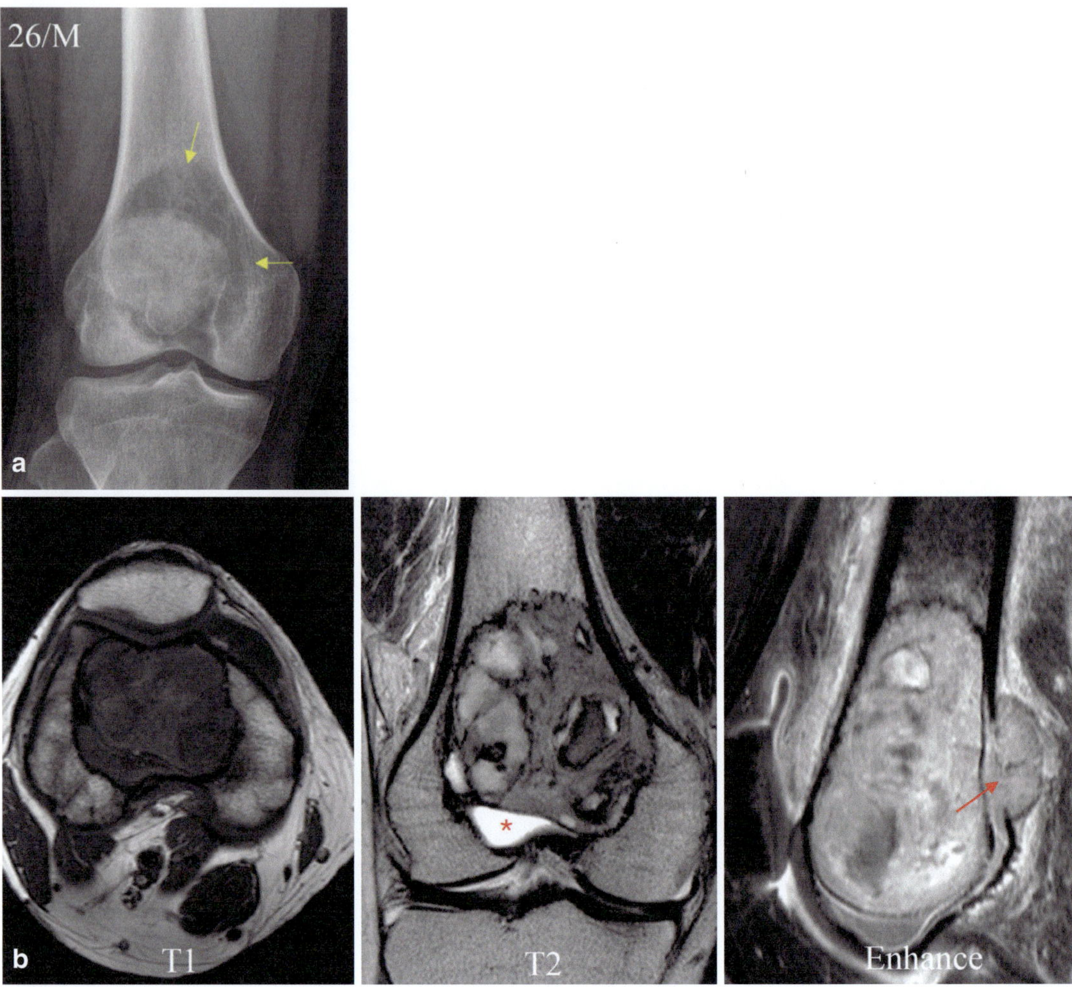

Fig. 1.4 (**a**) Radiograph taken for right knee of 9-month duration in 26-year-old young man shows a centrally located multi-lobulated geographic destruction with an ill-defined broad zone of transition (yellow arrows) in the epi-metaphysis of right distal femur. (**b**) MR images reveal a multi-lobulated intramedullary mass-like lesion with low SI on T1- and heterogeneous intermediate and high SI with a focal bright signals of cystic change (asterisk) on T2-weighted image. The main lesion and perilesional bone marrow and soft tissue edema are heterogeneously enhanced. There is posterior cortex breakage with a soft tissue mass, which is also similarly enhanced (red arrow). (**c**) Pinhole bone scan notes a peripheral increased uptake (yellow asterisk) with central very mild to no uptake (white asterisk). (**d**) A distinct soft and tan-brown tumor tissue is well visualized with focal dark red areas suggesting hemorrhage through the window on the cortex for curettage. (**e**) Extended curettage using high-speed bur and thick subchondral allo-chip bone graft to prevent damage of articular cartilage by the heat from cementation (yellow arrow) was performed, and the defect was filled with bone cement and screw fixation. (**f**) Radiograph at 3 years after surgery shows good maintenance with no evidence of local recurrence with no collapse of the articular cartilage and degenerative change of the joint (yellow arrow)

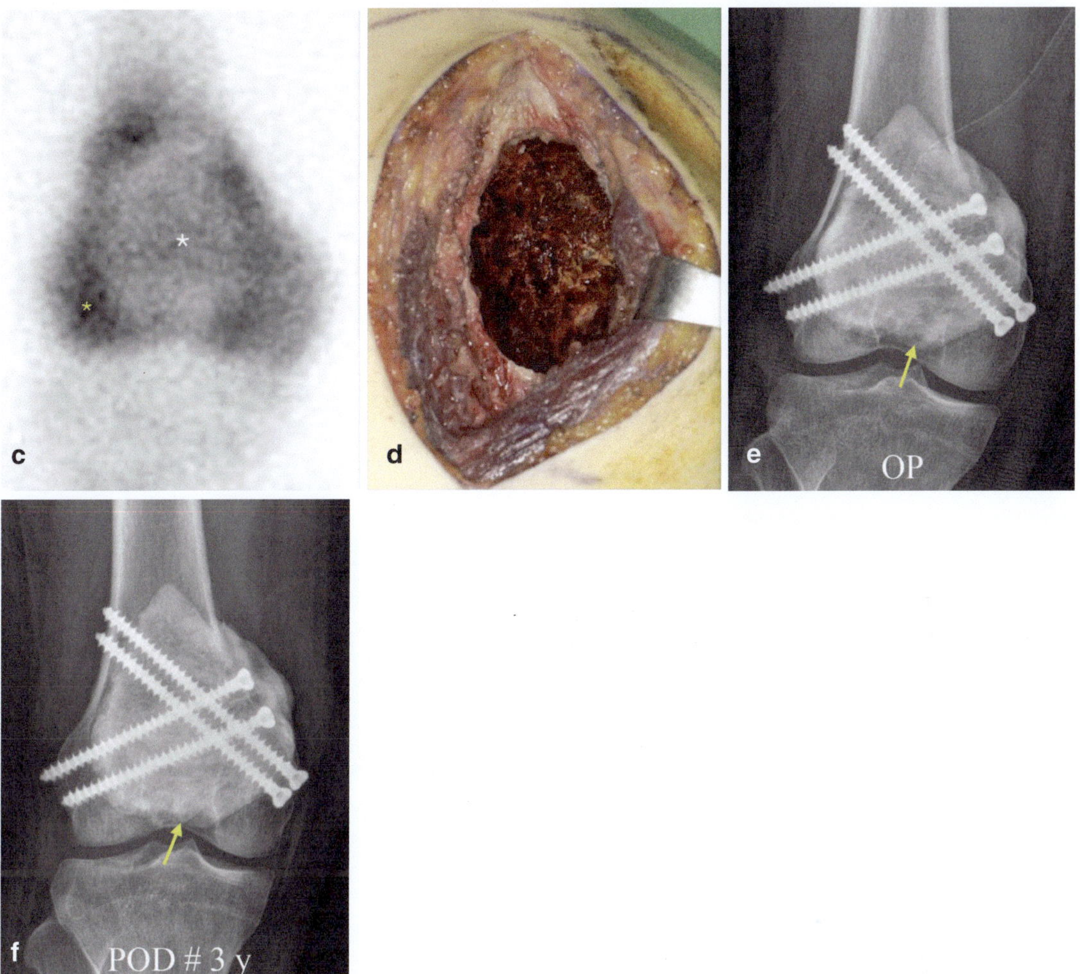

Fig. 1.4 (continued)

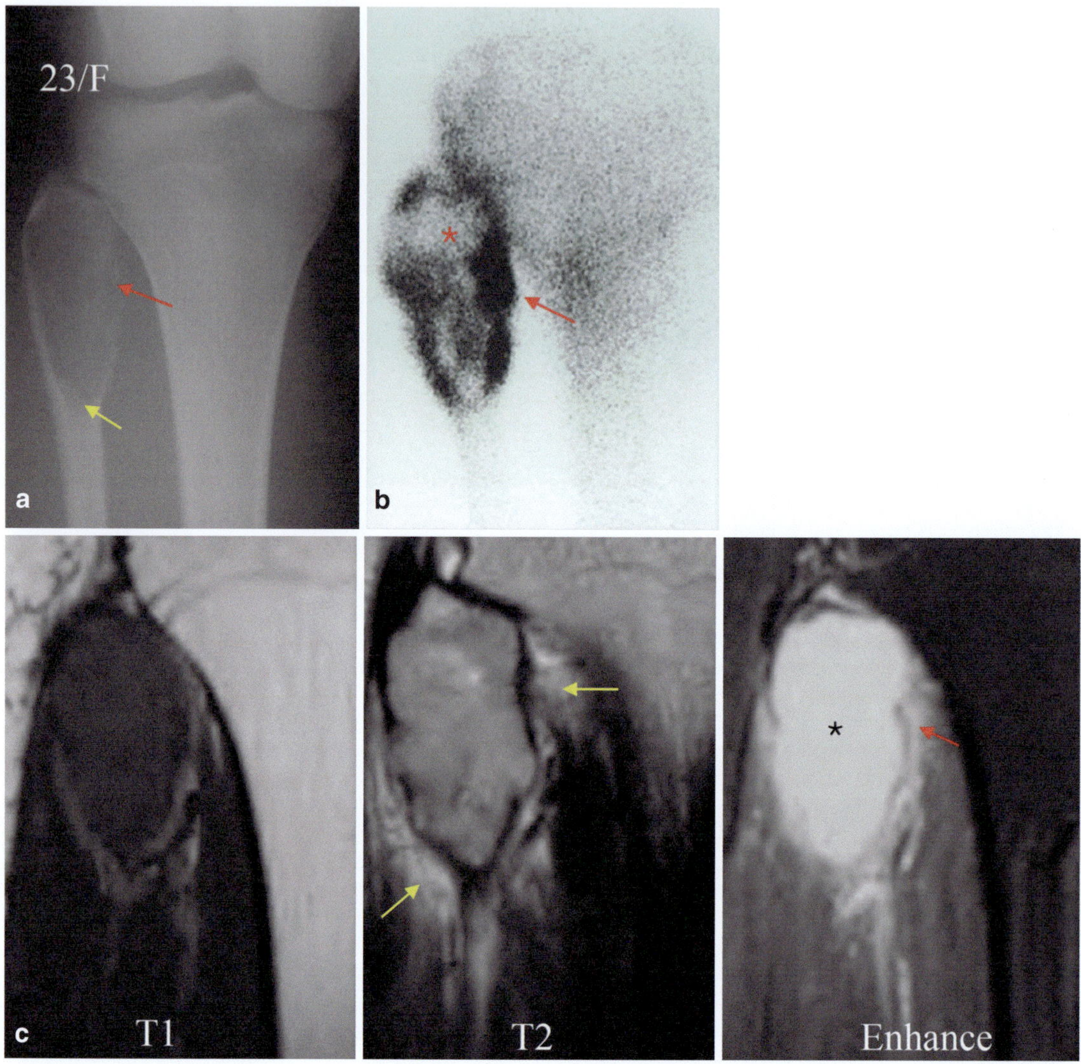

Fig. 1.5 (**a**) Radiograph taken for right knee pain of 5- to 6-month duration in 23-year-old young lady shows a relatively well-demarcated but no rim of sclerosis (yellow arrow), mildly expansile, geographic osteolytic lesion with suspicious cortical breakage (red arrow) affecting the epi-metaphyseal area of proximal fibula. (**b**) Pinhole bone scan typically shows a strongly increased uptake along the periphery of the lesion (arrow) with central photon defect (asterisk). (**c**) MR images demonstrate an expansile intramedullary mass-like lesion with low SI on T1-weighted image and intermediate to high SI on T2-weighted image. There is no discernible cortical breakage, but marked soft tissue edema (yellow arrows). The main lesion (asterisk) as well as soft tissue edema (arrow) is homogeneously well enhanced. (**d**) Follow-up radiograph at 6 years after en bloc resection under a histologic confirmation of GCT notes no evidence of local recurrence. (**e**) Another radiograph taken for right knee pain of 2-month duration in 25-year-old man shows an ill-defined lesion with moth-eaten margin (yellow arrow), irregular thinning of the cortex, and a possible cortical breakage (red arrow). (**f**) MR images reveal a mildly expansile mass lesion with central area of low to intermediate SI on T1-weighted image and intermediate to high SI on T2-weighted image, which is surrounded by thick dark signals on both sequences. There is a mild soft tissue extension though cortical breaches (yellow arrow) as well as prominent edema in the surrounding soft tissues (red arrow). The bony lesion as well as soft tissue mass (red arrow) is well enhanced by contrast media. (**g**) Chest CT scan notes a focal irregular consolidation and peripheral linear increased opacities in the lung, suggesting an implantation of GCT. However, a lung biopsy confirmed unexpectedly a primary adenocarcinoma of the lung. (**h**) Follow-up radiograph at 2 years after en bloc resection under a histologic diagnosis of GCT shows no evidence of local recurrence

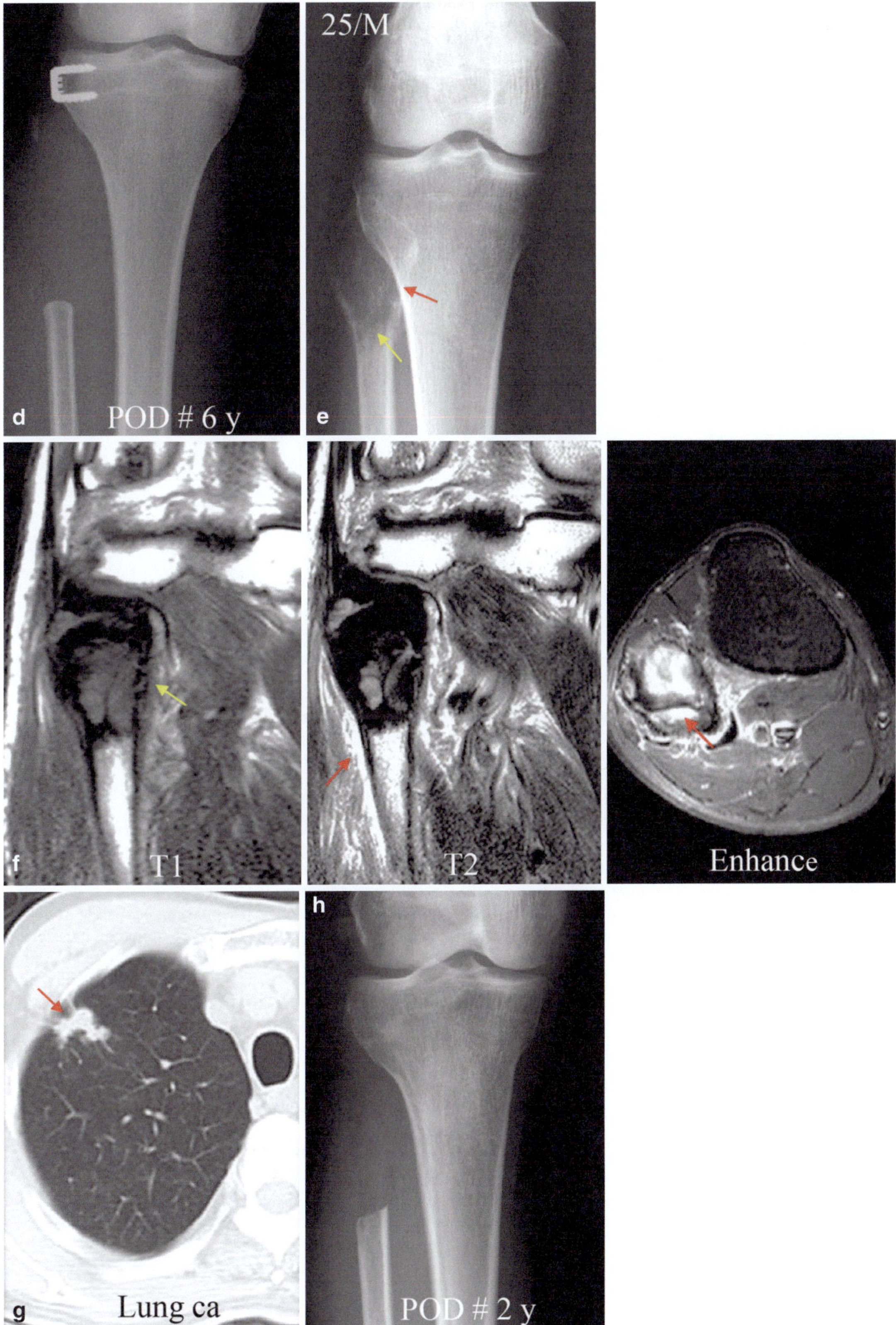

Fig. 1.5 (continued)

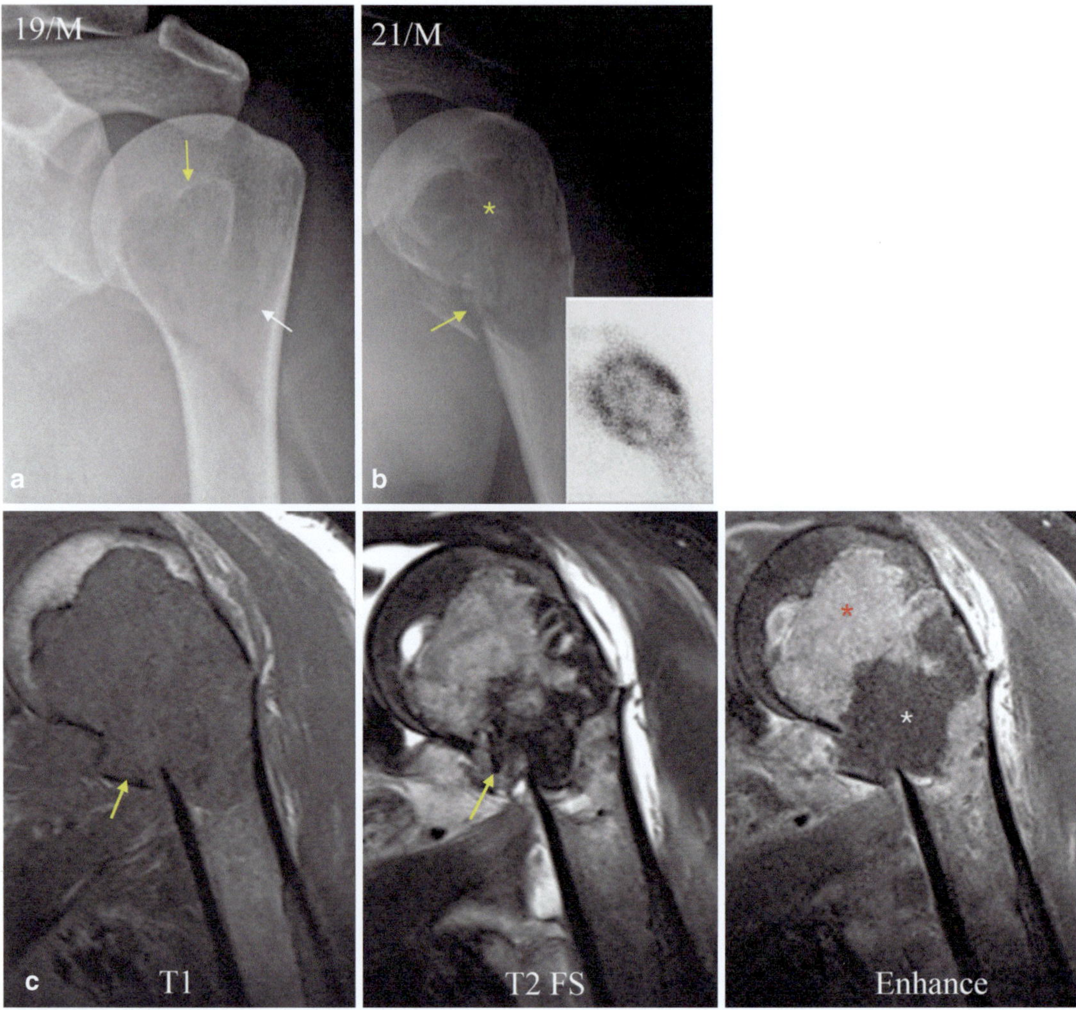

Fig. 1.6 (**a**) Radiograph taken for left shoulder pain of 2-year duration in 19-year-old young man shows an ill-defined multi-lobulated hazy radiolucent lesion mostly with broad transitional zone (white arrow) and focally with incomplete thin rim of sclerosis (yellow arrow) in the humeral head and neck. However, the lesion was not recognized by the primary physician probably due to poor quality of the radiograph. The patient was managed by pain killer and steroid injection. (**b**) Radiograph taken for sudden aggravation of the pain after slip 2 years later notes a progression of the lesion (asterisk) with comminuted pathologic fracture (red arrow). Pinhole bone scan an increased uptake in the periphery with central photon defect (inset). (**c**) MR images demonstrate a well-defined intramedullary mass-like lesion with intermediate SI on T1-weighted image and heterogeneous high SI with low signal areas on fat saturated T2-wighted image. Pathologic fracture is noted with surrounding soft tissue inflammation and fluid collection (arrows). The upper part of lesion is diffusely enhanced (red asterisk), but lower part is not enhanced (white asterisk), suggesting a possible extensive necrosis by fracture. (**d**) PET/CT scan notes a hypermetabolic lesion (SUVmax 8.8), suggesting more likely malignant tumor. (**e**) Trocar biopsy was performed under guide of C-arm image intensifier. (**f**) Microscopic examination shows round to oval mononuclear stromal cell proliferation with evenly scattered multinucleated giant cells reflecting an enhanced upper part of the lesion on MRI, which is indicative of conventional GCT (top), and focus of viable tumor cells in a background of prominent hemorrhage (bottom). Note extensive necrotic area probably by fracture reflecting a non-enhanced lower part (inset). (**g**) Extended curettage using high-speed bur and cryosurgery with liquid nitrogen was performed. (**h**) Follow-up radiograph at 3 years after surgery reveals no evidence of local recurrence

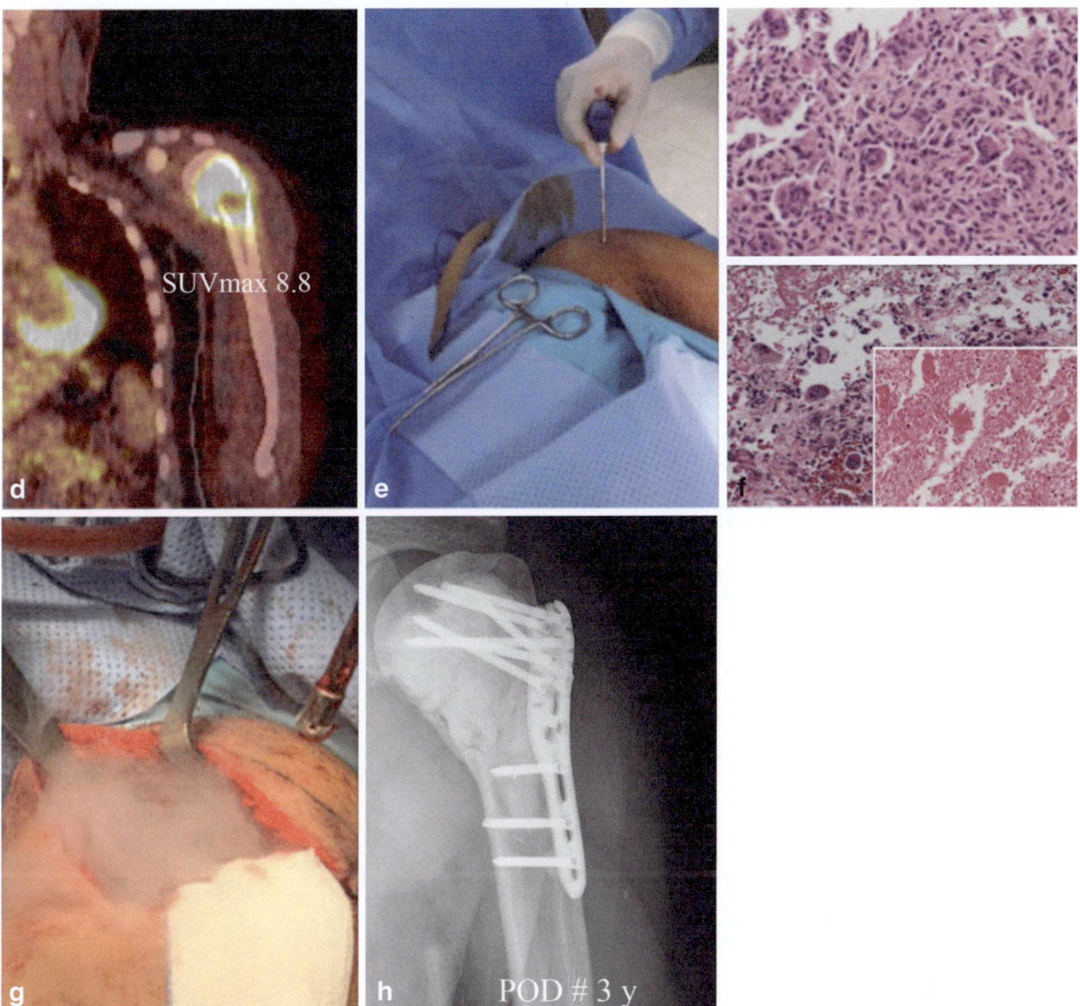

Fig. 1.6 (continued)

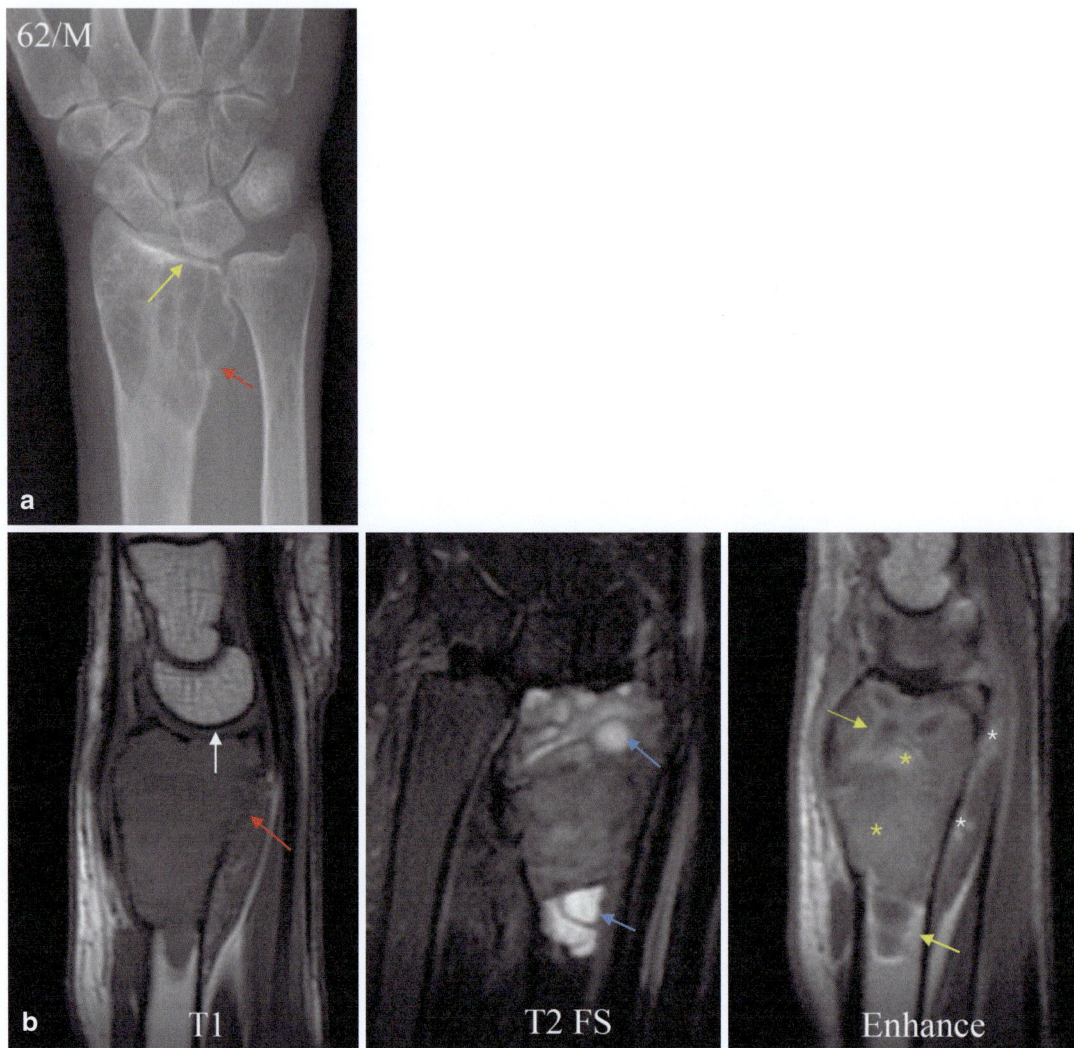

Fig. 1.7 (**a**) Radiograph taken for left wrist pain of 7-month duration in 62-year-old man shows a relatively well-defined multi-lobulated osteolytic lesion without a rim of surrounding sclerosis in the epi-metaphysis of distal radius. There is mild focal expansion and cortical breakage (red arrow). The lesion reaches subchondral bone abutting the border of articular cartilage (yellow arrow). (**b**) MR images demonstrate a mildly expansile mass-like lesion with no surrounding rim of sclerosis. There are cortical destruction and soft tissue extension (red arrow), and the lesion irregularly perforates the articular cartilage and eventually spread into the joint space (white arrow). The SI is low on T1-weighted image and heterogeneous intermediate and high SI with bright signals of cystic change (blue arrows) on fat saturated T2-weighted image. The central solid lesion is diffusely enhanced (yellow asterisks), and peripheral cystic wall as well as septa is also enhanced (yellow arrows). The soft tissue mass is focally enhanced (white asterisks). (**c**) With a pathologic confirmation of GCT, wide resection and reconstruction using an allograft harvested from a young child that was only available in the bone bank at that time. (**d**) Immediate postoperative radiograph reveals a good match and rigid fixation using plate with minimal gap between the host bone and allograft (white arrow). You can see the growth plate of the allo-graft is still open (red arrow). (**e**) Follow-up radiograph at 4 months after surgery notes a volar slippage of the allograft epiphysis from the growth plate with an angulation (red arrow). (**f**) Radiograph shows good anatomic reduction with screw fixation. (**g**) However, follow-up radiograph at 2 months after fixation reveals a re-slippage of the epiphysis (red arrow). (**h**) Follow-up radiograph at 2 years after autograft and additional plate fixation notes a good union of the epiphysis (red arrow) as well as junction between host bone and allograft (yellow arrow) with no evidence of local recurrence

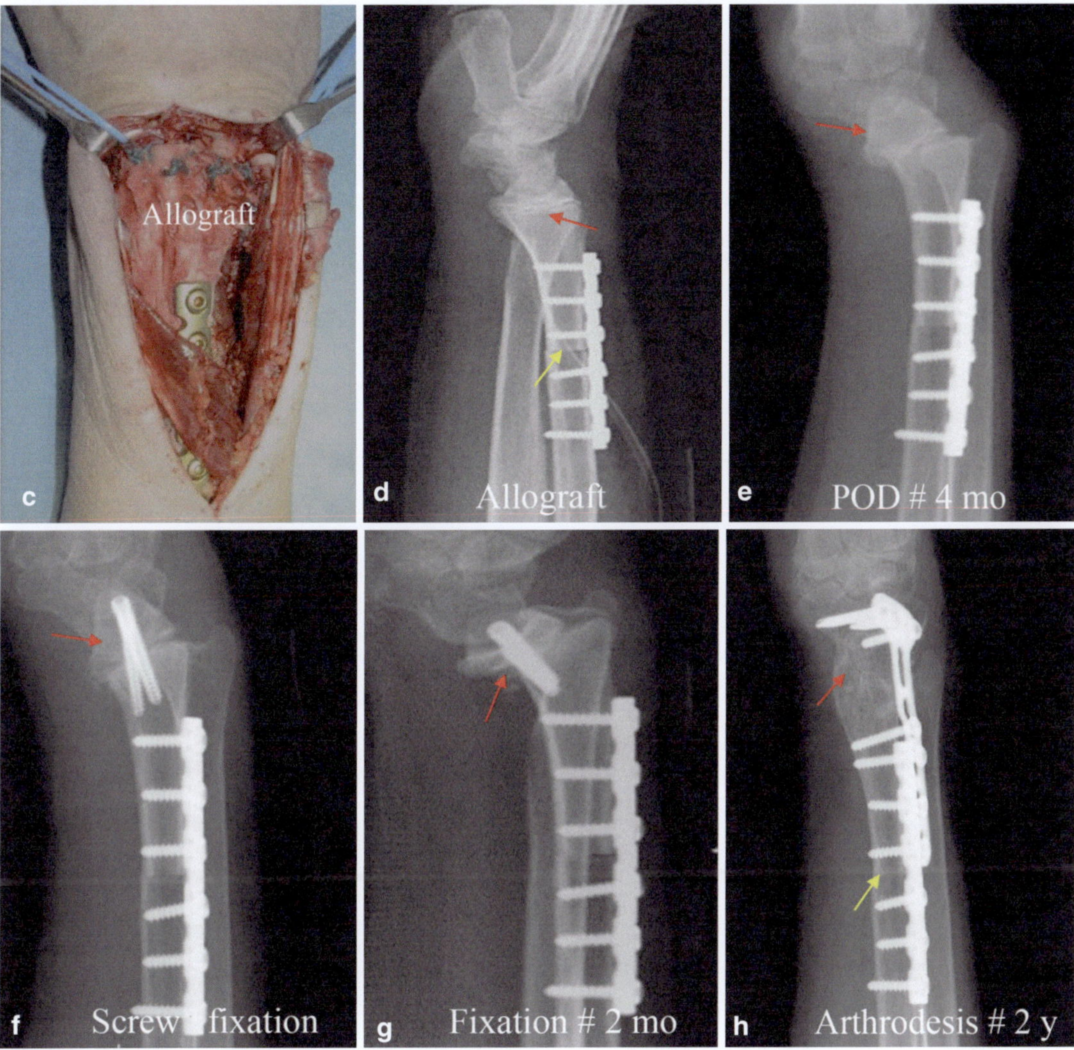

Fig. 1.7 (continued)

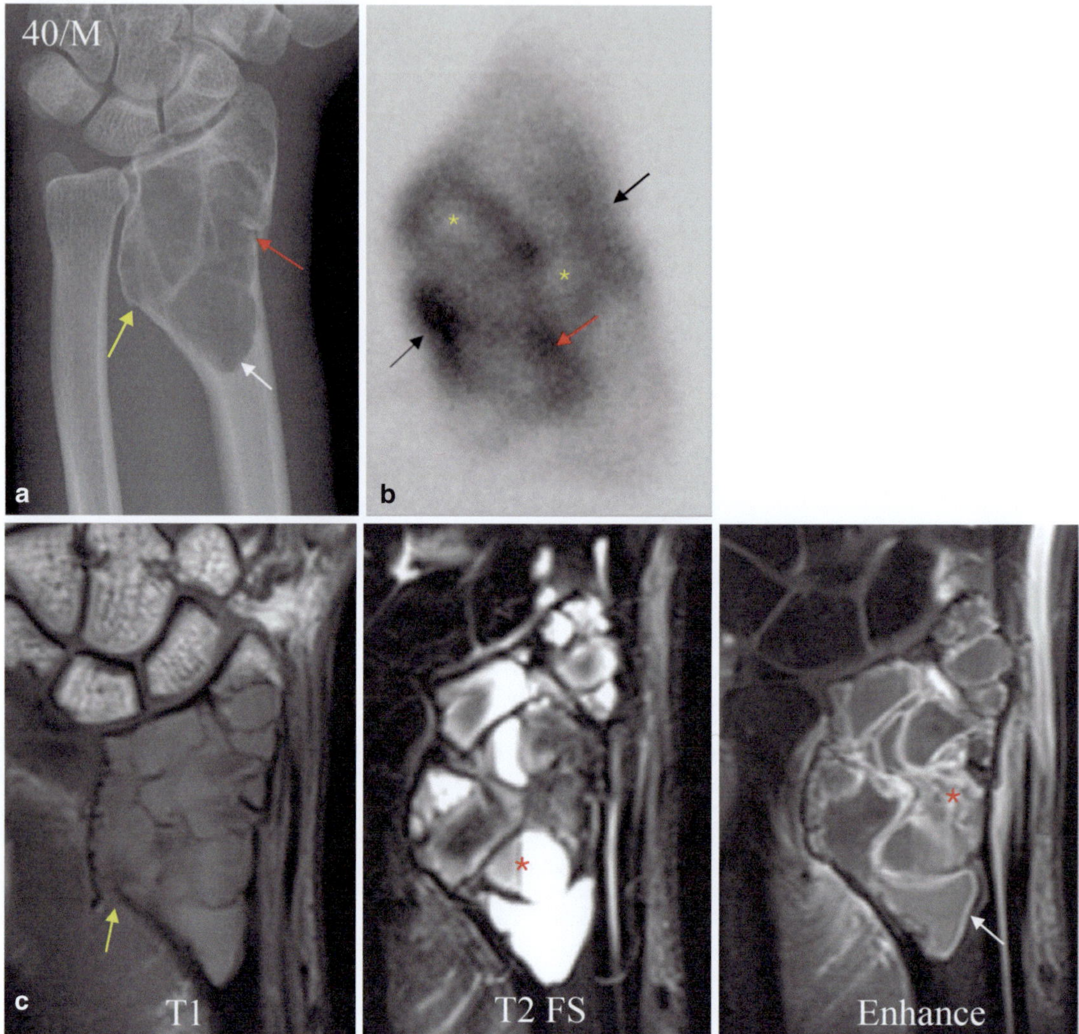

Fig. 1.8 ***GCT with secondary ABC*** (**a**) Radiograph taken for right wrist pain by twisting the bottle cap to open (sprain injury) in 40-year-old man shows a well-defined multi-lobulated geographic destruction with a narrow transition but no discernible sclerotic rim (white arrow) affecting the epi-metaphysis of distal radius. There is focal ballooning with diffuse cortical thinning (yellow arrow) and non-displaced pathologic fracture (red arrow). (**b**) Pinhole bone scan reveals an increased uptake along the outer shell (black arrows) and septa (red arrow) with internal void areas (asterisks). (**c**) MR images demonstrate a multi-lobulated mass lesion with a focal bulging and cortical thinning but no surrounding scelrotic rim. There is cortical discontinuity indicating a pathologic fracture (yellow arrow). The SI is intermediate on T1-weighted image and heterogeneous low and intermediate with multiple bright signal of cystic change on T2-weighted image. Note a fluid-fluid level (asterisk) indicating secondary ABC change. The lesion is heterogeneously enhanced in solid portion (asterisk) and thinly enhanced along the periphery and septa in the cystic areas (yellow arrow). (**d**) Tan-brown colored tissue (white asterisk) and dark red colored hemorrhage (yellow asterisk) are visualized through the window for curettage. Extended curettage using high-speed bur followed by cryosurgery with liquid nitrogen and allo-chip bone graft was performed. (**e**) Microscopic examination. (Left) Middle-power magnification shows proliferation of round to oval mononuclear stromal cell with scattered multi-nucleated giant cells indicative of GCT. There are spicules of reactive woven bone in the periphery (black asterisk) as well as an area foam cells (inset), reflecting the tan-brown tumor tissue. (Middle) Another area revels secondary ABC change with dilated vasculature and massive hemorrhage, reflecting the dark red tissue. (Right) In addition, there are irregular primitive woven bone spicules rimmed by prominent osteoblasts (arrow) and injury vessels, which begin to connect to each other forming circles, indicating a fracture callus of about 10–14 day's estimated age. Clinically, the biopsy specimen was obtained during surgery on 11 days after sprain injury. (**f**) Follow-up radiograph at 5 years postoperatively shows no evidence of local recurrence

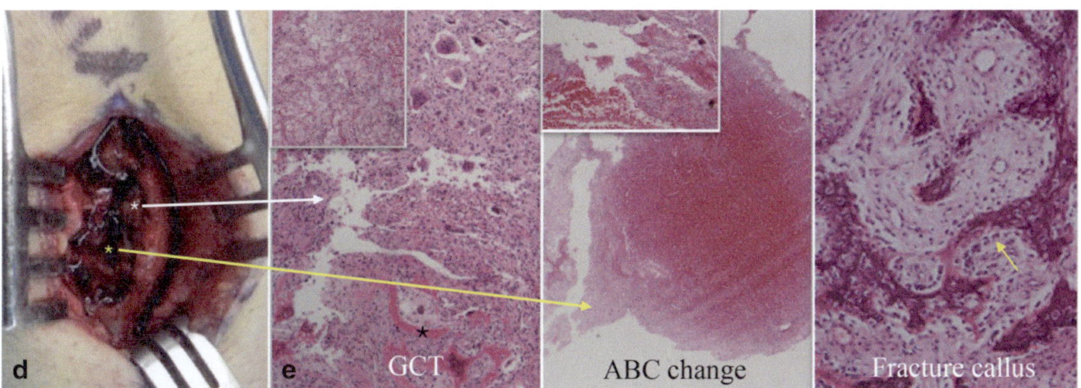

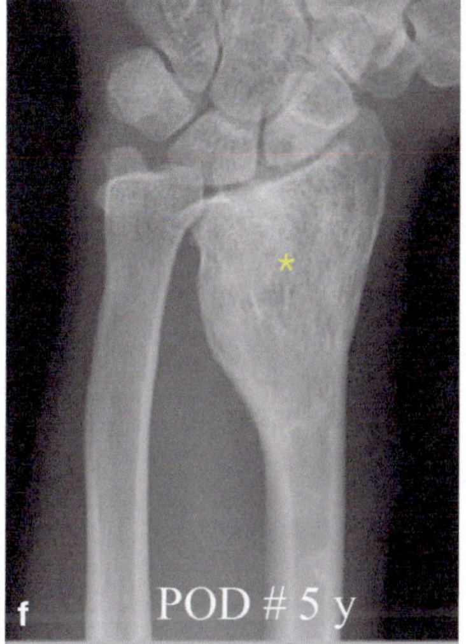

Fig. 1.8 (continued)

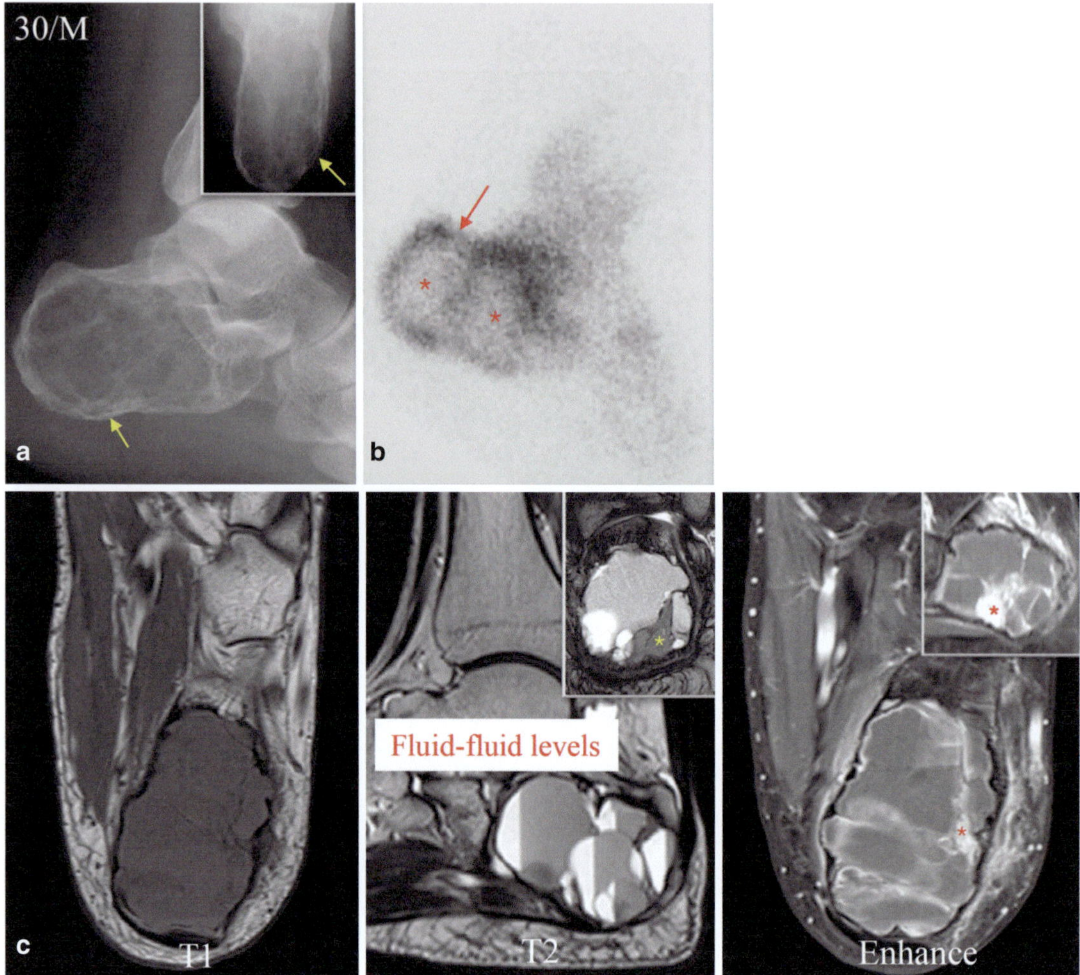

Fig. 1.9 ***Rare location of calcaneus with secondary ABC*** (**a**) Radiograph taken for left heel pain of 2-year duration in 30-year-old man shows a multichambered mildly expansile osteolytic lesion with internal trabeculations, so-called "*bubbly appearance*," and scalloping with irregular thinning of the cortex (arrows) in the entire calcaneus. (**b**) Pinhole bone scan reveals a peripherally increased uptake (red arrow) with central photopenic or void areas, so-called "*doughnut*" sign (asterisks). (**c**) MR images demonstrate a multi-lobulated cystic lesion with significant irregular thinning but no clear breakage of the cortex. The SI is low on T1-weighted image and multiple fluid-fluid levels on T2-weighted image with a focal solid area of intermediate SI (asterisk in inset), suggesting a secondary ABC with underlying solid bone tumor more likely than a primary ABC. The lesion is thinly enhanced along the periphery and septa in the cystic area with a well-enhanced focal solid area (red asterisks). (**d**) Aspiration before surgical procedure notes fresh blood suggesting more likely ABC rather than other cysts. (**e**) Microscopic examination shows two different solid and cystic components. (Left) Solid component notes an area of oval to polygonal mononuclear cells with scattered multinucleated giant cells (yellow asterisk) and adjacent areas producing abundant collagen material with general reduction of the multinucleated giant cells (yellow asterisk), indicating GCT. (Right) Another cystic area shows a multi-lobulated cyst-like wall architecture with fibrous septa of variable thickness consisting of bland fibroblast-like cells, woven bone formation, hemosiderin pigments, and multinucleated cells, indicative of ABC. (**f**) Extended curettage using high-speed bur and allo-chip bone packing was performed. (**g**) Follow-up radiograph at 2 years after surgery reveals consolidation of the lesion with no evidence of recurrence

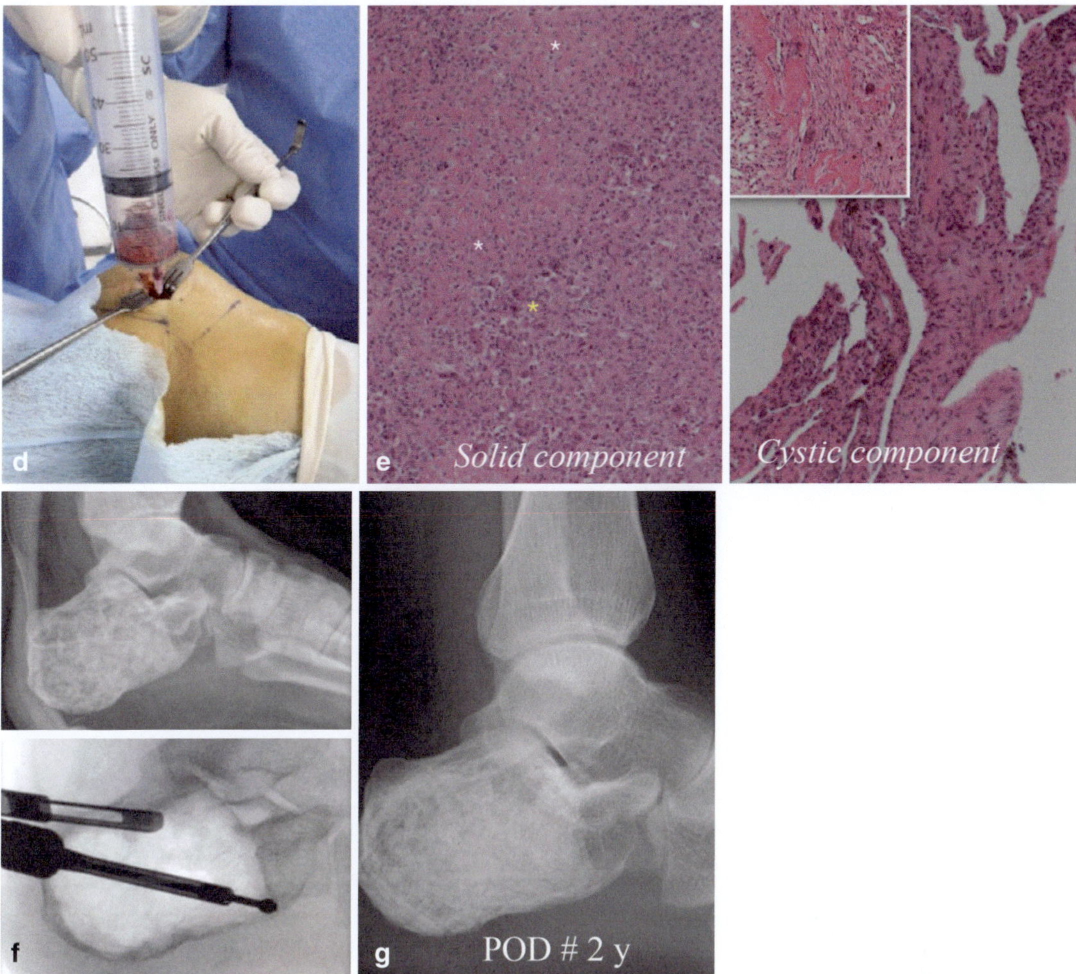

Fig. 1.9 (continued)

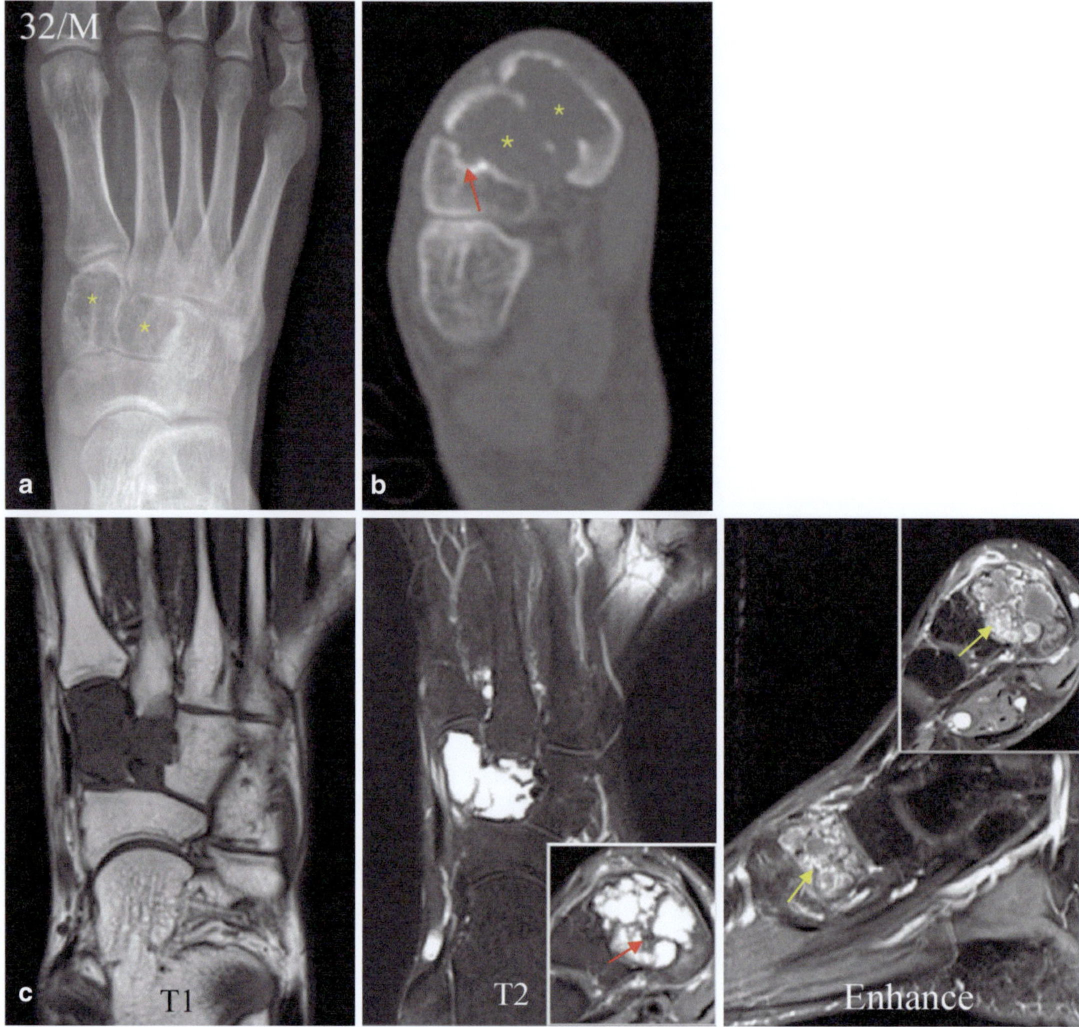

Fig. 1.10 ***Rare multicentric locations of foot with secondary ABC*** (**a**) Radiograph taken for right foot pain of 6-month duration in 32-year-old man shows multi-lobulated osteolytic lesions with a marked cortical thinning in the medial and intermediated cuneiforms (asterisks). (**b**) CT scan reveals an expansile osteolytic lesions with cortical destruction in the medial and intermediated cuneiforms (asterisks). The lateral cuneiform is focally eroded with surrounding reactive sclerosis (red arrow). (**c**) MR images demonstrate a multi-lobulated lesion with low SI on T1-weighted image and bright SI with focal low to intermediate signal (red arrow), suggesting mostly cystic lesion with a small solid component on T2-weighted image. The lesion notes peripheral and septal enhancement with multiple internal focal enhancement (arrows), which is more clearly indicating a pre-existing solid tumor component. (**d**) Microscopic examination demonstrates a typical finding of GCT (left) associated with secondary ABC (right). (**e**) Extended curettage using high-speed burr and anhydrous ethanol adjuvant treatment through the large window was performed. (**f**) The defect was filled with bone cement. (**g**) Follow-up radiograph at 3 years after surgery shows no peri-cement radiolucency indicating a local recurrence

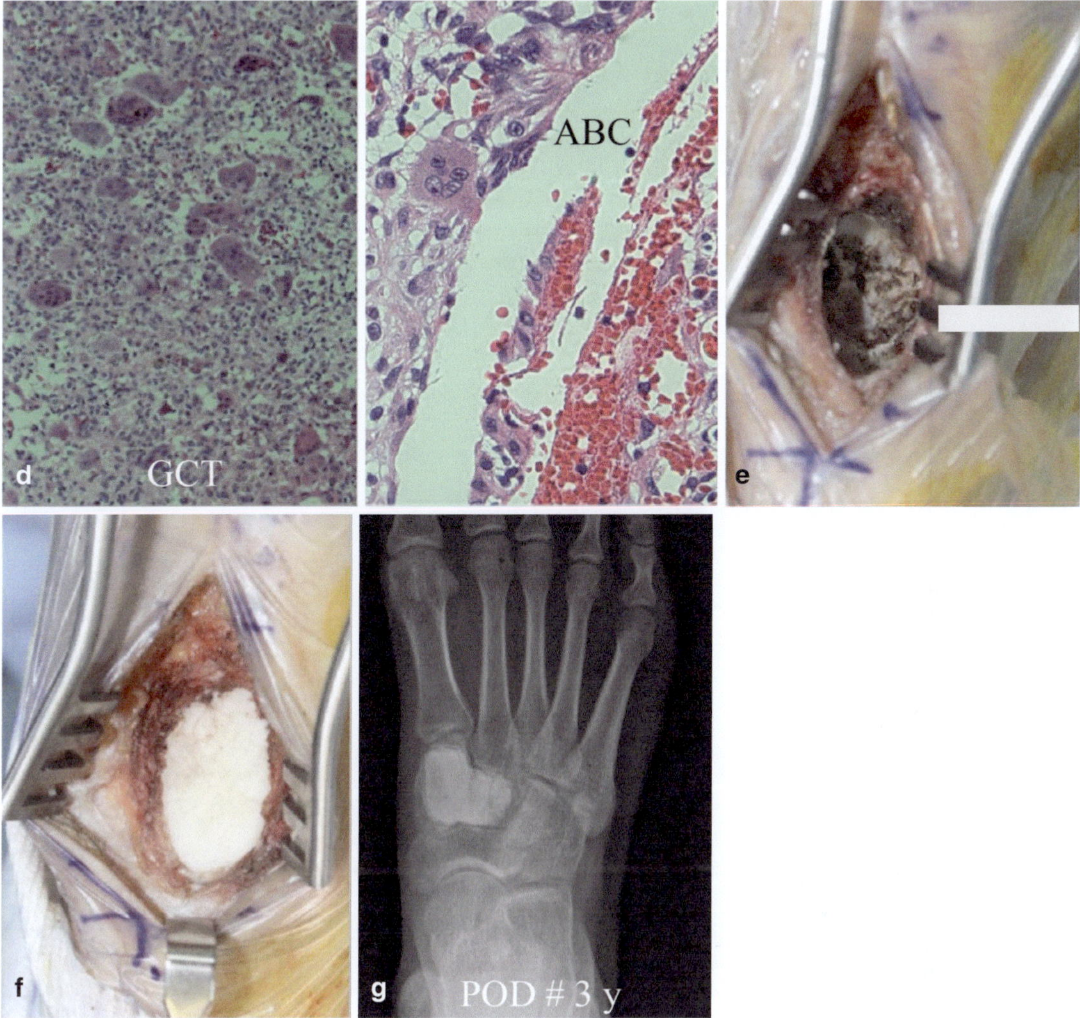

Fig. 1.10 (continued)

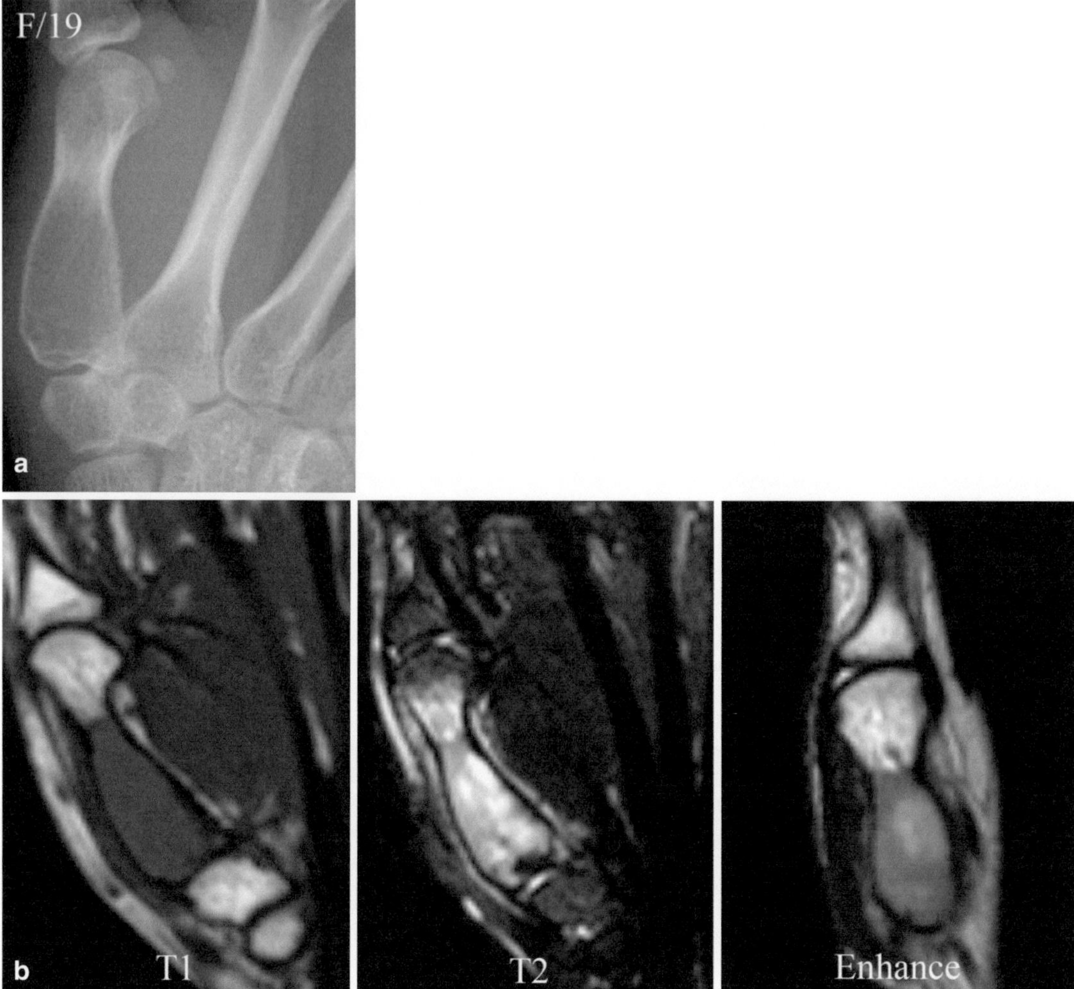

Fig. 1.11 ***Rare location of hand*** (**a**) Radiograph taken for right hand of 1-month duration in 19-year-old young lady shows a mildly expansile radiolucent lesion with cortical thinning affecting proximal two thirds of the first metacarpal bone. The lesion is well defined with narrow transitional zone but no rim of sclerosis. (**b**) MR images demonstrate a well-defined mass-like lesion with mild expansion but no discernible cortical breakage. The SI is low SI on T1-weighted image and intermediate SI with focal bright signals on T2-weighted image. The lesion is heterogeneously enhanced. (**c**) Bone scan reveals a homogeneous strong uptake with milder distal uptake. (**d**) Microscopic examination. (Left) Lower-power magnification notes neoplastic component of round to oval, short spindle, mononuclear cells and nonneoplastic component of diffusely scattered, and numerous multinucleated giant cells. There is no evidence of reactive granulation tissue or focal hemorrhage, which is usual finding of giant cell reparative granuloma. (Right) Higher-power magnification shows that the nuclei of the giant cells are identical to those of mononuclear stromal cells. (**e**) Follow-up radiograph at 3 months after curettage and allo-chip bone graft shows a consolidation of the lesion with no evidence of local recurrence

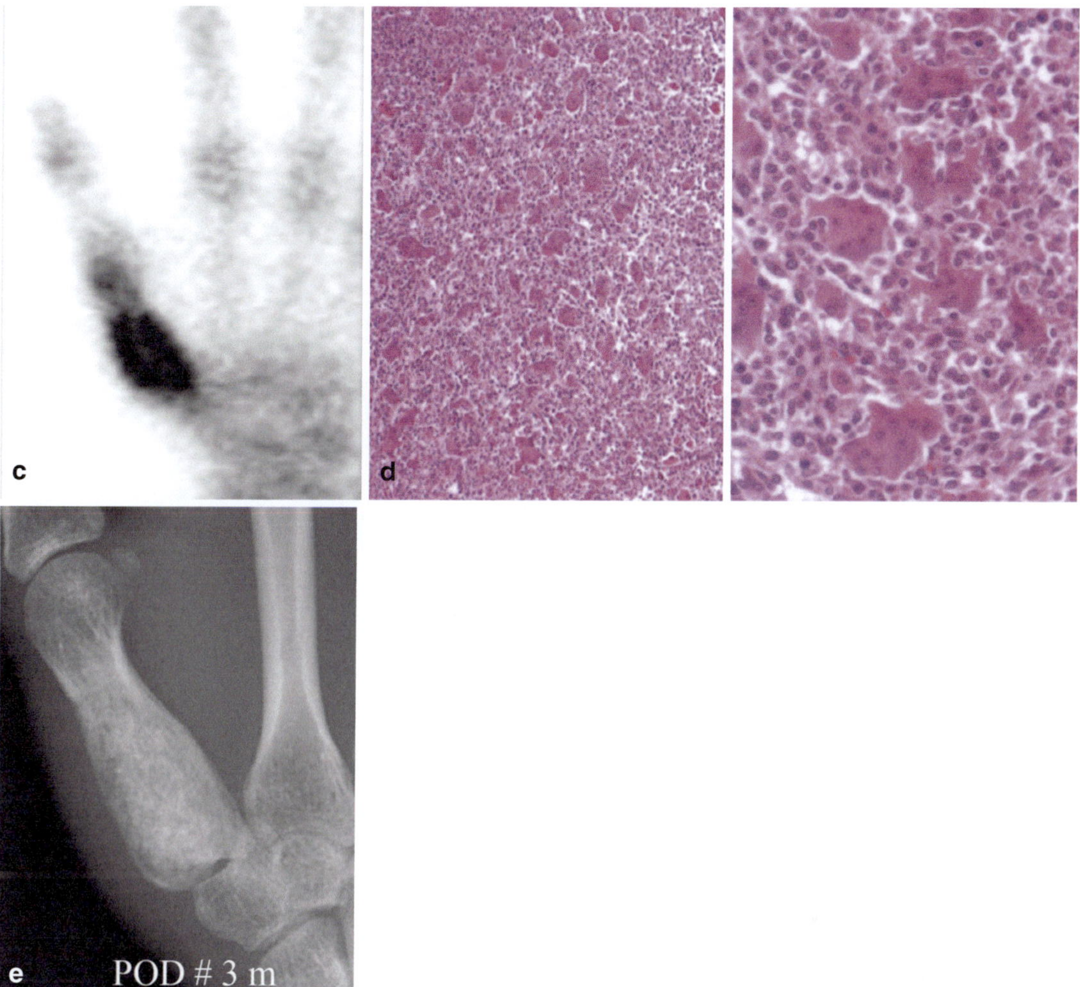

Fig. 1.11 (continued)

1.6 Clinical Features

Pain with or without local swelling is the most common symptom. Adjacent joint swelling or limitation of motion is frequently presented. Rarely, pathologic fracture is associated especially in GCT affecting the distal femur. Multifocal GCTs of bone without pre-existing Paget's disease are exceedingly rare only accounting for less than 1% of all cases of GCT of bone [11–14]. When diaphysis of long bone is involved or multiple bones are affected, GCT of hyperparathyroidism (brown tumor) being histologically identical to GCT of bone should be excluded by laboratory examination including calcium, phosphate, and parathyroid hormone. There have been several reports regarding the occurrence or progression of GCT during pregnancy. The rapid progression or growing of GCT with an aggressive behavior during pregnancy has been sporadically documented in the literature [15–17] (Fig. 1.12). However, it may be coincidental to find GCT in pregnant women because affected patients are often of childbearing age, the age in which tumors show a high incidence in the general population [18]. When GCT affects sacrum during pregnant, the delay in detection due to vague pain, discomfort, and numbness around the pelvis being misinterpreted as symptoms of pregnancy allow unexpected growth leading surgical management difficulty [19]. Rarely, tumors with a histology identical to GCT of bone may primarily occur

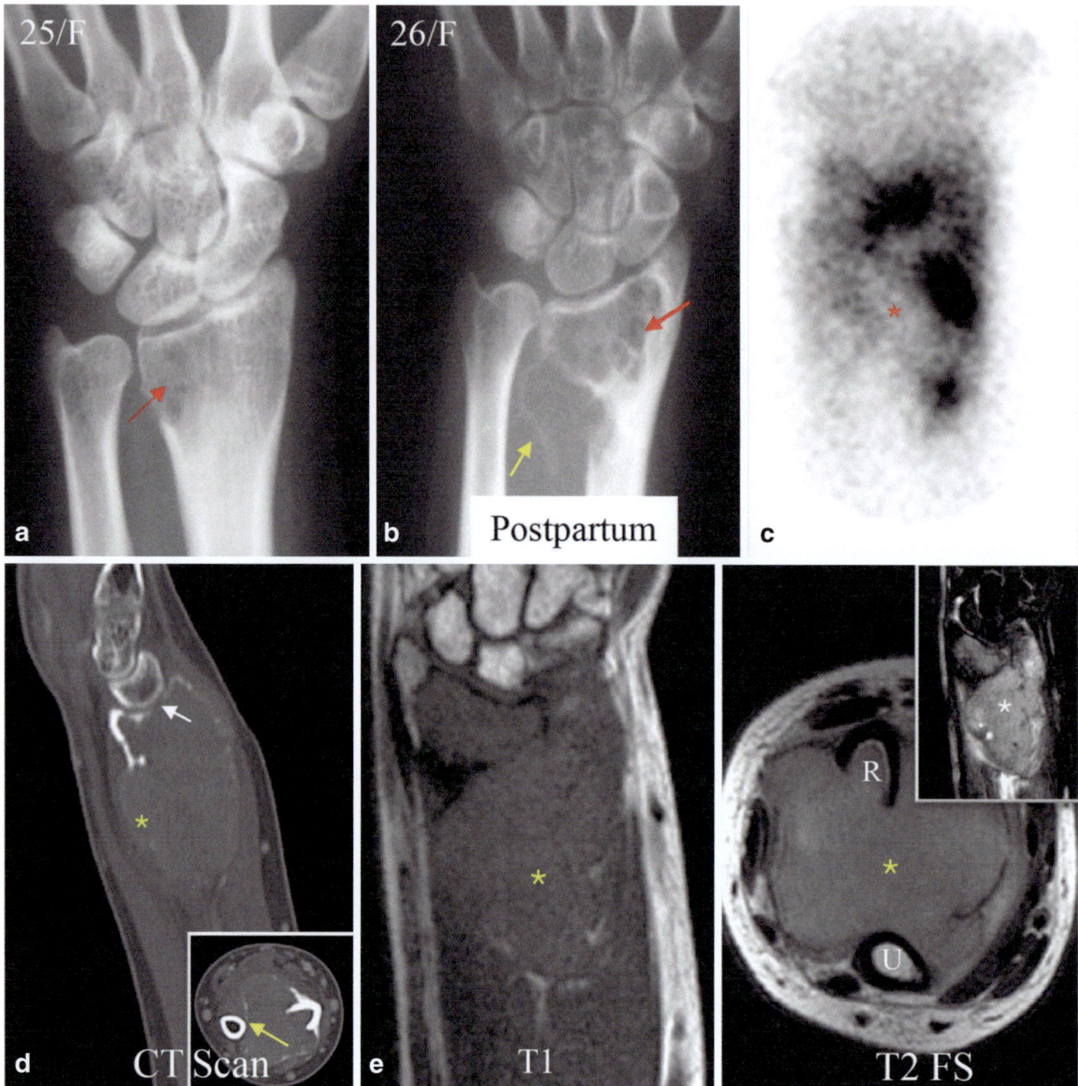

Fig. 1.12 ***Pregnancy related progression.*** (**a**) Radiograph taken for right wrist swelling of 3-month duration in 25-year-old young lady shows an ill-defined, eccentric, radiolucent lesion with broad transitional zone mainly in the epiphysis of distal radius (red arrow). Incision biopsy confirmed conventional GCT. She was pregnant at that time and did not want further evaluation and management until delivery. (**b**) Radiograph immediately after her delivery reveals significant progression of the lesion with an enlarged, multilobulated, "soap-bubble" appearance (red arrow) extending to metaphysis and a part of diaphysis. The medial cortical is markedly destructed, and tumor extends into the adjacent soft tissue forming a mass surrounded by thin new bone formation (yellow arrow). (**c**) Pinhole bone scan notes heterogeneous strong and intermediate uptake with central photon defect area (asterisk). (**d**) CT scan demonstrates a medullary mass lesion with marked expansion, cortical destruction, and soft tissue mass formation (asterisk) as well as breakage of articular cartilage (white arrow). The soft tissue mass is large enough to abut the cortex distal ulna (arrow in inset). (**e**) MR images demonstrate a large, ill-defined, multi-lobulated intramedullary mass lesion (asterisks) with low SI on T1-weighted image and heterogeneous intermediate and focal high SI on fat saturated T2-weighted image. Note cortical destruction of radius (R) with a huge soft tissue mass formation (yellow asterisk) abutting to the cortex of distal ulna (U) on T2-weighted axial image. (**f**) Wide resection followed by reconstruction with vascularized fibula autograft (long red arrow) was performed. (**g**) Follow-up radiograph taken for right wrist swelling at 1 year after initial surgery shows a dense shadow of soft tissue swelling (yellow arrow) as well as external erosion of distal ulna (red arrow), suggesting a local recurrence probably in the soft tissue. (**h**) CT scan confirms a low density of large soft tissue mass surrounding the distal ulna (asterisk). (**i**) Excision of soft tissue mass with curettage of the externally eroded ulna followed by allo-chip bone graft (arrow) and plate fixation was performed. (**j**) Follow-up radiograph at 2 years after re-operation reveals consolidation of the erosion by bone graft (arrow) with no evidence of local recurrence

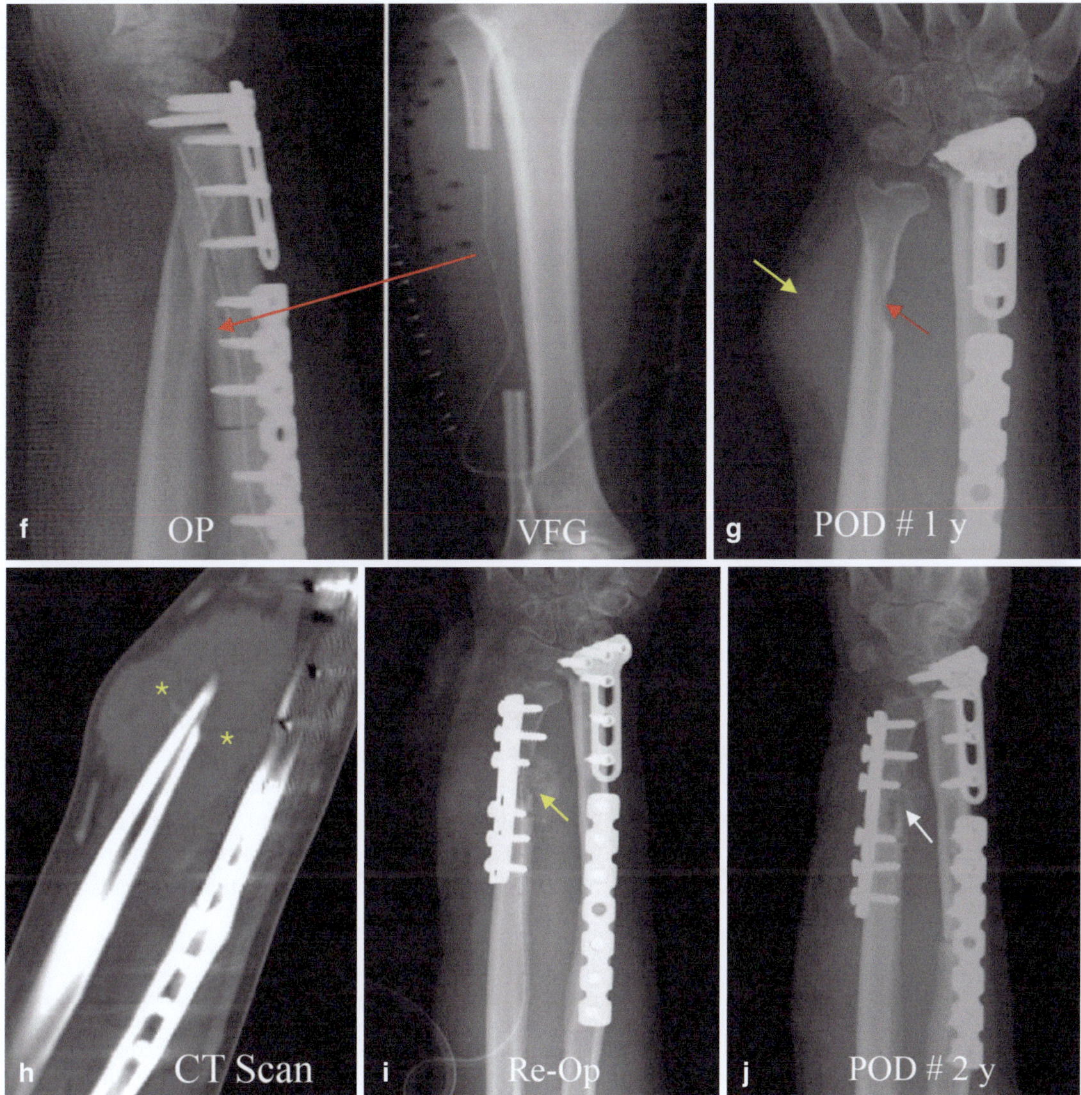

Fig. 1.12 (continued)

within the soft tissues, which can be divided into benign and malignant variants [20–22].

1.7 Grading System

A histological grading of GCT of long bone was first devised by Jaffe and colleagues [23], which has subsequently proved to be unreliable to predict prognosis. Later, Enneking and colleagues [24, 25] proposed a surgical staging system based on clinical, radiographic, and pathological criteria for all benign and malignant tumors of bone. Benign bone tumors can be inactive or quiescent, active, or aggressive. Inactive tumors (Stage 1) occupy for less than 10% of cases and characterized by a lytic defect limited to the medullary cavity with minimal or no cortical involvement, which is surrounded by a complete rim of sclerosis. Active tumors (Stage 2) are the most common representing for about 70% and typified by a thinned or scalloped, expanded cortex without clear margin. Aggressive tumors (Stage 3) account for about 20% and characterized by a lytic defect with ill-defined margins and cortical destruction often with a naked soft tissue mass formation simulating malignant bone tumors. More later, Campanacci et al. [3] also suclassified the GCT into three grades depending on their radiographic appearance: a grade 1 lesion (latent) has a well-defined margin and an intact cortex; a grade 2 lesion (active) has a relatively well-defined margin but no radiopaque rim, and the cortex is thinned and moderately expanded; and a grade 3 lesion (aggressive) has indistinct borders and cortical destruction [6, 9].

1.8 Radiologic Findings

When affecting long bones, the growth plate is almost always closed although it can be rarely opened (Fig. 1.1e). The lesion typically appears as a well-defined, eccentric or sometimes centric, purely osteolytic, geographic destruction in the epiphysis of the long bones usually with significant metaphyseal extension in most cases [1–8]. The lesion is usually larger with or without surrounding rim of sclerosis, and the cortex is often expanded with focal destruction at least suggesting locally aggressive lesion in the contrary to CB, which is usually smaller and usually with a complete thin rim and confined to the epiphysis without change of bone contour. However, rare cases of GCT can present the findings of internal sclerotic rim and outer reactive new bone formation highly suggesting benignancy (Fig. 1.1e). If the lesion purely involves meta-diaphysis or diaphysis without epiphyseal involvement, GCT of hyperparathyroidism (brown tumor), giant cell-rich osteosarcoma, or Paget's disease should be carefully excluded. Osteolysis is often prominent depending on the number and activity of the osteoclast-like giant cells. Fine to coarse trabeculations are commonly seen in the radiolucent lesion as honeycomb-like or multi-lobulated appearance. The lesion is often well demarcated by complete rim of sclerosis indicating benign tumor in some cases (Figs. 1.1e and 1.3a) or incomplete rim mimicking a locally aggressive or even malignant lesion in other cases (Figs. 1.1a and 1.6a). The lesion may be centrally located and ill-defined with a broad zone of transition sometimes by moth-eaten destruction lacking a discernible surrounding rim of sclerosis, which may more likely mimic a malignant tumor (Figs. 1.4, 1.5, 1.12, 1.13, 1.14). However, some of them may show a thin sclerotic rim on lateral view (Fig. 1.13a) or MRI (Figs. 1.4b, 1.13b, 1.14b). The lesion often reaches subchondral bone and abuts a border of the articular cartilage (Figs. 1.7 and 1.8) and eventually spreads into the

Fig. 1.13 ***Denosumab management of the recurrent GCT*** (**a**) Radiograph taken for right knee pain on exercise in 28-years-old young lady shows a relatively well-defined, centrally located, large, osteolytic lesion with a narrow transitional zone but no discernible rim of sclerosis (white arrows) in the epi-metaphysis of the distal femur. However, the distal margin is clearly marginated with a rind of sclerosis on lateral view (inset). (**b**) MR images reveal a well-defined, multi-lobulated medullary mass-like lesion with low and intermediate SI on T1-weighted image and heterogeneous intermediate and high SI on T2-weighted image. Note dark signal of a complete reactive sclerotic rim on both sequences (yellow arrows). Post contrast image notes heterogeneous internal (red arrow) and thin peripheral (yellow arrow) enhancement. Perilesional bone marrow is also diffusely enhanced (asterisks). (**c**) Microscopic examination notes round to oval spindle stromal cells with diffusely scattered osteoclast-like multinucleated giant cells, indicative of GCT. (**d**) Follow-up radiograph at 5 years after extended curettage and cementation shows radiolucent areas around the cement (arrows), suggesting a possible local recurrence. (**e**) MR image shows a dark signal mass of previously inserted cement (asterisk) with adjacent focal solid lesions with heterogeneous enhancement (white arrows). CT scan reveals more clearly peri-cement multiple radiolucent areas (yellow arrows), indicating a local recurrence. (**f**) The recurred tumor tissue was thoroughly removed by extended curettage after removal of the cement. (**g**) Follow-up radiograph after six cycles of denosumab treatment for 3 months notes that the radiolucency becomes hazier and denser (asterisk) than that of the pre-denosumab treatment, suggesting an exuberant new bone formation. Extended curettage followed by cementing was performed again (inset). (**h**) Microscopic examination. (Left) Medium-power magnification shows an abundant new bone formation with striking loss of multinucleated giant cells, reflecting the post-denosumab treatment sclerotic change on radiograph. (Right) Higher-power magnification reveals, however, no change in number of mononuclear stromal cells, indicating denosumab selectively targets non-neoplastic giant cells but limited inhibitory effect on neoplastic stromal cells. (**i**) Follow-up radiograph at 3 years after re-operation shows no evidence of local recurrence

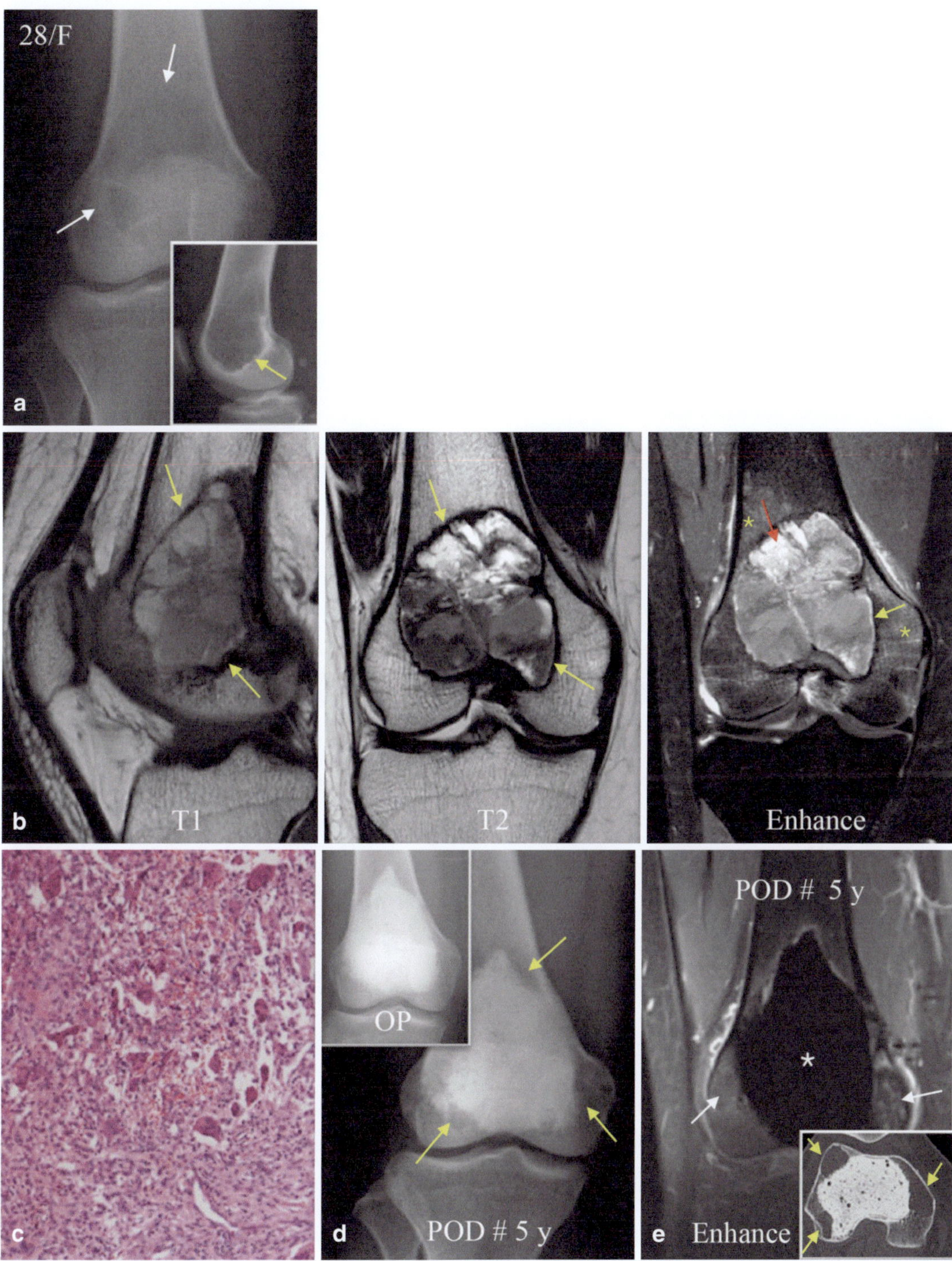
28/F
a
b
T1
T2
Enhance
c
OP
d
POD # 5 y
POD # 5 y
e
Enhance

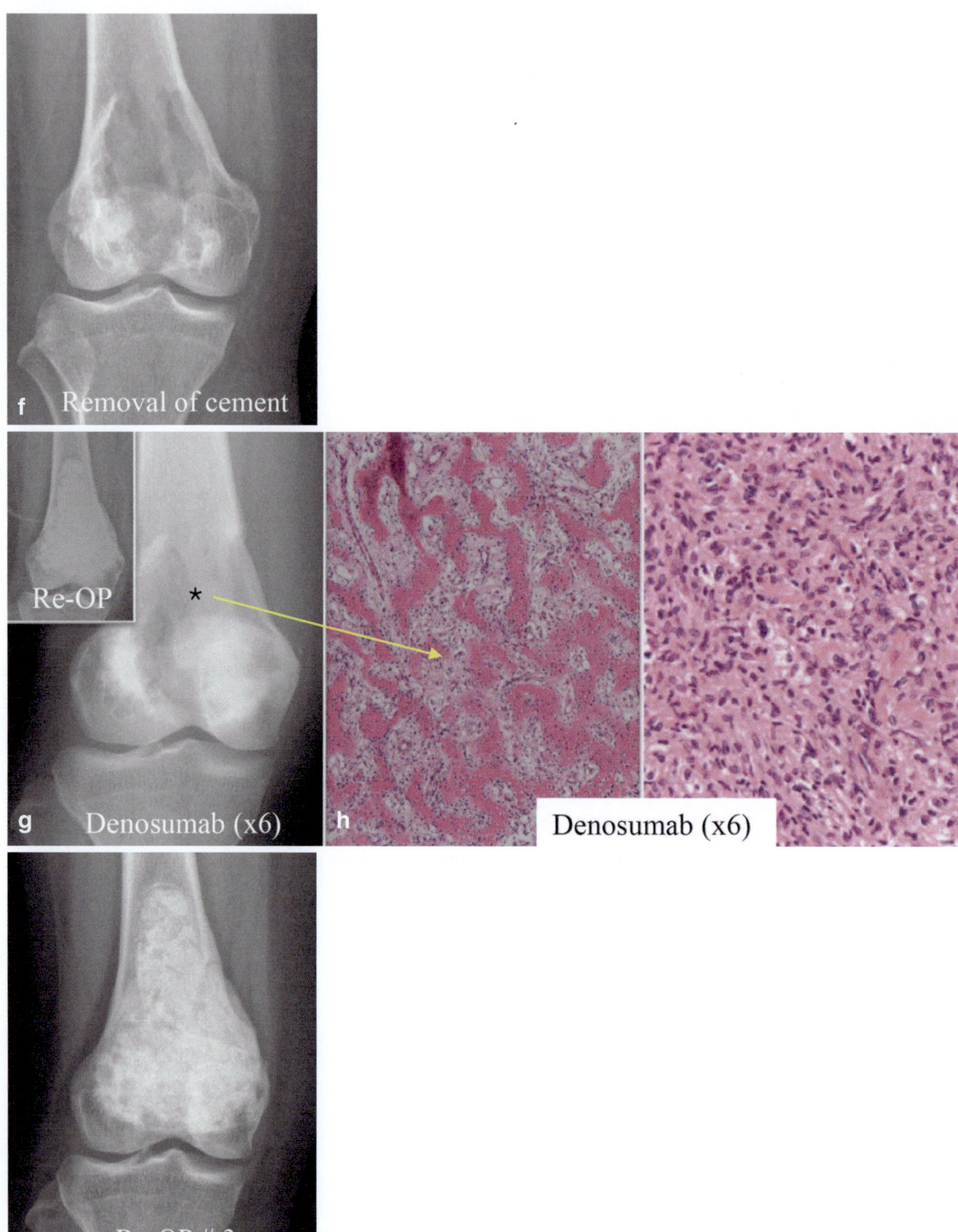

Fig. 1.13 (continued)

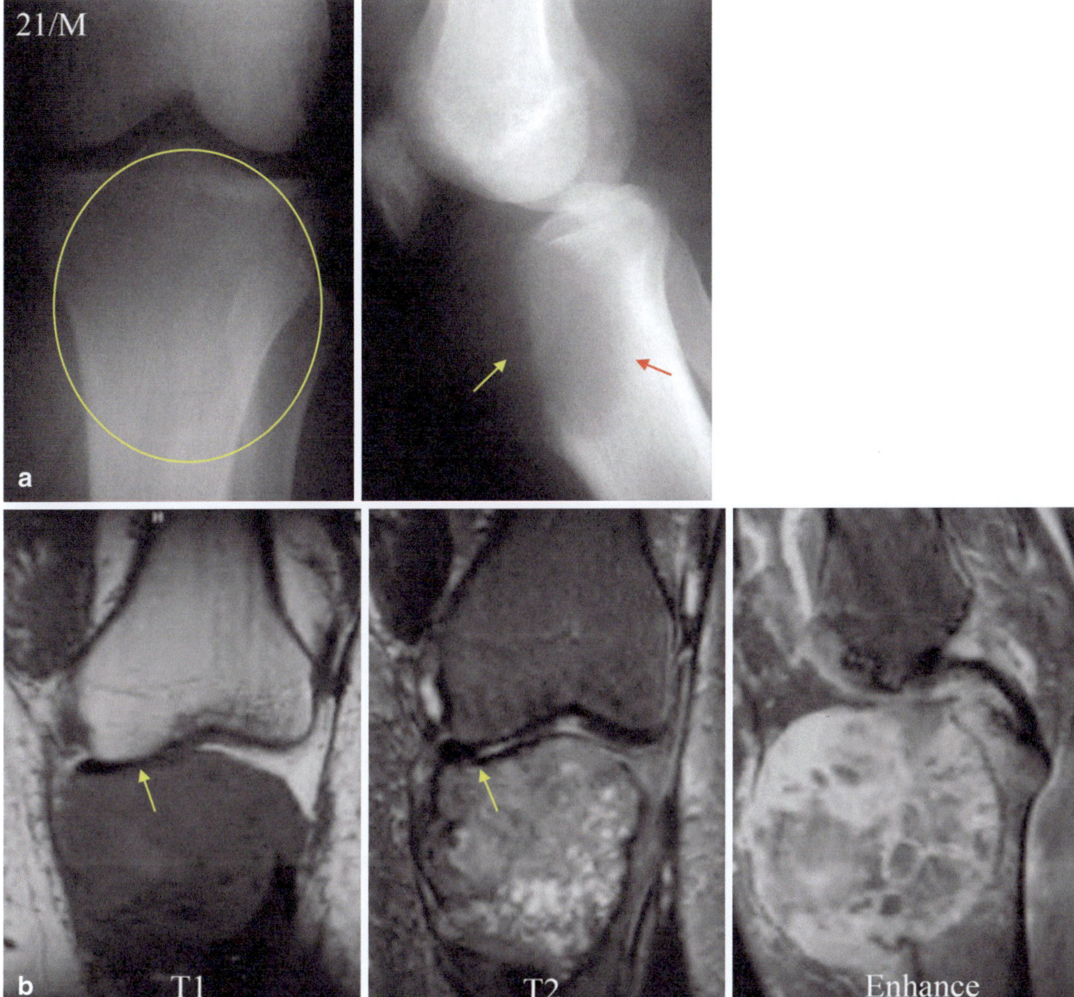

Fig. 1.14 ***Soft tissue recurrence with pulmonary implant*** (**a**) Radiograph taken for left knee swelling of 5 months' duration in 21-year-old young man shows a large ill-defined, hazy radiolucent lesion (red circles) in the epi-metaphysis of proximal tibia. The quality of radiography is very hazy and poor because of severe obesity of the patient over 130 kg in weight. But lateral view reveals a clearer osteolytic lesion with broad zone of transition (red arrow) and anterior cortical destruction with naked huge soft tissue mass (yellow arrow), suggesting locally aggressive GCT or even malignant tumor. (**b**) MR images reveal a huge multi-lobulated expansile mass-like lesion abutting to subchondral bone with low SI on T1-weighted image and heterogeneous intermediate and high SI on T2-weighted image. However, there is no definite destruction of articular cartilage and joint extension (yellow arrows). The bone lesion as well as soft tissue mass is heterogeneously enhanced. (**c**) Extended curettage using high-speed burr with fibula allograft and iliac crest autograft was performed under a pathologic diagnosis of GCT with secondary ABC (inset). (**d**) Seven months later, local recurrence occurred and second extended curettage using chemical cauterization with 99% alcohol was done. (**e**) At 6 months after second surgery, chest radiograph and CT scan notes a clearly discernable nodule (yellow arrows), which was surgically resected after pathologic confirmation of GCT by CT guided biopsy. (**f**) Two years later, follow-up radiograph shows a well-circumscribed, sclerotic soft tissue mass (red arrow), which was excised and pathologically proven as local recurrence of GCT in the soft tissue. (**g**) Follow-up radiograph at 16 years after initial surgery reveals no evidence of local recurrence and another pulmonary implantation. Note severe degenerative change of the knee joint (arrow), but he is free of knee pain

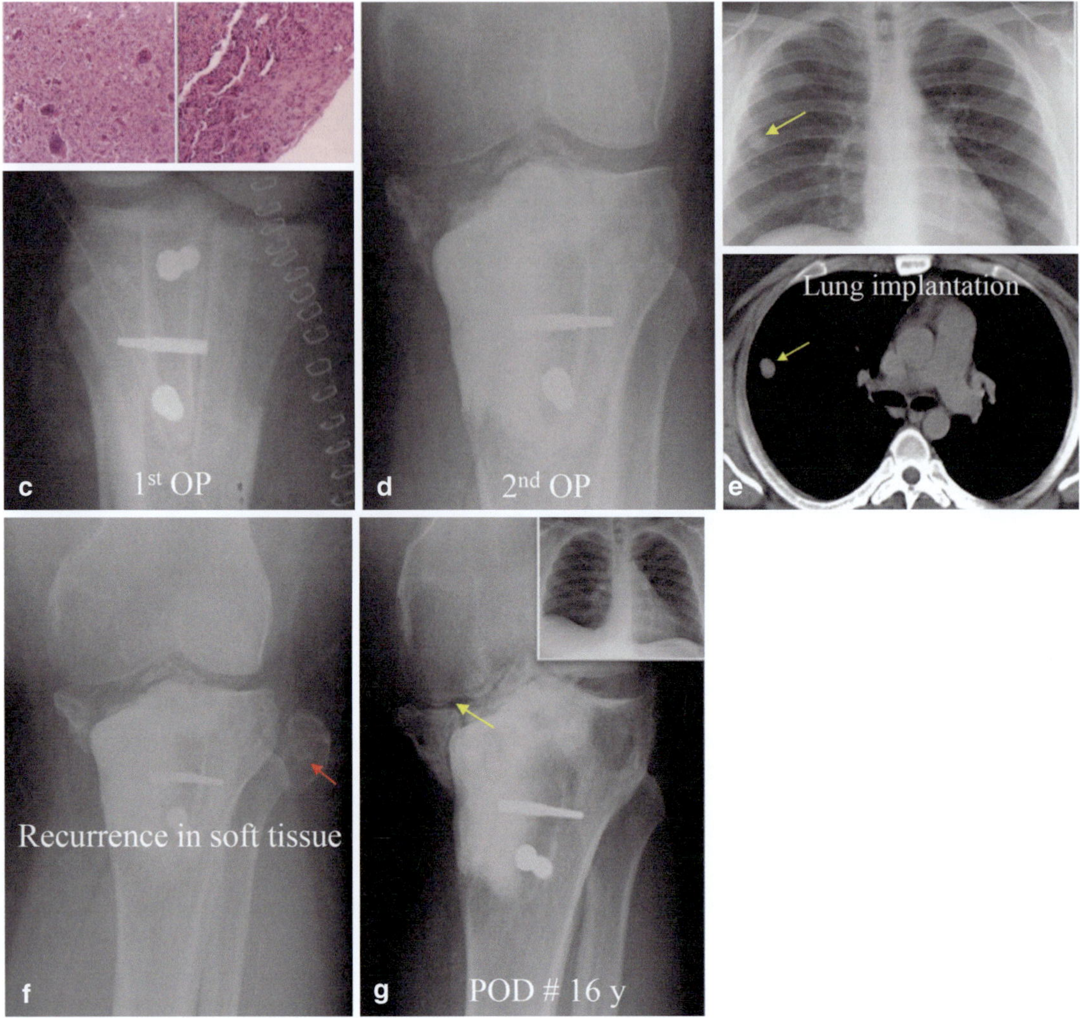

Fig. 1.14 (continued)

joint space. The cortex can be eroded or beached by the tumor in association with elevation of the periosteum resulting in a thin periosteal shell of reactive bone. The periosteal new bone formation may suggest a benignancy despite the local aggressiveness (Figs. 1.3, 1.2, and 1.15). However, more aggressive GCT can destroyed the cortex and periosteum invading into adjacent soft tissue without reactive bone formation simulating malignant tumor (Fig. 1.1a). Even rarely, incomplete rim of reactive sclerotic bone formation may herald a malignant transformation of the pre-existing GCT (Fig. 1.16). **Bone scan** usually shows intensely increased uptake, often increased uptake in the periphery of the lesion with central weaker uptake or photon defect appearing as "*doughnut*" shape. It may fail to detect soft-tissue tumor extension and thus is less useful in planning surgical management but useful to detect extremely rare multifocal GCTs. **CT scan** usually depicted as eccentrically located solitary lucent bone lesion with no matrix mineralization. It can more clearly present cystic changes, cortical thinning or destruction, periosteal reaction, and soft tissue extension than plain radiograph. **MR images** shows the extent of the intramedullary mass-like lesion, cortical involvement, destruction with soft tissue exten-

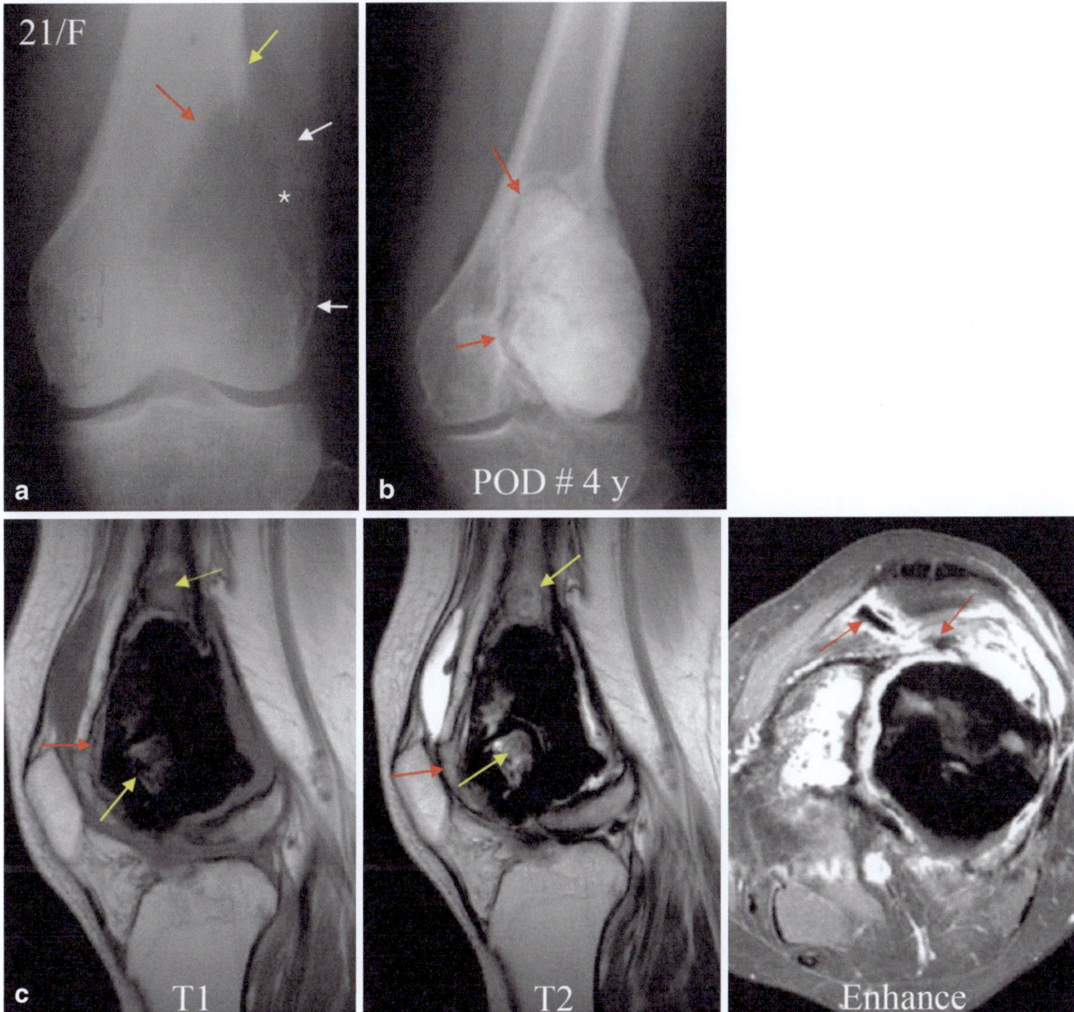

Fig. 1.15 ***Bony local recurrence with pulmonary implantation*** (**a**) Radiograph taken for left knee pain of 3-month duration in 21-year-old young lady shows an ill-defined, eccentric, geographic destruction with a wide transitional zone (red arrow) in the epi-metaphysis of right distal femur. There is a significant cortical destruction with soft tissue extension (asterisk). Note Codman's triangle (yellow arrow) and thin surrounding periosteal shell of reactive bone (white arrows), suggesting probable locally aggressive benignancy or low-grade malignancy rather than high-grade sarcoma. (**b**) Radiograph taken for recurrent knee pain at 4 years after extended curettage with bone cementing under a pathologic diagnosis of GCT shows a circumferential radiolucent line around the cement, suggesting a local recurrence (arrows). (**c**) MR images reveal small solid lesions around and within the dark signal of cement (yellow arrows) with heterogeneous SI on both T1- and T2-weighted images, which are irregularly enhanced. Intra-articular lesion as well as synovium is also enhanced. Several irregular black signal foci (red arrows) are seen in the patellofemoral joint space representing intra-articular leakage of bone cement particles through the joint destruction. (**d**) Removal of cement followed by extended curettage using high-speed bur through a large window with re-cementing and plate fixation for prevention of postoperative pathologic fracture was performed. (**e**) On 2 weeks after second surgery, chest radiograph taken for chest pain with severe dyspnea notes a large amount of pleural effusion at right lower lung field. (**f**) Follow-up CT after chest tube drainage demonstrates reduced effusion and a well-defined hypodense lesion with dot-like hyperdense nodule (arrow) in the right lower lobe. (**g**) Three-dimensional helical CT/angiography shows a well-defined oval and hypervascular mass with feeding and draining vessels (arrow) in the right lower lobe, highly suggestive of an arteriovenous malformation. However, thoracotomy finding was a solid mass of 2 cm in diameter, having feeding vessels and large blood clots in the right lower lobe. Wedge resection including the mass was performed. The mass was histologically proven to be a GCT of benign nature. (**h**) Radiograph at 16 years after re-operation reveals no evidence of local recurrence. She is doing well with no apparent recurrence in the bone and chest

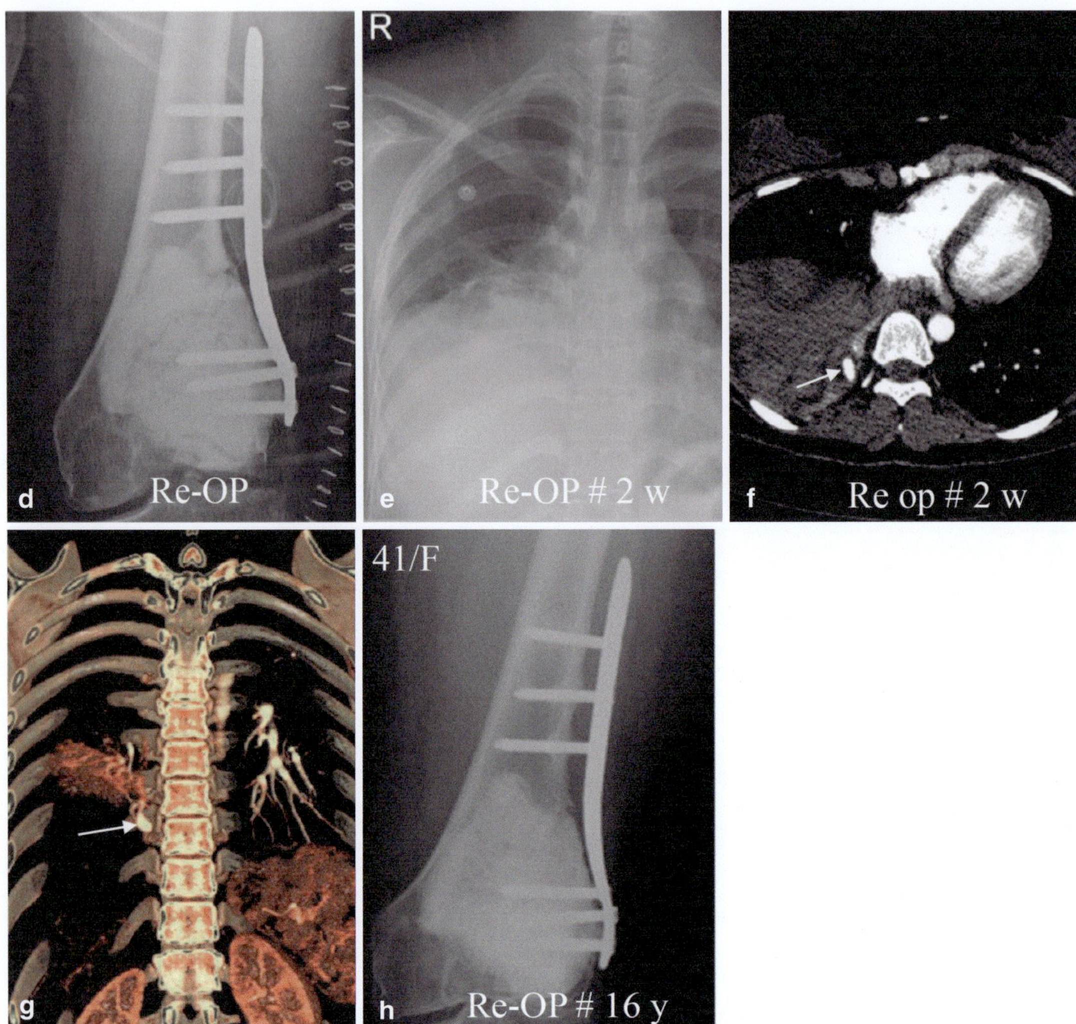

Fig. 1.15 (continued)

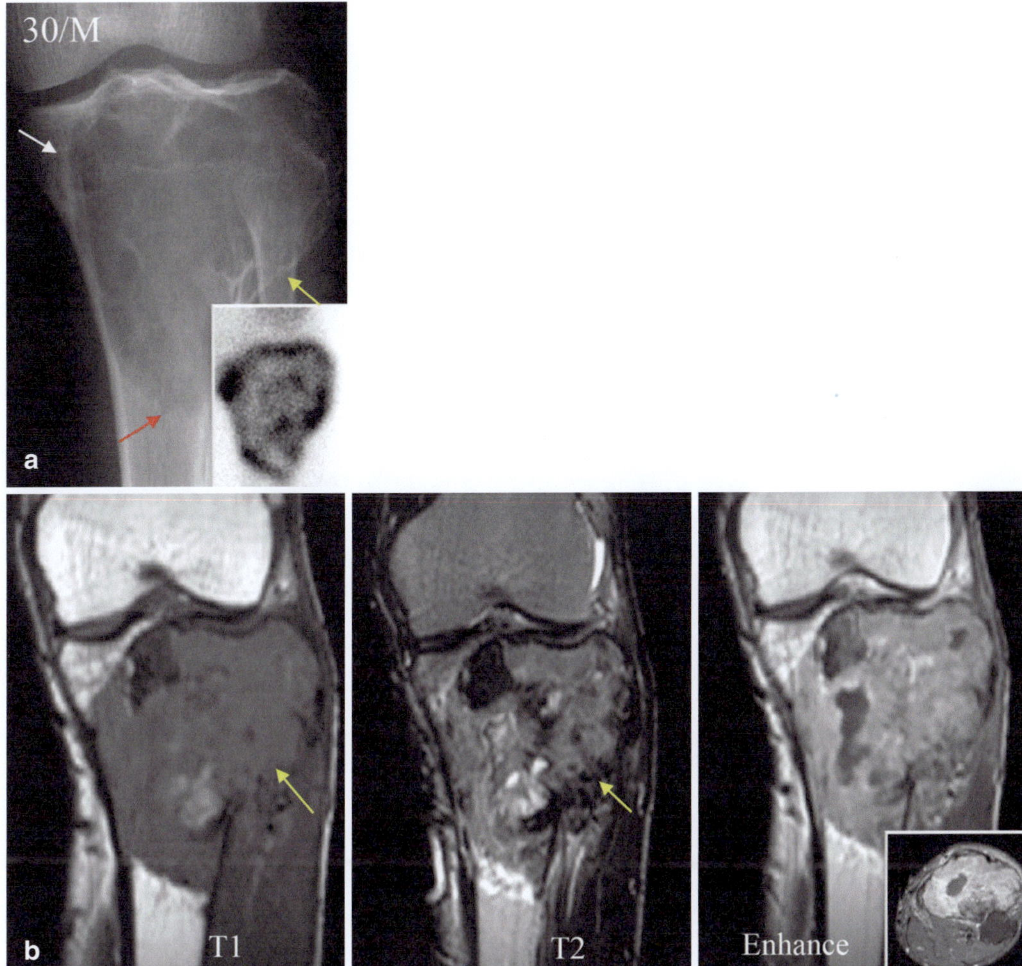

Fig. 1.16 ***Malignant transformation in a recurrent GCT*** (**a**) Radiograph taken for left knee pain of 1 year's duration in 30-year-old man shows a large multichambered geographic destruction with focal ballooning and cortical thinning as well as possible cortical breakage (yellow arrow) in epimetaphysis of proximal tibia. The margin is abutting to the subchondral area and ill-defined with a wide transitional zone with no sclerotic margin distally (red arrow) and focal incomplete rim of sclerosis proximally (white arrow), suggesting locally aggressive or malignant change of pre-existing benign tumor, or even primary malignant tumor. Pinhole bone scan notes densely increased uptake at periphery and septa of the lesion with internal photon defect areas (inset). (**b**) MR images reveal a large intramedullary mass-like lesion with focal ballooning, cortical breakage, and tumor extension to soft tissue (arrows). The SI is heterogeneous low and intermediate SI on T1-weighted image and mixed intermediate and high SI with internal dark and focal bright signals on T2-weighted image. The lesion is heterogeneously enhanced with non-enhancing areas. (**c**) Extended curettage using high-speed bur followed by cementing after subchondral bone graft with plate fixation was performed with a pathologic diagnosis of conventional GCT (inset). (**d**) Follow-up radiograph taken for recurrent knee pain at 10 years after surgery demonstrates radiolucent areas around the cement (red arrows) with collapse of medial condyle and marked varus deformity of the knee compared to immediate postoperative radiograph (yellow lines), suggesting a local recurrence. (**e**) Follow-up pinhole scan notes strong (yellow asterisks) at the peri-cement radiolucent areas on radiograph. There is also small area of milder uptake (white arrow). (**f**) Bone SPECT also shows an increased uptake at the same areas (yellow arrows) and adjacent soft tissue (white arrow), suggesting a possible bony recurrence with soft tissue extension. (**g**) PET/CT scan also shows intense FDG uptake around the previous surgical area. (**h**) Incision biopsy was performed in the radiolucent area under a guidance with C-arm image intensifier (inset). Microscopic examination. (Left) Lower-power magnification reveals a high cellularity of spindle cells with pleomorphic and atypical nuclei. (Right) Higher-power magnification notes highly bizarre anaplastic nuclei with mitoses, indicating high-grade sarcoma. The final diagnosis is a malignant transformation to undifferentiated pleomorphic sarcoma from a recurrent GCT at 10 years after initial surgery. (**i**) Follow-up radiograph at 4 years after wide resection and reconstruction with tumor prosthesis reveals good maintenance with no local recurrence nor pulmonary metastasis

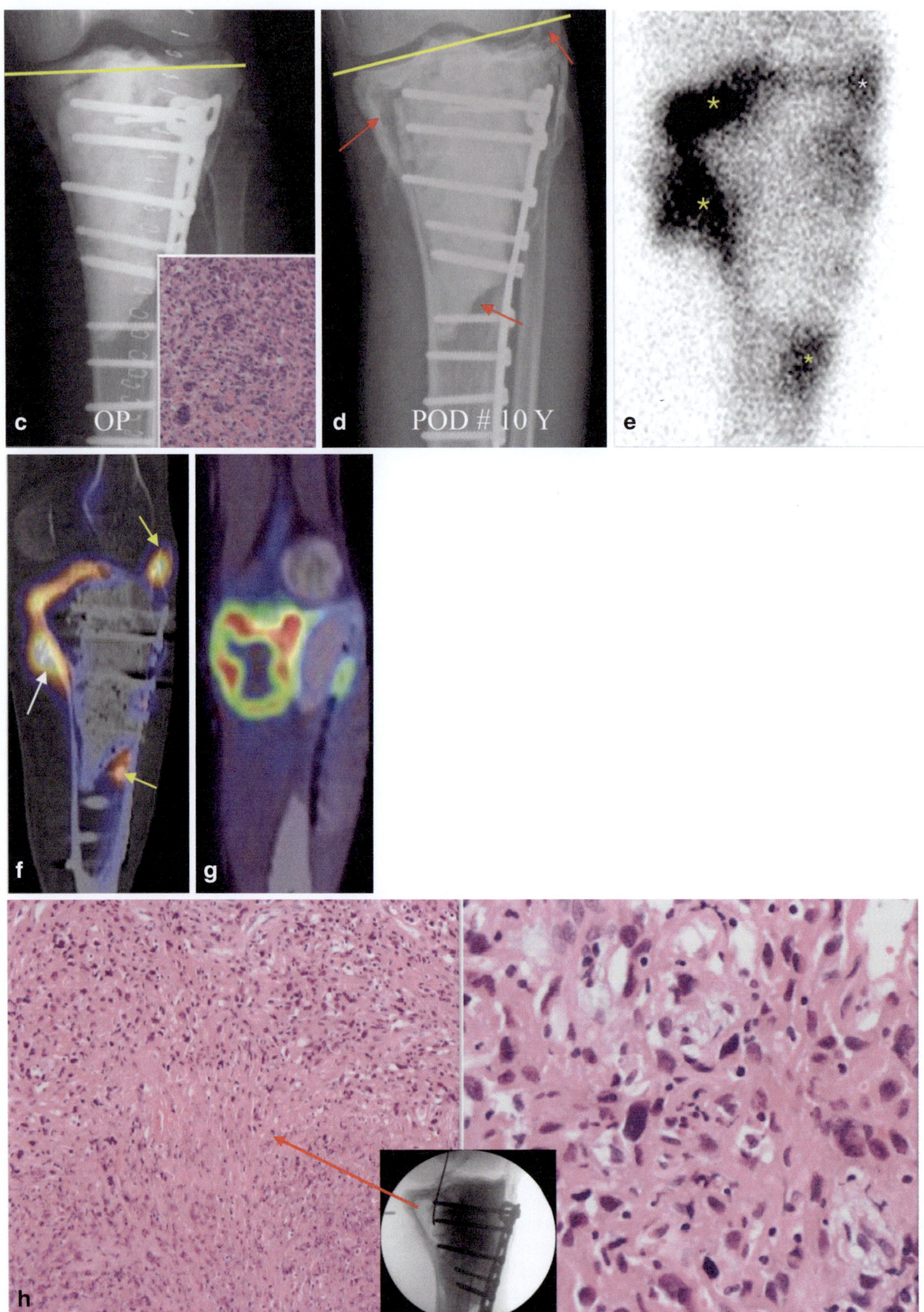

Fig. 1.16 (continued)

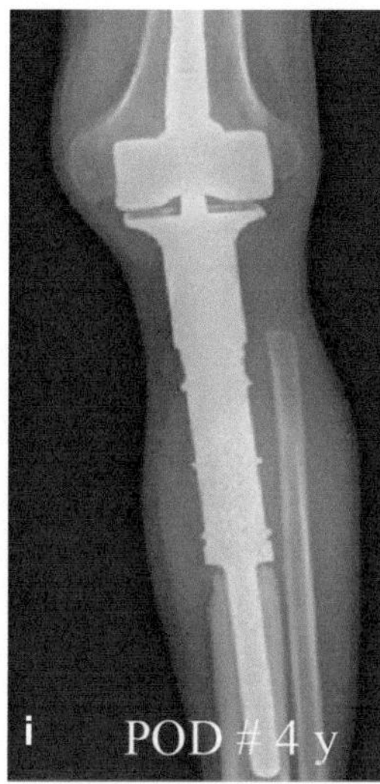

Fig. 1.16 (continued)

sion, and secondary changes such as hemorrhagic areas, fluid-fluid levels indicating secondary aneurysmal bone cyst (ABC), and surrounding bone marrow edema. Signal intensity (SI) is low to intermediate on T1-weighted image and heterogeneous low to intermediate with high signals on T2-weighted image. There can be a variety of areas with mixed signals of high and variable degree of low intensity depending on a degree of cellularity, collagen or hemosiderin deposition, fibrosis, and recent hemorrhage on T2-weighted image. The lesion can be well defined by a surrounding thin rim of dark signal suggesting benignancy, but the sclerotic rim can be absent or incomplete suggesting a local aggressiveness (Figs. 1.7b and 1.8c). The cortex is often broken and the lesion forms a large soft tissue mass simulating a malignant tumor (Figs. 1.1c and 1.4b). Cystic degeneration is commonly associated, and fluid-fluid levels can be well visualized on T2-weighted image, suggesting associated secondary ABC (Figs. 1.8c and 1.9c). High signals in adjacent bone marrow represent peri-tumoral inflammation and edema. The solid component of lesion is well enhanced by contrast medium, which helps to differentiate GCT with secondary ABC change from primary ABC without pre-existing solid lesion (Fig. 1.10c).

1.9 Histologic Findings

GCT is histologically typified by *neoplastic component* of round to oval, short spindle, mononuclear cells in the moderately vascular stroma and *nonneoplastic component* of diffusely scattered, varying number of osteoclast-like multinucleated giant cells (Fig. 1.17a). The nuclei of mononuclear stromal cells are identical to those of giant cells. Bi-nucleated or tri-nucleated cells can be observed that suggest a gradual merge of mononuclear cells to multinucleated cells with variable number of nuclei (Fig. 1.17b). There can be rich in vascular trees of varying size including "*staghorn*" pattern between those cells as in hemangiopericytoma. Occasionally, intravascular involvement of tumor cells can be observed (Fig. 1.17b), but it seems to be not significant for predicting prognosis [2, 4]. Mitotic activity of mononuclear cells is almost always present. However, there is no mitotic activity within multinucleated giant cells. Those typical findings can be altered by secondary changes such as hemorrhage, hemosiderin deposits, aggregation of foamy macrophages, necrosis, ABC changes, and reactive bone formation. Some cases may present a varying degree of collagen deposition with a general reduction in number of multinucleated giant cells (Figs. 1.9e and 1.17c). Tumor itself does not produce bone or cartilage matrix, but varying proportion of reactive osteoid or woven bone is often presented usually in the periphery of the tumor (Figs. 1.8e and 1.17c). Less than 10% of GCT are rich in fibrohistiocytic tissues and even xanthoma cells with fatty change, hemorrhage, necrosis, reparative tissues, and variable sized areas (usually small) of conventional GCT often with markedly reduced number of giant cells, so-called "*fibrous histiocytoma-like variant*" *or ancient GCT* (Fig. 1.18), which would be expected for a longstanding form of GCT [4]. On occasion, fibrohistiocytic reaction can be arranged in storiform pattern that may be so prominent to replace the pre-existing GCT with variable degree of reduced number of giant cells, simulating benign fibrous histiocytoma or non-

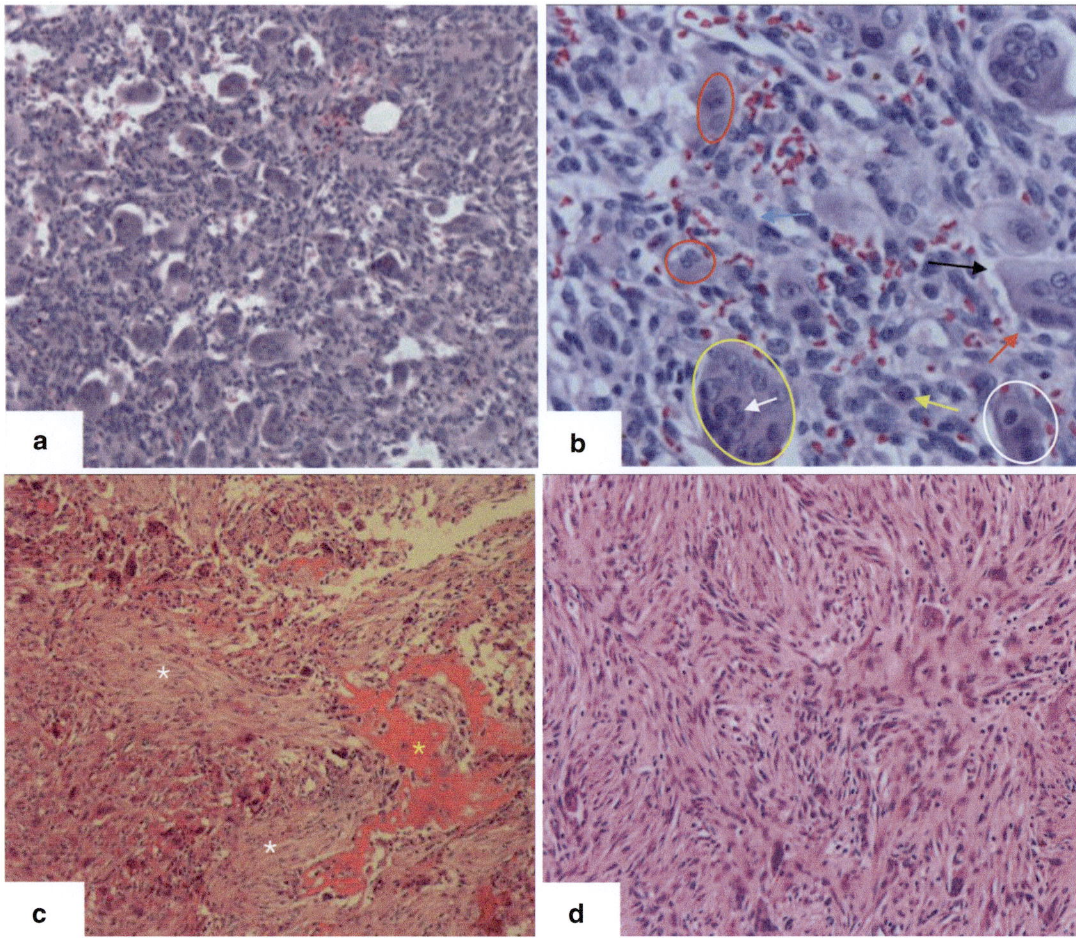

Fig. 1.17 ***Microscopic features***. (**a**) Low-power magnification shows typical two parts of "*neoplastic component*" of round to oval, short spindle, mononuclear cell and "*nonneoplastic component*" of diffusely scattered numerous multinucleated giant cells. (**b**) Medium-power magnification reveals mononuclear cells as well as bi-nucleated (red circles) or tri-nucleated cells (white circle), suggesting a gradual merge of mononuclear cells finally to multinucleated cells (yellow circle) in the hypervascular and hemorrhagic stroma. The nuclei of multinucleated cells (white arrow) are identical to those of mononuclear cells (yellow arrow). There are rich in vascular trees of varying size including "*staghorn*" pattern between those cells as in hemangiopericytoma (black arrow) often with intravascular extension of the tumor cells (red arrow). (**c**) Focal collagenized foci are seen with no giant cells in them (white asterisks), and reactive woven bone spicules are deposited in the periphery of the tumor (yellow asterisk). (**d**) An area with predominant histiocytic cells arranged in storiform pattern with scattered multinucleated giant cells simulating non-ossifying fibroma is associated. (**e**) Areas of foam cells and prominently collagenized stroma (inset) are seen. Often, scanty to no giant cells can be seen in elderly patients. (**f**) Focal or massive hemorrhage is often observed (asterisks), and necrosis may be rarely presented. The number of multinucleated giant cells is considerably small, and a few ghostlike outlines of the giant cells are visible in this area. Biopsy specimen obtained from the lesion associated with pathologic fracture present an area of massive to total necrosis (inset). (**g**) A variable estimated aged callus ascribed to microfracture or concealed stress fracture should be recognized. This area shows woven bone trabeculae rimmed by a single row of osteoblast, which begin to connect together forming variable-sized circles, indicating a callus with estimated age of 2–3 weeks. This kind of callus is no more considered as a malignant tumor, but it can make a diagnosis complicated if not recognized as callus. (**h**) Areas with dilated, thick, blood vessel walls with red blood cells, indicating secondary ABC are seen in this filed

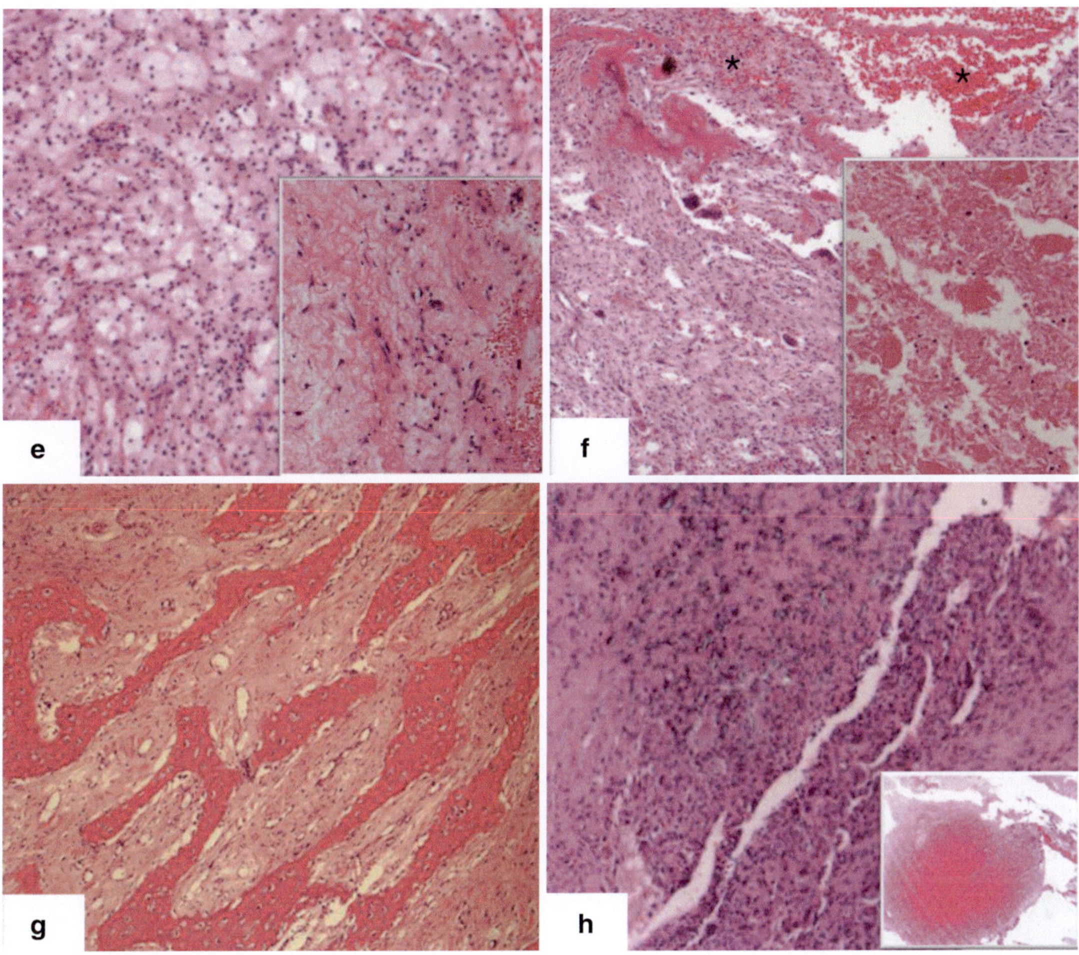

Fig. 1.17 (continued)

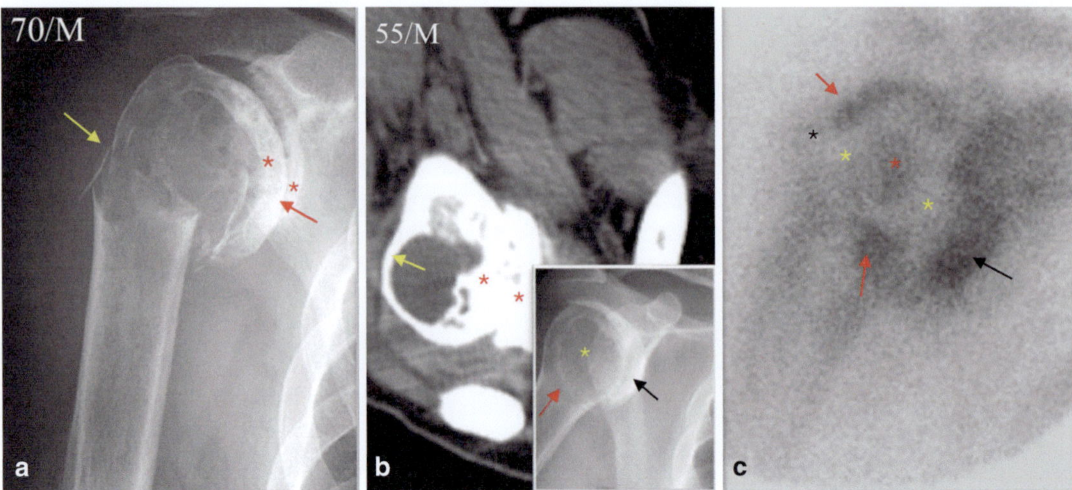

Fig. 1.18 ***"Fibrous histiocytoma-like variant" or "Ancient" GCT*** (**a**) Radiograph taken for right shoulder after slip in 70-year-old man shows an ill-defined multi-septate geographic destruction with significant cortical thinning and pathologic fracture (yellow arrow) in the head and neck of humerus. There is also marked subchondral sclerotic change in the humeral head and scapular glenoid (asterisks) with severe narrowing of the joint space, which indicate a severe degenerative arthritis. (**b**) Retrospective review of chest CT scan taken for fever study 10 years ago when the patient was 60 years old already notes a well-defined geographic destruction with cortical erosion and thinning (yellow arrow) and significant degrative change of the shoulder joint (asterisks). Chest radiograph (inset) also noted a well-defined lucent lesion (yellow asterisk) with a thin rim of sclerosis (red arrow) and same sclerotic change in the shoulder joint (black arrow). Those findings were not recognized by the primary physician at that time. (**c**) Bone scan reveals a heterogeneous peripheral weak uptake (red arrows) with mostly void uptake suggesting cystic change (yellow asterisks) and focal area of central weak uptake (red asterisk) suggesting pre-existing solid tumor. There is more intense uptake at gleno-humeral joint (black arrow) indicating degrative arthritic change. (**d**) MR images demonstrate multi-lobulated lesion occupying almost whole humeral head and neck (yellow asterisks) with low SI on T1-weighted image (left inset) and heterogeneous high SI with focal areas of low and intermediate signals on fat saturated T2-weighted image, indicating mostly cystic lesion with internal focal solid lesion. The central solid area is focally enhanced (arrow). There is also small multiple focal enhancement in other cut level (right inset). (**e**) Microscopic examination. (Left) Low-power magnification shows mostly nonspecific degenerative cystic structure and small area of GCT with focal calcification (red circle). (Middle) Focal areas of solid component with round to oval spindle cells and few scattered degenerated multinucleated cells (inset) with focal calcification (black circles) are observed in association with area of hemorrhage, fibrin deposition, and inflammatory exudate within fibrinous granular background (yellow circle), suggesting an early callus estimated age of a few days. (Right) In addition, large foci of collagen deposition are observed with scanty degenerated multinucleated giant cells (yellow arrows) as well as foam cells in other filed (inset). In correlation of patient's age and imaging findings including radiographs, CT, MRI and bone scintigraphy, a diagnosis of "*fibrous histiocytoma-like variant*" or "*ancient*" GCT with huge degenerative cyst was rendered. (**f**) Follow-up radiograph taken at 4 years after curettage, cementing and plate fixation notes good maintenance with no evidence of local recurrence

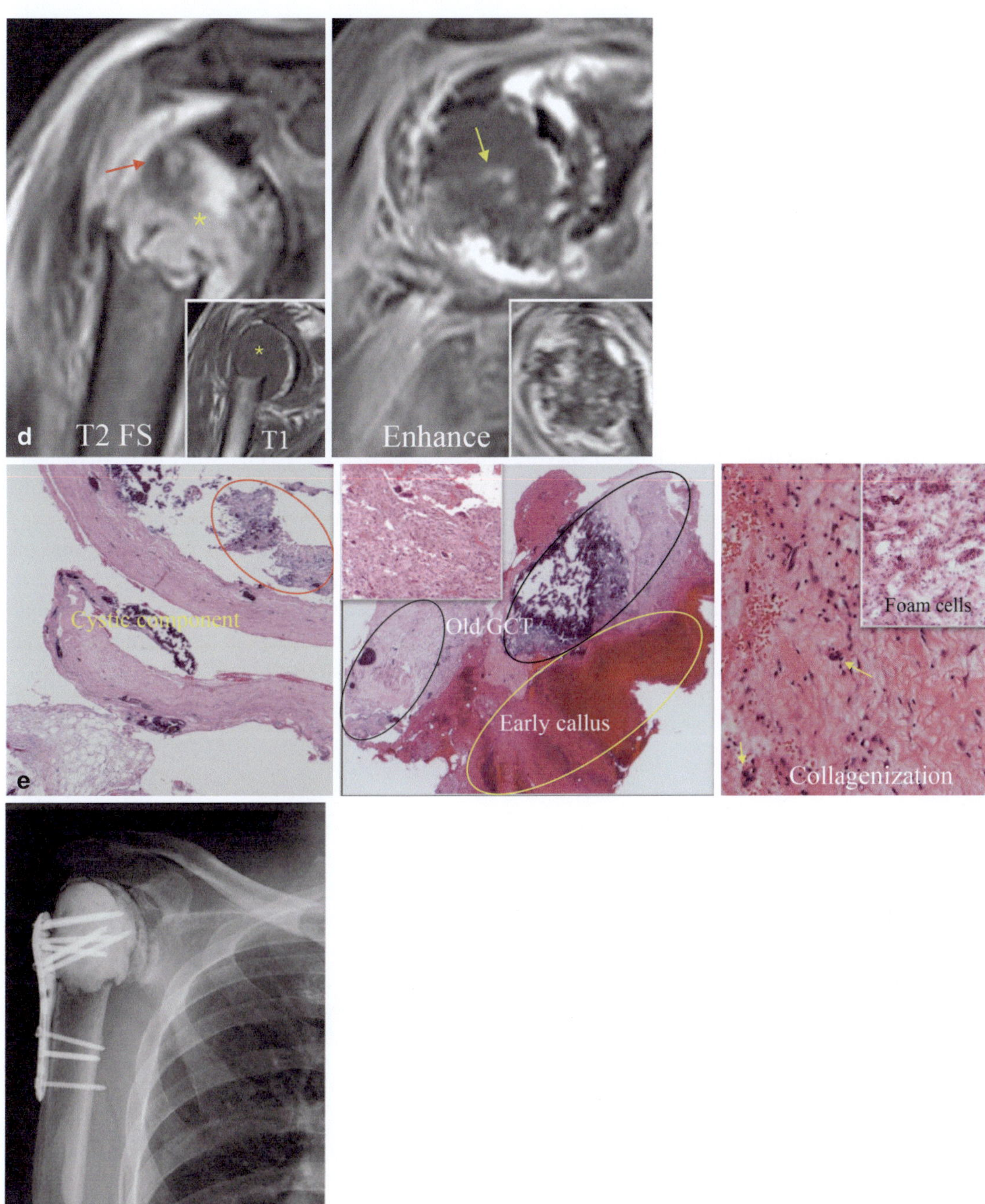

Fig. 1.18 (continued)

ossifying fibroma (Fig. 1.17d). In such cases, patient's age and location of the lesion as well as radiographic findings should be correlated for a correct diagnosis. A few cases of elderly patients may also show foci of foam cells with collagenized stroma and considerable reduction of the sprinkled giant cells (Fig. 1.17e). Focal or massive hemorrhage is often observed, and necrosis may be rarely presented without fracture (Figs. 1.6f and 1.17f). They usually result from fracture or mechanical compression, but quite extensive hemorrhage and necrosis can present without any obvious reason [1]. Some ghostlike outlines of the multinucleated giant cells are still easily seen in the necrotic area (Fig. 1.17f). Callus of varying estimated age by microfracture or pathologic fracture can be observed in addition to the tumor itself (Fig. 1.17g). Microscopic foci of ABC can be frequently observed. Secondary ABC change with large, dilated, thick-walled blood containing cyst-like structure (Fig. 1.17h) is seen in less than 10% of GCTs [1]. In extremely rare cases, bizarre nuclear changes without abnormal mitosis representing degenerative phenomenon can be also observed as in various other benign bone tumors [1, 5, 26]. The bizarre nuclear can occur after gelfoam embolization done a few days before surgery for reduction of perioperative bleeding (Fig. 1.19). They histologically simulate malignant tumor but do not indicate aggressive behavior. Very rarely, a frank malignancy can be associated with conventional GCT as either primary or secondary form. Primary malignant GCT is extremely rare and present at first diagnosis, which consists of an area or a nodule of high-grade pleomorphic mononuclear with a continuum of benign GCT (Fig. 1.20) [23]. Secondary malignant GCT (malignant change) occurs at the site of previously documented or treated GCT with single or multiple local recurrence, and the preexisting benign GCT may or may not be evident (Fig. 1.16). It may be transformed into osteosarcoma, undifferentiated pleomorphic sarcoma, or fibrosarcoma [1, 27].

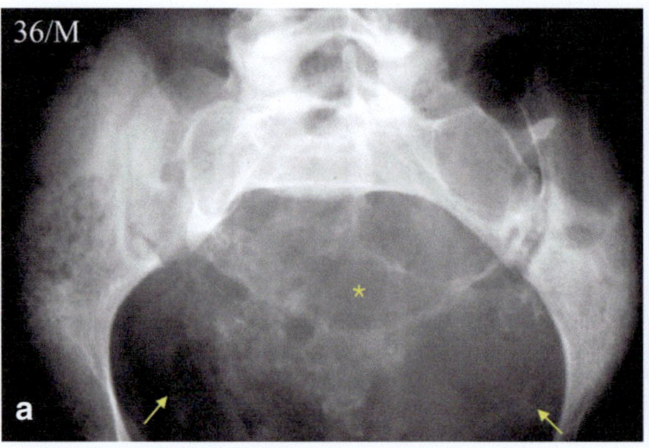

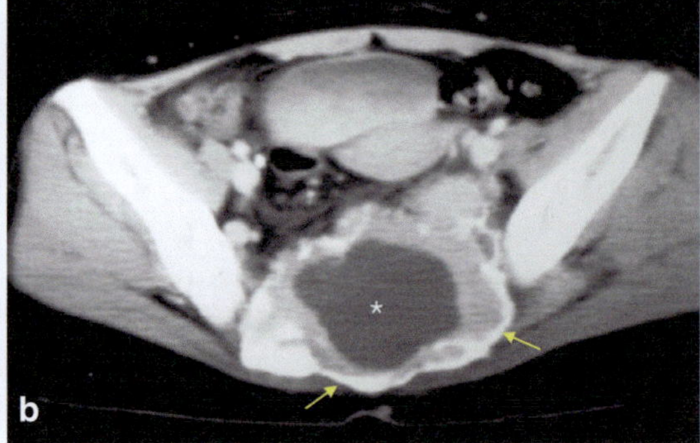

Fig. 1.19 ***"Pseudoanaplastic" GCT*** (**a**) Radiograph taken for sacral pain in 36-year-old man shows a huge, expansile geographic destruction in the sacrum (asterisk). A hint of probable benignancy despite the huge size and locally aggressive nature is noted by a hazy sclerotic rim of reactive new bone (yellow arrows). (**b**) CT scan reveals a well-defined huge osteolytic lesion (asterisk) with irregular cortical thinning but no discernible destruction (yellow arrows). Gelfoam embolization was performed to reduce perioperative bleeding before surgery, and thorough curettage was performed. (**c**) Microscopic examination notes round to oval, short spindle, mononuclear stromal cells with diffusely sprinkled osteoclast-like multinucleated giant cells, indicating conventional GCT in this field. (**d**) Higher-power examination of another field shows tons of large and bizarre atypical nuclei resembling a high-grade sarcoma. However, nuclei are somewhat smudged, and a single abnormal mitosis is not found in any of the slides. Gelfoam embolization was believed to be the cause the significant degenerative nuclear change mimicking a malignancy. In correlation of radiographic finding of a hazy sclerotic rim of reactive new bone as well as CT scan finding of a well-defined lesion with no cortical destruction suggesting a benignancy, the final diagnosis of "*pseudoanaplastic*" GCT was rendered. He is free of local recurrence and pulmonary metastasis at the final follow-up at 5 years after curettage. (Courtesy by Prof. JM Mirra)

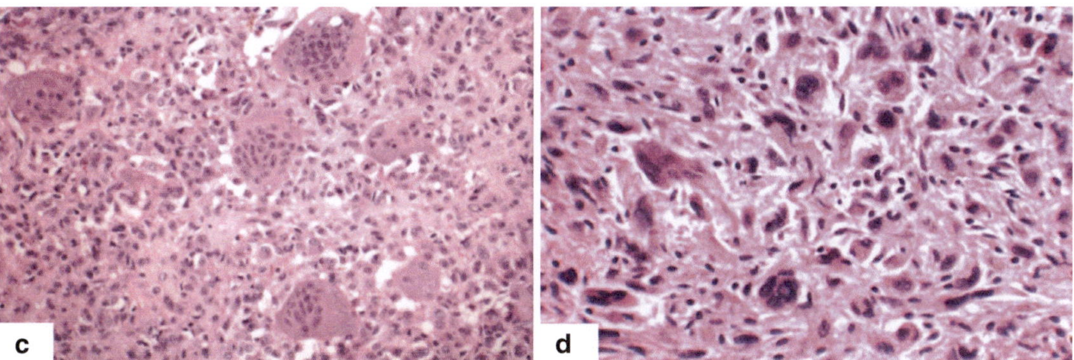

Fig. 1.19 (continued)

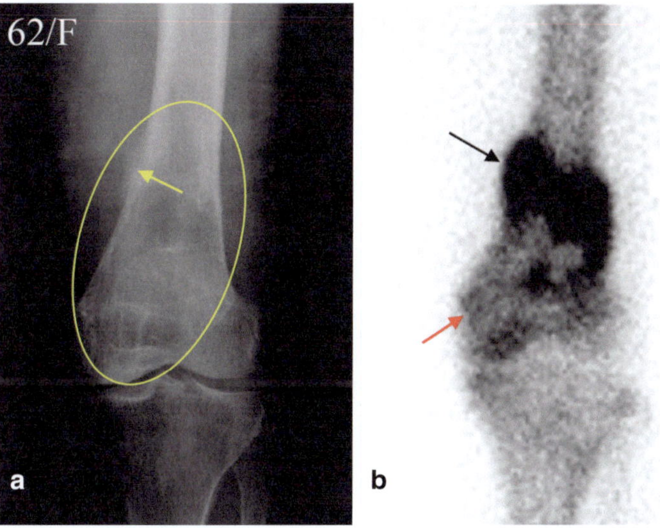

Fig. 1.20 ***Primary, de novo, malignant GCT*** (**a**) Radiograph taken for left knee pain of 2-month duration in 62-year-old woman shows an ill-defined osteolytic lesion (circle) with moth-eaten destruction and broad transzonal zone. There are suspicious cortical breakage and soft tissue extension with new bone formation (arrow) in the epi-metaphysis of distal femur. (**b**) Bone scan shows homogeneous strong uptake mainly in the metaphysis (black arrow) and milder uptake in the epiphysis (red arrow) with central void area. (**c**) MR images demonstrate an ill-defined intramedullary mass-like lesion with focal cortical destruction and soft tissue extension (yellow arrows), suggesting locally aggressive or malignant tumor. There is a focal epiphyseal invasion (red arrow). The SI is low and intermediate SI on T1-weighted image and heterogeneous intermediate and high SI with internal dark signal on T2-weighted image. The bony (red arrow) and extraosseous lesion (yellow arrow) are heterogeneously well enhanced. However, she refused further evaluation and management for personal reason. (**d**) Radiograph taken for severe aggravation of the pain after slip at 3 months after initial visit notes a pathologic fracture. (**e**) Microscopic examination. (Left & Middle) Medium-power magnification notes an area with proliferation of bland round to oval mononuclear stromal cells and scattered multinucleated giant cells indicating benign GCT, and juxtaposed area with highly pleomorphic mononuclear cells with bizarre-looking giant cells indicative of malignant GCT. (Right) Higher-power magnification of malignant-looking area shows more prominent atypism and pleomorphism with bizarre nuclei as well as abnormal mitoses (black arrows). (**f**) Follow-up radiograph at 7 years after wide resection and reconstruction with tumor prosthesis shows no evidence of local recurrence

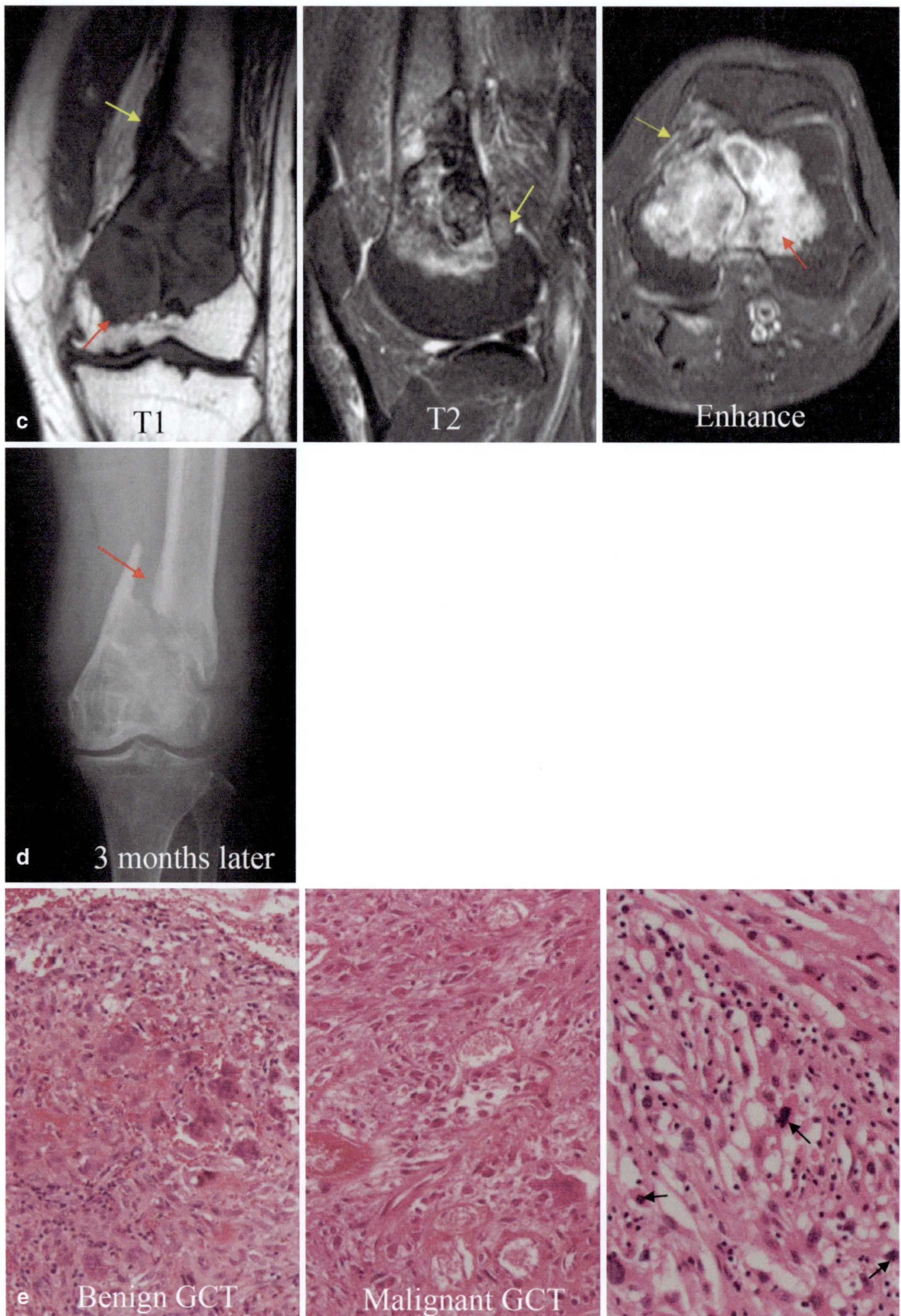

Fig. 1.20 (continued)

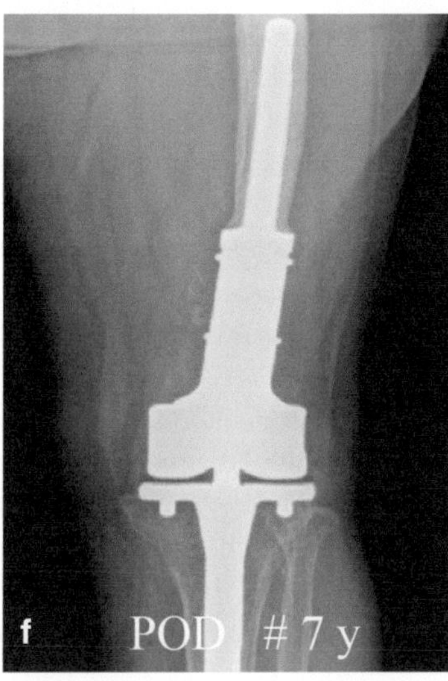

Fig. 1.20 (continued)

1.10 Management

Thorough curettage with filling the defect is a standard option of management. Curettage can be extended by a combination of the use of surgical, chemical, or thermal adjuvants. The adjuvant therapy may include high-speed burr, liquid nitrogen (cryotherapy), phenol, ethanol, and argon-beam coagulation to extend killing of tumor cells. The bone defect after curettage is usually filled using autologous bone grafts, allograft, and PMMA bone cement with or without internal fixation. Bone cement is useful for reconstruction of a larger defect with advantages including immediate mechanical stability to permit early weight bearing and immediate rehabilitation as well as feasible detection of local recurrence by radiolucency between the lesion and cement (Figs. 1.13d, 1.15b, and 1.16d). Although the cement produce heat during polymerization, it cannot deliver the heat deeply seated tumors effectively and selectively. Some authors suggested that the polymerization heat alone has no necrotizing effect, although hot toxic chemicals during polymerization may inhibit bone blood perfusion and remodeling [28, 29]. However, the heat from the bone cement can damage the articular cartilage, and thus thick subchondral bone graft before cementing is necessary to protect the articular cartilage (Fig. 1.4e). En bloc resection is indicated for an extensive destruction with cortical destruction and poor residual bone stock, impossible joint salvage, and for expendable bone such as fibular head or distal ulna (Fig. 1.5). Transarterial embolization, which may kill the tumor cells by blocking oxygen and nutrition, often performed prior to surgery for a huge sacral tumor or cases in which surgical management is not possible. The preoperative embolization may lead marked nuclear degeneration and pleomorphism but no definite abnormal mitosis, so-called *"pseudoanaplastic" GCT*, which can be mistaken for malignancy (Fig. 1.19). Radiotherapy can be considered in unresectable in the axial skeleton, recurrent or incompletely resected cases. It may provide a suitable alternative to mutilating surgery if sufficient dose can be delivered [30]. Recently, RANK/RANKL ligand inhibitor, specifically forbidding tumor-associated bone lysis, is used for patients with recurrent, unrespectable, metastatic GCT or for patients in whom surgery would be morbid. Denosumab, currently approved by the FDA and European Medical Agency (EMA) for osteoporosis and also for management of skeletal related events in bone metastases from solid tumors, is an effective and useful drug for managing GCT of bone [31]. Several studies reported histologic response to denosumab including complete absence or marked regression of the giant cells as well as stromal tumor cells and reactive bone formation. Radiologic changes reported to include reduction in tumor size, arrest of lysis with central sclerosis and surrounding new bone formation, and shrinkage of soft tissue mass. Those changes can facilitate surgical resection of locally advanced GCT. Several authors reported a clinical beneficial response to denosumab, particularly in terms of pain control and improvement in function and mobility [32–35]. However, more recent studies reported a higher recurrence rate in patient treated with curettage and malignant change of GCT after denosumab therapy [36–38]. Denosumab selectively targets nonneoplastic osteoclastic giant cells with limited inhibitory effect on neoplastic stromal cells (Fig. 1.13h), which may continuously proliferate on cessation of the drug. There is still a controversy regarding optimal dose, duration, or interval between treatment, to date. The common side effects include fatigue, muscle pain, arthralgia, extremity and back pain, headaches, and nausea. Atypical femur fracture, peripheral neuropathy, skin rash, abnormal serum electrolyte, and jaw osteonecrosis have been also reported. Malignancy in GCT should be treated as other primary bone sarcomas.

1.11 Clinical Course and Prognosis

Grading system of GCT is not valuable for prognosis [2]. High rate of local recurrence has been reported up to 40–50% of GCT after simple curettage [1, 3–5, 39, 40]. However, extended curettage with abovementioned local adjuvants has been reported to improve tumor control with the recurrence rate to below 10% [1, 40, 41]. Cryosurgery using liquid nitrogen was reported to be effective adjunct with local recurrence of 2.3% in a long-term follow-up series [42]. Most recurrence occurs within the first 3 years after initial surgical treatment. Thus, patients should be carefully monitored especially in the first 3 years [41, 43]. The rate of pulmonary metastasis, so-called "*benign pulmonary implants*" by Mirra [44], has been reported in 1–4% of patients [1, 5, 45, 46]. The pulmonary nodules usually grow slowly and are generally cured by simple surgical resection (Fig. 1.15). However, rare patients can suffer multiple disseminated lung nodules and die of disease [7, 46]. Although correlation between tumor growth and pregnancy has not yet been clarified, pregnancy seems to accelerate GCT growth and aggressiveness (Fig. 1.12) as well as increasing chance of local recurrence and pulmonary metastases probably due to alterations of endocrinologic, immunologic, and angiogenic environments in a literature review. The authors emphasized a multidisciplinary approach to offer the best treatment for mother and child's health in case of GCT during pregnancy [47]. Malignant change is the most serious complication of GCT. Malignant change can occur much frequently following radiation therapy, usually 5 years or more after the initial radiation exposure [1], and less commonly in locally recurred tumors after surgical removal. It usually occurs after many years or even decades following multiple local recurrences but can be rarely complicated after a single local recurrence (Fig. 1.16). GCT may undergo malignant change to *fibrosarcoma, undifferentiated pleomorphic sarcoma, or osteosarcoma*. Even malignant change can be identified at the time of initial diagnosis of conventional GCT [1]. It may undergo malignant change to fibrosarcoma, undifferentiated pleomorphic sarcoma, or osteosarcoma. In a comprehensive analysis of four large series of patients with malignant GCT that provided data on 2315 patients with GCT, the cumulative incidence of malignancy was 4.0%. The incidence of primary malignancy was 1.6% (0–9.5%) compared with 2.4% (1.1–5.1%) for secondary malignancy [27]. The authors confirmed that most malignant GCT of bone is secondary and occurs following radiation. To date, the prognosis of malignant GCT is not fully understood because of the rarity. Since Thomas et al. reported a high-grade sarcoma arising in benign GCT following treatment with denosumab therapy [32], several studies reported drug-related malignant transformation of benign GCT following treatment with denosumab therapy [37, 48–51].

References

1. Czerniak B. Giant-cell lesions. In: Dorfman HD, Czerniak B, editors. Dorfman and Czerniak's bone tumors. 2nd ed. Amsterdam: Elsevier; 2016. p. 692–759. (eBook).
2. Unni KK, Inwards CY. Giant cell tumor. In: Unni KK, Inwards CY, editors. Dahlin's bone tumors. 6th ed. Philadelphia: Lippincott Williams & Wilkins; 2010. p. 225–42.
3. Manaster B, Doyle AJ. Giant cell tumors of bone. Radiol Clin North Am. 1993;31(2):299–323.
4. Mirra JM. Giant cell tumors. In: Mirra JM, editor. Bone tumors: clinical, radiologic, and pathologic correlation. 2nd ed. Philadelphia: Lea & Febiger; 1989. p. 942–1020.
5. Turcotte RE, Wunder JS, Isler MH, et al. Giant cell tumor of long bone: a Canadian Sarcoma Group study. Clin Orthop Relat Res. 2002;397:248–58.

6. Campanacci M, Baldini N, Boriani S, Sudanese A. Giant-cell tumor of bone. J Bone Joint Surg. 1987;69(1):106–14.
7. Dahlin DC, Cupps RE, Johnson EW Jr. Giant-cell tumor: a study of 195 cases. Cancer. 1970;25(5):1061–70.
8. Wilde GE, Gakhal MS. Radiological reasoning: imaging of a talar mass. Am J Roentgenol. 2011;196(6 Suppl):WS47–52. https://doi.org/10.2214/AJR.09.7195. PMID: 21606240.
9. Campanacci M. Giant cell tumor (giant cell tunor of bone, osteoclastoma). In: Bone and soft tissue tumors. Clinical features, imaging, pathology and treatment. 2nd ed. Wien: Springer; 1999. p. 99–142.
10. Hoch B, Inwards C, Sundaram M, Rosenberg AE. Multicentric giant cell tumor of bone: clinicopathologic analysis of thirty cases. J Bone Joint Surg. 2006;88(9):1998–2008.
11. Dahlin DC. Caldwell Lecture. Giant cell tumor of bone: highlights of 407 cases. Am J Roentgenol. 1985;144(5):955–60.
12. Sim FH, Dahlin DC, Beabout JW. Multicentric giant-cell tumor of bone. J Bone Joint Surg Am. 1977;59(8):1052–60.
13. Peimer CA, Schiller AL, Mankin HJ, Smith RJ. Multicentric giant-cell tumor of bone. J Bone Joint Surg Am. 1980;62(4):652–6.
14. Bacchini P, Bertoni F, Ruggieri P, Campanacci M. Multicentric giant cell tumor of skeleton. Skeletal Radiol. 1995;24(5):371–4.
15. Murshed KA, Elsayed AM, Szabados L, Rashid S, Ammar A. Locally aggressive giant cell tumor of bone with pulmonary distant metastasis and extrapulmonary seeding in pregnancy. J Am Acad Orthop Surg Glob Res Rev. 2020;4(1):e19.00161. https://doi.org/10.5435/JAAOSGlobal-D-19-00161.
16. Kim JA, Park JS, Park SY, Jin W, Park YK, Han CS, et al. Aggressive behavior of a giant cell tumor involving the metacarpal bone during pregnancy: case report. J Korean Soc Radiol. 2011;64(5):509–13.
17. Ross AE, Bojescul JA, Kuklo TR. Giant cell tumor: a case report of recurrence during pregnancy. Spine. 2005;30(12):E332–E5.
18. Turcotte RE, Sim FH, Unni KK. Giant cell tumor of the sacrum. Clin Orthop. 1993;291:215–21.
19. Komiya S, Zenmyo M, Inoue A. Bone tumors in the pelvis presenting growth during pregnancy. Arch Orthop Trauma Surg. 1999;119(1):22–9.
20. Salm R, Sissons H. Giant-cell tumours of soft tissues. J Pathol. 1972;107(1):27–39.
21. O'Connell JX, Wehrli BM, Nielsen GP, Rosenberg AE. Giant cell tumors of soft tissue: a clinicopathologic study of 18 benign and malignant tumors. Am J Surg Pathol. 2000;24(3):386–95.
22. Oliveira AM, Dei Tos AP, Fletcher CD, Nascimento AG. Primary giant cell tumor of soft tissues: a study of 22 cases. Am J Surg Pathol. 2000;24(2):248–56.
23. Jaffe HL, Lichtenstein L, Portis RB. Giant cell tumor of bone. Its pathologic appearance, grading, supposed variants and treatment. Arch Pathol. 1940;30(5):993–1031.
24. Enneking WF, Spanier SS, Goodman MA. A system for the surgical staging of musculoskeletal sarcoma. Clin Orthop. 1980;153:106–20.
25. Enneking WF. A system of staging musculoskeletal neoplasms. Clin Orthop. 1986;204:9–24.
26. Bahk WJ, Mirra JM. Pseudoanaplastic tumors of bone. Skeletal Radiol. 2004;33(11):641–8.
27. Palmerini E, Picci P, Reichardt P, Downey G. Malignancy in giant cell tumor of bone: a review of the literature. Technol Cancer Res Treat. 2019;18:1533033819840000.
28. Malawer M, Marks M, McChesney D, Piasio M, Gunther S, Schmookler B. The effect of cryosurgery and polymethylmethacrylate in dogs with experimental bone defects comparable to tumor defects. Clin Orthop Relat Res. 1988;226:299–310.
29. Stürup J, Nimb L, Kramhøft M, Jensen JS. Effects of polymerization heat and monomers from acrylic cement on canine bone. Acta Orthop Scand. 1994;65(1):20–3.
30. Kriz J, Eich HT, Muecke R, Buentzel J, Mueller R-P, Bruns F, et al. Radiotherapy for giant cell tumors of the bone: a safe and effective treatment modality. Anticancer Res. 2012;32(5):2069–73.
31. Gaston CL, Grimer RJ, Parry M, Stacchiotti S, Dei Tos AP, Gelderblom H, et al. Current status and unanswered questions on the use of Denosumab in giant cell tumor of bone. Clin Sarcoma Res. 2016;6(1):1–6.
32. Thomas D, Henshaw R, Skubitz K, Chawla S, Staddon A, Blay J-Y, et al. Denosumab in patients with giant-cell tumour of bone: an open-label, phase 2 study. Lancet Oncol. 2010;11(3):275–80.
33. Chawla S, Henshaw R, Seeger L, Choy E, Blay J-Y, Ferrari S, et al. Safety and efficacy of denosumab for adults and skeletally mature adolescents with giant cell tumour of bone: interim analysis of an open-label, parallel-group, phase 2 study. Lancet Oncol. 2013;14(9):901–8.
34. Luengo-Alonso G, Mellado-Romero M, Shemesh S, Ramos-Pascua L, Pretell-Mazzini J. Denosumab treatment for giant-cell tumor of bone: a systematic review of the literature. Arch Orthop Trauma Surg. 2019;139(10):1339–49.
35. Borkowska A, Goryń T, Pieńkowski A, Wągrodzki M, Jagiełło-Wieczorek E, Rogala P, et al. Denosumab treatment of inoperable or locally advanced giant cell tumor of bone. Oncol Lett. 2016;12(6):4312–8.
36. Errani C, Tsukamoto S, Leone G, Righi A, Akahane M, Tanaka Y, et al. Denosumab may increase the risk of local recurrence in patients with giant-cell tumor of bone treated with curettage. J Bone Joint Surg. 2018;100(6):496–504.
37. Aponte-Tinao LA, Piuzzi NS, Roitman P, Farfalli GL. A high-grade sarcoma arising in a patient with recurrent benign giant cell tumor of the proximal tibia while receiving treatment with denosumab. Clin Orthop Relat Res. 2015;473(9):3050–5.

38. Agarwal MG, Gundavda MK, Gupta R, Reddy R. Does denosumab change the giant cell tumor treatment strategy? Lessons learned from early experience. Clin Orthop Relat Res. 2018;476(9):1773.
39. Larsson S, Lorentzon R, Boquist L. Giant-cell tumor of bone. A demographic, clinical, and histopathological study of all cases recorded in the Swedish Cancer Registry for the years 1958 through 1968. J Bone Joint Surg Am. 1975;57(2):167–73.
40. Resnick D, Kyriokos M, Greenway GD. Giant cell tumor. In: Resnick D, Kransdorf MJ, editors. Bone and joint imaging. 3rd ed. Philadelphia: Elsevier Saunders; 2005. p. 1164–7.
41. Campanacci M. Simple bone cyst. Bone and soft tissue tumors. New York: Springer; 1999. p. 791–811.
42. Malawer MM, Bickels J, Meller I, Buch RG, Henshaw RM, Kollender Y. Cryosurgery in the treatment of giant cell tumor: a long term followup study. Clin Orthop Relat Res. 1999;359:176–88.
43. McDonald DJ, Sim F, McLeod R, Dahlin D. Giant-cell tumor of bone. J Bone Joint Surg Am. 1986;68(2):235–42.
44. Mirra JM, Ulich T, Magidson J, Kaiser L, Eckardt J, Gold R. A case of probable benign pulmonary "metastases" or implants arising from a giant cell tumor of bone. Clin Orthop Relat Res. 1982;162:245–54.
45. Klenke FM, Wenger DE, Inwards CY, Rose PS, Sim FH. Giant cell tumor of bone: risk factors for recurrence. Clin Orthop. 2011;469(2):591–9.
46. Dominkus M, Ruggieri P, Bertoni F, Briccoli A, Picci P, Rocca M, et al. Histologically verified lung metastases in benign giant cell tumours-14 cases from a single institution. Int Orthop. 2006;30(6):499–504.
47. Formica VM, Bruno V, Di Uccio AS, Cocca E, Rossi B, Zoccali C. The giant cell tumor during pregnancy: a review of literature. Orthop Traumatol Surg Res. 2023;109:103396. https://doi.org/10.1016/j.otsr.2022.103396. Epub ahead of print. PMID: 36087835.
48. Rutkowski P, Ferrari S, Grimer RJ, Stalley PD, Dijkstra SP, Pienkowski A, et al. Surgical downstaging in an open-label phase II trial of denosumab in patients with giant cell tumor of bone. Ann Surg Oncol. 2015;22(9):2860–8.
49. Broehm CJ, Garbrecht EL, Wood J, Bocklage T. Two cases of sarcoma arising in giant cell tumor of bone treated with denosumab. Case Rep Med. 2015;2015:767198. https://doi.org/10.1155/2015/767198. Epub 2015 Dec 22.
50. Park A, Cipriano CA, Hill K, Kyriakos M, McDonald DJ. Malignant transformation of a giant cell tumor of bone treated with denosumab: a case report. JBJS Case Connect. 2016;6(3):e78. https://doi.org/10.2106/JBJS.CC.16.00024. PMID: 29252655.
51. Tsukamoto S, Righi A, Vanel D, Honoki K, Donati DM, Errani C. Development of high-grade osteosarcoma in a patient with recurrent giant cell tumor of the ischium while receiving treatment with denosumab. Jpn J Clin Oncol. 2017;47(11):1090–6.

2 Brown Tumor of Hyperparathyroidism

2.1 Definition

Brown tumor is rare one of the manifestations of hyperparathyroidism (HPT), which represents an osteolytic bone lesion consisting of a brownish mass of nonneoplastic reactive tissue that arises from excessive activation of osteoclast activity by increased secretion of parathyroid hormone (PTH). It can result primarily from neoplasm or diffuse hyperplasia of parathyroid gland or secondary to renal disease.

2.2 Synonym

Osteitis fibrosa cystica.

2.3 Incidence

The skeletal lesions of HPT including brown tumor becomes rarer due to routine check of serum calcium levels allowing to an earlier diagnosis of HPT [1, 2]. Brown tumor have mildly higher frequency in primary than secondary HPT. However, secondary HPT is much more common than primary HPT; thus, most brown tumors are associated with secondary HPT [3].

2.4 Age

Patients are mostly adult in fourth and sixth decades of life.

2.5 Locations

It usually occurs in jawbones, rib, clavicle, pelvic girdle, and tubular bones of the extremities. When long tubular bone is affected, it often occurs in the diaphysis. The lesion may be solitary or often multiple.

2.6 Clinical Manifestations

Clinical manifestations include slow-growing mass or swelling, diffuse skeletal pain, and pathological fracture. The bone pain is relatively milder and is often incidentally found on radiograph for other reasons. Patient may present constitutional symptoms of weakness, weight loss, polyuria, and recurrent stone formation by HPT. The most common cause of primary HPT is parathyroid adenoma causing the hypersecretion of PTH [4].

W.-J. Bahk, *Diagnosis and Management of Primary Bone Tumors*,
https://doi.org/10.1007/978-981-99-5498-8_2

2.7 Radiologic Findings

Bony manifestations of HPT are typified by decalcification of bone including diffuse osteopenia, subperiosteal bone resorption, pathological fractures, brown tumor, terminal acrosteolysis, and skull lesions (Fig. 2.1). When the giant cell-rich lesion affects purely diaphysis of long bone or multiple locations, brown tumor of HPT should be included for differential diagnosis because pure diaphyseal location in conventional GCT does not virtually exist and multifocal GCT of bone without underlying Paget's disease is extremely rare. Brown tumor is usually a well-defined, single, or multi-lobulated, expansile radiolucent lesion with little reactive bone formation but occasional intralesional trabeculations. The cortex is often thinned but is usually not penetrated. The characteristic "*tunneling*" bone resorption of cortex as well as lacelike irregularity is often seen in the phalanges and distal phalangeal tuft (Fig. 2.1g). The skull lesions are characterized by granular decalcification, well-known "*salt-and-pepper*" sign or "*pepper pot*" skull or homogeneous ground glass-like appearance. However, multiple, round to oval, focal, or diffuse osteosclerotic changes can be rarely reported [5–7] (Fig. 2.1j). The mechanism and pathogenesis of the osteosclerotic lesions is still unknown. However, the phenomenon may result from a prolonged osteoclastic activity producing the catabolic effect of the PTH toward the anabolic effect, which leads an exaggerated osteoblastic activity, particularly in younger patients with high bone turnover rate [5, 7]. **MR images:** The appearance depends on the proportion of its

Fig. 2.1 (**a**) Radiograph taken for right shoulder pain by moving a heavy object incidentally shows a well-defined osteolytic lesion with significant cortical thinning and thin sclerotic rim in the whole head of humerus. With shaft of humerus protruding into the expanded area (asterisk) with buttress of periosteal reaction, so-called Codman's triangle (blue arrow), overall appearing "*finger-in-the-balloon*" shape as seen in aneurysmal bone cyst. Without Codman's triangle, the finding may indicate pathologic fracture with marked impaction (asterisk). Other small radiolucent lesions with surrounding sclerosis are also incidentally observed in the clavicles and second rib (yellow arrows). (**b**) MR images reveal a well-defined intramedullary mass-like lesion with low and intermediate SI on T1-weighted image and heterogeneous high SI with focal bight signal on T2-weighted image, with a thin dark signal of sclerotic rim on both sequences. The lesion is well enhanced along the periphery indicating a cystic component (yellow arrow) with inner heterogeneous enhancement of solid component (red arrows). (**c**) Bone scan demonstrates heterogeneously strong uptake along the periphery with central photon defect in the humeral lesion. In addition, multiple strong uptake is also seen in the skull and sternum with small focal uptake in the left femoral neck and proximal tibia, indicating a multifocal lesion. However, there is no increased uptake in other areas, including clavicles, ribs, and hands in which radiolucent lesion or bone resorption is observed on radiographs. (**d**) Microscopic examination notes numerous multinucleated giant cells in a background of mononuclear oval to spindle stromal cells with hemorrhage and hemosiderin pigments, being identical to conventional GCT of bone (Left). Another field consists of reparative granulation tissue with abundant proliferating vessels and spicules of reactive woven bone (Right). (**e**) Parathyroid subtraction scan shows a hot uptake, suggesting a parathyroid adenoma. Serum calcium level was 13.4 mg/dl (normal; 8.2–10.2) and parathyroid hormone was 763.3 pg/ml (normal; 15–65), indicating primary hyperparathyroidism. Parathyroidectomy followed by curettage, allo-chip bone graft, and K-wire fixation for the humeral lesion was performed. (**f**) Follow-up radiograph at 8 years after surgery reveals no evidence of local recurrence with a mild deformity but normal articulation (red arrow). Note spontaneous healing of other lesions of clavicle and second rib (yellow arrow). (**g**) Radiographs of hands show a resorption of the distal phalangeal tufts (blue arrows) and subperiosteal resorption along the distal radial aspects of the middle phalanges (yellow arrows). Note typical "*tunneling*" bone resorption of the cortex (red arrows). Geographic destruction surrounded by a thin sclerotic rim is also noted in the capitate (black arrow). Not all of these findings are reflected as increased uptake on bone scan. (**h**) Subperiosteal bone resorption is also in medial aspect of proximal tibia (blue arrow). (**i**) Bubbly osteolytic lesions with rim of sclerosis in the iliac wing and ischial body become hazy on radiograph at 8 years after parathyroidectomy. (**j**) In addition, diffusely scattered round to oval sclerotic foci which is unusual finding in HPT seem to be reduced in number

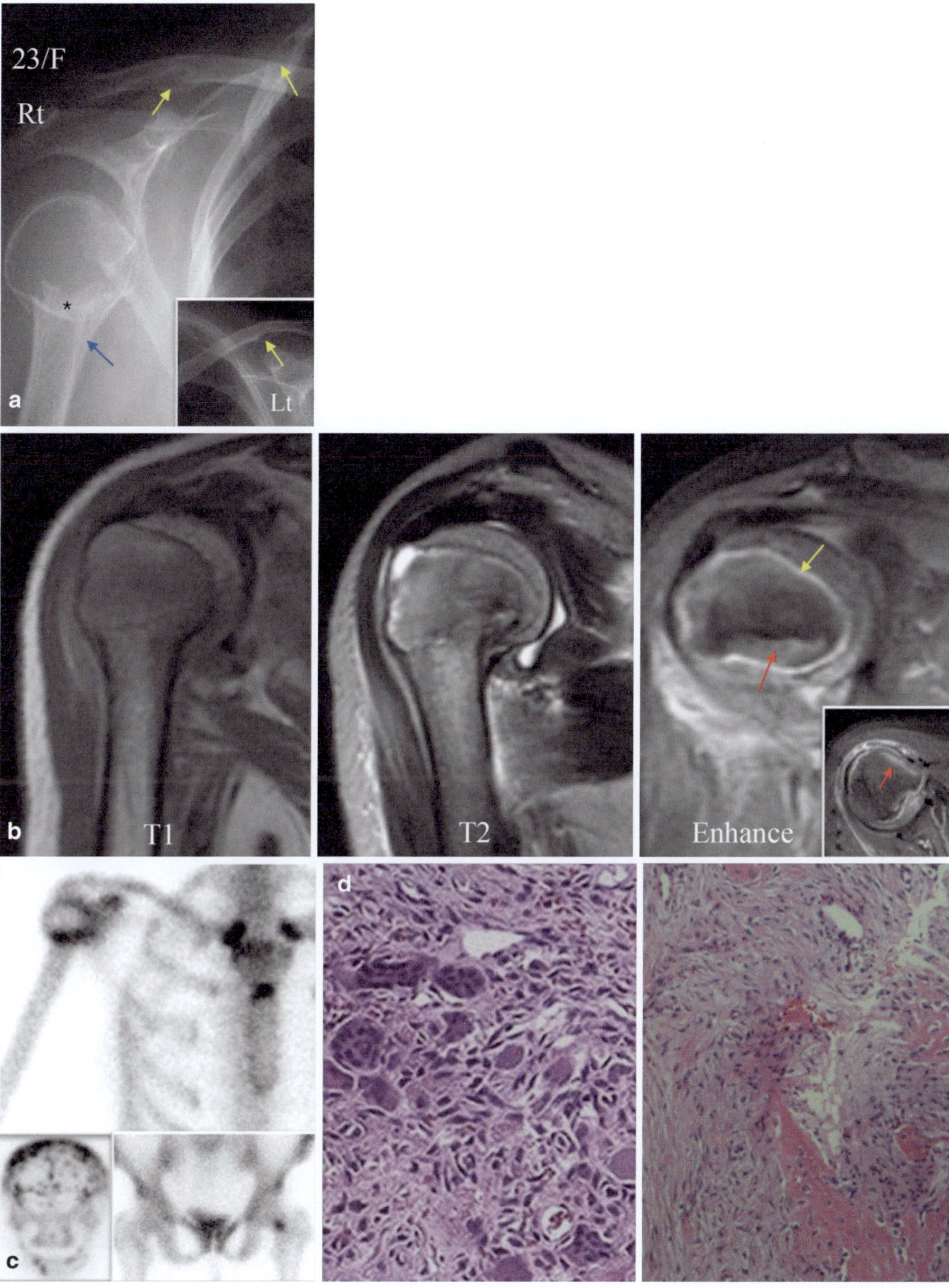

23/F
Rt
*
Lt
a
b
T1
T2
Enhance
c
d

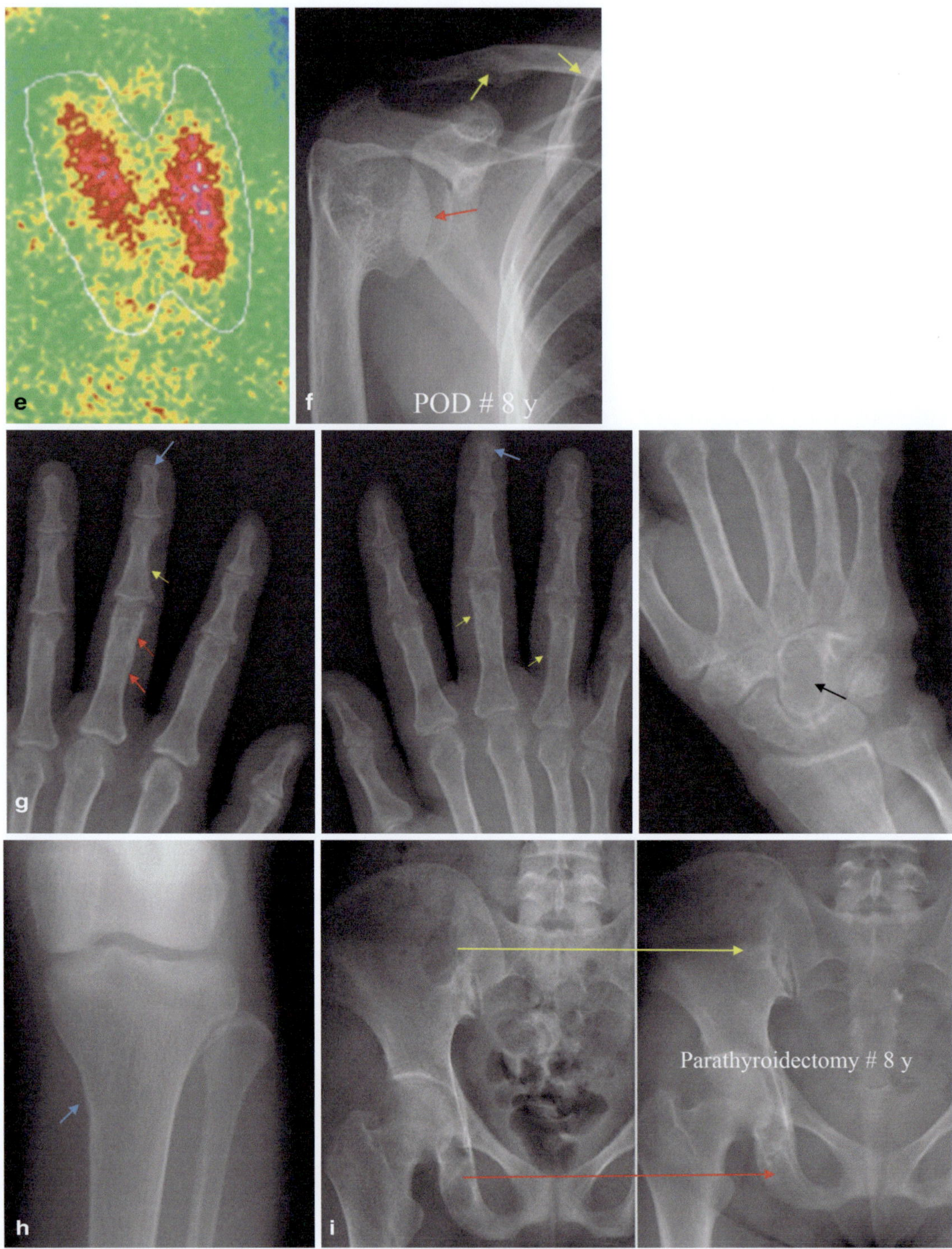

Fig. 2.1 (continued)

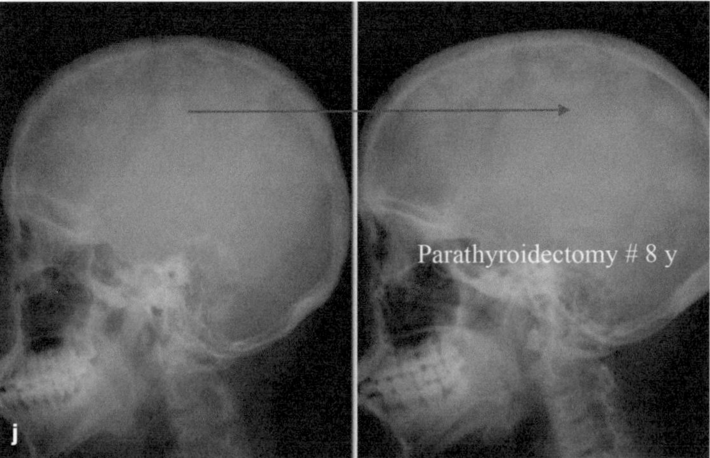

Fig. 2.1 (continued)

solid and cystic components. Solid components show heterogeneous low to intermediate SI on T1- and T2-weighted images, while the cystic components present high SI on T2-weighted images. The solid component as well as septa is heterogeneously enhanced (Fig. 2.1b). **Bone scan** is useful to detect other bone involvement with varying degree of increased uptake. However, some lesions are not detected due to no increased uptake (Fig. 2.1c).

2.8 Histologic Findings

Brown tumor is characterized by numerous multinucleated giant cells in a background of mononuclear oval to spindle stromal cells, which is indistinguishable from conventional GCT. A brownish mass consists of a combination of various stages of hemorrhage, hemosiderin pigments, reparative granulation tissue with proliferating vessels, pronounced new bone formation (Fig. 2.1d), or even fracture callus from repeated microfracture. Hemosiderin imparting the brown color is not a distinctive feature of brown tumors and is seen in conventional GCT as well. The brown tumor of hyperparathyroidism can be easily misdiagnosed from conventional GCT only with a histologic examination but no laboratory findings of elevated blood calcium and parathyroid hormone levels or parathyroid subtraction scan (Fig. 2.1e). Therefore, correlation with radiographic, clinical findings and laboratory findings is essential for a correct diagnosis.

2.9 Management

Since bone healing is compromised by an abnormally increase function of parathyroid, the underlying disease needs to be controlled medically or surgically prior to surgical management of bone lesion. Parathyroidectomy usually result in spontaneous healing in primary cases. Surgical curettage and bone grafting or cementing is necessary when the lesion is large with pathologic fracture, impending fracture or increasing pain.

2.10 Clinical Course

Once the underlying metabolic condition is corrected, bone healing with sclerosis is usual if the lesion not complicated by cyst formation.

References

1. Grulois V, Buysschaert I, Schoenaers J, Debruyne F, Delaere P, Poorten VV. Brown tumour: presenting symptom of primary hyperparathyroidism. B-ENT. 2005;1(4):191–5. PMID: 16429752.
2. Heath H III, Hodgson SF, Kennedy MA. Primary hyperparathyroidism. Incidence, morbidity, and potential economic impact in a community. N Engl J Med. 1980;302:189–93.
3. Hayes C, Conway W. Hyperparathyroidism. Radiol Clin N Am. 1991;29(1):85–96.
4. Parisien M, Silverberg SJ, Shane E, Dempster DW, Bilezikian JP. Bone disease in primary hyperparathyroidism. Endocrinol Metab Clin N Am. 1990;19(1):19–34.
5. Fujino Y, Inaba M, Nakatsuka K, Kumeda Y, Imanishi Y, Tahara H, et al. Primary hyperparathyroidism with multiple osteosclerotic lesions of the calvarium. J Bone Miner Res. 2003;18:410–2.
6. Shetty S, Kapoor N, Naik D, Paul TV. Focal osteosclerosis of the skull in primary hyperparathyroidism. Cancer Res. 2014;2014:bcr2014204236.
7. Chopra S, Manchanda S, Kothari D, Kulshreshtha B. Multiple osteosclerotic lesions of skull in two cases with co-existing hyperparathyroidism and vitamin D deficiency. J Indian Acad Clin Med. 2012;13(4):349–51.

3 Giant Cell Reparative Granuloma

3.1 Definition

Giant cell reparative granuloma (GCRG) is a rare benign giant cell-rich tumorlike reactive lesion with a predilection for craniofacial skeleton (*gnathic*) and small bones of the hands and feet (*extragnathic*). It is not a true neoplasm, but rather a reactive process. Early in 1953, Jaffe [1] first described GCRG as a benign nonneoplastic process peculiar to jawbones related to intraosseous hemorrhage, which contains multinucleated giant cells in a predominantly fibroblastic stroma. Years later, Ackerman and Spjut [2] reported two similar lesions describing as a rare, benign, nonneoplastic lesion involving small bones of the hands, and they named it "*giant cell reaction*". Decades later, Lorenzo and Dorfman [3] reported eight additional cases involving hands and feet with high recurrence rate of 50% of their cases, and added the term "reparative" to "giant cell reaction" to represent a reactive process to hemorrhage. They also prefer to designate these lesions as "extragnathic GCRG". Sanerkin and colleagues [4] reported non-cystic lesion involving the spines and ethmoid, with morphologic similarity to that in aneurysmal bone cyst (ABC) and overlapped histology with GCRG. They regarded this lesion as a variant of ABC devoid of a cystic "blowout" and referred to it as a "*solid ABC*." There has been some controversy regarding the nomenclature of the particular lesion. More recently, GCRG is regarded as synonymous with solid variant of ABC in extragnathic sites because of indistinguishable morphologic findings and high rate of positive USP6 gene rearrangements as in ABC [5].

3.2 Possible Pathogenesis

Lorenzo and Dorfman also noted that the overlapping morphologic features with similar biologic behavior of high recurrence with ABC and hypothesized that these lesions may be related responses to intraosseous hemorrhage [3]. Clonal mutation or cytogenetic abnormalities such as *USP6* gene rearrangement, which was identified only in primary ABC with positive rate of 70% but not in secondary ABC [6–8], is also identified in GCRG involving the hands and feet. Agaram et al. [5] reported the *USP6* gene rearrangements were identified in about 90% of GCRGs, 60% of primary ABCs, but none of GCT. However, no abnormalities were identified in the gnathic lesions. Thus, they suggested terminology of GCRG should be limited to lesions from gnathic location.

W.-J. Bahk, *Diagnosis and Management of Primary Bone Tumors*,
https://doi.org/10.1007/978-981-99-5498-8_3

3.3 Synonym

Central giant cell lesion/giant cell lesion of small bones/giant cell reaction/giant cell granuloma or cyst.

3.4 Incidence

GCRG is very rare.

3.5 Age

Most patients are young to middle-aged adults between second and third decades of life [3, 9, 10]. Up to 74% of patients are reported to be under 30 years of age at presentation [11]. However, the ages reported in the literature are widely ranging from 3 to 76 years [12–16].

3.6 Location

GCRG mostly arises in jaw bones (mandible > maxilla) followed by in short tubular bones of hands and feet. Although extremely rare in the long tubular bones, it has been sporadically reported [16–20].

3.7 Clinical Features

Pain with or without swelling of variable duration ranging between several weeks to years is the most common presentation. Rarely, it is incidentally discovered on radiographs taken for other reasons. Some patients may give a history of minor trauma [3]. Significant enlargement during pregnancy has been described, presumably related to hormonal stimulation [21]. GCRG has also been described in association with enchondromatosis, fibrous dysplasia, Paget disease, and Goltz syndrome [22–25].

3.8 Radiologic Findings

In craniofacial bone, the lesion presents a round or oval radiolucent area with minimal reactive sclerosis and expansion with marked cortical thinning. But the cortex is typically intact without periosteal reaction. In the short tubular bones of hands and feet, it usually involves meta-diaphysis or diaphysis, even the entire bone. Generally, it does not cross the open growth plate but can extend occasionally to epiphysis in the skeletally mature patients. It begins as a small round to oval radiolucent lesion and gradually becomes larger occasionally with fine trabeculations producing "*honeycomb*" appearance. The margin is usually distinct with or without a surrounding thin reactive sclerosis. The contour of short tubular bone can be expanded with significantly thinned, but the cortex is usually intact (Fig. 3.1a and 3.2a). A periosteal reaction is usually absent. **MR images** shows nonspecific findings of an intramedullary mass-like lesion. SI is low to intermediate SI on T1-weighted image and heterogeneous low to intermediate SI with variable degree of high signal depending on the amount of secondary histologic changes such as hemosiderin and fibrosis, or even recent hemorrhage on T2-weighted image (Fig. 3.1b and 3.2b). The lesion is diffusely well enhanced by the contrast medium. **Bone scan** shows a homogeneous increased uptake or peripherally increased uptake with central photon defect appearing as "*doughnut*" shape (Fig. 3.1c).

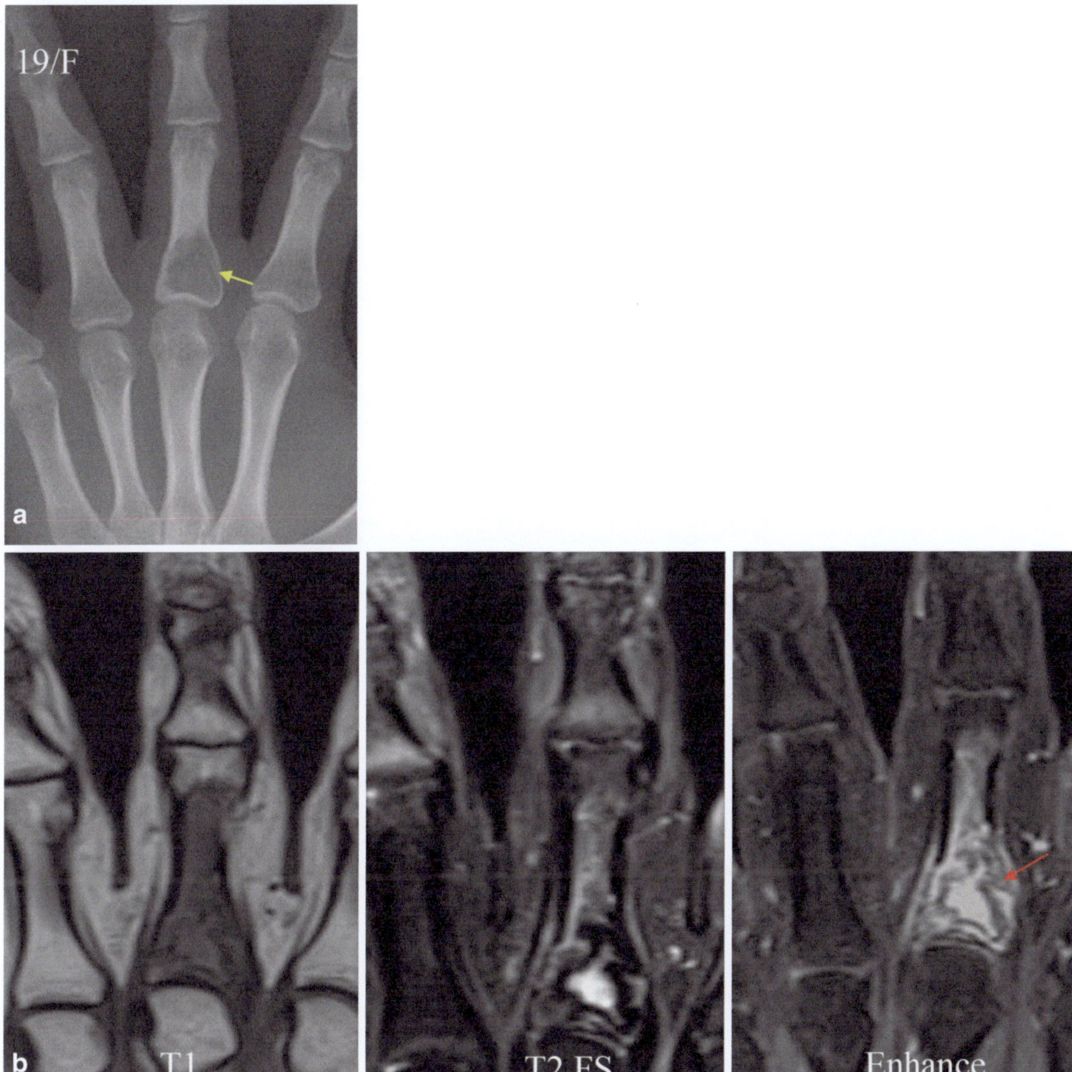

Fig. 3.1 (**a**) Radiograph taken for left middle finger pain of 1-year duration in 19-year-old girl shows a well-defined radiolucent lesion with marked cortical thinning and mild expansion as well as suspicious pathologic fracture (arrow) in the proximal one third of the proximal phalanx. The margin of the lesion is distinct with no surrounding rim of sclerosis. There is no periosteal reaction (**b**) However, MR images demonstrate a well-defined intramedullary mass-like lesion in most of the proximal phalanx. The SI is low to intermediate SI on T1-weighted image and heterogeneous intermediate SI with focal high and bright signal on fat saturated T2-weighted image. Non-displaced fracture is noted with hemorrhage (red arrow). The lesion is diffusely well enhanced by the contrast medium. (**c**) Pinhole bone scan reveals a marginal strong uptake and internal photon defect, so-called "*donut appearance*." (**d**) Microscopic examination. Low-grade magnification shows an overall shape of granuloma with high cellularity and multinucleated giant cells. Higher-magnification notes that the lesion consists of high cellularity of bland spindle-shaped stromal cells arranged in fascicular to whirling pattern, collagenous stroma, and osteoclast-type giant cells as well as prominent hemorrhage. The giant cells tend to aggregate around areas of stromal hemorrhage (inset). (**e**) Curettage and allo-chip bone graft was performed. (**f**) Follow-up radiograph at 5 years after surgery notes consolidation of the lesion with no evidence of local recurrence

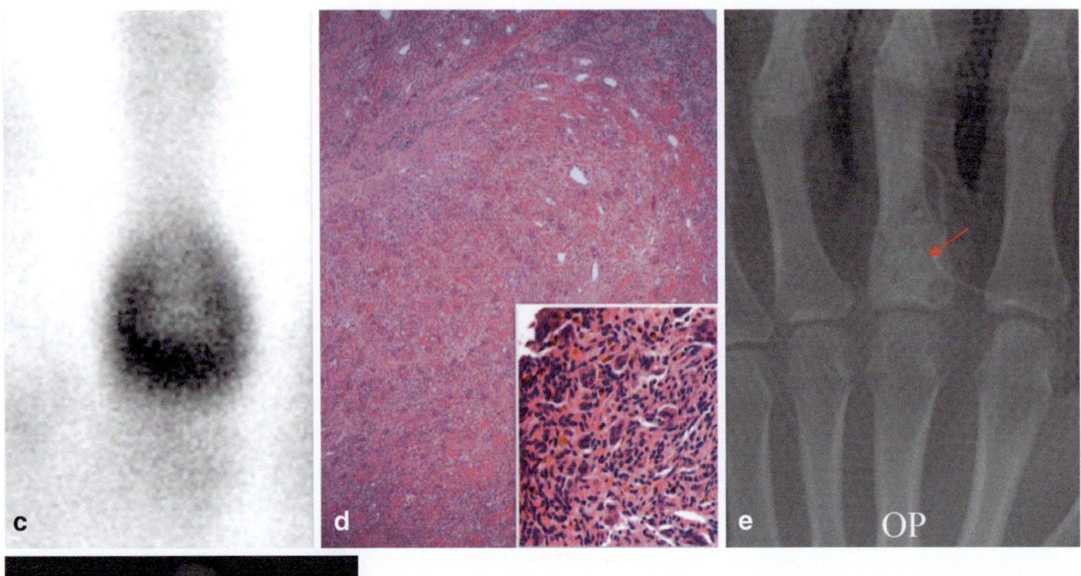

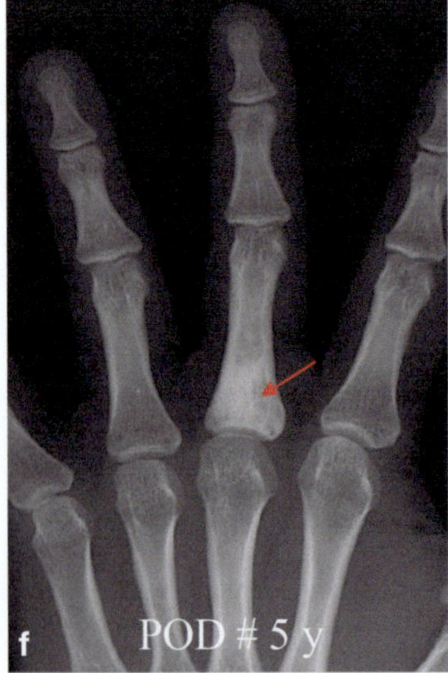

Fig. 3.1 (continued)

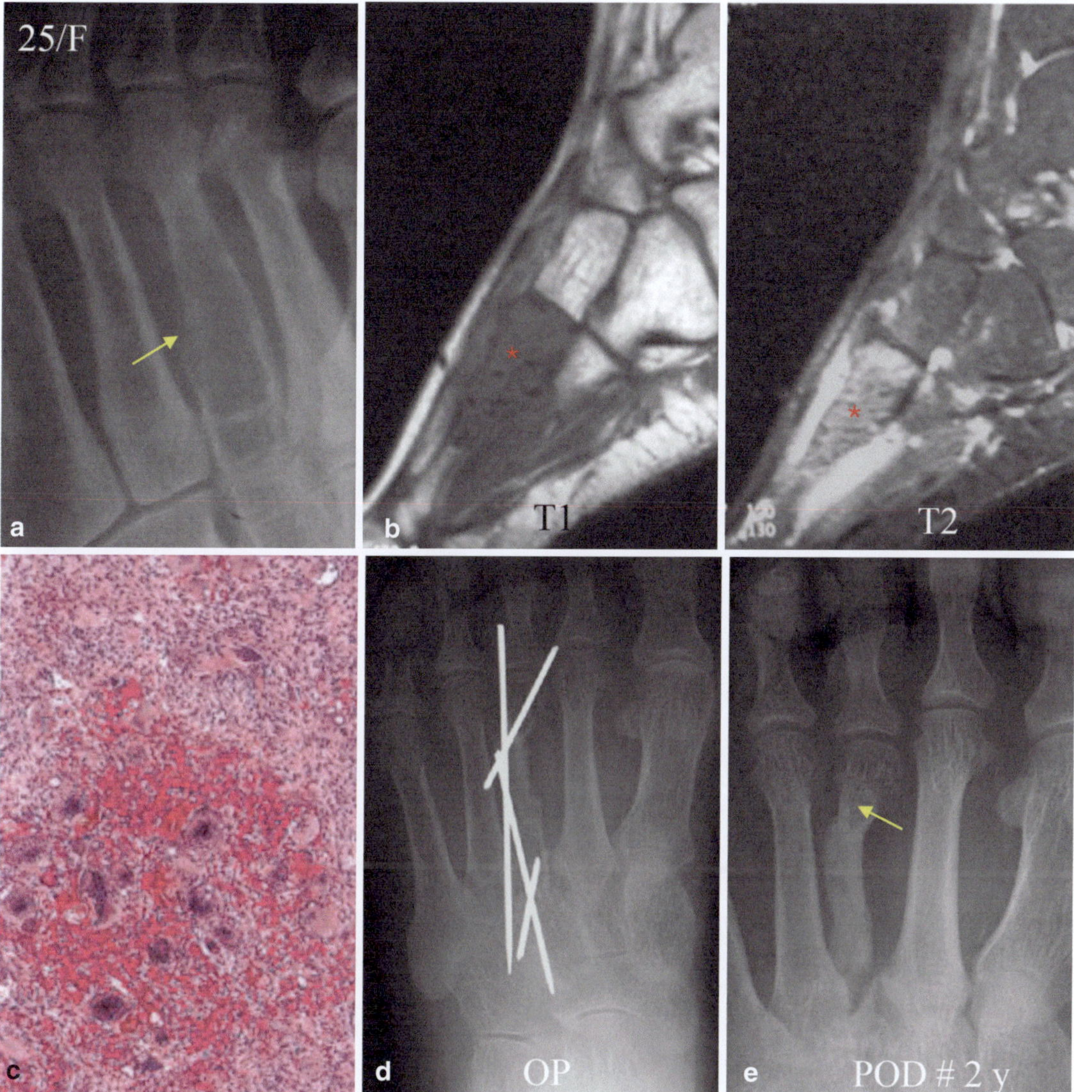

Fig. 3.2 (**a**) Radiograph taken for left foot pain of 1-month duration in 25-year-old lady shows relatively ill-defined radiolucent lesion with irregular severe cortical thinning and diffuse expansion (arrow) in the third metatarsal bone. (**b**) MR images demonstrate a well-defined medullary mass-like lesion with low SI on T1-weighted image and heterogeneous intermediate and high SI on T2-weighted image affecting the two thirds of the metatarsal bone (asterisks). (**c**) Microscopic examination reveals moderate to high cellularity of fibroblastic cells within abundant collagenous stroma with quite extensive hemorrhage in which the multinucleated giant cells are unevenly distributed and aggregated in small clusters. (**d**) Segmental resection and autogeneous strut iliac bone grafting fixed using K-wires was performed. (**e**) Follow-up radiograph at 2 years after surgery notes union of the graft with some shortening and mild bending but no evidence of local recurrence. She is free of symptoms

3.9 Histologic Findings

GCRG is histologically heterogeneous and represents with microscopic presentations overlapping to those of GCT or solid ABC. GCRG is typified by a nodular or granulomatous appearance produced by fibrous stroma with plump, bland fibroblasts, and multinucleated giant cells (Fig. 3.3a, b). The lesion is composed of moderate to high cellularity of spindled fibroblasts arranged in fascicular to whirling pattern and varying amount of collagen with diffusely scattered areas of hemorrhage (Fig. 3.1d). Another key feature is the presence of unevenly distributed multinucleated giant cells forming clusters separated by bundles of scar-like stromal tissue. In general, the multinucleated giant

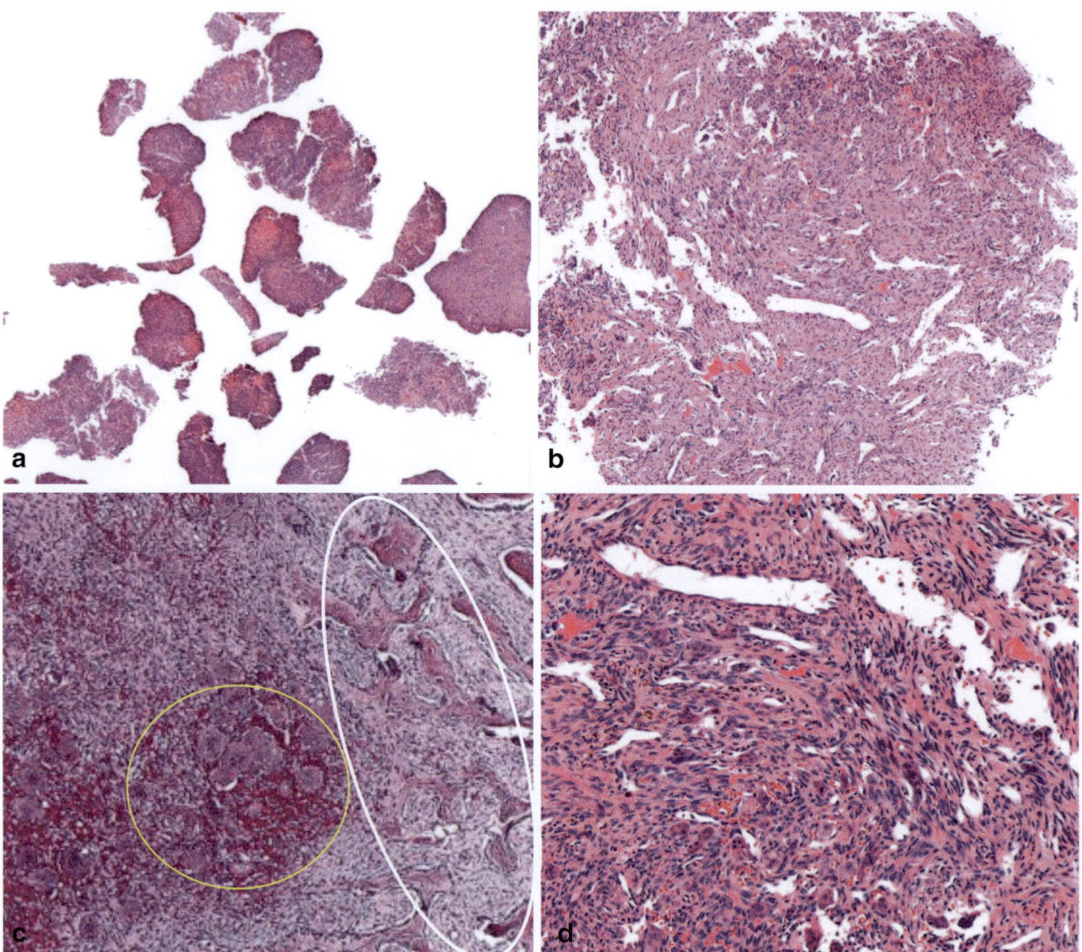

Fig. 3.3 *Microscopic features*. (**a**) Scanning view shows multiple tiny nodular masses with high cellularity, which are severely fragmented and separated by curettage. (**b**) Low-power magnification reveals a well-circumscribed mass consisting of spindle-shaped stromal fibroblasts within vascular and collagen-rich stroma with clustered multinucleated giant cells, multiple areas of hemorrhage, reactive bone formation, and inflammatory cells. (**c**) Characteristically, middle-power magnification notes multinucleated giant cells to aggregate in clusters around areas of prominent hemorrhage (yellow circle) and juxtaposed area of high cellular spindle-shaped fibroblasts arranged in fascicular to whirling pattern. Note abundant reactive bone spicules with prominent osteoblastic rimming (white circle). (**d**) Higher-power magnification shows fibrous stroma spindle-shaped fibroblasts with clusters of giant cells around fresh and old hemorrhage with hemosiderin pigmentation and prominent dilated vascular spaces lined with fibrocellular stroma and osteoclasts. Some authors may call the vascular spaces as the "aneurysmal sinusoids" in solid ABC

cells tend to aggregate in small clusters around areas of hemorrhage often juxtaposed with fibrous stroma area (Fig. 3.2c and 3.3c) and are usually less numerous than those in GCT. Often, there are secondary changes such as reactive woven bone with prominent osteoblastic rimming, which can be quite extensive enough to obscure other elements of the lesion as well as scattered inflammatory cells and hemosiderin pigmentation. Often, small blood channels or hemorrhagic cyst formation is seen with similarity to solid ABC (Fig. 3.3d).

3.10 Management

Thorough curettage with or without bone graft is the choice of treatment (Fig. 3.1e and 3.2d).

3.11 Prognosis

After curettage and bone graft, varying rate of high rate of local recurrence has been reported, ranging from 18 to 50% [3, 15, 26, 27]. However, most recurred lesions are controlled by another curettage and bone graft [3, 14, 28]. Digital or ray amputation may be necessary, particularly in multiple recurrent cases or lesions destroying most or all of the short bone of the hand and feet.

References

1. Jaffe HL. Giant-cell reparative granuloma, traumatic bone cyst, and fibrous (fibro-osseous) dysplasia of the jawbones. Oral Surg Oral Med Oral Pathol. 1953;6(1):159–75.
2. Ackerman LV, Spjut J. Giant cell reaction in tumors of bone and cartilage. In: Spjut HJ, Dorfman HD, Fechner RE, Ackerman LV, editors. Atlas of tumor pathology. Sect. II, Fascicle 4, Series 1. Washington, DC: Armed Forces Institute of Pathology; 1962. p. 282, 344–5.
3. Lorenzo JC, Dorfman HD. Giant-cell reparative granuloma of short tubular bones of the hands and feet. Am J Surg Pathol. 1980;4(6):551–64.
4. Sanerkin N, Mott M, Roylance J. An unusual intraosseous lesion with fibroblastic, osteoclastic, osteoblastic, aneurysmal and fibromyxoid elements. "Solid" variant of aneurysmal bone cyst. Cancer. 1983;51(12):2278–86.
5. Agaram NP, LeLoarer FV, Zhang L, Hwang S, Athanasian EA, Hameed M, et al. USP6 gene rearrangements occur preferentially in giant cell reparative granulomas of the hands and feet but not in gnathic location. Human Pathol. 2014;45(6):1147–52.
6. Oliveira AM, Perez-Atayde AR, Inwards CY, Medeiros F, Derr V, Hsi B-L, et al. USP6 and CDH11 oncogenes identify the neoplastic cell in primary aneurysmal bone cysts and are absent in so-called secondary aneurysmal bone cysts. Am J Pathol. 2004;165(5):1773–80.
7. Oliveira AM, Hsi BL, Weremowicz S, Rosenberg AE, Cin PD, Joseph N, et al. USP6 (Tre2) fusion oncogenes in aneurysmal bone cyst. Cancer Res. 2004;64(6):1920–3.
8. Oliveira AM, Perez-Atayde AR, Dal Cin P, Gebhardt MC, Chen CJ, Neff JR, et al. Aneurysmal bone cyst variant translocations upregulate USP6 transcription by promoter swapping with the ZNF9, COL1A1, TRAP150, and OMD genes. Oncogene. 2005;24(21):3419–26.
9. D'alonzo RT, Pitcock JA, Milford LW. Giant-cell reaction of bone: report of two cases. J Bone Joint Surg. 1972;54(6):1267–71.
10. Panico L, De Rosa N, D'Antonio A, De Rosa G, Passeretti U. Giant cell reparative granuloma of the distal skeletal bones. Virchows Arch. 1994;425(3):315–20.
11. Waldron CA, Shafer WG. The central giant cell reparative granuloma of the jaws. An analysis of 38 cases. Am J Clin Pathol. 1966;45(4):437–47.
12. Caskey PM, Wolf MD, Fechner RE. Multicentric giant cell reparative granuloma of the small bones of the hand. A case report and review of the literature. Clin Orthop Relat Res. 1985;193:199–205.
13. Forouhar FA, Phelan NP, Benton DC. Giant cell reparative granuloma of the small bones of the hands and feet: a report of three cases. Ann Clin Lab Sci. 2000;30(3):272–7.
14. Ratner V, Dorfman HD. Giant-cell reparative granuloma of the hand and foot bones. Clin Orthop Relat Res. 1990;260:251–8.
15. Wold LE, Dobyns JH, Swee RG, Dahlin DC. Giant cell reaction (giant cell reparative granuloma) of the small bones of the hands and feet. Am J Surg Pathol. 1986;10(7):491–6.
16. Subasi M, Kapukaya A, Buyukbayram H, Bukte Y. Giant-cell reparative granuloma of the tibia. Acta Orthop Belg. 2003;69(4):363–7.
17. Hermann G, Abdelwahab I, Klein M, Berson B, Lewis M. Case report 603. Giant cell reparative granuloma of the distal end of right femur. Skelet Radiol. 1990;19(5):367–9.
18. Thomas I, Chow C, Cole W. Giant cell reparative granuloma of the humerus. J Pediatr Orthop. 1988;8(5):596–8.
19. Yamaguchi T, Dorfman HD. Giant cell reparative granuloma: a comparative clinicopathologic study of lesions in gnathic and extragnathic sites. Int J Surg Pathol. 2001;9(3):189–200.

20. Oda Y, Tsuneyoshi M, Shinohara N. "Solid" variant of aneurysmal bone cyst (extragnathic giant cell reparative granuloma) in the axial skeleton and long bones. A study of its morphologic spectrum and distinction from allied giant cell lesions. Cancer. 1992;70(11):2642–9.
21. Fechner RE, Fitz-Hugh GS, Pope TL. Extraordinary growth of giant cell reparative granuloma during pregnancy. Arch Otolaryngol. 1984;110(2):116–9.
22. Oda Y, Iwamoto Y, Ushijima M, Masuda S, Sugioka Y, Tsuneyoshi M. Case report 877: giant cell reparative granuloma arising in enchondromatosis. Skelet Radiol. 1994;23(8):669–71.
23. De Smet AA, Travers H, Neff JR. Case report 207: giant cell reparative granuloma of left femur arising in polyostatic fibrous dysplasia. Skelet Radiol. 1982;8(4):314–8.
24. Upchurch KS, Simon LS, Schiller AL, Rosenthal DI, Campion EW, Krane SM. Giant cell reparative granuloma of Paget's disease of bone: a unique clinical entity. Ann Intern Med. 1983;98(1):35–40.
25. Selzer G, David R, Revach M, Cvibah TJ, Fried A. Goltz syndrome with multiple giant-cell tumor-like lesions in bones: a case report. Ann Intern Med. 1974;80(6):714–7.
26. Biscaglia R, Bacchini P, Bertoni F. Giant cell tumor of the bones of the hand and foot. Cancer. 2000;88(9):2022–32.
27. Fechner RE, Mills SE. Tumors of the bones and joints, atlas of tumor pathology, third series, fascicle 8. Bethesda: Armed Forces Institute of Pathology; 1993. p. 179.
28. Bertoni F, Biscaglia R, Bacchini P. Giant cell reparative granuloma of the phalanx of the hand with aggressive radiographic features. Skelet Radiol. 1998;27(10):584–7.

Part II

Hematopoietic Tumors

4 Langerhans Cell Histiocytosis

(***histio-*** "tissue" + ***cytes*** "cells" + ***-osis*** "a process")

4.1 Definition

Langerhans cell histiocytosis (LCH) of bone is a rare abnormal clonal proliferation of Langerhans cells within bone. *Langerhans cells* are type of dendritic cells containing organelles called Birbeck granules, which regulate the immune system, and are normally found throughout the body, especially in the reticuloendothelial system (RES) including the skin, lymph nodes, spleen, lungs, liver, and bone marrow. LCH can involve any such organs causing single or multifocal within a single system (most frequently bone), or disseminated multisystemic disease.

4.2 Possible Pathogenesis

Nowadays, after decades of debate on the pathogenesis, a neoplastic mechanism is now favored on the basis of LCH cell clonality [1]. LCH is a disease caused by somatic mutations at critical stages of myeloid differentiation that result in cellular transformation as in other myeloid disorders [2]. Mutations of the BRAF V600E, MAP2K1, RAS, and ARAF genes may make the Langerhans cells grow continuously and multiply to accumulate these cells, which destroy tissues and result in the lesions.

4.3 Synonyms

Eosinophilic granuloma/histiocytosis X.

4.4 Incidence

LCH of bone accounts for less than 1% of biopsied primary bone tumors, and monostotic type is two to three times more common than polyostotic type including those with extraosseous involvement [3, 4].

4.5 Age

The age of the patients varies widely from birth to the eight decades of life. But majority of patients (90%) with monostotic type present between 5 and 15 years [5]. About 80% of patients are younger than age years, and half of patients are children younger than age 10 years [6]. However, disseminated forms most commonly occur in infant.

4.6 Location

LCH can involve any of the mononuclear phagocyte system (RES). However, bone is by far the most common site for monostotic LCH and is

W.-J. Bahk, *Diagnosis and Management of Primary Bone Tumors*,
https://doi.org/10.1007/978-981-99-5498-8_4

also favorite location for disseminated variants. Peculiarly, LCH affects most commonly flat bones such as craniofacial bones as well as trunk bones including vertebra, pelvis, and ribs, representing about 70% of patients. The rest of monostatic lesions occurs in diaphysis or metaphysis of major long bones, most frequently the femur followed by the humerus, tibia, and forearm bones [4]. In long bones, LCH predominantly affects diaphysis and extends metaphysis but does not usually cross the growth plate [6], and long bone involvement is more common in children [7]. Small tubular bones of hands and feet are very rarely affected.

4.7 Clinical Features

Variable clinical symptoms may be presented depending on the affected organ. The most common symptom related to the involved bones is localized aching pain of short duration usually less than 2 months, tenderness, and swelling or palpable mass around the lesion. Pathologic fracture is rare. Spinal involvement causes back pain, stiffness, and scoliosis and even may lead to neurologic complication by vertebral collapse. The lesion in the craniofacial bones may cause loosening/loss of the teeth, oral ulcers, otitis media, diminished hearing, or exophthalmos. Symptoms of diabetes insipidus is the most common form of extraskeletal involvement, which usually develop within 3 years of initial diagnosis [8]. Organomegaly and lymphadenopathy may result from the tumor infiltration in the RES. Skin manifestations such as rashes, petechial, eczema, xanthomatosis, or soft-tissue nodules. Disseminated disease may produce severe complications including thrombocytopenia, anemia, pneumonia, chronic lung interstitial fibrosis, transverse myelitis, and biliary cirrhosis, which can be fatal [4, 9]. About 10% of the patients with unifocal lesion eventually progress to multifocal or extraskeletal disease [4, 10]. LCH may be associated with a nonspecific inflammatory response such as general weakness and mild fever with local redness. Particularly, when such clinical presentation is accompanied by leukocytosis and increased erythrocyte sedimentation rate (ESR), the localized osseous LCH is easily mistaken for osteomyelitis.

4.8 Radiologic Findings

Radiologic findings are widely variable depending on the affected bone and phases of the lesion. ***In early phase,*** the lesion is more aggressive-looking ill-defined small osteolytic destruction often with moth-eaten to permeative margin indicating a rapid growth. Cortical thinning or thickening, erosion or endosteal scalloping, intracortical tunneling, and even naked soft tissue mass can be observed simulating a malignant bone tumor. A varying size of soft tissue mass can be formed in 5–10% of patients [4]. One or multiple layered periosteal reaction of parallel laminations with various thicknesses, so-called "*onion-skinning*," can be seen mimicking malignant bone tumor such osteosarcoma or Ewing's sarcoma and acute osteomyelitis. The degree of periosteal reaction is often more extensive than would be expected from severity of cortical destruction (Fig. 4.1a). ***In mid-phase,*** the lesion is growing and becoming confluent to reach maximum size of geographic lesion with more clearly defined margin often surrounded by a surrounding sclerotic rim of reactive bone (Figs. 4.2a, 4.3b and 4.4a). The periosteal reaction is still prominent (Fig. 4.2e) or begin to be diminished (Fig. 4.3f). ***In late healing phase,*** the lesion is similar to that in the mid-phase with well-defined, blurred, and diminished lytic oval lesion and resolution of periosteal lamellation with better demarcation (Fig. 4.4f) or thicker rim of sclerosis. It will take several months to years to resolve spontaneously without surgical treatment (Figs. 4.1 and 4.2). With times, a dense thick periosteal new bone formation with thickening of the cortex is observed. Rarely, a "*sequestrum*" can be found, which is pathologically defined as a piece of devitalized bone that is separated from the surrounding bone during a process of necrosis. Radiologically, it refers to visible densification or nidus surrounded by relatively well-demarcated lucent lesion without referring

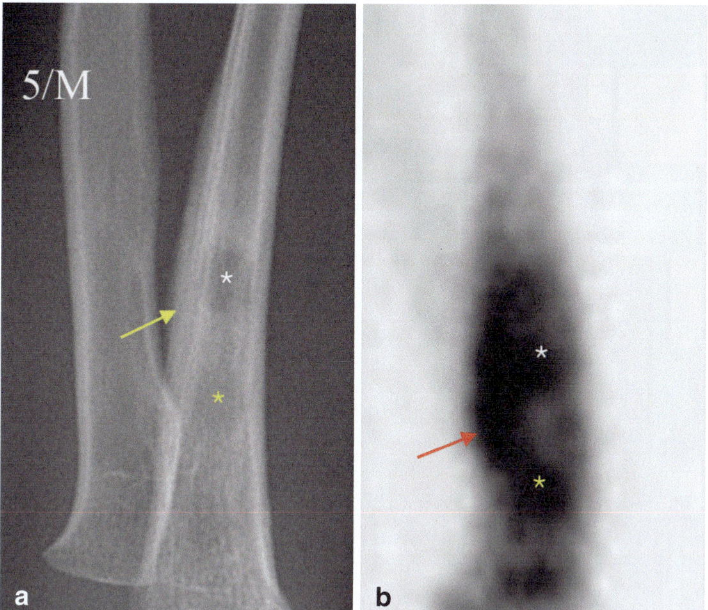

Fig. 4.1 (**a**) Radiograph taken for left proximal forearm pain of 2-month duration in 5-year-old boy shows two separated-looking, ill-defined, hazy, oval to round osteolytic lesions (asterisks) with multiple laminations of thick periosteal reaction, so-called "*onion skinning*" (yellow arrow) in the diaphysis of proximal ulna. The periosteal reaction is more extensive than expected from the severity of bone destruction. (**b**) Pinhole bone scan reveals strong uptake in both lesions (asterisks) and area of thick periosteal reaction (arrow). (**c**) MR images demonstrate well-defined two separated oval medullary lesions (asterisks) with low SI on T1-weighted image and heterogeneous intermediate and high SI on T2-weighted image, surrounded by dark signals of sclerotic rim on both sequences. There is multiple superficial endosteal scalloping with a deep invasion with no discernible soft tissue mass (inset). The lesions are well enhanced (red asterisks), and tumor deeply invading the cortex is also well enhanced (white arrow in inset). Perilesional bone marrow (red arrow) as well as adjacent soft tissue edema (yellow arrow) is also well enhanced. He was managed conservatively by intermittent use of painkiller with a histologic diagnosis of LCH. (**d**) Follow-up radiograph at 6 months notes disappearance of the lesions (asterisks) with thickening of the cortex (arrow). (**e**) Last follow-up radiograph at 18 months shows complete spontaneous healing of the lesions with remodeling of the cortex (arrow). (**f**) Another radiograph taken for left forearm pain of 4-day duration in 5-year-old girl reveals an ill-defined osteolytic lesion with a wide transzonal zone int the mid-shaft of radius. Note cortical destruction and limited soft tissue extension (red arrow) under the multiple layers of thickened periosteum (yellow arrow). (**g**) Bone scan and bone SPECT (inset) note mildly increased uptake only in the lesion, indicating a solitary lesion. (**h**) MR images demonstrate an intramedullary mass-like lesion with iso-intensity to surrounding muscle on T1-weighted image and high SI on T2-weighted image. Note cortical destruction with an extraosseous extension (yellow arrows) and multiple layers of paralleling periosteal reaction (red arrow). There are prominent perilesional bone marrow and surrounding soft tissue edema (asterisks) by inflammatory response to the tumor, mimicking locally aggressive lesion such as acute osteomyelitis or Ewing sarcoma. In addition, the lesion shows a thick peripheral enhancement (red arrow) with central non-enhancing dark signal (black arrow), suggesting an island of residual host bone or dead bone, so-called "*sequestrum*." The significant bone marrow and soft tissue edema are also strongly enhanced. These findings would suggest osteomyelitis with sequestrum or abscess rather than aggressive bone tumor. However, microscopic examination shows a diffuse proliferation of the Langerhans mononuclear cells with numerous scattered eosinophils, indicating LCH. She was managed conservatively without surgery. (**i**) Follow-up radiograph at 4 months after biopsy shows a complete resolution of the lesion with thickening of the overlying cortex. (**j**) Follow-up radiograph at 3 years after biopsy reveals complete healing of the lesion with no evidence of local recurrence

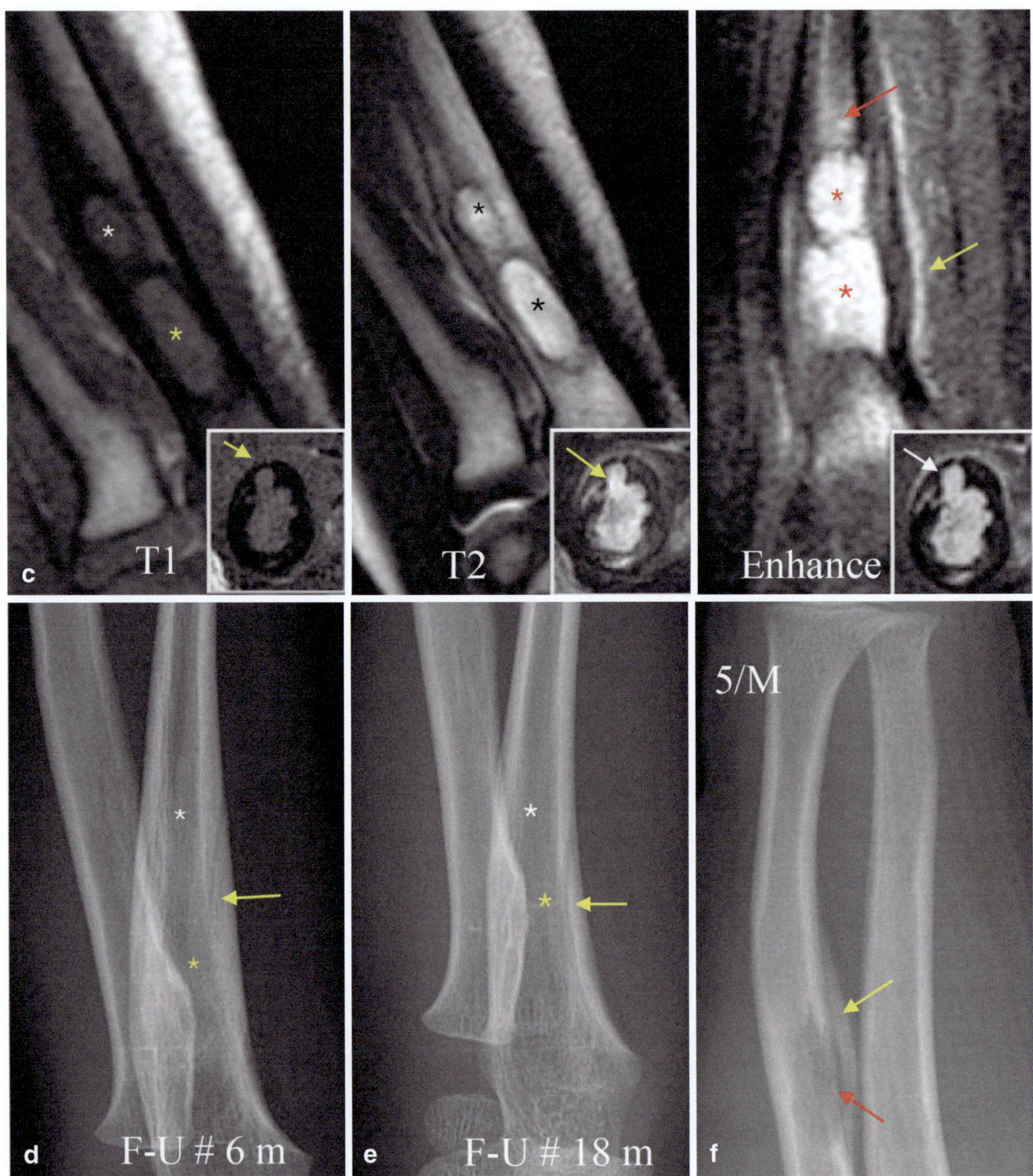

Fig. 4.1 (continued)

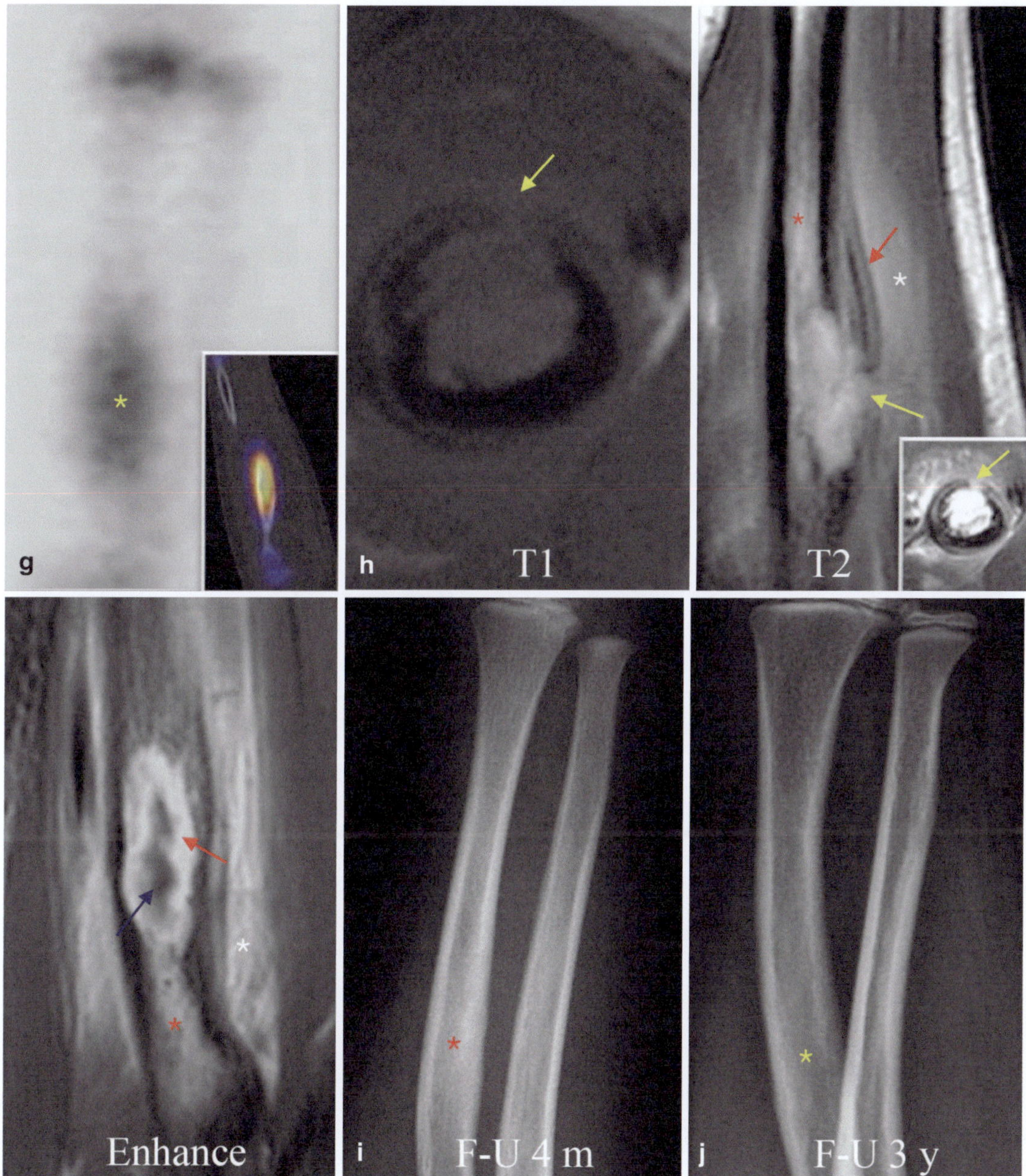

Fig. 4.1 (continued)

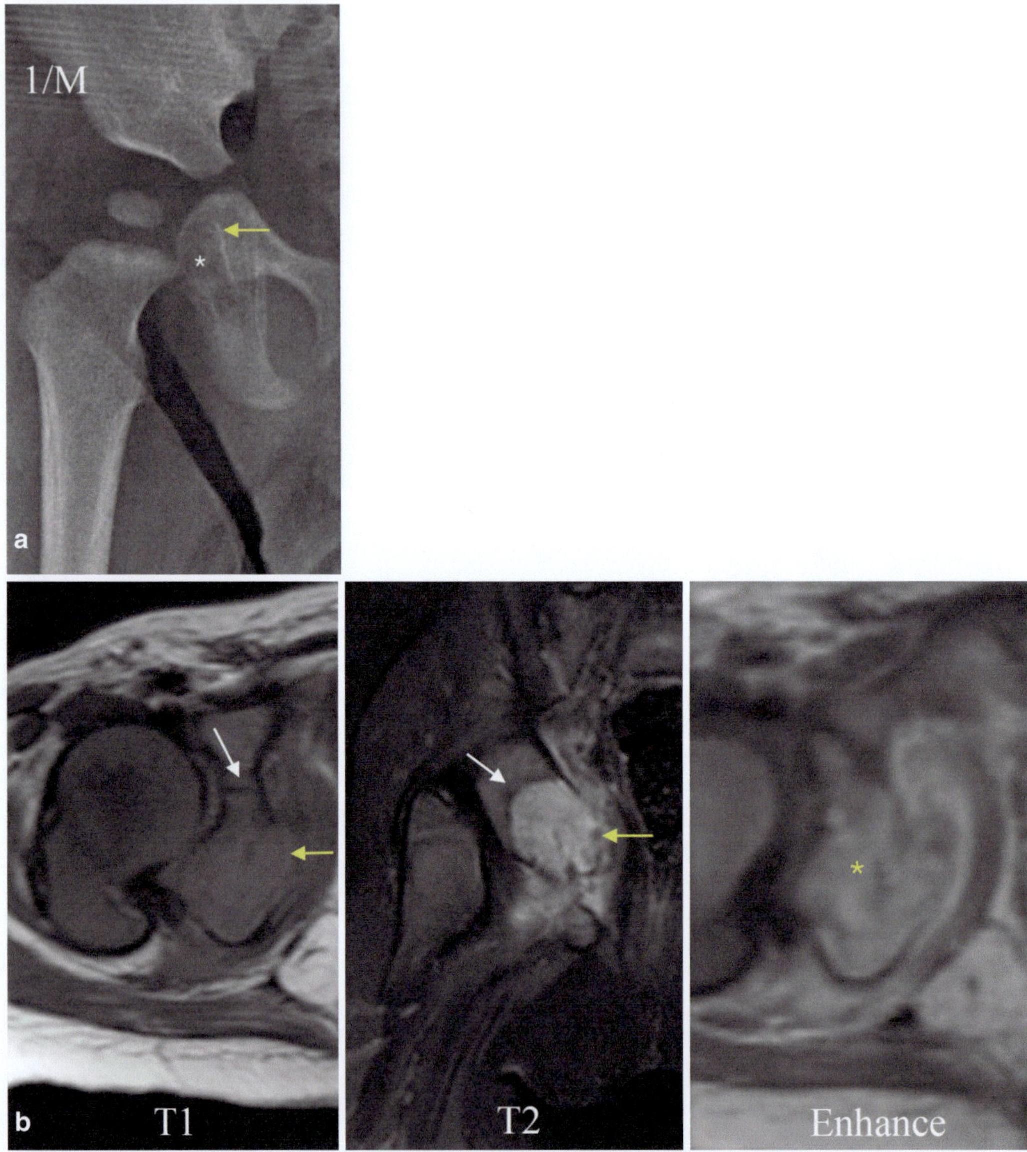

Fig. 4.2 (**a**) Radiograph taken for irritability by right hip motion during diaper change of 10-day duration in 12-month-old boy show a relatively well-defined osteolytic lesion (asterisk) surrounded by a thin sclerotic rim (arrow) affecting the ischium. (**b**) MR images demonstrate a well-defined intramedullary lobulated lesion with low SI on T1-weighted image and intermediate and high SI on T2-weighted image, which is surrounded by a dark signal of thin surrounding sclerosis (white arrows). There is focal cortical breakage and soft tissue extension (yellow arrows). The lesion is heterogeneously well enhanced by contrast medium (yellow asterisk). (**c**) Follow-up radiograph in 3 months after histologic confirmation of LHC by incision biopsy reveals consolidation of the lesion without any treatment. (**d**) Follow-up radiograph in 2 years after biopsy notes remodeling of the affected ischium with no recurrence. (**e**) Radiograph taken for left proximal thigh pain of 2-month duration in 12-year-old girl shows an ill-defined oval radiolucent lesion focally invading the cortex with a thick periosteal reaction (yellow arrow) and thin lamellated periosteal reaction (red arrow) in the diaphysis of proximal femur. (**f**) Bone scan reveals heterogeneously increased uptake mainly at thickened cortical area (arrow). (**g**) MR images demonstrate a relatively well-defined multi-lobulated mass-like lesion with heterogeneous low and high SI on both sequences. Note cortical perforation (red arrow) and multilayered periosteal reaction (yellow arrow). However, the lesion is still confined to the thickened cortex under the thick periosteum with no soft tissue extension. There is prominent perilesional bone marrow and adjacent soft tissue edema (asterisks), suggesting a diffuse inflammatory response to the tumor. The lesion and edema are heterogeneously enhanced. (**h**) Microscopic examination reveals clusters of loosely aggregated histiocytic-appearing Langerhans cells admixed with inflammatory cells, predominantly eosinophils, indicating LCH

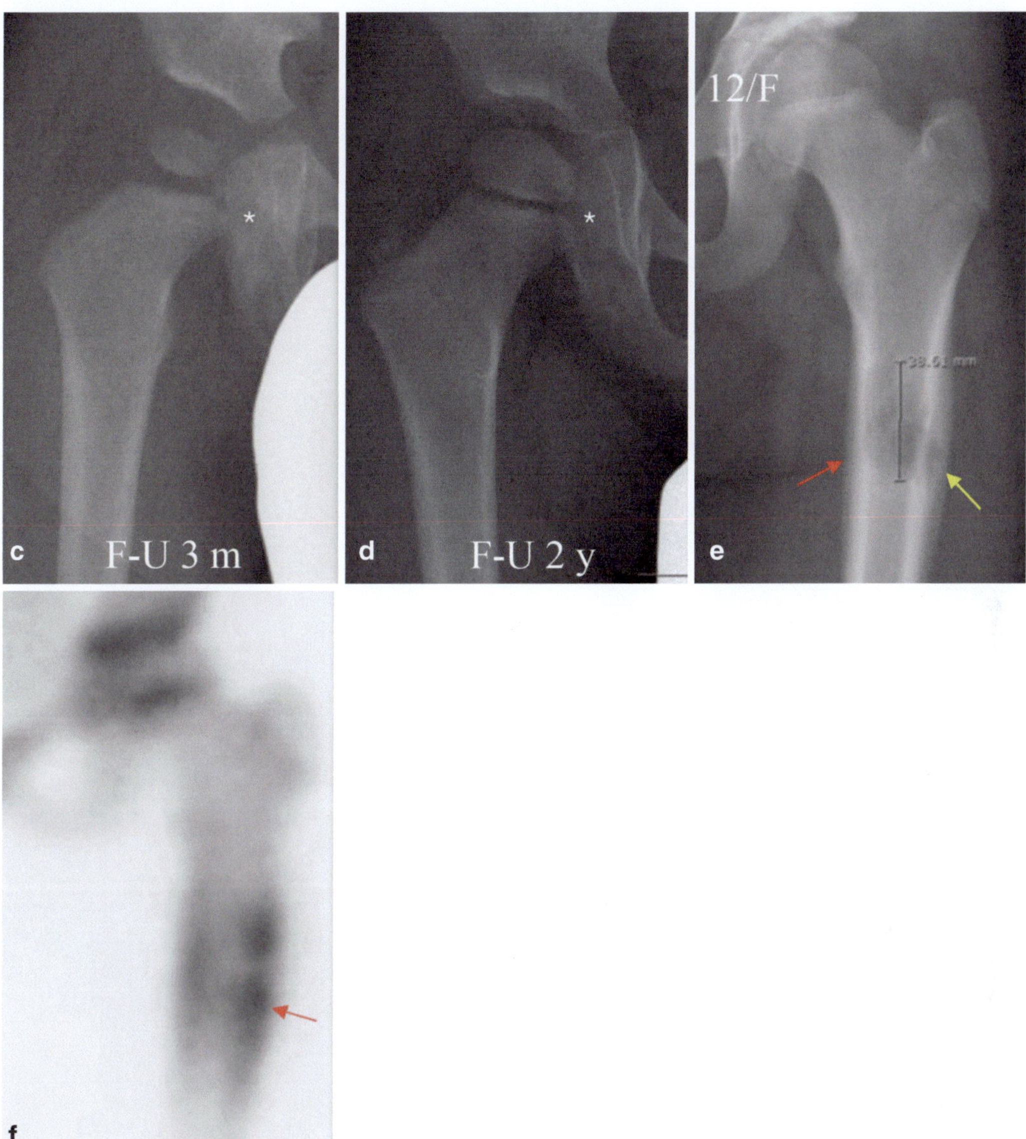

Fig. 4.2 (continued)

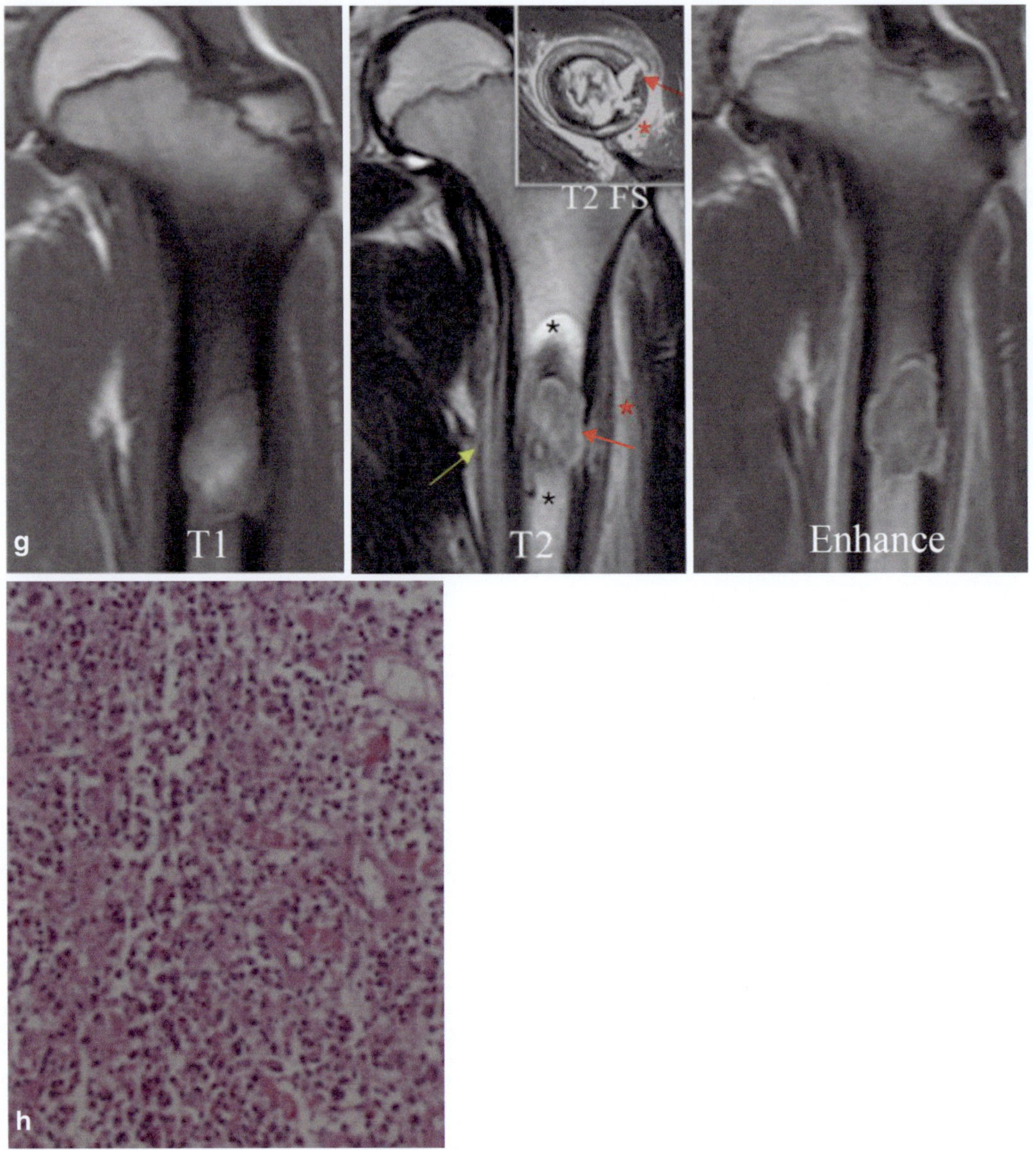

Fig. 4.2 (continued)

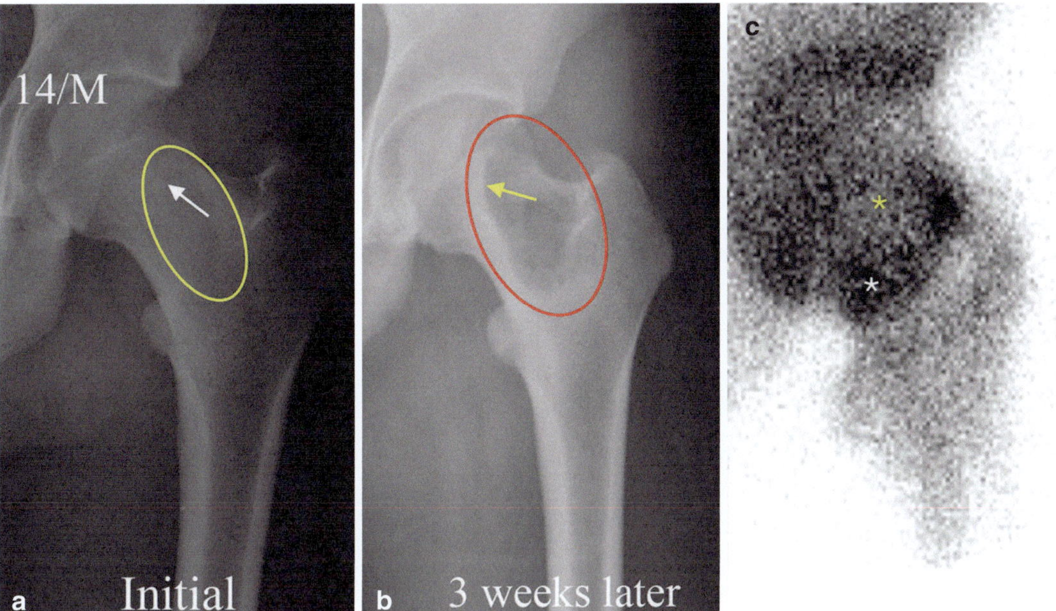

Fig. 4.3 (**a**) Radiograph taken for left hip pain of 5-day duration in 14-year-old boy shows a hazy, ill-defined, oval, osteolytic lesion (yellow circle) with hazy sclerotic rim (arrow) involving femoral neck. (**b**) Three weeks later, the lesion becomes larger and well-defined (red circle) with a clear thin rim of sclerosis (arrow). (**c**) Pinhole bone scan reveals strong uptake along the periphery (white asterisk) with mild uptake in the center of lesion (yellow asterisk). (**d**) MR images demonstrate a well-demarcated intramedullary lesion with low SI on T1-weighted image and high SI with focal low signal on fat saturated T2-weighted image, surrounded by a thin dark signal on both sequences (yellow arrows). The lesion is heterogeneously enhanced in the center with a peripheral thin enhancement (white arrow). (**e**) Radiograph at 6 months after curettage, all-chip bone graft, and fixation with compression hip screw to prevent fracture notes consolidation of the lesion (asterisk). (**f**) Radiograph taken for right thigh pain of 2-week duration in 14-year-old boy show an ill-defined, hazy, osteolytic lesion (asterisk) with cortical thickening and mild cortical erosion as well as a thin periosteal reaction (arrow), simulating osteomyelitis or aggressive bone tumor in the diaphysis of proximal femur. (**g**) However, pinhole bone scan reveals only mild uptake along the cortex (arrow) with central void area (asterisk), suggesting inactive lesion rather than active or aggressive lesion. (**h**) MR images notes a well-defined intramedullary lesion with intermediate SI on T1-weighted image and intermediate to high SI and focal dark signals on T2-weighted image, which is surrounded by a dark signal of thin surrounding sclerosis. There is a mild cortical scalloping with multiple thin layers of periosteal reaction (yellow arrow) and perilesional bone marrow edema (black asterisks). The lesion itself as well as edema is heterogeneously well enhanced. (**i**) Microscopic examination. (Left) Low-power magnification shows a diffuse proliferation of the mononuclear cells and eosinophils as well as several scattered multinucleated giant cells and prominent hemorrhage. (Right) Higher-power magnification reveals that the number of Langerhans cells seems to be reduced to that of eosinophils at a glance. The histiocytes begin to become degenerated and produce increasing number of foamy macrophages (arrows)

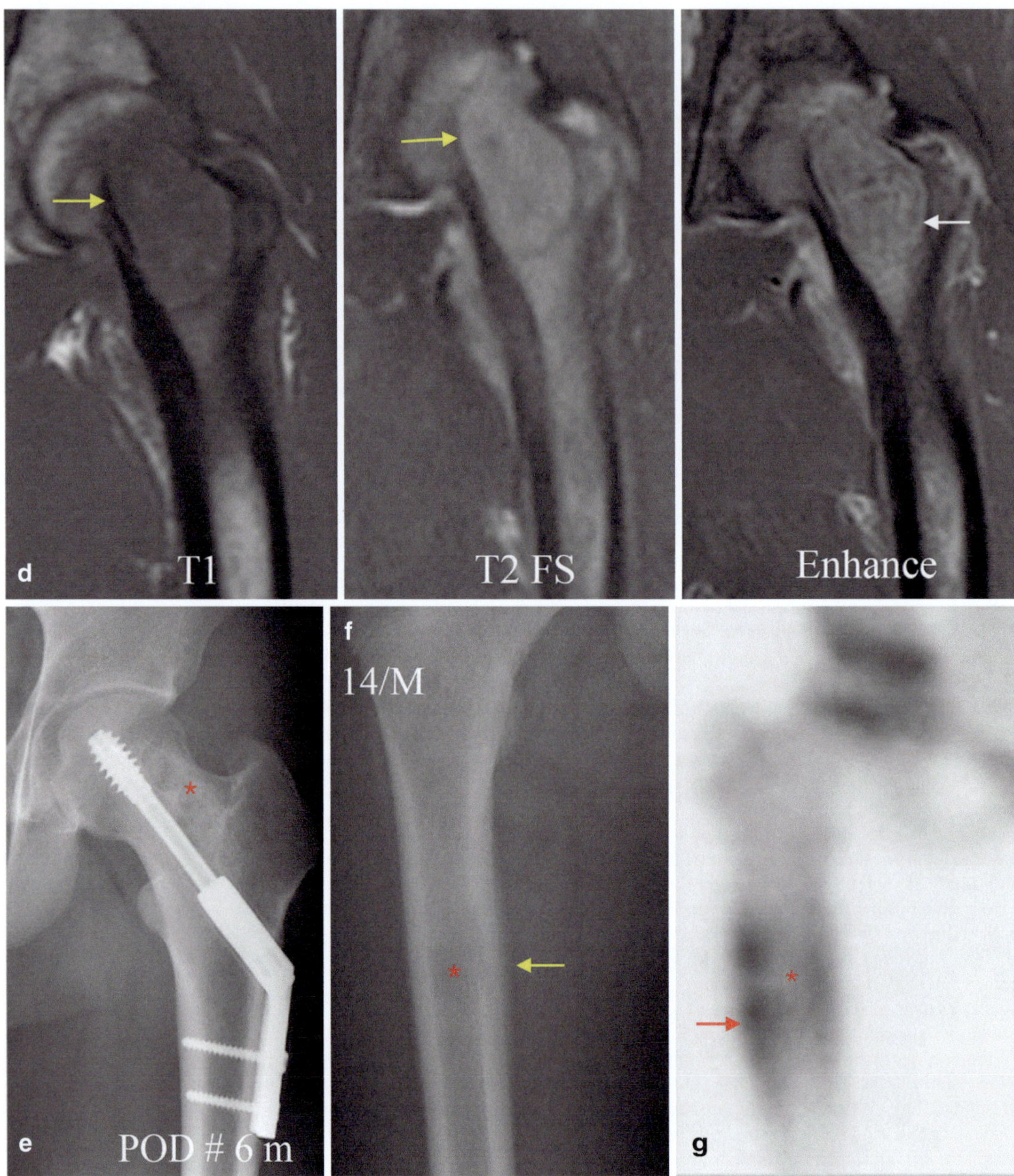

Fig. 4.3 (continued)

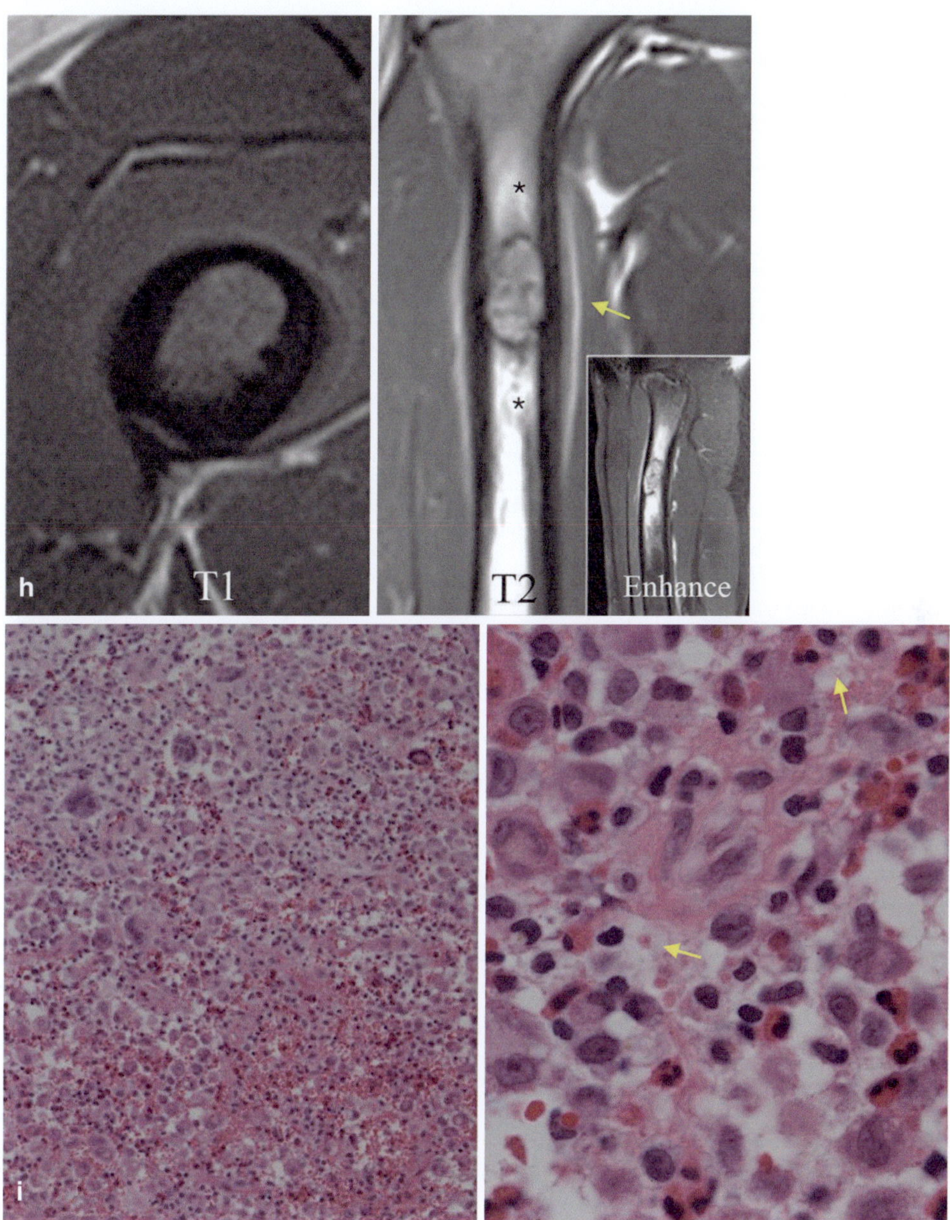

Fig. 4.3 (continued)

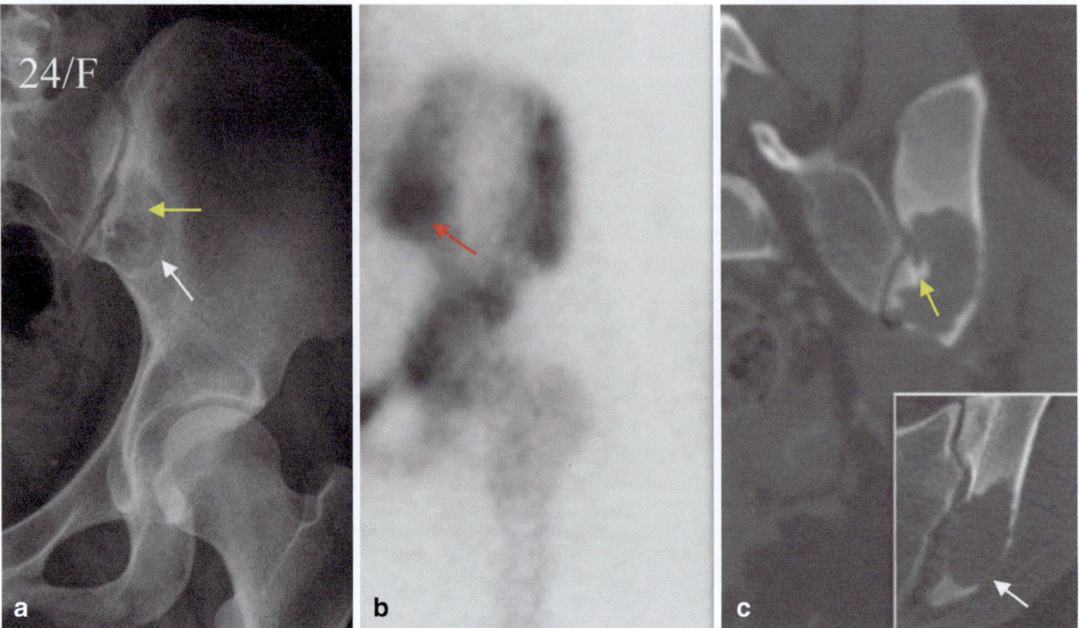

Fig. 4.4 (**a**) Radiograph taken for left buttock pain of 2-month duration in 24-year-old young lady shows a well-defined osteolytic lesion with internal bone opacity (yellow arrow) surrounded by a thin sclerotic rim (white arrow) in the left iliac bone adjacent to sacroiliac joint. (**b**) Bone scan reveals a focal moderate uptake in the lesion (red arrow). (**c**) CT scan notes an irregular dense bone density (yellow arrow) in the center of osteolytic lesion, indicating a so-called "*button sequestrum.*" There is focal cortical breakage but no discernible soft tissue extension (inset). (**d**) MR images demonstrate a well-defined lesion (asterisks) with low to iso SI on T1-weighted image and intermediate to high SI with focal bright signal on T2-wighted image, which is surrounded by a thin dark signal of sclerosis. There is significant peri-tumoral bone marrow (yellow arrow) and soft tissue edema (white arrow), suggesting prominent inflammatory response to the tumor. The lesion is only focally enhanced (arrow). Microscopically, there are markedly increased number of eosinophils with scanty number of Langerhans cells and prominent foam cells forming masses with fibrosis or scar tissue, indicating the late phase of LCH. (**e**) Follow-up radiograph at 3 years after curettage shows consolidation of the lesion (arrow). (**f**) Radiographs taken for right thigh pain for 1 month in 42-year-old man show an ill-defined multilobulated lesion with cortical invasion (red circle) in the diaphysis of proximal femur. Pinhole bone scan demonstrates an eccentric, inhomogeneous strong uptake in the lesion (inset). (**g**) MR images reveal an intramedullary lesion (asterisks) with cortical scalloping and focal breakthrough at posterolateral aspect but no clearly discernible invasion into surrounding soft tissue (red arrows). The SI is intermediate to high SI on T1-weighted image and heterogeneously high on fat saturated T2-weighted image. Note prominent bone marrow and soft tissue edema with inflammatory reaction (red asterisks). The lesion is focally and peripherally enhanced (blue arrow), and the inflammatory lesions with edema are diffusely enhanced (red asterisks). In consideration of age of 45 years and high serum C-reactive protein (CRP) level of 1.29 mg/dl (normal < 0.3), subacute osteomyelitis is suspected rather than LCH. (**h**) However, microscopic examination demonstrates masses of foamy histiocytes of varying size between collagen fibers, some bi- or multinucleated giant cells, and a few scattered eosinophils (yellow arrows), indicating LCH between mid-phase and late phase. Note many histiocytes converted into macrophages with pale or foamy cytoplasm (red arrows). Note area of extensive necrosis in other filed (inset). (**i**) Follow-up radiograph at 1 year after trocar biopsy still notes the lesion with some haziness (inset). However, radiograph at 3 years after biopsy shows complete healing of the lesion with normalization of the cortex (circle)

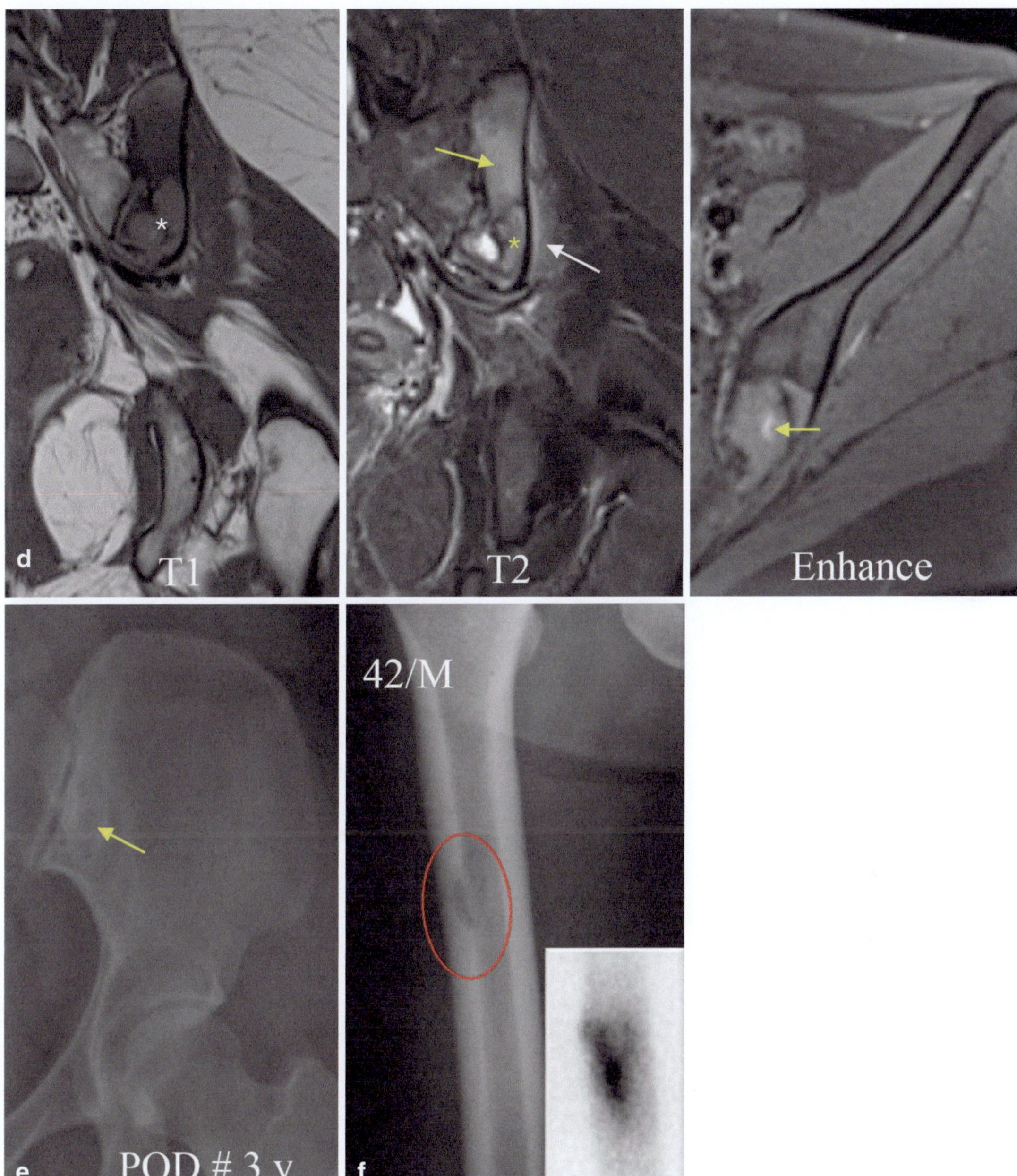

Fig. 4.4 (continued)

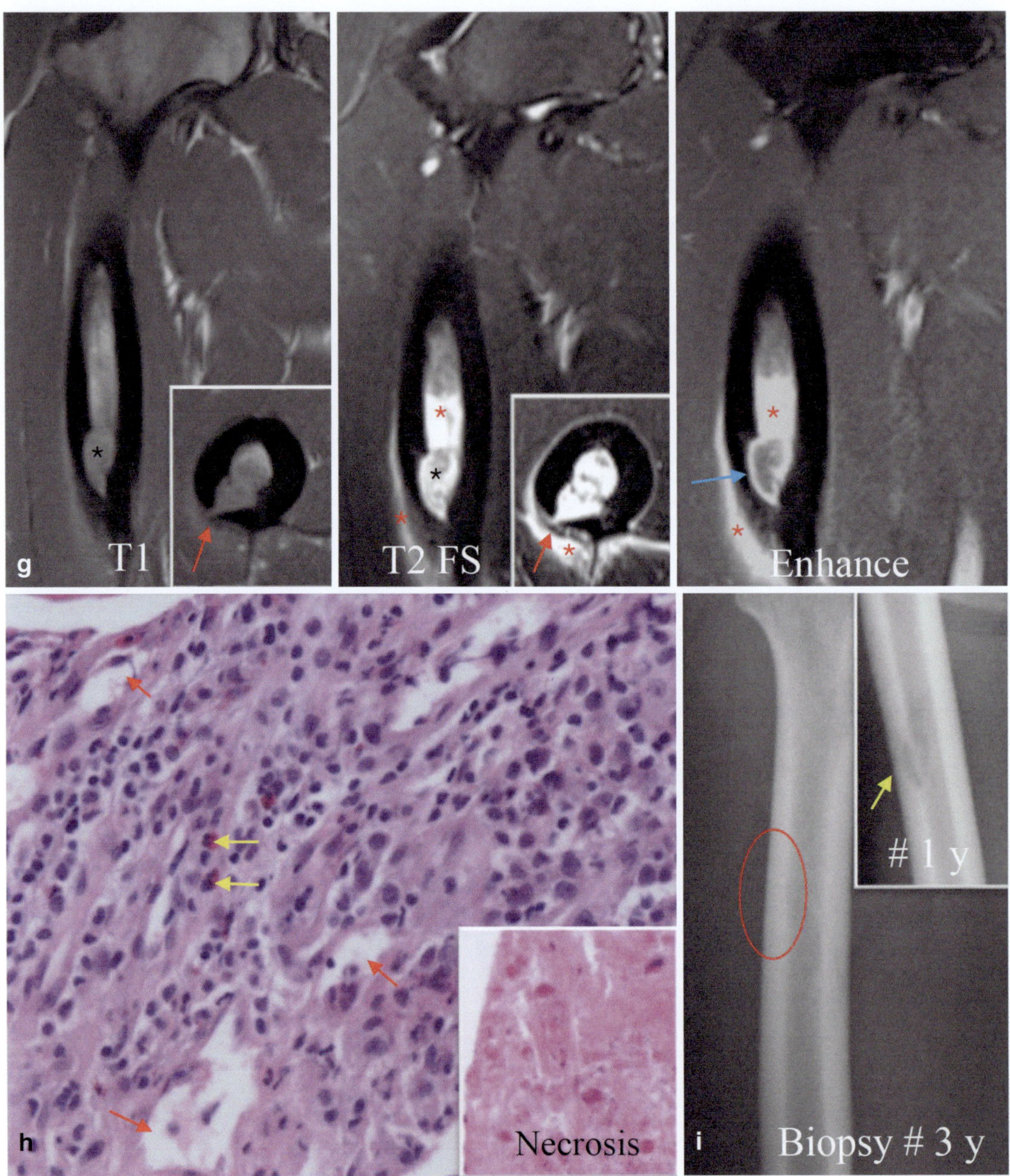

Fig. 4.4 (continued)

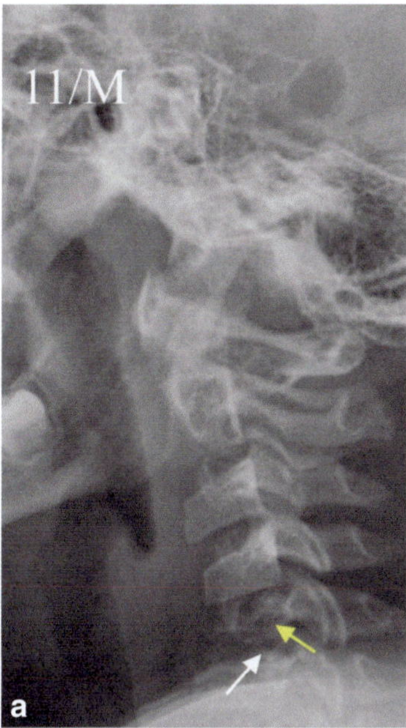

Fig. 4.5 (**a**) Radiograph taken for neck pain in 11-year-old boy shows a uniform destruction and collapse to a condensed wafer-thin body of the fifth cervical (C5) vertebra, so-called "*vertebra plana*" (yellow arrow). The disk space is, however, preserved well (white arrow). (**b**) MR images demonstrate a collapsed C5 body with marrow replacing lesion (yellow arrows) of low SI on T1-weighted image and heterogeneous high SI on T2-weighted image. However, the adjacent disk space is well preserved (white arrows). The lesion is well enhanced by the contrast medium (red arrow). (**c**) Follow-up radiograph at 3 months reveals slightly denser vertebral body but no recuperation of the height. (**d**) One year later, the lesion becomes denser with partial height recuperation. (**e**) Three years later, the spine body is markedly recovered to near normal shape and height. (**f**) Skull radiograph taken for a forehead mass of 2-month duration in 5-year-old girl shows irregular punched-out lesion outlined with "*double contour*" (red arrow) involving the frontal bone. (**g**) CT scan reveals a well-defined soft tissue mass with full thickness uneven destruction of the frontal bone. The outer table is more severely destroyed (red arrow) than inner table (yellow arrow) producing a typical "*double-contoured*" or "*beveled-edge*" appearance. (**h**) MR images demonstrate a multi-septated soft tissue mass with destruction of frontal bone (red arrows) with heterogeneous intermediate and high SI on T1-weighted image and heterogeneous high SI on T2-weighted FLAIR image. The bony lesion is focally enhanced (white arrow), and the soft tissue mass is peripherally enhanced (yellow arrow). (**i**) Dark yellowish to brownish soft tissue mass extended though the destructed frontal bone (black asterisk) is visible on operation filed. Skull bone defect with spared inner table is seen after excision of the mass and curettage (inset) under a histologic confirmation of LCH by frozen biopsy. She is doing well with no evidence of recurrence at 3 years after surgery

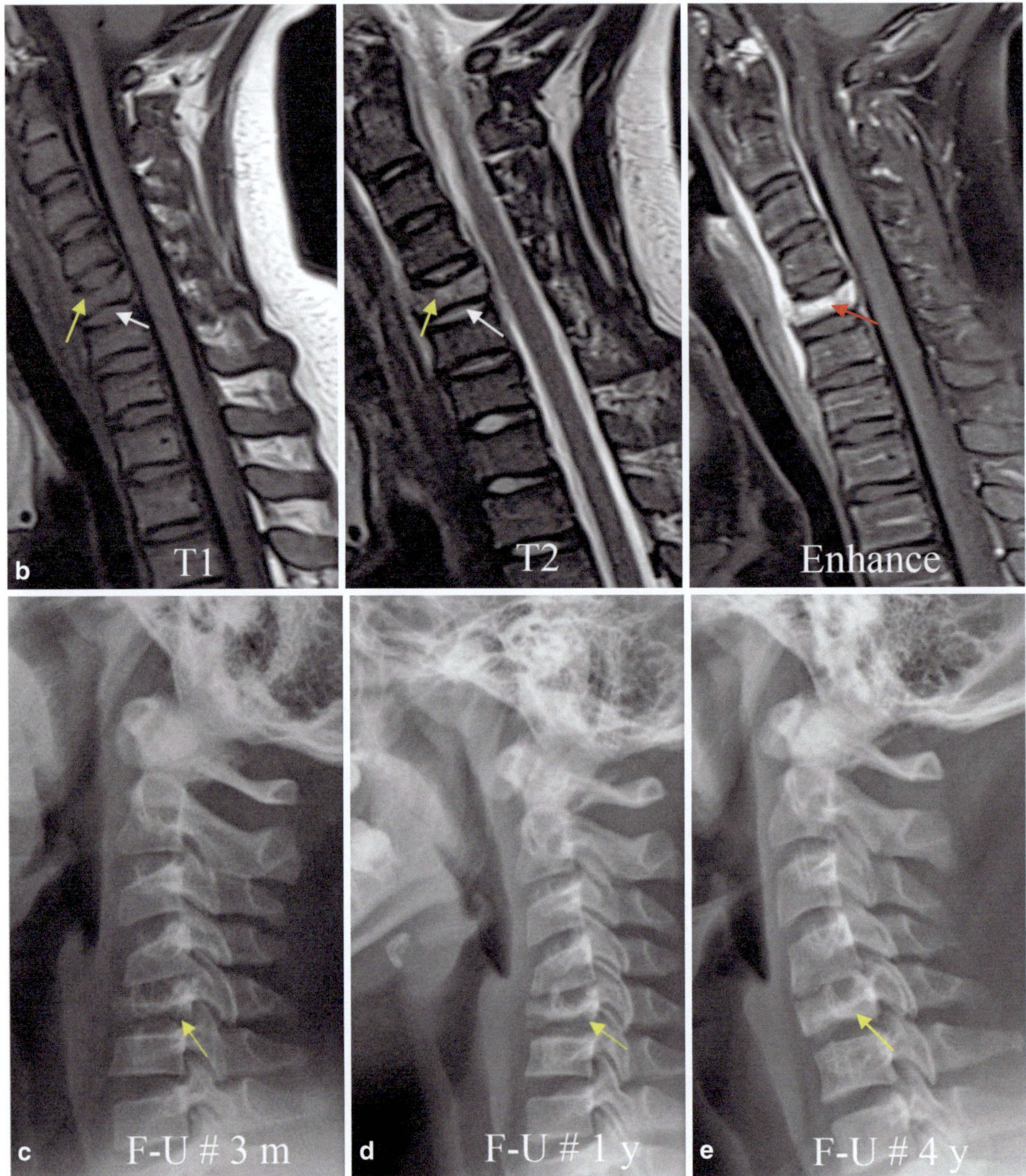

Fig. 4.5 (continued)

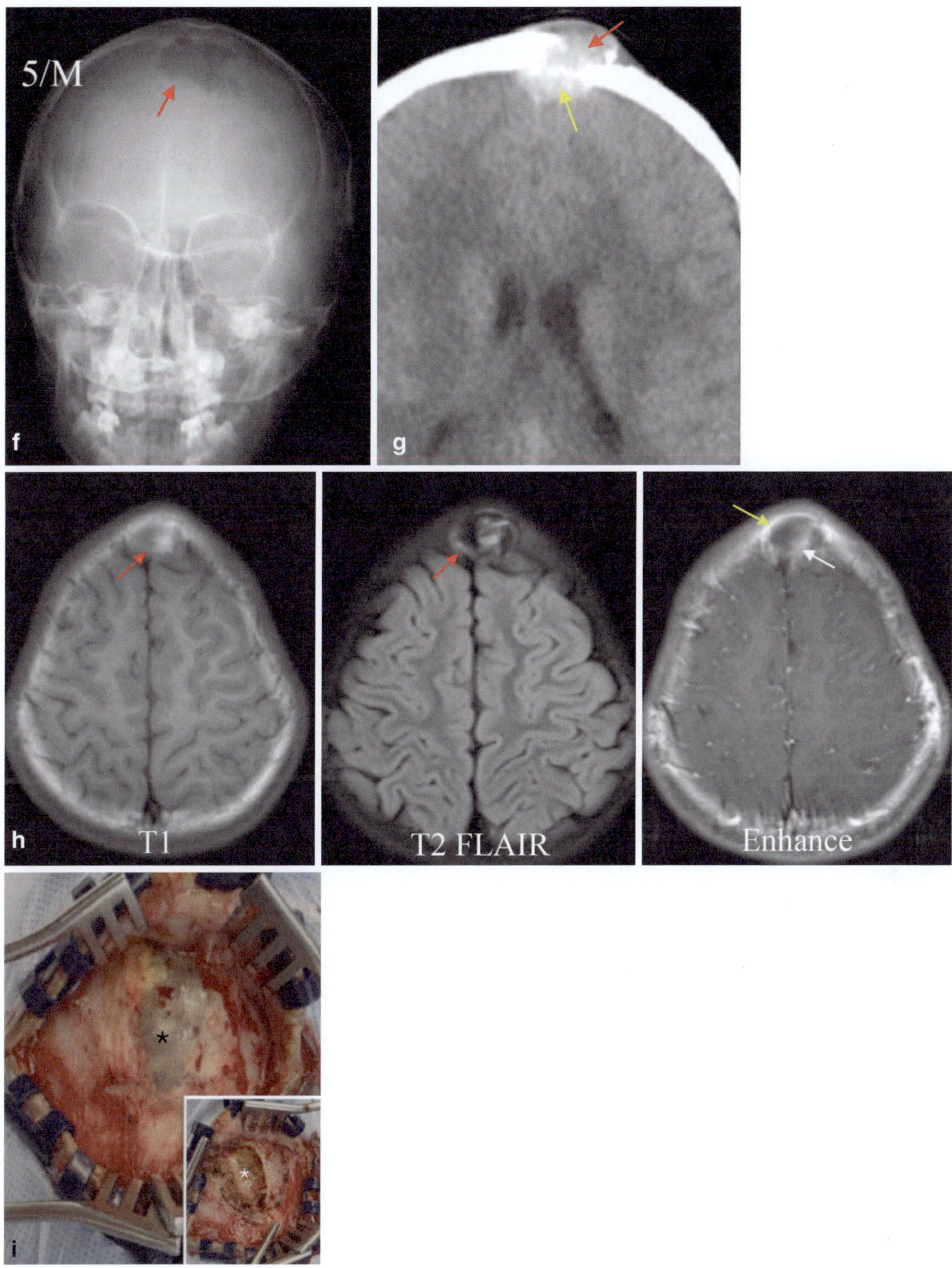

Fig. 4.5 (continued)

to the vascular status and can be also found in a variety of other bone lesions [11, 12]. When involving skull bones, the lesions are characteristically round to ovoid with a well-defined but no sclerotic margin, so-called "*punched-out*" appearance. The lesions asymmetrically destroyed the inner and outer tables of the skull (hole within a hole sign) with a characteristic "*double contour*" or "*beveled edges*" appearance (Fig. 4.5f, g). A small sequestrum appearing as a "*button*" of intact bone in the center of a circular radiolucent destruction, so-called "*button sequestrum*" coined by Wells [13], can be observed [12, 14, 15] (Fig. 4.4a, c). This type of sequestrum can be also seen in osteomyelitis, eosinophilic granuloma, fibrous tumor including fibrosarcoma, desmoplastic fibroma and malignant fibrous histiocytoma, or lymphoma [16]. Partially calcified intraosseous lipoma can also appear as a bone opacity surrounded by a relatively lucent area [10, 17]. It may also present in tuberculous osteitis, radiation necrosis, metastatic carcinoma, fibrous dysplasia, epidermoid and dermoid cyst, hemangioma, and meningioma [12]. Often, the affected spine in children is insidiously collapsed to a condensed wafer-thin body with intact the disk space, so-called "*vertebra plana*" (Fig. 4.5a). In contrast, the disk space is severely destructed in bacterial spondylitis. LCH is the most common cause of vertebra plana in children. **CT scan** shows similar findings to those of plain radiograph with better demonstration of cortical erosion and soft tissue extension suggesting more aggressive lesion. CT scan can more clearly visualize the "*button sequestrum*" (Fig. 4.4c) [16] and typical "*beveled-edge*" appearance (Fig. 4.5g). **Bone scan** notes variably increased or decreased uptake depending on the stage of the lesion (Figs. 4.1, 4.2, 4.3, and 4.4) and is valuable to find other asymptomatic lesions in polyostotic type. **MR images** demonstrate low to intermediate SI on T1-weighted image and high SI on T2-weighted images with diffuse or focal contrast enhancement (Figs. 4.1, 4.2, 4.3, 4.4, and 4.5). Occasionally, cortical invasion or perforation often with soft tissue mass can be observed (Fig. 4.1h). On occasion, a sequestrum may be difficult to identify on MRI. The sequestrum would appear as a low-intensity fragment on T1-weighted imaging, and sequestrum itself does not enhance, but surrounding granulation tissue is well enhanced (Fig. 4.1h). Perilesional marrow and adjacent soft tissue edema or inflammation is often considerable, which can be mistaken for locally aggressive lesion or osteomyelitis particularly when nonspecific inflammatory symptoms such as general weakness, mild fever with local redness, and abnormal lab findings are associated.

4.9 Histologic Findings

LHC basically consists of two types of cells, pathognomonic and clonal histiocytic-appearing "*Langerhans cells*" and "*eosinophils*". In addition to these two basic cells, variable degree of other types of inflammatory cells is frequently admixed. ***In incipient phase,*** low- and medium-power magnification demonstrates loose nests or clusters of loosely aggregated histiocytic-appearing Langerhans cells and inflammatory cells, predominantly eosinophils as well as neutrophils, lymphocytes, or plasma cells (Fig. 4.6a, b). On higher-power magnification, the hallmark Langerhans cells present oval to vesicular or reniform (kidney-shaped) nuclei of varying size and blue or red colored (amphophilic or neutrophilic) to pale cytoplasm with more or less distinct border. Characteristically, Langerhans cells have deeply indented or linear grooves that traverse length of nuclei, so-called "*coffee-bean*" appearance (Fig. 4.6c, d). The eosinophils are small and bi-lobulated with pink or orange-colored granules and eccentrically located dark nuclei. The proportion of Langerhans cells and eosinophils is varying from case to case and even from field to field in same case. In contrast to amphophilic or pale Langerhans cells, eosinophils are darker and present arranged in sheets or focal clusters. Ordinary non-Langerhans histiocytes with neither linear grooves nor reniform nuclei are also seen in some cases, which can merge to become multinucleated cells (Fig. 4.6e). Multinucleated giant cells are often seen, especially around the necrotic or hemor-

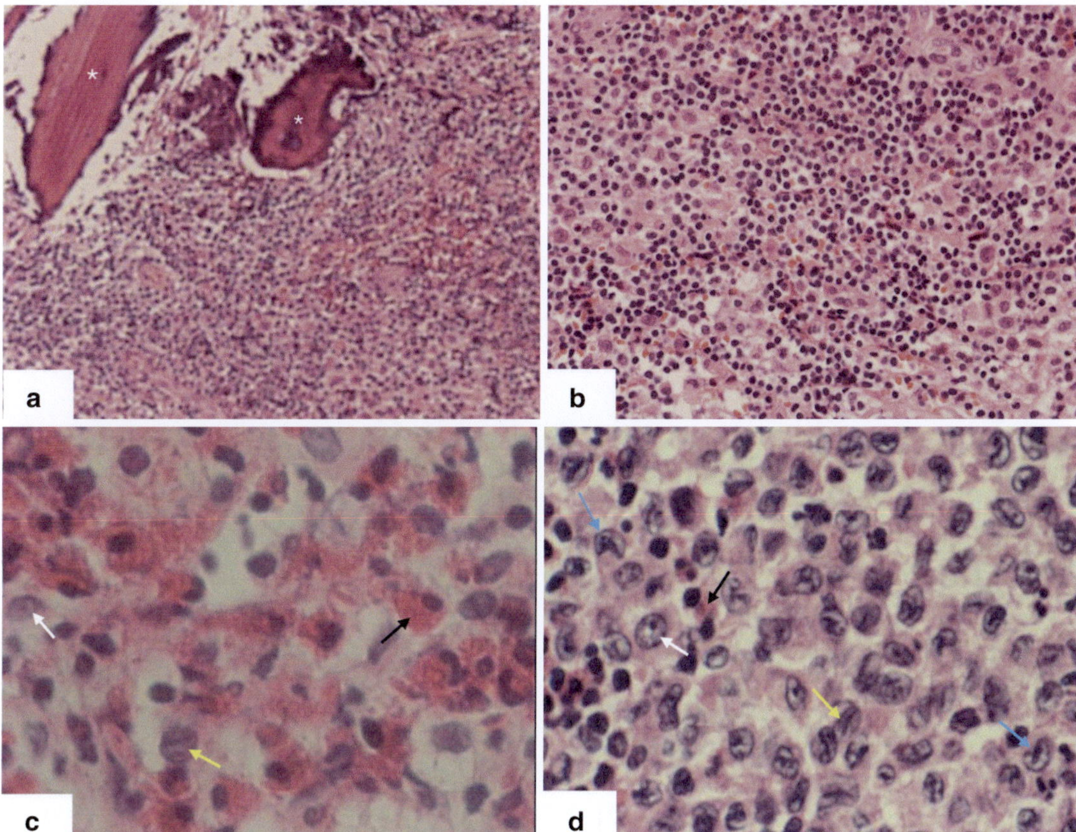

Fig. 4.6 ***Microscopic features***. (**a**) Low-power magnification shows clusters of loosely aggregated small bluish to purple round cells as well as pinkish to orange-colored eosinophilic cells. Some pieces of host lamellar bone are seen in this curetted specimen (asterisks). (**b**) Medium-power magnification reveals histiocytic appearing cells admixed with hemorrhage and inflammatory cells, predominantly eosinophils as well as some neutrophils, lymphocytes, and plasma cells. (**c**, **d**) Higher-power magnification demonstrates the clonal Langerhans cells, the hallmark of LCH, and eosinophils. Nuclei of the Langerhans cells are oval to vesicular typically with deeply indented or linear grooves that traverse length of nuclei appearing as a "*coffee-bean*" (yellow arrows) and granular eosinophilic to clear cytoplasm having more or less distinct border. Reniform (kidney-shaped) nuclei are also seen (blue arrows). Ordinary non-Langerhans histiocytes with round to oval nuclei without linear grooves are observed (white arrows). Varying number of eosinophils with eccentric nucleus and eosinophilic cytoplasm are seen scattered (black arrows). The proportion of Langerhans cells and eosinophils may vary from case to case and even from field to field in same case. The eosinophils are very high in number in a case (**c**) but scanty in another case (**d**). (**e**) Ordinary non-Langerhans mononuclear histiocytes gradually merge into larger cells and finally become to multinucleated giant cells. Note similar shape of round to oval nuclei in individual cells indicating that each mononuclear cell merges into multinucleated cells with varying number of nuclei (insets). (**f**) A large number of multinucleated giant cells are scattered throughout the lesion simulating GCT at a glance in this particular case. However, higher-power magnification reveals characteristic Langerhans cells with "*reniform*" nuclei (blue arrow) or "*coffee-bean*" appearance (yellow arrow), and ordinary non-Langerhans histiocytes without linear grooves (white arrow) admixed with eosinophils (black arrow), typically indicative of LCH (inset). (**g**) A nest with histiocytic-appearing small round cells extended through the broken cortex makes a naked soft tissue mass (white circle) and the cells invades into the surrounding muscles (M) reflecting extraosseous extension on MR image (Fig. 4.1h). (**h**) Necrotic area (N) is seen adjacent to nests with living cells (L). But necrosis does not herald aggressive clinical course. In practice, the lesion with this large area of necrotic area is completely healed on follow-up radiograph at 3 years after biopsy even without any treatment (Fig. 4.4i). (**i**) With time, the number of Langerhans cells is gradually decreased, and eosinophils become more prominent. Note varying size of the prominent foamy macrophages, which are produced by histiocytes converting the ingested debris into lipid. The number of foam cells is significantly increased to form masses with fibrosis or scar tissue in the late phase. (**j**) Langerhans cells express CD1a, Langerin, and S100 protein

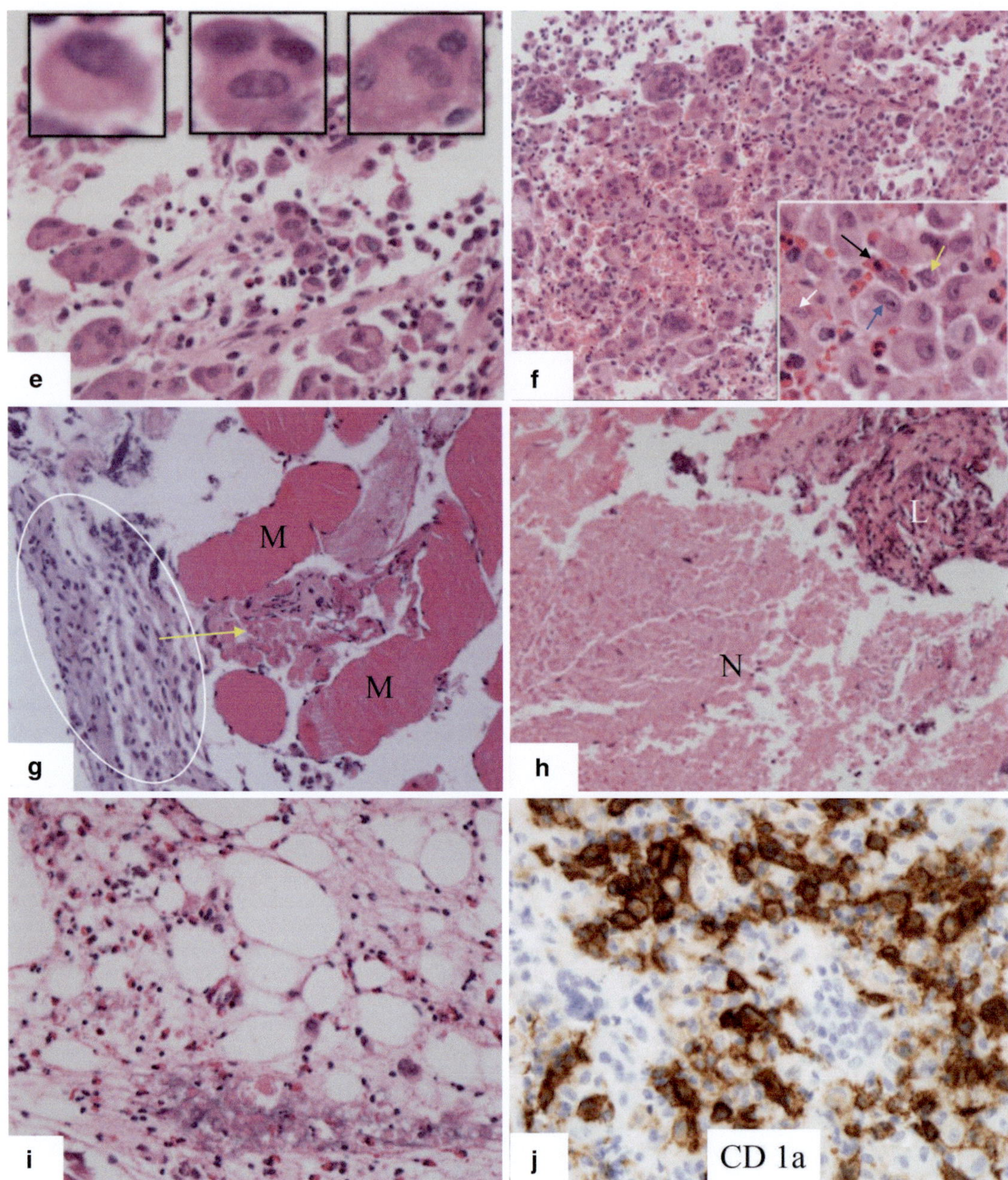

Fig. 4.6 (continued)

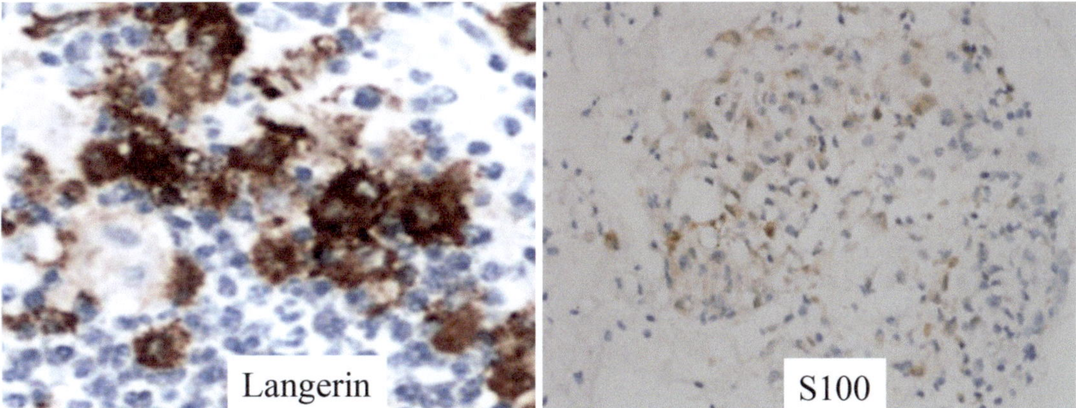

Fig. 4.6 (continued)

rhagic areas probably related to resorption of the materials. Rare cases are dominated by numerous giant cells mimicking neoplastic giant cell tumor (Fig. 4.6f). The tumor may be extended to soft tissue or even surrounding muscle through the cortical breakage (Fig. 4.6g). Mitoses are rare and typical. ***In mid-phase,*** the number of Langerhans cells is gradually reduced to that of eosinophils. The histiocytes begin to become degenerated and to convert the ingested debris into lipid making foamy or pale cytoplasm (foam cells) (Fig. 4.3i). The ratio of the foam cells and non-lipid laden cells is increased with times. Necrotic area can be seen adjacent to nests with living cells (Fig. 4.6h), but it does not herald aggressive nature. ***In late phase,*** the number of foam cell is gradually increasing to form masses with fibrosis or scar-like tissue. With times, the scar tissues become more abundant with scattered foam cells between collagen fibers (Fig. 4.6i). The Langerhans cells are significantly reduced in number up to absent. All other elements can be markedly diminished to totally disappear in very late phase.

4.10 Special Stains

Langerhans cells express CD1a, Langerin and S100 protein (Fig. 4.6j). CD1a and Langerin are specific for Langerhans cells. However, S100 is nonspecifically present in Langerhans cells and cells from neural crest (Schwann cells and melanocytes), chondrocytes, adipocytes, myoepithelial cells, macrophages, and dendritic cells.

4.11 Management

LCH of bone can be managed with several options depending on site and size of lesion, age of patient, and number of the lesion. Symptomatic lesion can be managed either by painkiller or local corticosteroid injection after histologic confirmation. Most of simple skeletal lesions are spontaneously healed over a period of months to years, and healing may be initiated from the biopsy itself (Figs. 4.1e, j, 4.2c, and 4.4j). Asymptomatic lesion can be observed with periodic follow-up. Surgical decompression and fusion with instrumentation may be indicated for spine lesions with rapidly progressive neurologic sign or cord compression not responding to irradiation. Scaglietti et al. [18] first reported the use of intralesional methylprednisolone injection in bone cysts with good results and considered it may favor a progressive process of repair in other bone lesions including LCH and nonossifying fibroma. Radiofrequency ablation has been also introduced for selective patients [19]. Simple curettage or bone graft with or without internal fixation is indicated for persisted symptomatic lesion or pathologic fracture. Low-dose irradiation therapy can be for selective lesions at difficult site in adult. Systemic disease can be progressive and may require chemotherapy.

4.12 Clinical Course

Prognosis is excellent with a very low rate of recurrence and little complications when the disease is confined to the skeleton, especially when it is a solitary lesion. The majority of such lesions would be spontaneously resolved by fibrosis and ossification within 1–2 years (Figs. 4.1 and 4.2). Vertebra plana can be spontaneously healed, and the height is partially to near totally recovered with growth in immature children (Fig. 4.5).

References

1. Tran G, Huynh TN, Paller AS. Langerhans cell histiocytosis: a neoplastic disorder driven by Ras-ERK pathway mutations. J Am Acad Dermatol. 2018;78(3):579–90.e4.
2. Berres ML, Merad M, Allen CE. Progress in understanding the pathogenesis of Langerhans cell histiocytosis: back to Histiocytosis X? Br J Haematol. 2015;169(1):3–13.
3. David R, Oria RA, Kumar R, Singleton EB, Lindell MM, Shirkhoda A, et al. Radiologic features of eosinophilic granuloma of bone. Am J Roentgenol. 1989;153(5):1021–6.
4. Mirra JM. Eosinophilic granuloma. In: Mirra JM, editor. Bone tumors: clinical, radiologic, and pathologic correlation. 2nd ed. Philadelphia: Lea & Febiger; 1989. p. 1023–60.
5. Stull M, Kransdorf M, Devaney K. Langerhans cell histiocytosis of bone. Radiographics. 1992;12(4):801–23.
6. Ewton A. Hematopoietic tumors. In: Dorfman HD, Czerniak B, editors. Dorfman and Czerniak's bone tumors. 2nd ed. Amsterdam: Elsevier; 2016. p. 817–902. (eBook).
7. Huvos AG. Bone tumors. 2nd ed. Philadelphia: Saunders; 1991. p. 695–771.
8. Kilpatrick SE, Wenger DE, Gilchrist GS, Shives TC, Wollan PC, Unni KK. Langerhans' cell histiocytosis (histiocytosis X) of bone a clinicopathologic analysis of 263 pediatric and adult cases. Cancer. 1995;76(12):2471–84.
9. Mickelson MR, Bonfiglio M. Eosinophilic granuloma and its variations. Orthop Clin North Am. 1977;8:933–45.
10. Resnick D, Kransdorf MJ. Langerhans cell histiocytosis. In: Resnick D, Kransdorf MJ, editors. Bone and joint imaging. 3rd ed. Philadelphia: Elsevier Saunders; 2005. p. 674–9.
11. Jennin F, Bousson V, Parlier C, Jomaah N, Khanine V, Laredo J-D. Bony sequestrum: a radiologic review. Skelet Radiol. 2011;40(8):963–75.
12. Sholkoff SD, Mainzer F. Button sequestrum revisited. Radiology. 1971;100(3):649–52.
13. Wells PO. The button sequestrum of eosinophilic granuloma of the skull. Radiology. 1956;67(5):746–7.
14. Krasnokutsky MV. The button sequestrum sign. Radiology. 2005;236(3):1026–7.
15. Rosen IW, Nadel HI. Button sequestrum of the skull. Radiology. 1969;92(5):969–71.
16. Helms CA, Jeffrey RB, Wing VW. Computed tomography and plain film appearance of a bony sequestration: significance and differential diagnosis. Skelet Radiol. 1987;16(2):117–20.
17. Kaplan PA, Helms CA, Dussault R, Anderson MW, Major NM. Foot and ankle. In: Kaplan PA, Helms CA, Dussault R, Anderson MW, Major NM, editors. Musculoskeletal MRI. Philadelphia: Saunders; 2001. p. 424.
18. Scaglietti O, Marchetti P, Bartolozzi P. Final results obtained in the treatment of bone cysts with methylprednisolone acetate (depo-medrol) and a discussion of results achieved in other bone lesions. Clin Orthop Relat Res. 1982;165:33–42.
19. Corby RR, Stacy GS, Peabody TD, Dixon LB. Radiofrequency ablation of solitary eosinophilic granuloma of bone. Am J Roentgenol. 2008;190(6):1492–4.

5 Plasma Cell Myeloma/Multiple Myeloma

(***multiplex*** "multiple" + ***myelos*** "marrow" + ***ōma*** "forming")

5.1 Definition

Plasma cells are a type of white blood cells derived from mature B-lymphocytes in the bone marrow, which play an important role in protecting the body against infection and disease by producing immunoglobulins, also known as antibodies, consisting of two heavy chains and two light chains. *Heavy chains* consist of IgG, IgA, IgM, IgD, and IgE, and two types of *light chain* are termed as kappa and lambda. Myeloma can be presented by combination of the type of heavy and light chains: IgG kappa, IgG lambda, IgA kappa, or IgA lambda. Plasma cell neoplasms can be differentiated to two different forms of plasma cell: myeloma (PCM)/multiple myeloma (MM) and solitary plasmacytoma. PCM is a multifocal, monoclonal neoplastic proliferation of plasma cells in the bone marrow producing abnormal immunoglobulin, so-called myeloma protein (M-protein) or paraprotein, which can also damage extraskeletal multiple organs.

5.2 Synonym

Myelomatosis/Kahler disease; no more used.

5.3 Incidence

PCM is the most common primary malignant bone tumor in adults, accounting for about 1–2% of all malignant neoplasms, more than 10% of all hematologic malignancies, and 15% of the malignant bone tumors [1–4].

5.4 Age

Majority (more than 90%) of the patients are older than 40 years of age with a peak age between seventh and eighth decades of life [2]. The risk of developing PCM is gradually increased as people become older. However, the incidence rate has been increased in younger age of 25–49 years by an analysis of a population-based state registry in the United States from 1995 to 2014 [5].

5.5 Location

Any bone containing red marrow in the adult can be affected, but the axial skeleton is involved more frequently than the appendicular skeleton. The skull, vertebral bodies, ribs, pelvis, clavicle,

W.-J. Bahk, *Diagnosis and Management of Primary Bone Tumors*,
https://doi.org/10.1007/978-981-99-5498-8_5

scapula, and long bones above elbow or knee corresponding to the predominant hematopoietic marrow are most commonly affected. In the long bone, the lesion is usually in the metaphysis and diaphysis but rarely in the epiphysis. Thoracic spines are more frequently involved than cervical or lumbar spines, and the lesion primarily affects body of the spines.

5.6 Clinical Features and Diagnostic Analysis

Diagnostic analysis for plasma-cell disorders includes clinical features, physical examination, bone lesion and/or bone marrow biopsy, laboratory studies including blood chemistry and complete blood count, immunoelectrophoresis (IEP)/immunofixation electrophoresis (IFE), evaluation of the urine for M protein, and imaging studies. A monoclonal gammopathy of undetermined significance (MGUS) or monoclonal gammopathy, unattributed/unassociated (MG[u]), is typified by serum M-protein concentration of <30 g/L and lesser than 10% plasma cells in the bone marrow with no evidence of PCM, other B-cell proliferative disorders, or amyloidosis [6]. In a large series, cumulative probability of progression to PCM, primary systemic amyloidosis, or other related plasma-cell proliferative disorders was 10% at 10 years, 21% at 20 years, and 26% at 25 years with overall progression risk of approximately 1% per year [7]. PCM/MM can be subclassified to asymptomatic and symptomatic form. *"Smoldering"* myeloma is an asymptomatic plasma-cell proliferative disorder associated with a high risk of progression to symptomatic PCM. It is characterized by serum M-protein level over 30 g/L or more than 10% plasma cells in the bone marrow without anemia, hypercalcemia, renal insufficiency, and skeletal lesions [6, 8]. A large series reported that the risk of progression to symptomatic form of PCM was 10% per year for the first 5 years, 5% per year for the next 3 years, and then 1–2% per year for the next 5 years [9]. Some patients remain free of progression for several years. *"(Symptomatic) PCM"* can be diagnosed when there are serum M-protein greater than 3 g/dL and more than 10% clonal plasma cells in the bone marrow with symptoms related to end organ damage, so-called "CRAB" (increased **C**alcemia, **R**enal insufficiency, **A**nemia, **B**one pain) [10]. The patients usually present with a triad of (1) clinical symptoms of bone pain produced by multifocal osteolysis, (2) microscopic findings of proliferation of atypical plasma cells, and (3) monoclonal gammopathy on IEP. The abnormal clone of plasma cells proliferates in the bone marrow and frequently invades the adjacent bone, producing extensive skeletal destruction. The patients may present various clinical presentations including bone problems of multifocal bone pain frequent with pathologic fracture (Figs. 5.1, 5.2, 5.3 and 5.4), spinal cord compression causing radiating pain, severe muscle weakness or paralysis, and a history of frequent infection such as pneumonia due to reduced immunity. General weakness or weight loss is often associated initially or during the disease. Laboratory findings include anemia, hypercalcemia, reverse A/G ratio (low albumin and high globulin), proteinuria, and Bence-Jones proteinuria. Proteinuria is noted in most patients (about 90%), but Bence-Jones proteinuria is identified in half of the patients [4, 11]. Renal insufficiency can be resulted by higher calcium levels in the blood related to bone destruction, and amyloidosis may be accompanied by M-proteins. IEP shows dominant monoclonal component spikes and decreased normal polyclonal immunoglobulins due to the suppression of the benign polyclonal populations of normal plasma cells by the expending clones of myeloma cells. Systemic amyloidosis can be associated at presentation or sometime during the course of the myeloma in 7–15% of the patients [4, 12]. The cause of the myeloma is unclear. Exposure to radiation, herbicides, insecticides, benzene, petroleum products, engine gasoline, and diesel exhaust was suggested possibly to play a role [9]. Very rarely, PCM may be associated with ***p***olyneuropathy, ***o***rganomegaly, ***e***ndocrinopathy, ***m***onoclonal gammopathy, and ***s***kin changes, so-called *"POEMS"* syndrome (Fig. 5.5). Initial presentation can be tingling sense of the extremities, muscle weakness, and gait disturbance in the setting of the syndrome. Recently, Dispenzieri [13] suggested diagnostic criteria based on a composite of clinical and laboratory findings and mandatory major criteria of typical demyelinating polyneuropathy and monoclonal plasma cell proliferative disorder (almost always λ), at least one of other three major criteria including Castleman disease, sclerotic bone lesions and increased levels of vascular endothelial growth factor (VEGF), and minor criteria including organomegaly (splenomegaly, hepatomegaly, lymphadenopathy), extravascular volume over-

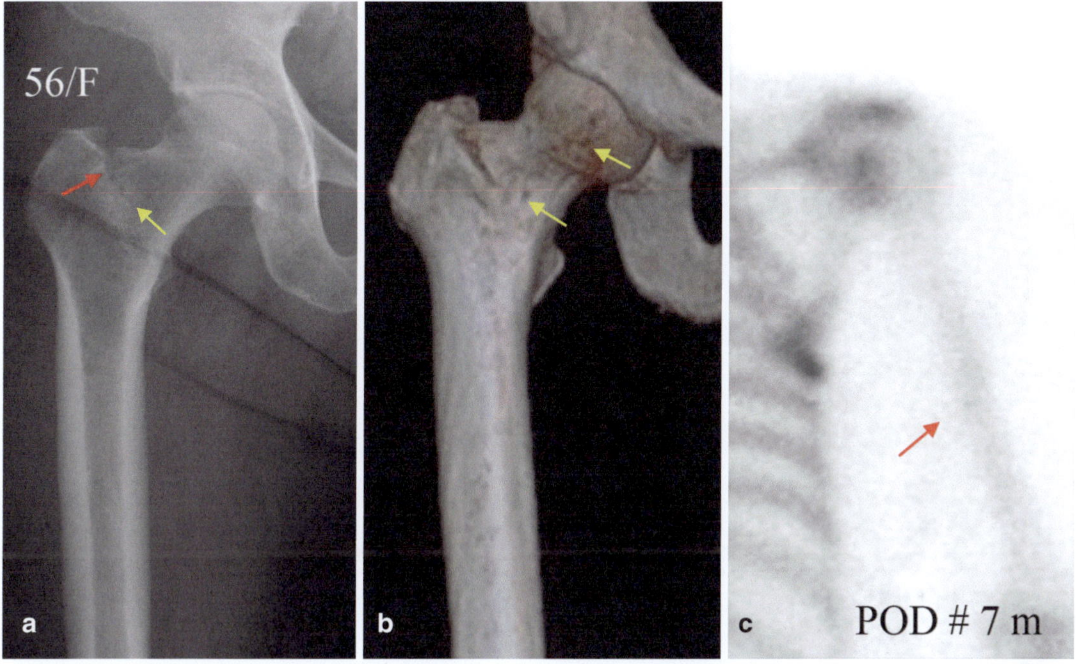

Fig. 5.1 ***Pathologic fracture with initially unrecognized PCM*** (**a**) Radiograph taken for right hip pain after slip on ice in 56-year-old woman shows an incomplete fracture at base of femoral neck (red arrow). There are a few indiscernible tiny holes (yellow arrows), which were not recognized at that time by the initial hip surgeon. (**b**) 3D CT scan clearly reveals the incomplete fracture line with a few tiny holes (yellow arrows), which were also not recognized. (**c**) Bone scan taken for early detection of avascular necrosis of femoral head at 7 months after surgery shows mild uptake in the fracture site and multiple ribs suggesting multiple rib fracture by slip. However, there is incidentally found subtle to no abnormal uptake in left humerus (red arrow). (**d**) Follow-up radiograph at 10 months after cannulated screw fixation notes radiologic union of fracture and clearer variable-sized numerous hole-like lesions (yellow arrows) with endosteal scalloping (white arrow) in the femur shaft. (**e**) Follow-up radiograph at 17 months after surgery shows more definite cortical infiltration (yellow arrow) and deeper erosion (white arrow). (**f**) Follow-up bone scan taken for multiple bone pain at 17-month surgery reveals more clearly increased uptake in the left humerus (red arrow) as well as additional other ribs and right ilium. (**g**) Radiograph shows numerous, variable-sized *"punched-out"* lesions in the left entire humerus with angulation and visible callus indicating old fracture (yellow arrow). Radiograph of contralateral right humerus also reveals similar lesion but no fracture. These features may suggest a probable progression of asymptomatic myeloma to disseminated symptomatic PCM. (**h**) Serum IEP reveals a prominent monoclonal band in the gamma globulin region with high concentration of M-protein (3.5 g/dL), and IFE indicates a monoclonal gammopathy of IgG/kappa isotype. Urine IEP reveals a faint monoclonal band in the gamma region, and IFE indicates Bence-Jones protein of kappa type. Microscopic examination shows plasma cell replacement of bone marrow suggesting PCM. On bone marrow examination, mature and immature plasma cells are increased in number up to 40% of all nucleated elements. (**i**) Follow-up radiograph at 4 months after surgery shows radiologic union of pathologic fracture with callus (arrow). She was transferred to department of hematology for BMT

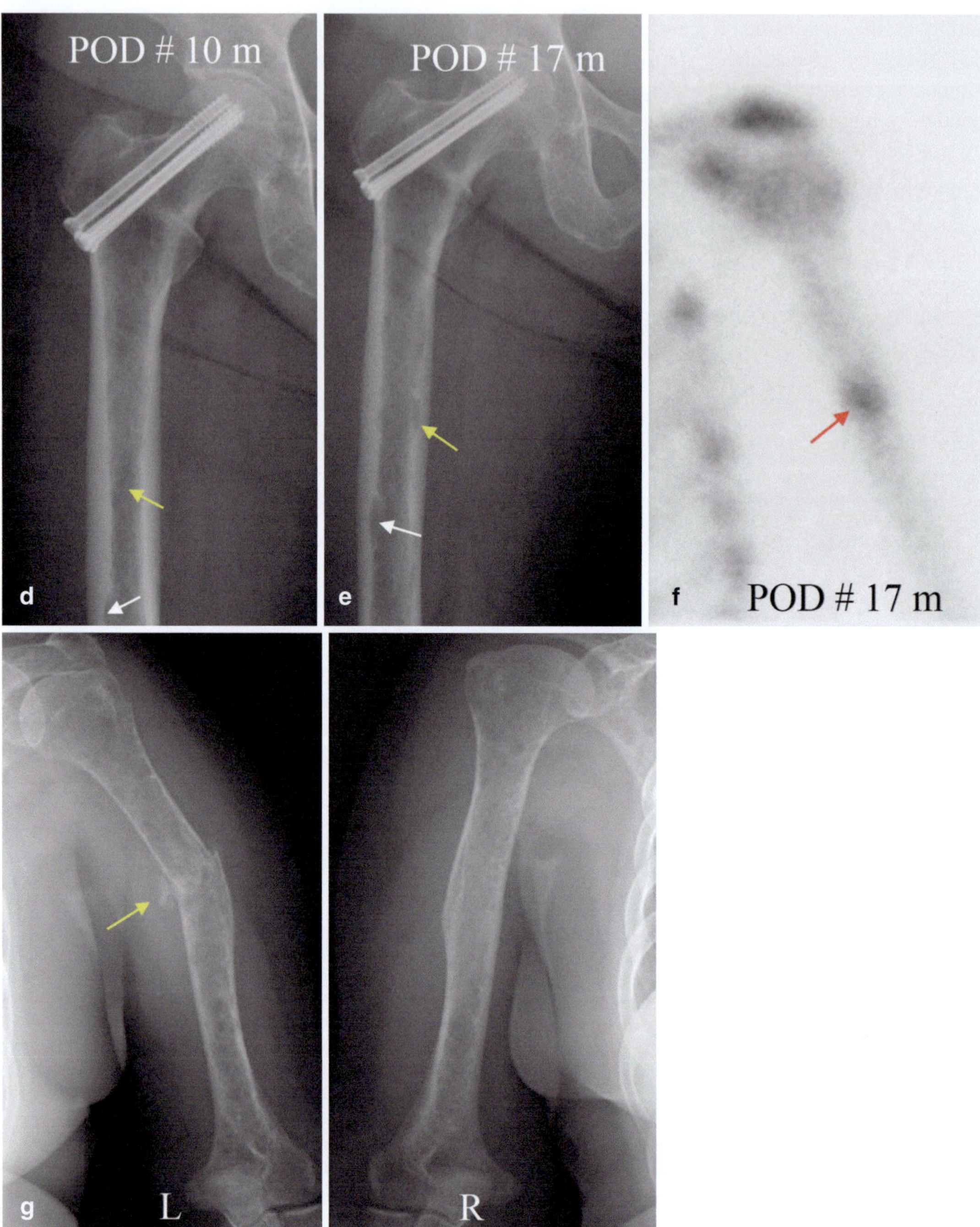

Fig. 5.1 (continued)

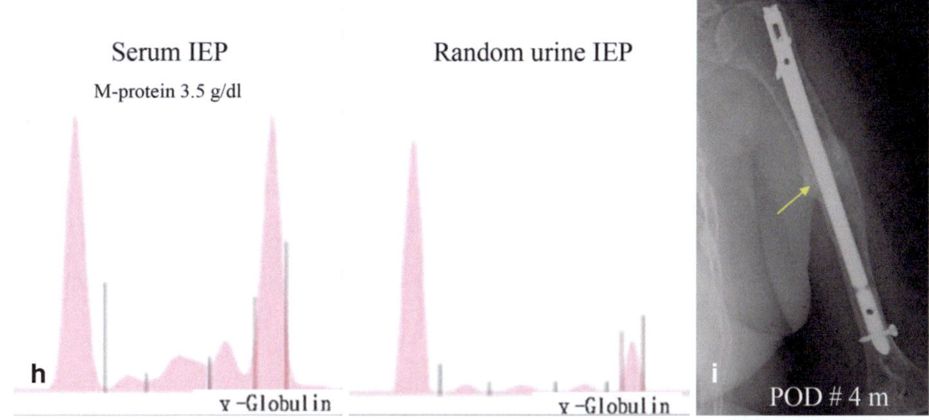

Fig. 5.1 (continued)

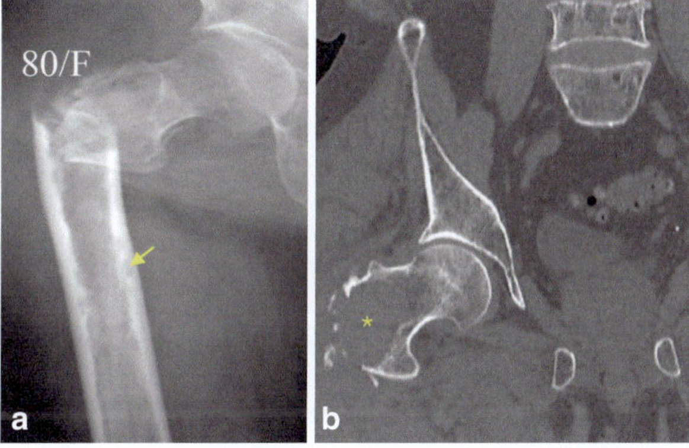

Fig. 5.2 ***Initially unrecognized PCM***. (**a**) Radiograph taken for right hip pain by fall from a bed in 80-year-old woman shows intertrochanteric fracture with significant angulation of right femur. Note pre-exisitng lesion with irregular endosteal scalloping as well as intramedullary and intracortical multiple small radiolucent holes (yellow arrow), suggesting a pathologic fracture. (**b**) CT scan reveals an intramedullary geographic destruction with cortical scalloping in the fracture area (asterisk). There are other additional lesions with multiple tiny holes in intertrochanteric and neck areas as well as pelvic bone and vertebral bodies. (**c**) MR images demonstrate a space-occupying lesion with low SI on T1-weighted image and intermediate and focal high SI on T2-weighted image. The lesion is peripherally enhanced with focal internal enhancement (arrow). (**d**) Retrospective review of scanogram taken for total knee replacement 3 months before fracture notes a geographic destruction with endosteal scalloping in the trochanteric area of right femur (circle), which was not recognized by the knee surgeon. Magnification view shows a clearly visible geographic destruction in the trochanteric area (asterisk) and endosteal scalloping in the shaft (yellow arrow), definitely indicating a pre-existing aggressive tumor. (**e**) Bone scan shows multiple increased uptake in the sternum, ribs, T5 vertebra, right proximal femur, and left ischial tuberosity, suggesting a multi-focal bone tumor. (**f**) PET/CT scan demonstrates multiple hypermetabolic lesions in the trochanteric area of right femur (SUVmax 20.1), left sphenoid sinus (SUVmax 18.8), and other multiple bones. Right destroyed lung with mediastinal shifting (blue arrow) is due to previous lung lobectomy for tuberculosis. (**g**) Serum IEP shows a prominent monoclonal band in the gamma globulin region with a low concentration of M-protein (0.8 g/dL), and IFE indicates a monoclonal gammopathy of IgG/kappa isotype. Urine IEP reveals a monoclonal band in the gamma region, and IFE indicates Bence-Jones protein of kappa type. (**h**) Wide resection followed by reconstruction with tumor prosthesis was done. (**i**) Microscopic examination of resected femur specimen shows both areas of myeloma and fracture callus. (a) Tumor lesion consisting of plasmatoid cells replaces the bone marrow space. (b) Higher-power magnification shows that tumoral plasma cells are varying from normal to pleomorphic looking. (c) Masses of myeloma cells (M) are infiltrating and replacing the normal bone marrow elements (BM). (d) Mature woven to lamellar bone spicules with prominent osteoblastic rimming are scattered with injury vessels in the bland fibrous stroma, suggesting a fracture callus with an estimated age of 2–3 weeks. Practically, surgical management was performed at 16 days after fracture. (e) Bone spicules in the femoral head are significantly thinned with normal bone marrow but no myeloma cells, indicating a significant osteoporotic change. (f) IHC stains for CD38 and CD 138, reliable marker for plasma cells, are positive

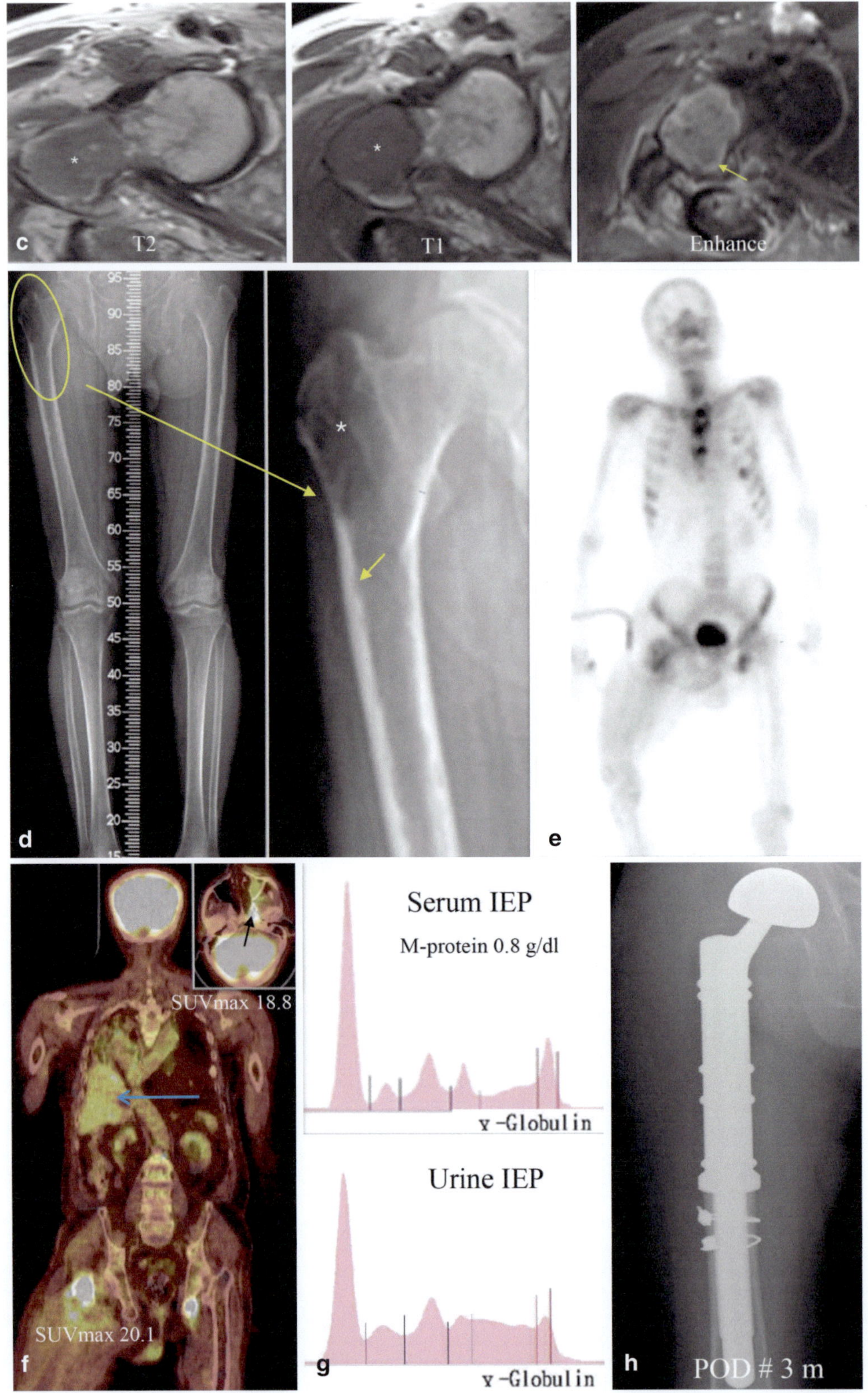

Fig. 5.2 (continued)

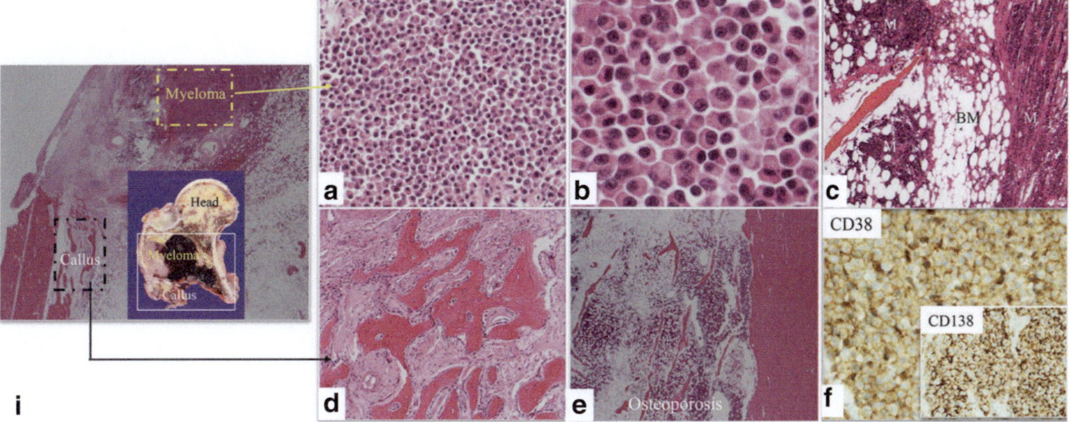

Fig. 5.2 (continued)

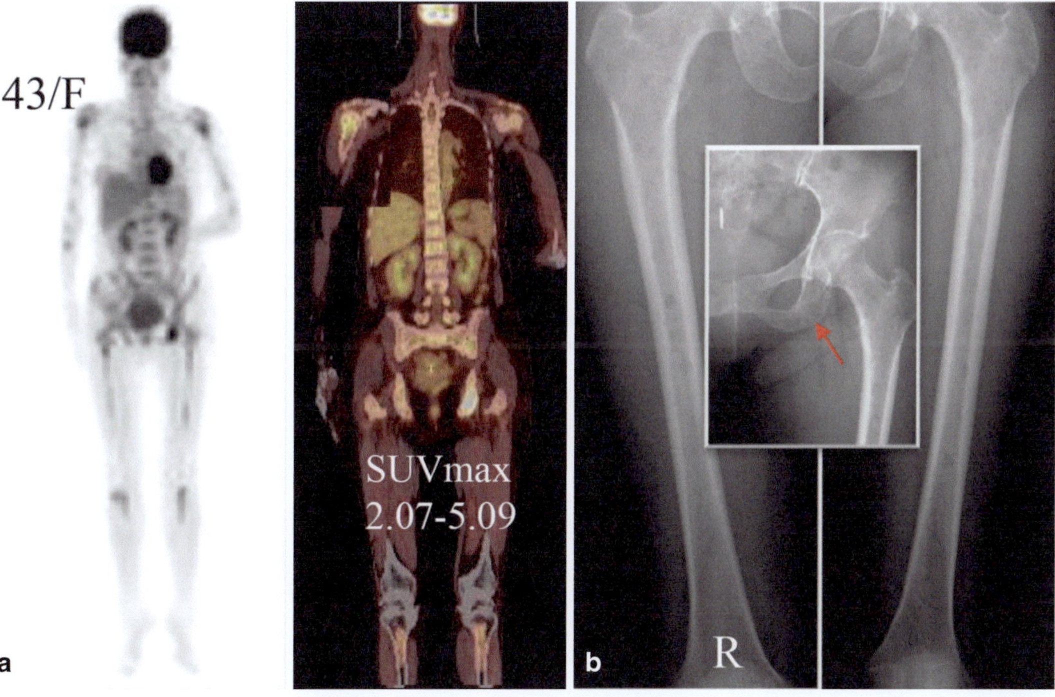

Fig. 5.3 (**a**) ***PCM incidentally found with multiple bone lesions*** (**a**) PET/CT scan taken for 4–5 kg weight loss and malaise of 3-month duration in 43-year-old woman incidentally shows multiple osteolytic bone lesions in both humerus, forearm bones, femur, and tibia as well as spines and pelvic bones, probably in the skull with varying degree of FDG uptake (SUVmax 2.07–5.09). However, there is no hypermetabolic activity in the ribs and sternum. (**b**) Corresponding radiographs reveal numerous varying sized *"punched-out"* lesions involving long bones of upper and lower extremities and skull vault. However, the spines show only diffuse osteopenia with no discernible lesions despite the increased FDG uptake (yellow circle). In addition, there are expansile bubbly osteolytic lesions involving left ischium (red arrow) and variable-sized geographic destructive lesions affecting left distal humerus and right proximal radius (yellow arrows). (**c**) Bone scan reveals increased uptake in right fibula head and shaft, left distal humerus, sternum, and both multiple ribs. Other bone lesions detected in PET/CT scan and radiographs show no abnormal uptake, but there are increased uptakes in both multiple ribs and along the sternum with internal cold uptake (inset), which were not detected on PET/CT scan. (**d**) CT scan images clearly show additional destructive lesions with expanded bone contour affecting sternoclavicular joints (red circle), sternal manubrium (yellow arrow), multiple ribs (white arrow), and vertebral bodies (red arrows). (**e**) The impending fractures of humerus and radius were managed with preventive nailing. Findings of bone marrow biopsy and urine/serum IEP confirmed a diagnosis of PCM. She was transferred to department of hematology for BMT.

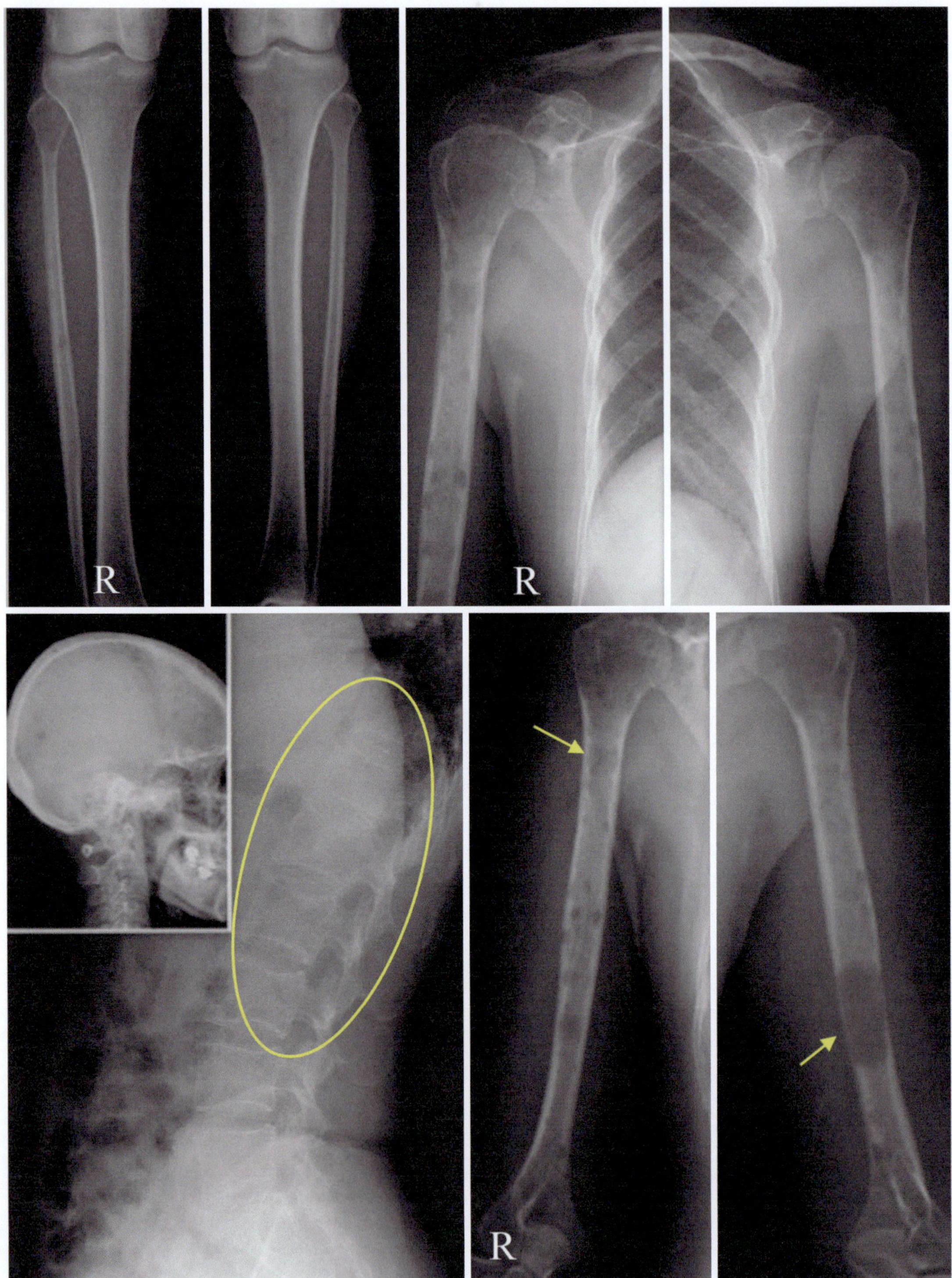

Fig. 5.3 (continued)

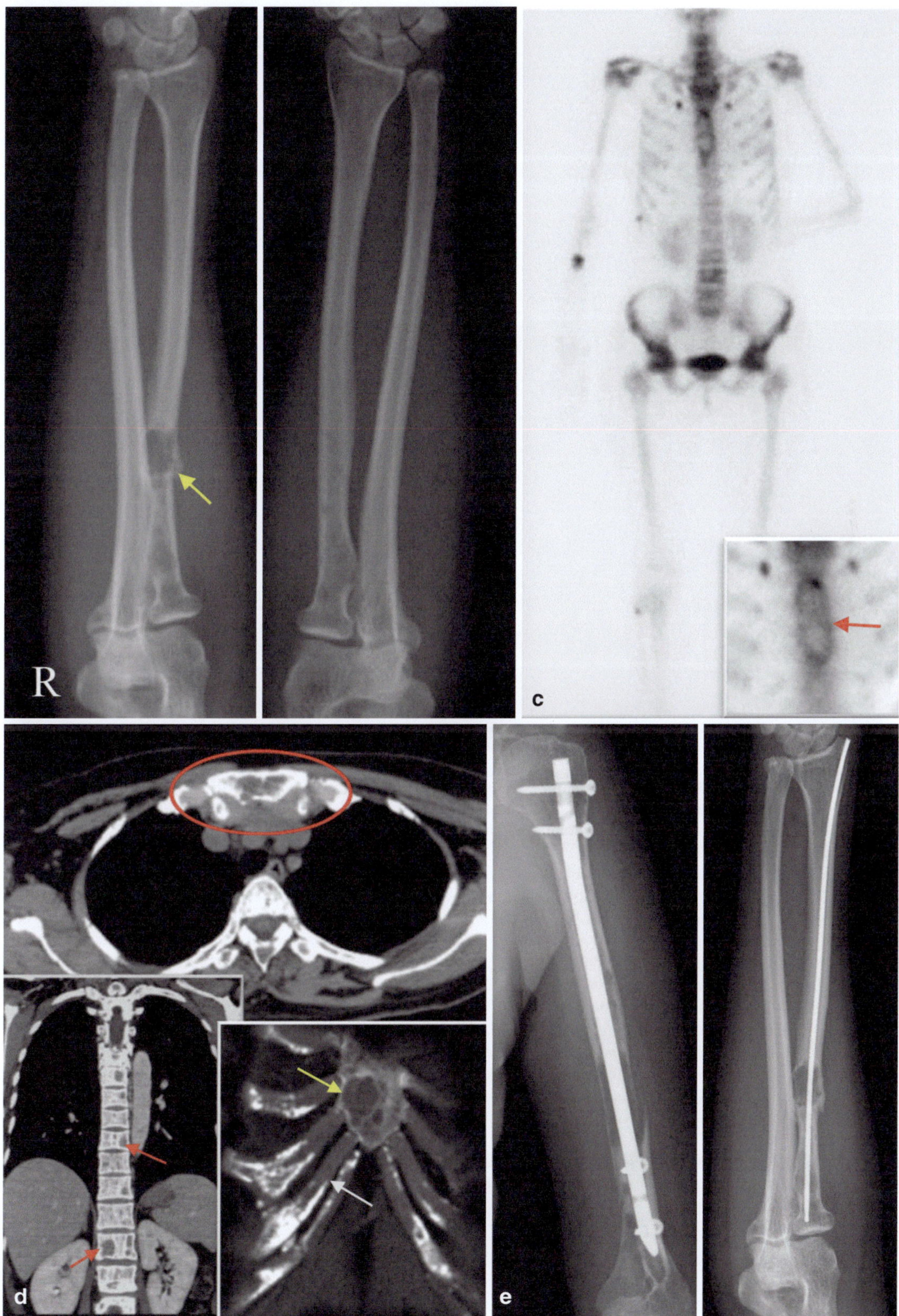

Fig. 5.3 (continued)

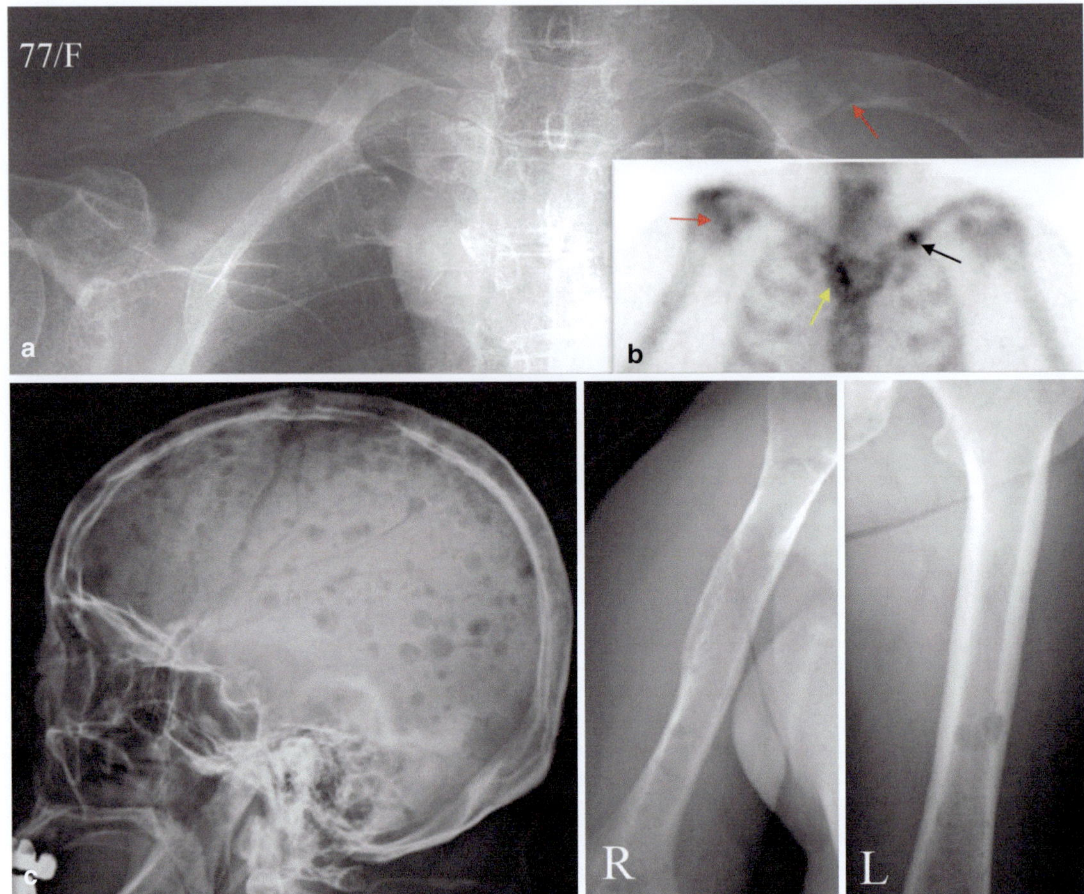

Fig. 5.4 (**a**) Radiograph taken for both clavicle pain of 1-month duration with aggravation of left clavicle pain for 3 days in 77-year-old woman shows multi-lobulated, bubbly, osteolytic lesions with expansion of the clavicle contour. Angulation with cortical breakage indicating pathologic fracture is seen in the left clavicle (red arrow). (**b**) Bone scan reveals no uptake in the clavicle lesions but focal hot uptake at fracture site (black arrow). In addition, there are moderate focal uptakes in the shoulder joint (red arrow) and sternal manubrium (yellow arrow). There are no clear uptakes in the long bones and the skull vault. (**c**) However, radiographs note typical multiple *"punch-out"* lesions in the skull and right humerus and left femur in which no uptake is seen on bone scan. (**d**) PET/CT scan demonstrates a focal high FDG uptake in the left fractured clavicle (SUVmax 6.28) as well as the sternum and right scapula (SUVmax 2.5–3.2). Extraskeletal FDG-avid lesion is not found. CT scans reveal destructive lesion with cortical breakage of corresponding bones (arrows). (**e**) Serum IEP shows a prominent monoclonal band in the gamma globulin region with a high concentration of M-protein (4.3 g/dL) (Top). IFE indicated a monoclonal gammopathy of IgG/lambda isotype. Urine IEP showed a prominent monoclonal band in the gamma region and Bence-Jones proteinuria of lambda type. Bone marrow biopsy showed that mature and immature plasma cells were increased in number up to 10% of all nucleated elements. Microscopic examination of resected left clavicle for pain control showed diffuse monotonous plasma cells consistent with PCM. The serum level of M-protein has been significantly decreased to zero with chemotherapy (Bottom). (**f**) Four years later, radiograph taken for severe pain of right shoulder shows a pathologic fracture in the proximal humerus (arrow). (**g**) Follow-up radiograph at 3 months after intramedullary nailing shows radiologic union with abundant callus formation (red arrow). However, she was transferred for hospice care due to rapid progression of disease with severe general weakness

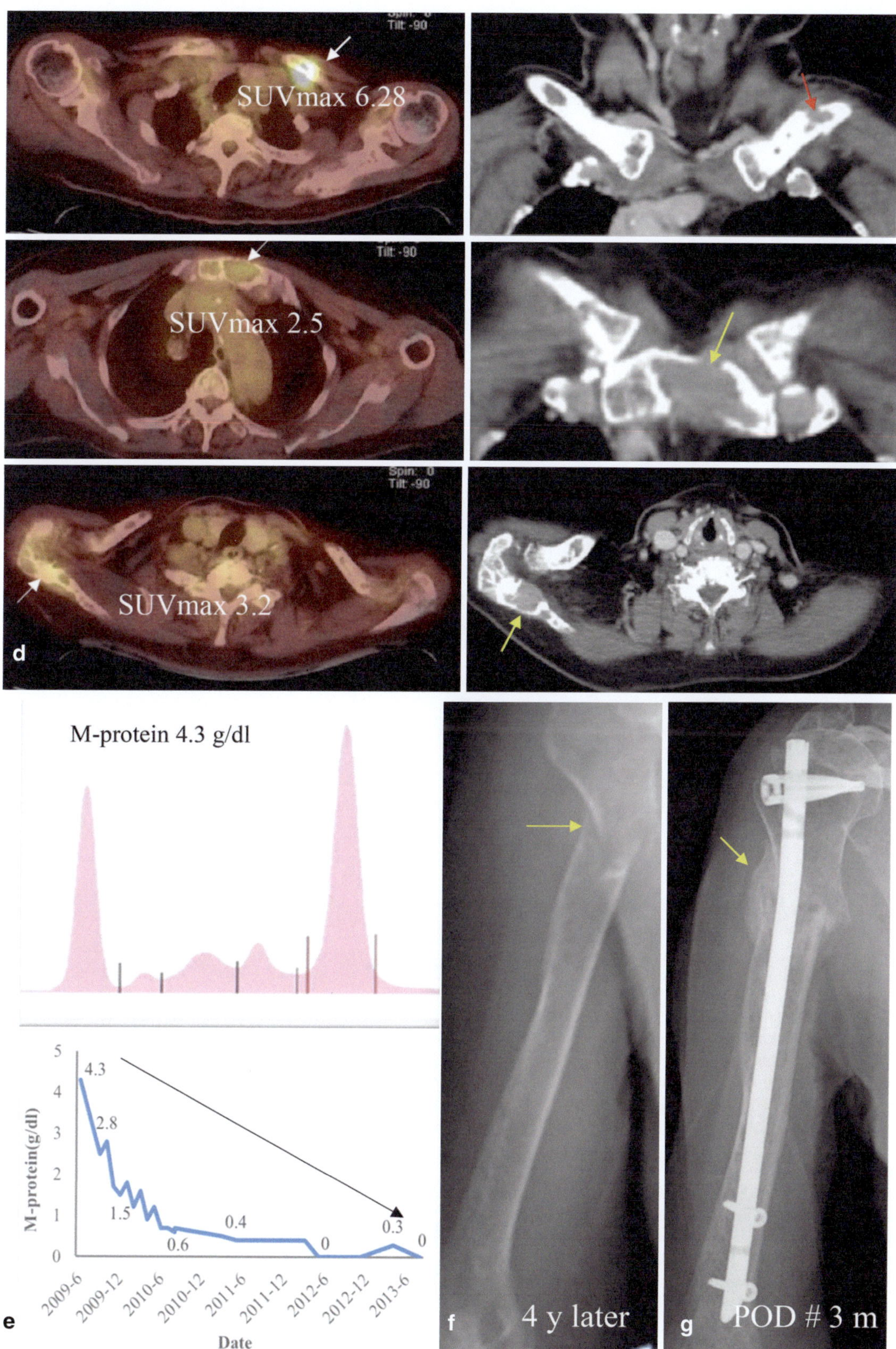

Fig. 5.4 (continued)

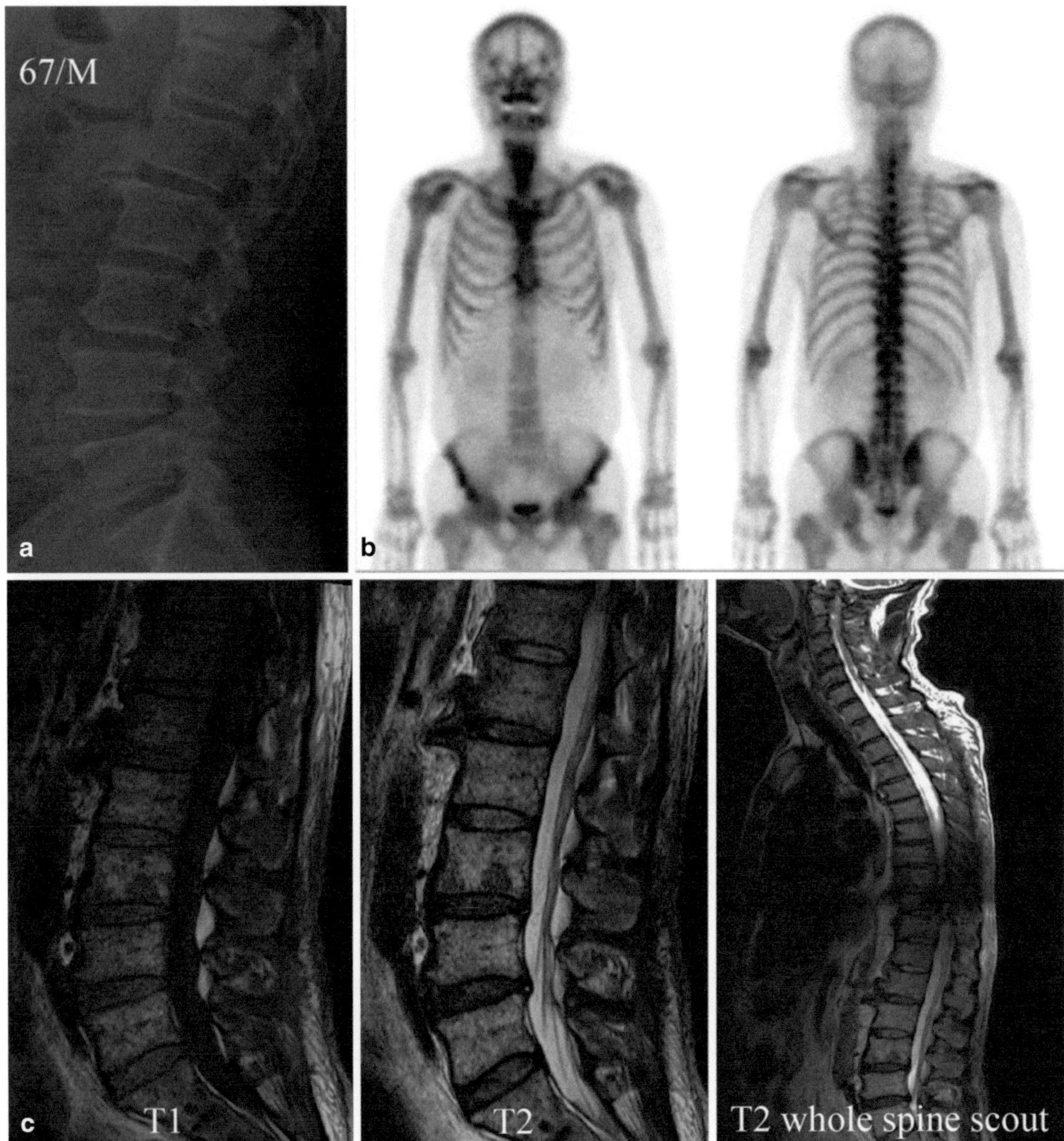

Fig. 5.5 ***POEMS syndrome*** (**a**) Radiograph taken for generalized weakness and tingling sense of both legs with walking disturbance as well as abnormal posture of back of 4-month duration in 67-year-old man shows only diffuse mild osteopenia but no definite marrow lesion. (**b**) However, bone scan reveals diffusely increased uptake in sternum and multiple vertebral bodies, suggesting a possible infiltrative hematologic disease. (**c**) MR images demonstrate numerous variable-sized bone marrow replacing lesion with low to intermediate SI on both T1- and T2-weighted images in all lumbar spines. T2-weighted whole spine scout image also notes similar bone marrow replacing lesions in almost entire vertebral bodies, suggesting a probable marrow infiltrating disease. A diagnosis of *"POEMS"* was confirmed by the presence of both *"mandatory major criteria"* of the presence of a monoclonal plasma cell disorder and peripheral polyneuropathy by EMG, one of *"other three major criteria"* including increased serum level VEGF. Two of *"six minor criteria"* including angiofollicular lymphadenopathy and thrombocytopenia. Bone marrow biopsy showed low cellular bone marrow with significant plasmatoid cell proliferation presenting 20% of all nucleated elements. Serum and urine IEP revealed abnormal bi-clonal peaks expression of IgGλ and IgAλ indicating monoclonal gammopathy of IgG/lambda isotype. Peripheral sensorimotor polyneuropathy was confirmed by EMG. He had multiple lymphadenopathies, and serum VEGF was markedly increased up to 1720 pg/mL (normal 0–115 pg/mL). Among minor criteria, only thrombocytosis was present. Autologous BMT was performed. He is doing well with recovery of muscle power as well as gaining of near normal gait and back posture at 15 months after BMT

load (edema, pleural effusion, ascites), skin changes, endocrinopathy, thrombocytosis/polycythemia, and papilledema. The diagnosis may be missed if the entity of *"POEMS"* syndrome is not aware.

5.7 Radiologic Findings

Because PCM is usually multifocal and potentially affects every skeletal segment, whole-body imaging study including whole spines, skull, chest, pelvis, and long bones including humerus and femur as well as any symptomatic areas is required for evaluation of disease extension. Conventional radiographs still remain the gold standard approach for evaluation of bone involvement at diagnosis [14]. They can identify skeletal involvement in about 80% of the patients with advanced destruction affecting a minimum of 30–50% of the trabecular bone [15–17]. However, 12–25% of patients do not present discernible foci of bone destruction [4] (Fig. 5.6a). Thus, other imaging tools including bone scan, CT scan, MRI, and PET/CT scan are necessary to detect the lesions which are not seen on radiographs in the rest of patients (Fig. 5.6). But loss of much smaller amount can be readily detected as shallow endosteal scallops if the cortical bone is affected [18]. The radiological evidence of skeletal involvement can appear in four different appearances including 1) solitary deposit (plasmacytoma), 2) diffuse skeletal involvement (myelomatosis), 3) sclerosing, and 4) only osteopenia to osteoporosis [16]. The lesion is typified by multiple, well-defined, predominantly lytic or mixed lytic and blastic, round to oval, *"punched-out"* holes with endosteal scalloping when abutting the cortex. The hole lesion may exhibit variable size of destruction from tiny moth-eaten or permeative to large geographic or mixed pattern (Figs. 5.1, 5.2, 5.3, 5.4 and 5.7). There is no sclerotic halo due to low osteoblastic activity, which can be reflected frequent negative finding on bone scan despite the extensive bone destruction. Some other cases may reveal purely lytic appearance with trabeculated, reticulated, or soap bubble pattern. Erosion of cortex is often observed, but prominent periosteal new bone formation is rare. Impending or pathologic fracture of long bone or spinal compression fracture is frequently accompanied. When involving bones with a small caliber such as ribs and clavicles, the lesion can expand the bone contour (Fig. 5.4a). Only generalized osteopenia, or osteoporosis simulating aging process, particularly of spine, can be seen without discernible foci of bone destruction at presentation in about 15–20% of the patients [16, 19] (Fig. 5.5a). The osteopenia is often associated with collapse of vertebral bodies or vertebra plana. Rarely, the lesion may appear sclerotic and can be confused with osteopetrosis or osteoblastic metastasis if it is generalized. The rare multiple sclerotic lesions are usually in the setting of *"POEMS"* syndrome. **18F-FDG PET/CT scan** is a modality of choice in various phases of PCM with a high sensitivity and specificity both in the evaluation of bone marrow and extramedullary disease, ranging from 80% to 100% [20–22]. Increased uptake of FDG by the myeloma lesion corresponds to lytic bone lesion or soft tissue mass lesion seen on CT scan. It is also useful in differentiation between new active disease and treated inactive lesions to be the best tool for evaluating treatment response. However, it may fail to find some lesions in sternum or ribs (Fig. 5.3a) and other bones as well (Fig. 5.7c), which is detected on bone scan. In addition, FDG has some limitations, which are related to the physiological uptake in the bone marrow and brain to reduce its effectiveness. Several alternative PET tracers have been studied to improve the limitations [23]. A study on 46 patients by Zamagni and colleagues reported that PET/CT scans failed to show abnormal findings in of the spine and pelvis where MRI revealed a bone marrow involvement in 30% of patients. In contrast, the whole-body PET/CT scan detected the lesions located outside the MRI field of view in 35% of patients. They concluded PET/CT scan provides additional and valuable information for the assessment of PCM of bone in areas such as spine and pelvis not covered by MRI, with an accuracy up to 92% in both medullary and extramedullary

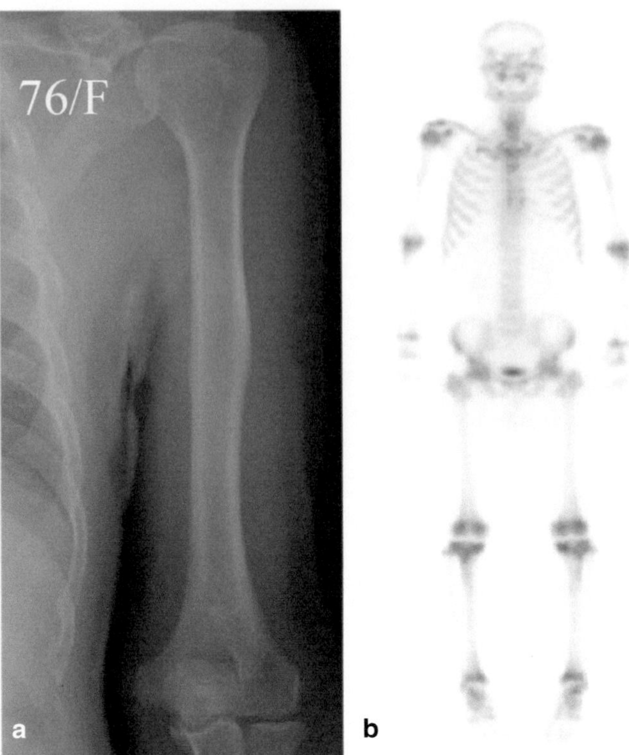

Fig. 5.6 (**a**) Radiograph taken for generalized ache with a particularly severe pain in left upper arm in 76-year-old man shows no definite abnormal bony abnormality. (**b**) Bone scan reveals also no remarkably abnormal uptake. (**c**) However, MR images demonstrate multiple well-defined numerous nodular lesions of varying size in the entire humerus shaft and glenoid of scapula with low SI on T1-weighted image and heterogeneous intermediate and high SI on fat saturated T2-weighted image. There are no definite cortical breakthrough and extracortical extension. Both lesions are heterogeneously enhanced (arrows). (**d**) PET/CT scan shows multiple hypermetabolic lesions in left humerus, C2, T10, L4 vertebral bodies, and left first rib. (**e**) CT scan reveals destructive lesions in the C2, T10, L4 vertebral bodies, left first rib, and left ilium (red arrows). (**f**) Serum IEP reveals a faint monoclonal band in the gamma globulin region with a high concentration of M-protein (3.1 g/dL), and IFE indicates a monoclonal gammopathy of IgG/kappa isotype. Urine IEP reveals a prominent monoclonal band in the beta region, and IFE indicates Bence-Jones protein of lambda type. Microscopic examination shows aggregation of numerous plasma cells admixed with some lymphocytes. Bone marrow biopsy shows mature and immature plasma cells, which are significantly increased in number up to 80% of all nucleated elements. He was transferred to department of hematology for BMT without surgical management

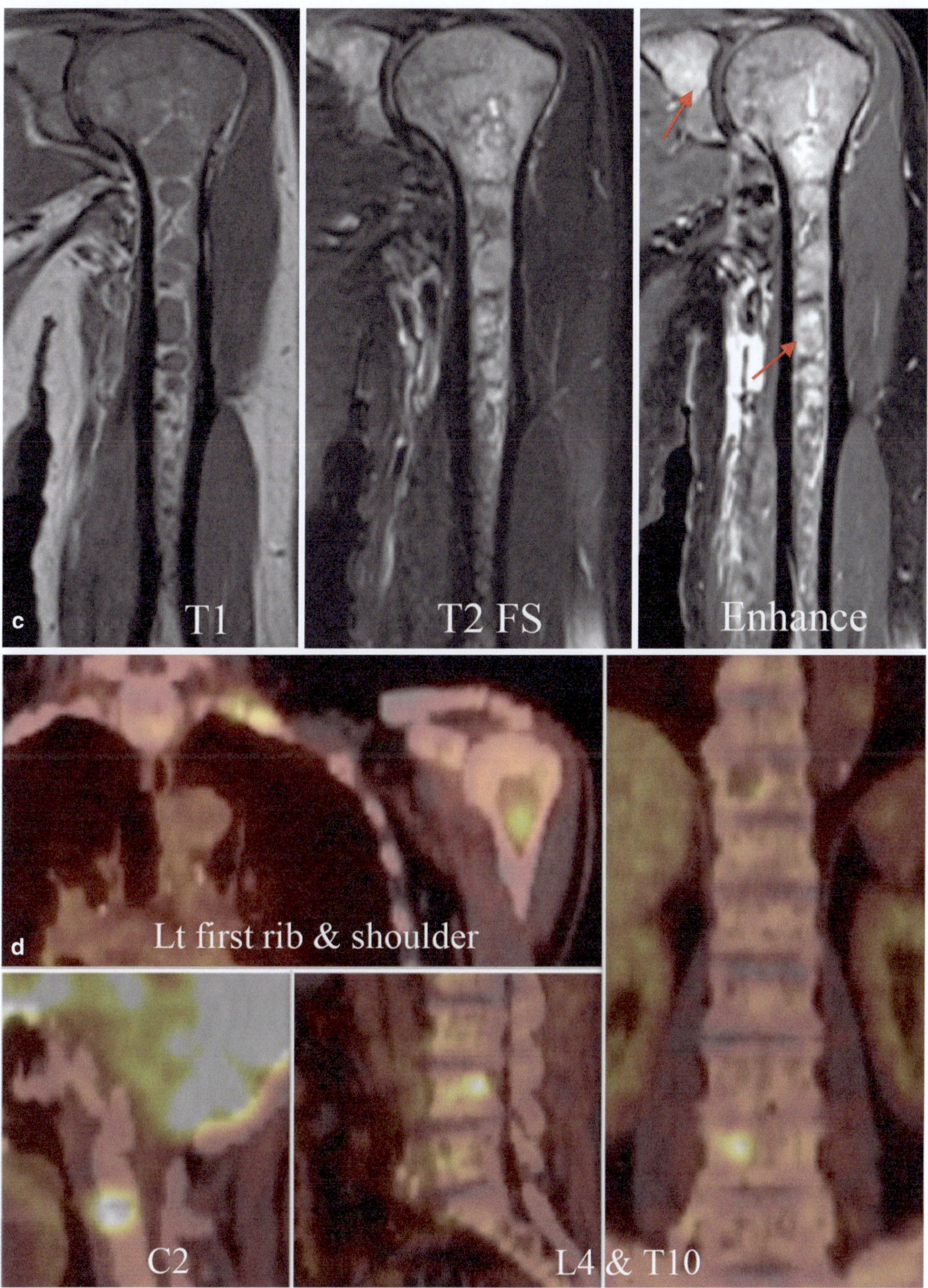

Fig. 5.6 (continued)

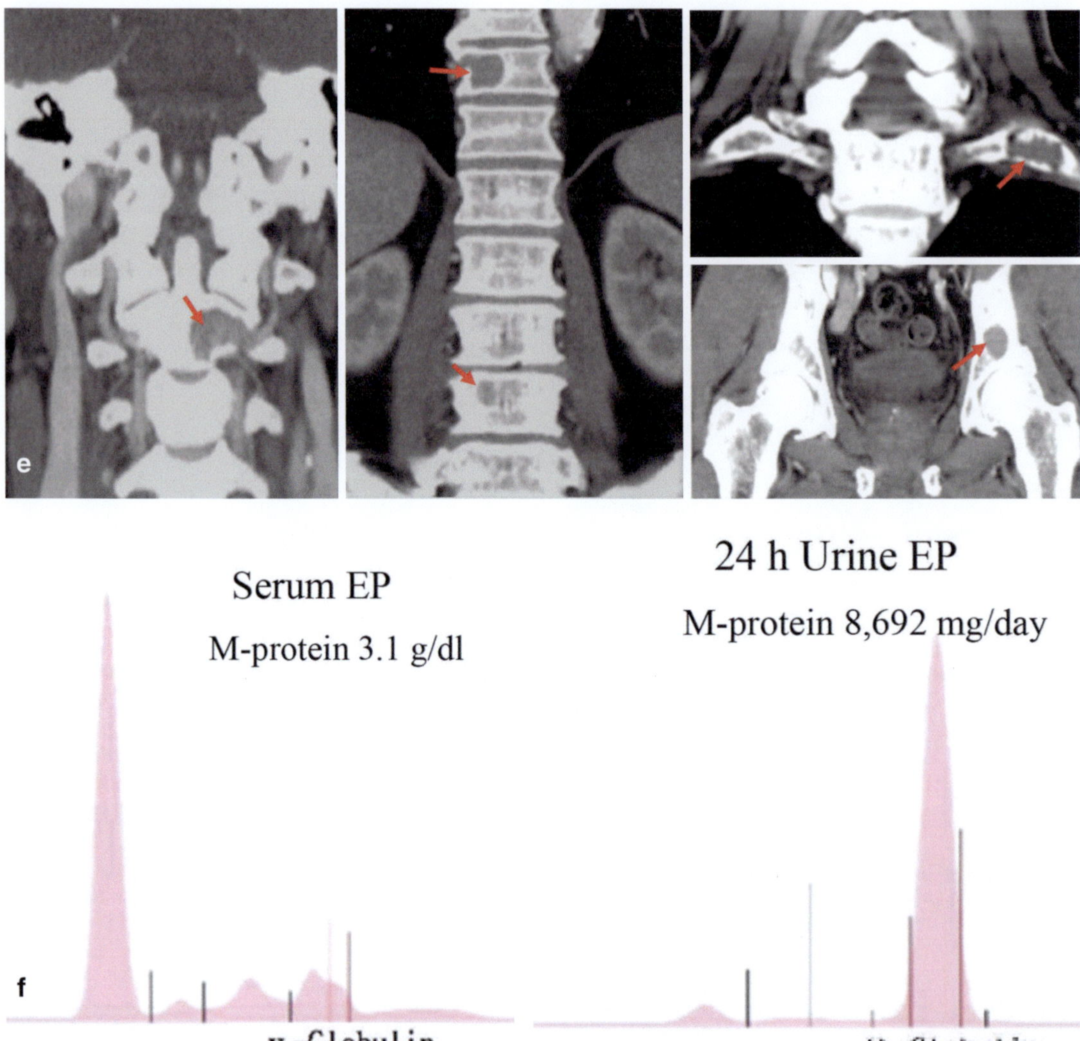

Fig. 5.6 (continued)

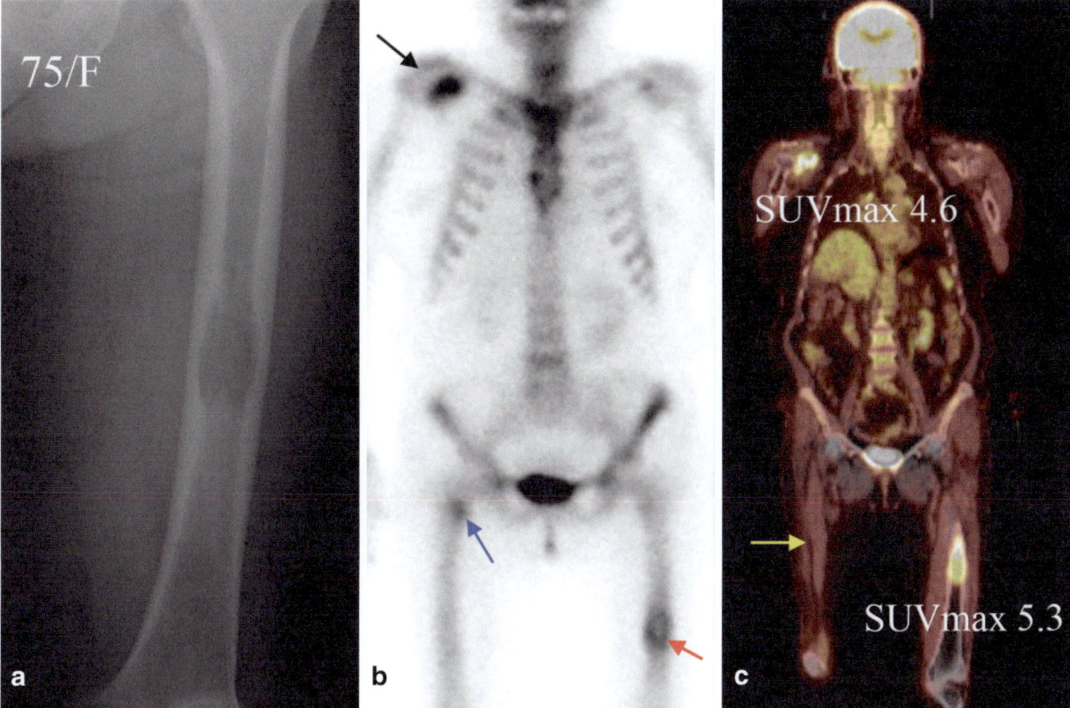

Fig. 5.7 (**a**) Radiograph taken for left thigh pain of several months duration in 75-year-old woman shows a geographic destruction and deep cortical erosion with a poorly defined margin in the mid-shaft of femur. (**b**) Bone scan reveals increased uptake with inner cold uptake in the left femoral shaft (red arrow) as well as stronger uptake of right scapular (black arrow) and milder focal uptake in the right proximal femur (blue arrow), suggesting multi-focal bone tumors. (**c**) PET/CT scan notes hypermetabolic activity in the left femoral shaft (SUVmax 5.3), right scapula (SUVmax 4.6) and milder activity in other multiple bones. However, there is no activity in right proximal femur (yellow arrow) in which focal uptake is seen on bone scan. (**d**) MR images demonstrate a well-defined intramedullary larger lesion eroding the lateral cortex and small to tiny multiple lesions (*combined focal and diffuse infiltration pattern*) with low SI on T1-weighted image and high SI with focal bright signals on fat saturated T2-weighted image. The lesions are well enhanced, and focal penetration through the entire thickness is clearly seen by contrast enhancement (arrow), heralding a impending fracture by trivial event. The well-enhanced small nodular lesions, which are seen proximally (circle), are not observed on other images including radiograph, bone scan, and PET/CT scan. (**e**) Immediate postoperative radiograph after prophylactic nailing notes a linear fracture lines, which may be produced by surgical procedure (arrows). PCM was confirmed by frozen biopsy during surgery, and postoperative chemotherapy was performed. (**f**) Radiograph of right femur with a focal uptake on bone scan shows no discernible lesion (inset). However, MRI reveals a large lesion in the trochanteric region and multiple small nodular lesions in the shaft of right proximal femur, with similar SI to the ipsilateral left femur lesion. (**g**) Additional shoulder MR images reveal multiple lesions with identical SIs observed in the proximal shaft of humerus as well as scapular glenoid and distal clavicle. (**h**) Follow-up radiograph at 3 years after surgery and chemotherapy shows complete healing of the lesion without local recurrence (yellow arrow). (**i**) Serum IEP shows a prominent monoclonal band in the gamma globulin region with a concentration of M-protein 2.0 g/dL, and IFE indicates a monoclonal gammopathy of IgG/kappa isotype. Urine IEP reveals a prominent monoclonal band in the gamma region, and IFE indicates Bence-Jones protein of kappa type. Microscopic examination shows a proliferation of dense plasmatoid cells. Bone marrow biopsy reveals that mature and immature plasma cells are increased in number to 25% of all nucleated elements. The serum level of M-protein has been significantly decreased to zero by chemotherapy but increased again 3 years after chemotherapy (Right). (**j**) MR images taken for newly developed back pain 2 years after chemotherapy demonstrate nodular lesions involving L2 and S3 vertebral body (yellow arrows) with low SI on T1-weighted image and intermediate SI on T2-weighted image. The lesions of L2 and S3 are well enhanced (arrows) suggesting extension of the PCM to the spines, but lesion-associated compression fracture in the L1 vertebral body is not enhanced suggesting (red arrows) suggesting severe osteoporosis being a probable cause of back pain. (**k**) The compression fracture was managed by vertebroplasty (red arrow), and back pain was improved. However, she suffered newly developed back pain, and MR images show another multiple spine metastasis 1 year later. She died of disease spread with increase of M-protein and aspiration pneumonia at 3 years after initial diagnosis of PCM

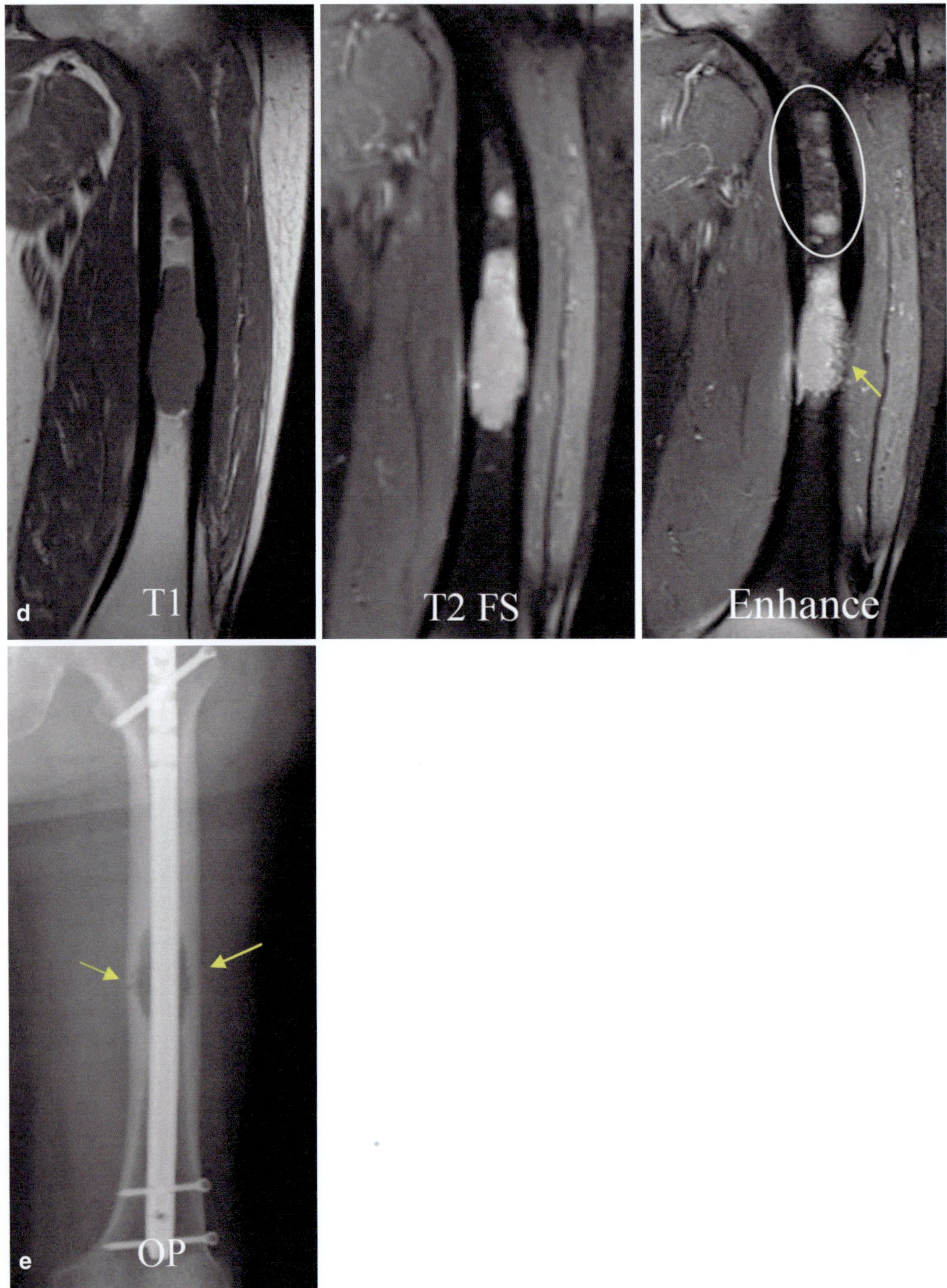

Fig. 5.7 (continued)

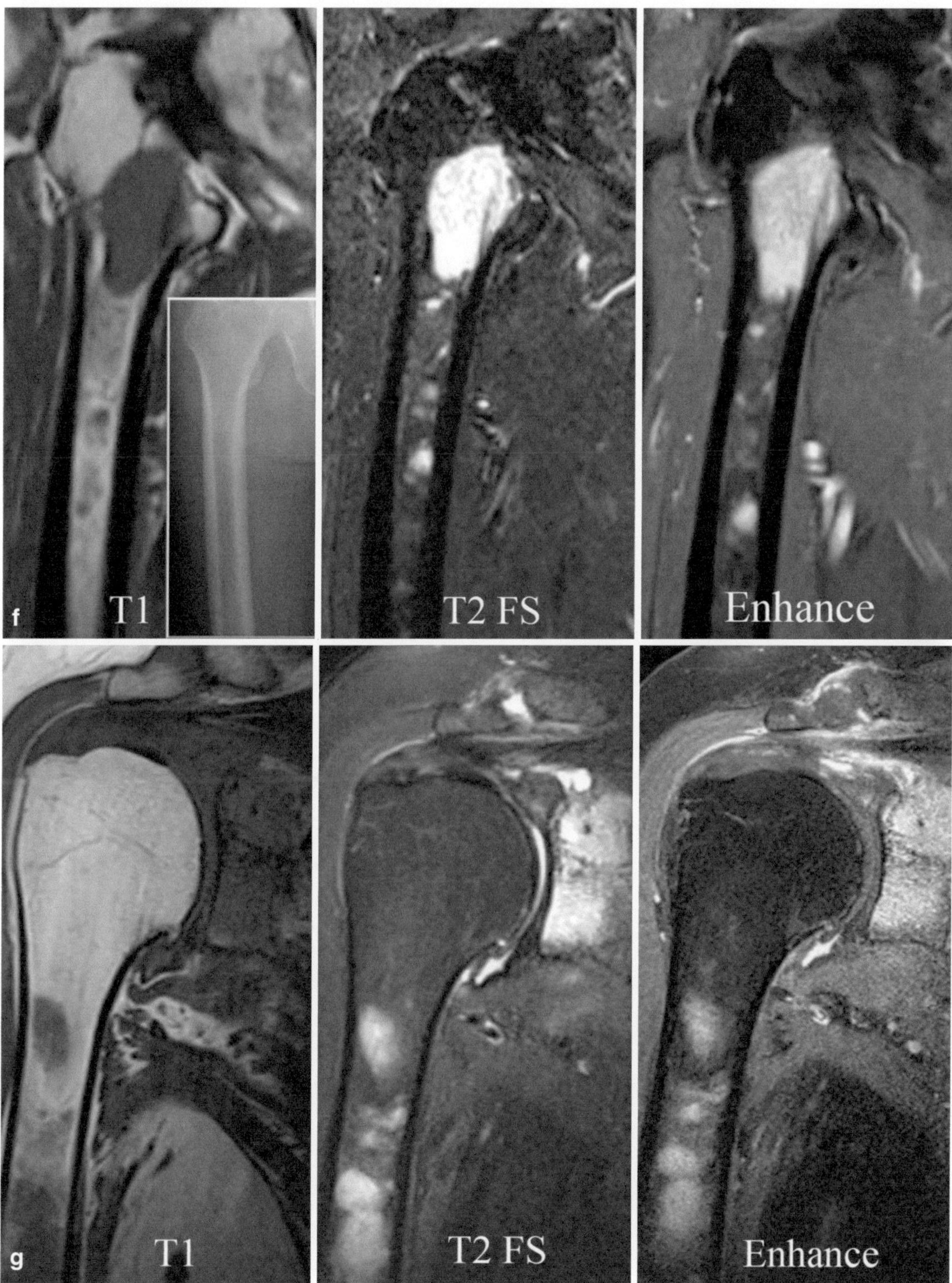

Fig. 5.7 (continued)

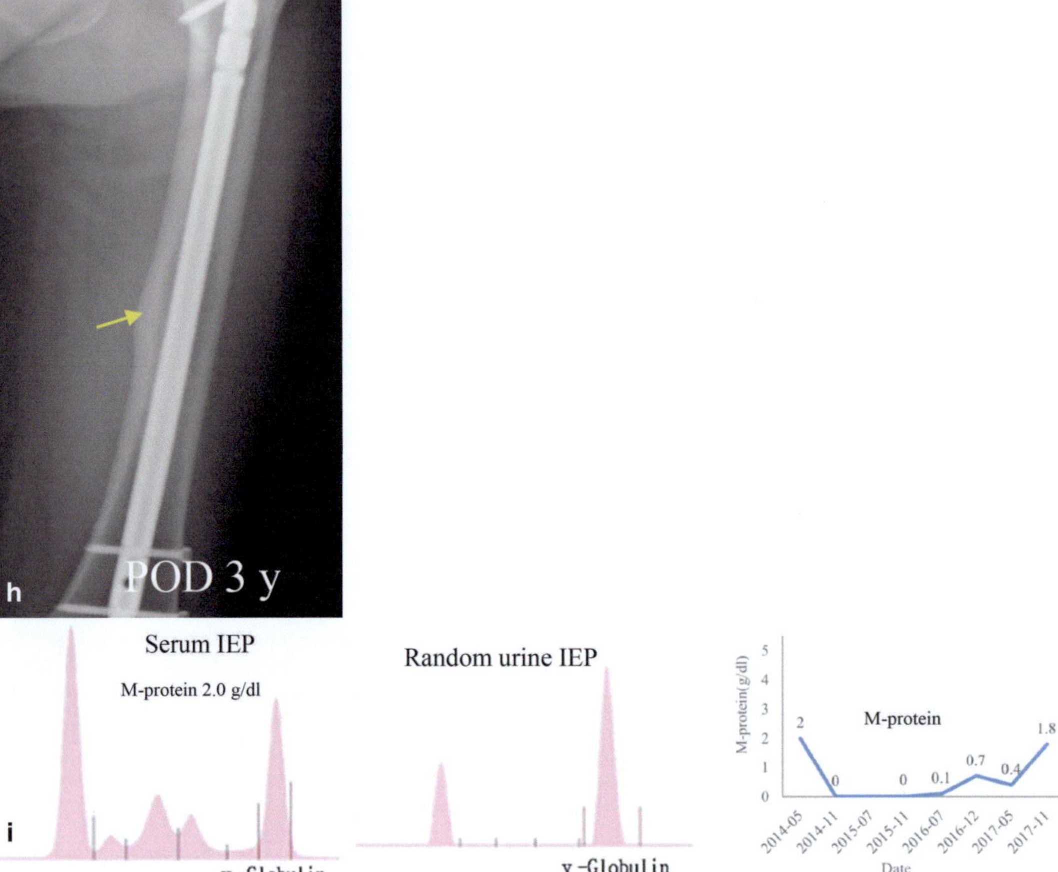

Fig. 5.7 (continued)

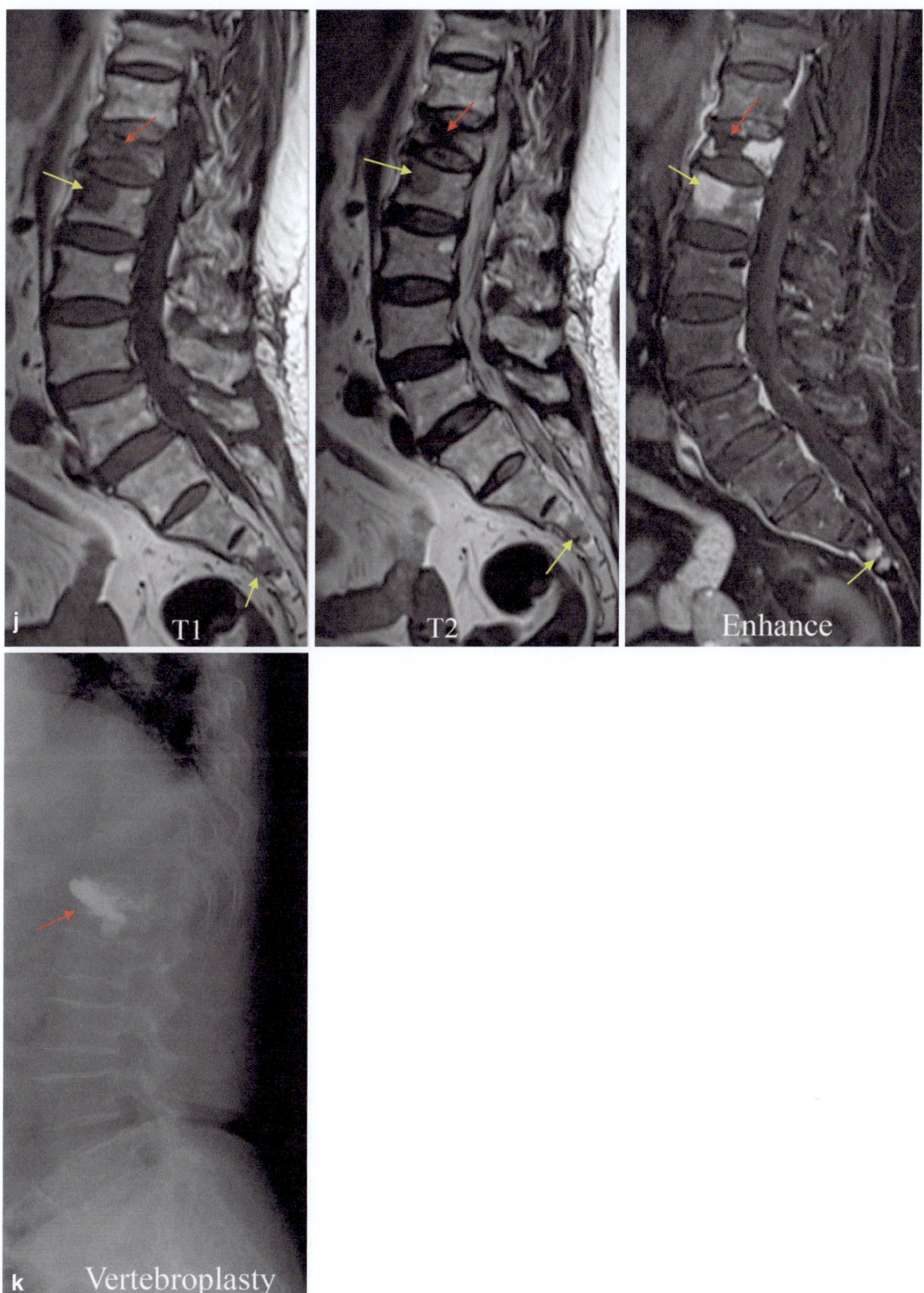

Fig. 5.7 (continued)

lesion by combining of both tools in the spine-pelvis [24]. **Bone scan** Radioisotope uptake is variable from hyperactive (hot) to normal or even decreased (photopenic or cold), depending on the osteoblastic activity. It is frequently negative despite the extensive bone involvement and/or destruction because of minimal new bone production (Figs. 5.4b and 5.6b). Thus, bone scan is usually not useful for the workup in suspected or established disseminated myeloma. However, it is occasionally useful to discover lesions in the ribs or sternum and even other bones, which are not detected on radiograph and even PET/CT scan (Fig. 5.7b). Therefore, bone scan and PET/CT scan can provide mutual aid as PET/CT scan and MRI do. **CT scan** can detect lesions with less than 5% trabecular bone destruction [25, 26]. Whole-body low dose (WBLD) CT scan is a reasonable and cost-effective initial imaging approach with low dose of radiation, which is more accurate than a whole body radiographs with a sensitivity up to 70% and specificity of 90% [27, 28]. It can detect the lesions particularly of ribs, sternum, and spines which are not discovered on radiograph, bone scan, or PET/CT scan (Fig. 5.3d). **MR findings** MR images are more sensitive in detecting PCM compared to the standard plain radiographs and bone scintigraphy [29, 30] (Figs. 5.6c and 5.7f). MRI is a standard method for bone marrow assessment before the mineralized bone tissue is destroyed [31]. It can effectively monitor the marrow changes during therapy, but abnormal signals persist despite the clinical response in some cases. MRI of the spine should be performed at the time point of initial diagnosis [32]. The signal intensity (SI) of the lesion is typically low on T1-weighted image and heterogeneous intermediate and high on T2-weighted image with varying degree of contrast enhancement depending on the vascularity of the lesion. Five different infiltration patterns have been described by Baur-Melnyk et al. [32]. The normal appearance of bone marrow is generally associated with low tumor burden almost exclusively in an early disease, and focal or diffuse involvements usually suggest a high tumor burden. (1) The *Normal* bone marrow signals can present despite the minor microscopic plasma cell infiltration and not exclude a diagnosis of PCM. (2) The *focal involvement pattern* usually consists of well-demarcated focal areas of decreased SI on T1-weighted image and increased SI on T2-weighted images with a varying degree of enhancement. (3) The *diffuse infiltration pattern*, a complete replacement of normal bone marrow by myeloma cells, shows diffusely and homogeneously decreased SI on T1-weighted image and diffusely or patchy likely increased SI on T2-weighted image with marked enhancement. (4) The *combined focal and diffuse infiltration pattern* reveals diffusely decreased SI with additional foci interspersed on T1-weighted image. Those foci are often better demarked on fat saturated T2-weighted image. (5) The *variegated or "pepper and salt" pattern* is typified by the presence of multiple foci of low SI on T1-weighted image and intermediate to high SI on T2-weighted images with varying degree of contrast enhancement. The focal and diffuse patterns can be also found in other hematological malignancies such as lymphoma and leukemia [32, 33].

5.8 Histologic Findings

PCM consists of monoclonal proliferation of malignant plasma cells, which replace the normal bone marrow and produce abnormal immunoglobulins. The degree of pleomorphism may vary depending on the level of differentiation. *"Well-differentiated"* myeloma is most common and is typified by near normal-looking plasma cells (Fig. 5.8a). It is impossible to distinct the tumor cells from normal plasma cells by cytology alone. *"Moderately differentiated"* myeloma presents a large number of more significant nuclear and cytoplasmic atypia, frequent bi-nucleated cells (Fig. 5.8b). *"Pleomorphic myeloma"* is rarest and is characterized by extremely anaplastic appearance with vesicular nuclei and prominent nucleoli but no abundant cytoplasm (Fig. 5.8c). Sometimes, it is impossible to distinguish from histiocytic lymphoma and others [1, 3]. The myeloma plasma cells are varying from mature normal looking to plasmablastic, immature, and

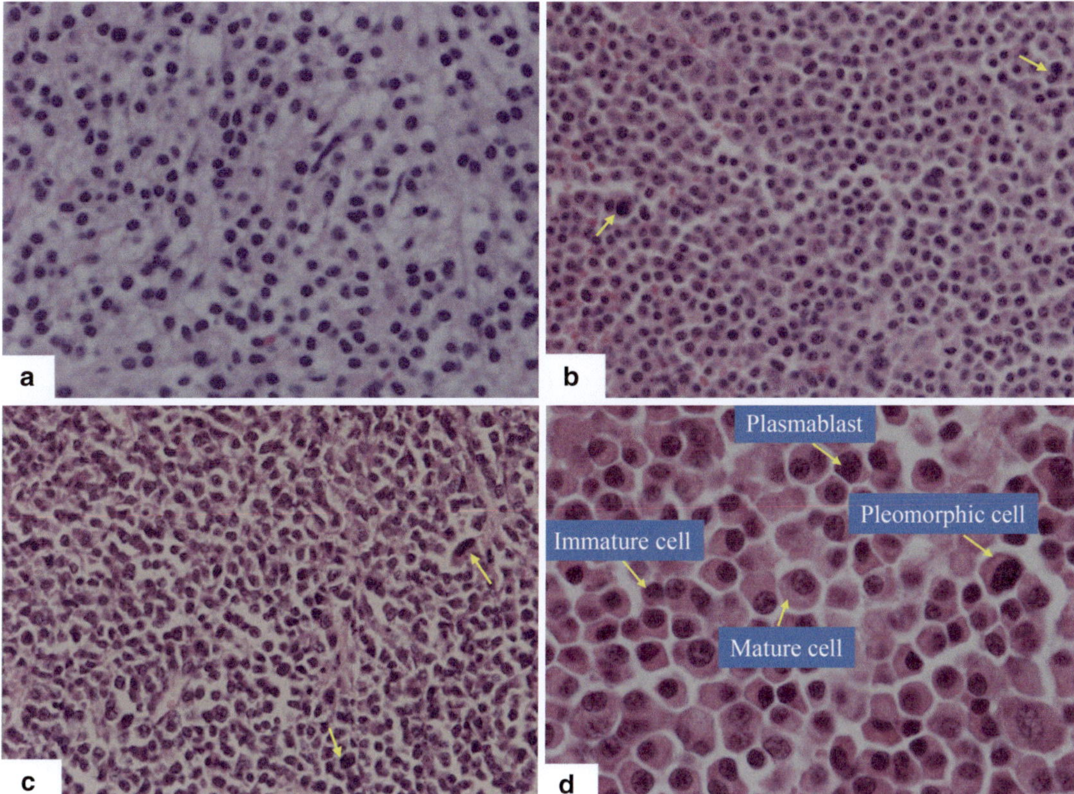

Fig. 5.8 ***Microscopic features***. (**a**) Well-differentiated myeloma consists of monotonous tumor cells with eccentric, round to oval nuclei, and abundant cytoplasm but no apparent nucleoli. The tumor cells are replacing the bone marrow space with remained fat marrow elements. (**b**) Moderately differentiated myeloma is composed of tumor cells with more prominent nucleoli and abundant cytoplasm, completely occupying the bone marrow space without remained marrow elements. Bi-nucleated large cells are frequently seen (yellow arrows). (**c**) In rare form of poorly differentiated myeloma, most cells are larger with vesicular nuclei and prominent nucleoli. However, cytoplasm is not that abundant as in well and moderately differentiated tumors. Note several bizarre pleomorphic cells (yellow arrows). (**d**) Myeloma cells demonstrate a wide spectrum of morphologic features depending on the degree of differentiation and are classified into *mature, plasmablast, immature, and pleomorphic* plasma cells. All of the cell types can be observed together as a mixed form in some cases. High-magnification views present comparable size and details of the four types of myeloma cells. (a) *Mature* plasma cells have round to oval, eccentric nucleus with coarse chromatin often appearing *"clock-face"* and *"perinuclear halo,"* but no prominent nucleoli. The findings are not discernible from normal plasma cells. (b) *Plasmablastic* myeloma cells are generally large with a vesicular chromatin and increased polymorphism resembling diffuse large B-cell lymphoma. (c) *Immature* plasma cells have more dispersed nuclear chromatin, higher nuclear/cytoplasmic ratio, and usually prominent nucleoli. (d) *Pleomorphic* myeloma cells are significantly bizarre and pleomorphic in size and shape with prominent nucleoli. (**e**) Round eccentric nucleus with coarse chromatin may have *"spoke-wheel"* or *"clock-face"* appearance. (**f**) A perinuclear halo or clearing (yellow double-headed arrows) which eccentrically dislodges the nucleus is observed in mature myeloma cells. It presents a large and extensive Golgi apparatus storing immunoglobulins before secreting but are not stained. It is more clearly visible in the bone marrow biopsy specimen with Wright stain (inset). There is basophilic cytoplasm outside the perinuclear clearing (black double-headed arrow). (**g**) The amorphous amyloid matrices (A) are focally deposited among myeloma cells (M). (**h**) ICH stains for CD38 and CD138, reliable markers of plasma cells, are positive. IHC for kappa reveals numerous kappa-positive cells, while IHC for lambda reveals only few scattered lambda-positive cells, indicating kappa isotype

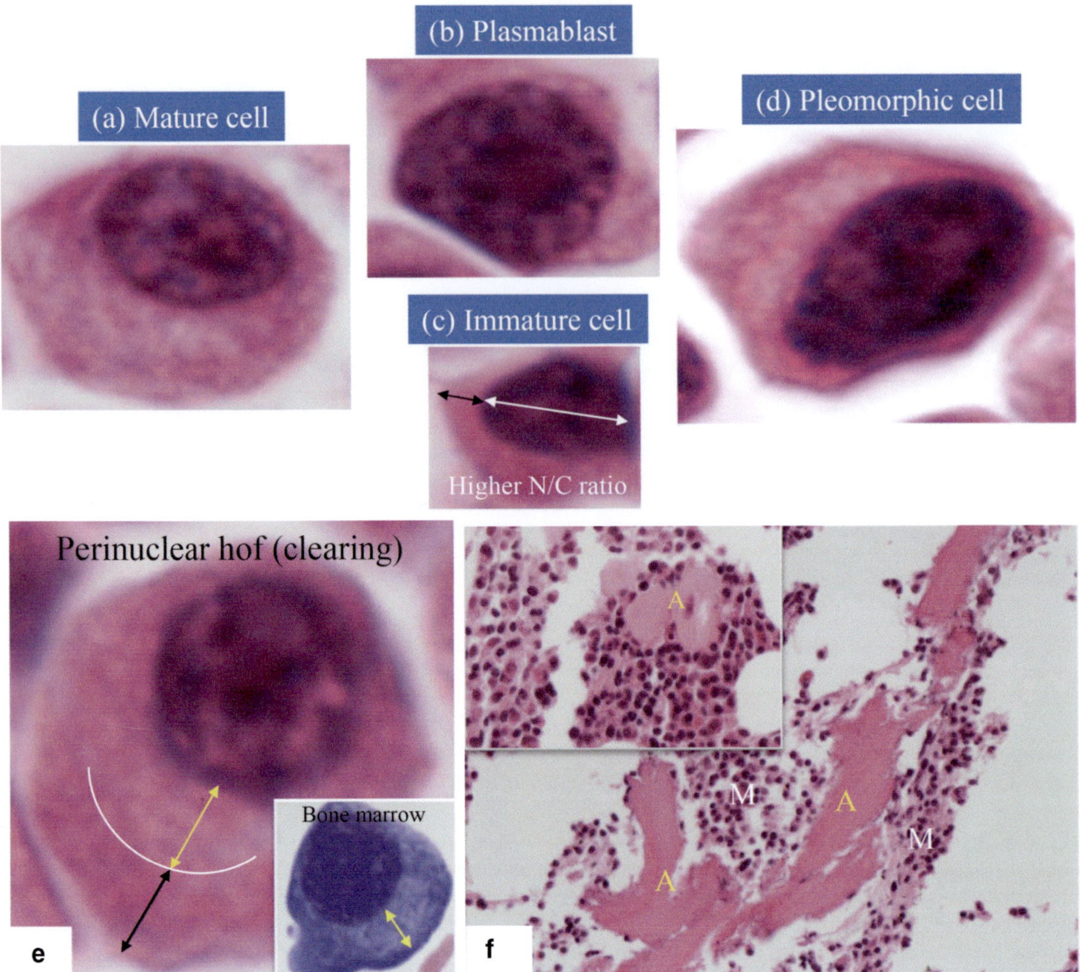

Fig. 5.8 (continued)

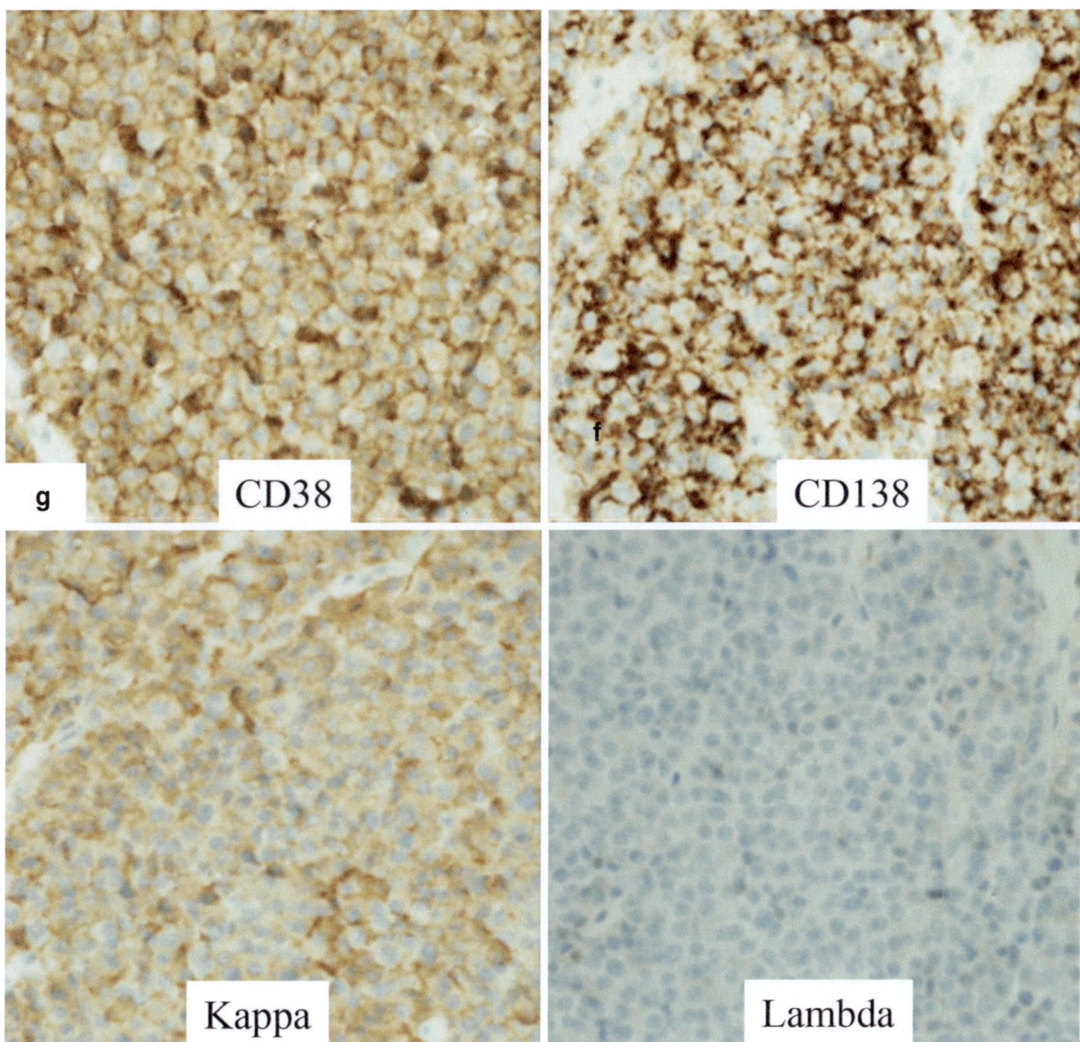

Fig. 5.8 (continued)

pleomorphic appearance (Fig. 5.8d). (a) *"Mature"* myeloma cells are usually indistinguishable from normal plasma cells, having a round to oval eccentric nucleus with coarse chromatin, sometimes so-called *"cart-wheel"* or *"clock-face"* looking (Fig. 5.8e), but no definite nucleoli. The cytoplasmic vacuoles increase in prominence by large and extensive Golgi apparatus storing immunoglobulins before secreting. They can also exhibit abundant basophilic cytoplasm with a *"perinuclear clearing (hof, halo)"* (the hollow in the cytoplasm that displace the nucleus) (Fig. 5.8f). (b) *"Plasmablastic"* myeloma cells are larger with nuclear polymorphism and mitotic figures resembling diffuse large B-cell lymphoma. (c) *"Immature"* myeloma cells have an irregular nucleus with more dispersed chromatin, a higher N/C ratio, and frequently prominent nucleoli. (d) *"Pleomorphic"* myeloma cells have bi- or multiple nuclei and significant pleomorphism in size and shape with prominent nucleoli [34]. On occasion, varying degree of amorphous amyloid matrix (para-amyloid or amyloid) can be focally or even extensively deposited among myeloma cells in some cases (Fig. 5.8g). They usually represent extracellular conglomerate deposits of globulins or other proteins, which present identical tinctorial property to intracellular "Russel bodies" [1].

5.9 Special Stains

Immunohistochemical stains (ICH) are mandatory to exclude other types of hematopoietic round-cell tumors. Positive stains for PCM include CD38 and CD 138. Kappa and lambda IHC stains and in situ hybridization (ISH) are useful tools for subclassification of PCM, kappa or lambda isotype (Fig. 5.8h). Detection of light chain restriction in CD138 positive plasma cells in bone marrow is a useful tool for simple, efficient, and accurate diagnosis of PCM [35, 36].

5.10 Management

There is no definite cure, but adequate treatments can slow down its progression and spread. Management includes local and systemic treatments. Local treatments include surgery and radiation therapy. Surgical treatment is sometimes needed for removal single lesion and for internal fixation of impending or pathologic fracture. Emergency surgical decompression with or without instrumentation is indicated for spinal cord compression causing severe muscle weakness or paralysis. Systemic treatments include chemotherapy and bone marrow transplant (BMT). Recent innovative therapeutic approach with new chemotherapy combinations, immunotherapy such as chimeric antigen receptor-T cell (CAR-T cell) therapy and bi-specific monoclonal antibodies (BiTEs), targeted small molecule inhibitors, and monoclonal antibodies would slow down its spread and improve quality of life and survival [37–39].

5.11 Clinical Course

PCM is generally progressive and incurable. Earlier in 1975, over 80% of the patients was reported to die most commonly due to infection and renal insufficiency with median survival of 20 months, and 66% of the patients were alive at 1 year and 18% at 5 years in a large series [4]. However, it is improved much nowadays. The overall 5-year survival rate in SEER stages was reported to be 78% for localized tumor (solitary plasmacytoma), 55% for distant tumor (multiple myeloma), and 56% for all SEER stages combined (American Cancer Society relying in SEER (Surveillance, Epidemiology, and End Results) between 2011 and 2017) [40].

References

1. Mirra JM. Myeloma. In: Mirra JM, editor. Bone tumors: clinical, radiologic, and pathologic correlation. 2nd ed. Philadelphia, PA: Lea & Febiger; 1989. p. 1121–46.
2. Ewton A. Hematopoietic tumors. In: Dorfman HD, Czerniak B, editors. Dorfman and Czerniak's bone tumors. 2nd ed. Philadelphia, PA: Elsevier; 2016. p. 817–902.
3. Unni KK, Inwards CY. Myeloma. In: Unni KK, Inwards CY, editors. Dahlin's bone tumors. 6th ed. Philadelphia, PA: Lippincott Williams & Wilkins; 2010. p. 191–200.
4. Kyle RA. Multiple myeloma: review of 869 cases. Mayo Clin Proc. 1975;50(1):29–40.
5. Sung H, Siegel RL, Rosenberg PS, Jemal A. Emerging cancer trends among young adults in the USA: analysis of a population-based cancer registry. Lancet Public Health. 2019;4(3):e137–e47.
6. The International Myeloma Working Group. Criteria for the classification of monoclonal gammopathies, multiple myeloma and related disorders: a report of the international myeloma working group. Br J Haematol. 2003;121:749–57.

7. Kyle RA, Therneau TM, Rajkumar SV, Offord JR, Larson DR, Plevak MF, et al. A long-term study of prognosis in monoclonal gammopathy of undetermined significance. N Engl J Med. 2002;346(8):564–9.
8. Kyle RA, Greipp PR. Smoldering multiple myeloma. N Engl J Med. 1980;302(24):1347–9.
9. Kyle RA, Rajkumar SV. Epidemiology of the plasma-cell disorders. Best Pract Res Clin Haematol. 2007;20(4):637–64.
10. Kyle RA, Rajkumar SV. Multiple myeloma. Blood. 2008;111:2962–72.
11. Perry M, Kyle R. The clinical significance of bence jones proteinuria. Mayo Clin Proc. 1975;50(5):234–8.
12. Merlini G, Bellotti V. Molecular mechanisms of amyloidosis. N Engl J Med. 2003;349(6):583–96.
13. Dispenzieri A. POEMS syndrome: 2021 update on diagnosis, risk-stratification, and management. Risk stratification, and management. Am J Hematol. 2021;96:872–88.
14. Ippolito D, Besostri V, Bonaffini PA, Rossini F, Di Lelio A, Sironi S. Diagnostic value of whole-body low-dose computed tomography (WBLDCT) in bone lesions detection in patients with multiple myeloma (MM). Eur J Radiol. 2013;82(12):2322–7.
15. Durie BG, Salmon SE. A clinical staging system for multiple myeloma correlation of measured myeloma cell mass with presenting clinical features, response to treatment, and survival. Cancer. 1975;36(3):842–54.
16. Angtuaco EJ, Fassas AB, Walker R, Sethi R, Barlogie B. Multiple myeloma: clinical review and diagnostic imaging. Radiology. 2004;231(1):11–23.
17. D'Sa S, Abildgaard N, Tighe J, Shaw P, Hall-Craggs M. Guidelines for the use of imaging in the management of myeloma. Br J Haematol. 2007;137(1):49–63.
18. Mulligan ME. Skeletal abnormalities in multiple myeloma. Radiology. 2005;234(1):313–4.
19. Collins C. Multiple myeloma. In: Husband J, Reznek R, editors. Imaging in oncology. 4 th ed. Boca Raton, FL: CRC Press; 2020; eBook ISBN9780203732656.
20. Cavo M, Terpos E, Nanni C, Moreau P, Lentzsch S, Zweegman S, et al. Role of 18F-FDG PET/CT in the diagnosis and management of multiple myeloma and other plasma cell disorders: a consensus statement by the international myeloma working group. Lancet Oncol. 2017;18(4):e206–e17.
21. van Lammeren-Venema D, Regelink JC, Riphagen II, Zweegman S, Hoekstra OS, Zijlstra JM. 18F-fluorodeoxyglucose positron emission tomography in assessment of myeloma-related bone disease: a systematic review. Cancer. 2012;118(8):1971–81.
22. Lu YY, Chen JH, Lin WY, Liang JA, Wang HY, Tsai SC, et al. FDG PET or PET/CT for detecting intramedullary and extramedullary lesions in multiple myeloma: a systematic review and meta-analysis. Clin Nucl Med. 2012;37(9):833–7.
23. Matteucci F, Paganelli G, Martinelli G, Cerchione C. PET/CT in multiple myeloma: beyond FDG. Front Oncol. 2021;10:622501.
24. Zamagni E, Nanni C, Patriarca F, Englaro E, Castellucci P, Geatti O, et al. A prospective comparison of 18F-fluorodeoxyglucose positron emission tomography-computed tomography, magnetic resonance imaging and whole-body planar radiographs in the assessment of bone disease in newly diagnosed multiple myeloma. Haematologica. 2007;92(1):50–5.
25. Amos B, Agarwal A, Kanekar S. Imaging of multiple myeloma. Hematol Oncol Clin North Am. 2016;30(4):843–65.
26. Chrzan R, Jurczyszyn A, Urbanik A. Whole-body low-dose computed tomography (WBLDCT) in assessment of patients with multiple myeloma–pilot study and standard imaging protocol suggestion. Pol J Radiol. 2017;82:356–63.
27. Ormond Filho AG, Carneiro BC, Pastore D, Silva IP, Yamashita SR, Consolo FD, et al. Whole-body imaging of multiple myeloma: diagnostic criteria. Radiographics. 2019;39(4):1077–97.
28. Bluemke DA, Kosmala A. Multiple myeloma and dual-energy CT: diagnostic accuracy of virtual noncalcium technique for detection of bone marrow infiltration of the spine and pelvis. Radiology. 2018;286:205–13.
29. Steinborn MM, Heuck AF, Tiling R, Bruegel M, Gauger L, Reiser MF. Whole-body bone marrow MRI in patients with metastatic disease to the skeletal system. J Comput Assist Tomogr. 1999;23(1):123–9.
30. Algra PR, Bloem JL, Tissing H, Falke T, Arndt J, Verboom L. Detection of vertebral metastases: comparison between MR imaging and bone scintigraphy. Radiographics. 1991;11(2):219–32.
31. Hillengass J, Landgren O. Challenges and opportunities of novel imaging techniques in monoclonal plasma cell disorders: imaging "early myeloma". Leuk Lymphoma. 2013;54(7):1355–63.
32. Baur-Melnyk A, Buhmann S, Dürr H, Reiser M. Role of MRI for the diagnosis and prognosis of multiple myeloma. Eur J Radiol. 2005;55(1):56–63.
33. Baur A, Stäbler A, Bartl R, Lamerz R, Reiser M. Infiltrationsmuster des Plasmozytoms in der Magnetresonanztomographie. Infiltration patterns of multiple myeloma in MRI. In RöFo-fortschritte auf dem gebiet der Röntgenstrahlen und der bildgebenden verfahren. Stuttgart, NY: Georg Thieme Verlag; 1996. 164(6): 457–463. DOI: https://doi.org/10.1055/s-2007-1015689.
34. Fujino M. The histopathology of myeloma in the bone marrow. J Clin Exp Hematop. 2018;58(2):61–7.
35. Nakayama-Ichiyama S, Yokote T, Hirata Y, Iwaki K, Akioka T, Miyoshi T, et al. Immunohistological diagnosis of plasma cell myeloma based on cytoplasmic kappa/lambda ratio of CD138-positive plasma cells. Leuk Lymphoma. 2012;53(11):2205–9.
36. Warnnissorn N, Treetipsatit J, Limvorapitak W. The cut-offs for kappa/lambda ratio in bone marrow immunohistochemistry for the diagnosis of multiple myeloma. Hematology. 2020;25(1):292–8.

37. Cohen AD, Garfall AL, Stadtmauer EA, Melenhorst JJ, Lacey SF, Lancaster E, et al. B cell maturation antigen–specific CAR T cells are clinically active in multiple myeloma. J Clini Invest. 2019;129(6):2210–21.
38. Zanwar S, Nandakumar B, Kumar S. Immune-based therapies in the management of multiple myeloma. Blood Cancer J. 2020;10(8):1–14.
39. Padala SA, Barsouk A, Barsouk A, Rawla P, Vakiti A, Kolhe R, et al. Epidemiology, staging, and management of multiple myeloma. Med Sci (Basel). 2021;9(1):3. https://doi.org/10.3390/medsci9010003; PMID: 33498356; PMCID: PMC7838784.
40. Huang C, Liu H, Jia L, Lu M, Hu S. Survival disparities in multiple myeloma by health insurance status among US non-elderly adults: a SEER-based comparative analysis. Acta Haematol. 2021;144(5):542–50.

6 Amyloidosis Associated with Plasma Cell Myeloma

(***Amylon*** "starch" + −**oid, *eidos*** "form" + −***osis*** "abnormal increase")

6.1 Definition

Amyloidosis is a rare disease resulted from abnormal amyloid deposition in body tissues and organs that can interfere with their normal function. Amyloid protein can be deposited either in a localized area, so-called *"localized amyloidosis"* or in the tissues throughout the body as a part of disseminated multi-organ involvement, referred to *"systemic amyloidosis"*, causing serious failure in any virtual organ of the body. In a large series, a systemic form represented a majority of the cases, and more than two-thirds are AL (amyloid light or formerly primary) amyloidosis occupying 70% of all cases. A localized form occupies about 20%, and most patients has the carpal ligament involvement. The rest of the cases representing 10% were familial, senile, and AA(secondary) amyloidosis [1]. The definition of organ involvement in systemic AL amyloidosis has been recently published, and a consensus conference has defined major criteria for seven main organ systems, including kidney, heart, liver, nerve, gastrointestinal tract, lung, and soft tissue [2]. However, bone disease was not included in the list of affected organs. Amyloid bone disease, so-called *"bone amyloidoma,"* has only been sporadically reported [3–6]. Bone amyloidosis produces an osteolytic lesion visible on radiograph, simulating bone tumor. Rarely, it may be diagnosed after emergency surgery of the spine [7, 8], or hip fracture [5, 9] (Figs. 6.1 and 6.2).

W.-J. Bahk, *Diagnosis and Management of Primary Bone Tumors*,
https://doi.org/10.1007/978-981-99-5498-8_6

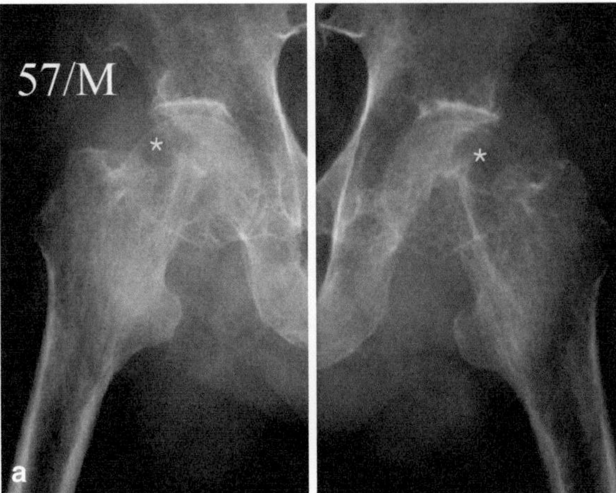

Fig. 6.1 ***AL amyloidosis associated with PCM*** (**a**) Radiographs taken for generalized weakness and multiple joint stiffness with walking difficulty of 5- to 6-month duration in 57-year-old man show diffuse *"punched-out"* lesions of both proximal femurs and acetabulum with geographic destruction in the femoral heads (asterisks). (**b**) MR images reveal a diffuse heterogeneous bone marrow replacement with numerous, variable-sized low SI on T1-weighted image and high SI on fat saturated T2-weighted images (yellow arrows) in both iliac wings and proximal femurs, which is heterogeneously enhanced by the contrast medium (white arrows), so-called *"salt and pepper"* appearance suggesting hematopoietic lesion such as PCM. Note another type of mass-like lesions with low SI both on T1- and T2-weighted images in both femoral heads (white asterisks) and peri-articular soft tissues (yellow asterisks), which are well enhanced (yellow arrows), suggesting a possible *amyloid arthroplasty associated PCM*. (**c**) Bone scan notes diffusely increased activity in the peri-articular areas in bilateral joints of extremities including shoulders, elbows, wrist, hands, hips, knees, ankles, and feet, suggesting disseminated arthroplasty rather than degenerative change. Focal activity is also seen in ribs. (**d**) PET/CT scan demonstrates hypermetabolic activity around both shoulders and hips including pelvic bones as well as peri-articular soft tissue and muscle and milder hypermetabolic activity at skull, both scapulae, ribs, vertebrae, and distal femurs (SUVmax 3.9–4.6), suggesting amyloidosis with PCM in consideration of MR findings. (**e**) Radiographs corresponding to increased uptake on bone scan and hypermetabolic areas on PET scan show diffuse radiolucent lesions of the joints as well as numerous *"punched-out"* lesions of the long bones. Geographic destruction is also noted in the humeral shaft (yellow arrow). (**f**) Microscopic examination of incision biopsy specimen right pelvic bone reveals dense aggregations of plasmatoid cell proliferation (P) and several small amorphous droplets (A) between the cells (Top). Higher-power view shows mature plasma cells with eccentric nuclei, indicating myeloma (inset). Specimen from soft tissue notes diffuse deposition of dense amorphous eosinophilic substance, suggesting localized amyloidosis (Bottom). (**g**) Serum IEP reveals a faint monoclonal band in the gamma globulin region with a very low concentration of M-protein (0.2 g/dL), and IFE indicates a monoclonal gammopathy of IgE/kappa isotype. Urine IEP shows a prominent monoclonal band in the gamma region, and IFE indicates Bence-Jones protein of kappa type. Bone marrow biopsy shows that mature and immature plasma cells are significantly increased in number up to 88% of all nucleated elements. Final diagnosis of *"AL amyloidosis"* associated with PCM is rendered. (**h**) Prophylactic IM nailing was performed for humeral shaft lesion (yellow arrow) to prevent pathologic fracture followed by autologous BMT. (**i**) Follow-up radiograph at 2 years after surgery shows no further progression of local disease (red arrow). (**j**) Two years later, radiograph taken for newly developed symptoms of shortening and weakness of left lower extremity by unknown reason shows a femur neck fracture with resorption of a part of femoral head (red arrow) and upward migration of the femur, suggesting old neglected fracture. (**k**) Follow-up radiograph at 2 years after total hip replacement shows good maintenance without evidence of infection and loosening. AL amyloidosis associated with PCM (**l**) (Left) Microscopic examination of resected femoral head reveals deposition of abundant amorphous pinkish material indicative of amyloidosis (A) and osteopenic bone spicules of femoral head (B). (Middle) Note prominent multinucleated giant cells (yellow arrows) reactive to the amyloid droplets (A) within stromal tissue and around the blood vessels (black arrows). (**m**) Polarized microscopic examination notes the typical apple-green birefringence of the deposits, and (Right) Polarized microscopic examination notes the typical apple-green birefringence of the deposits. He died of disease progression and sepsis at 5 years after BMT

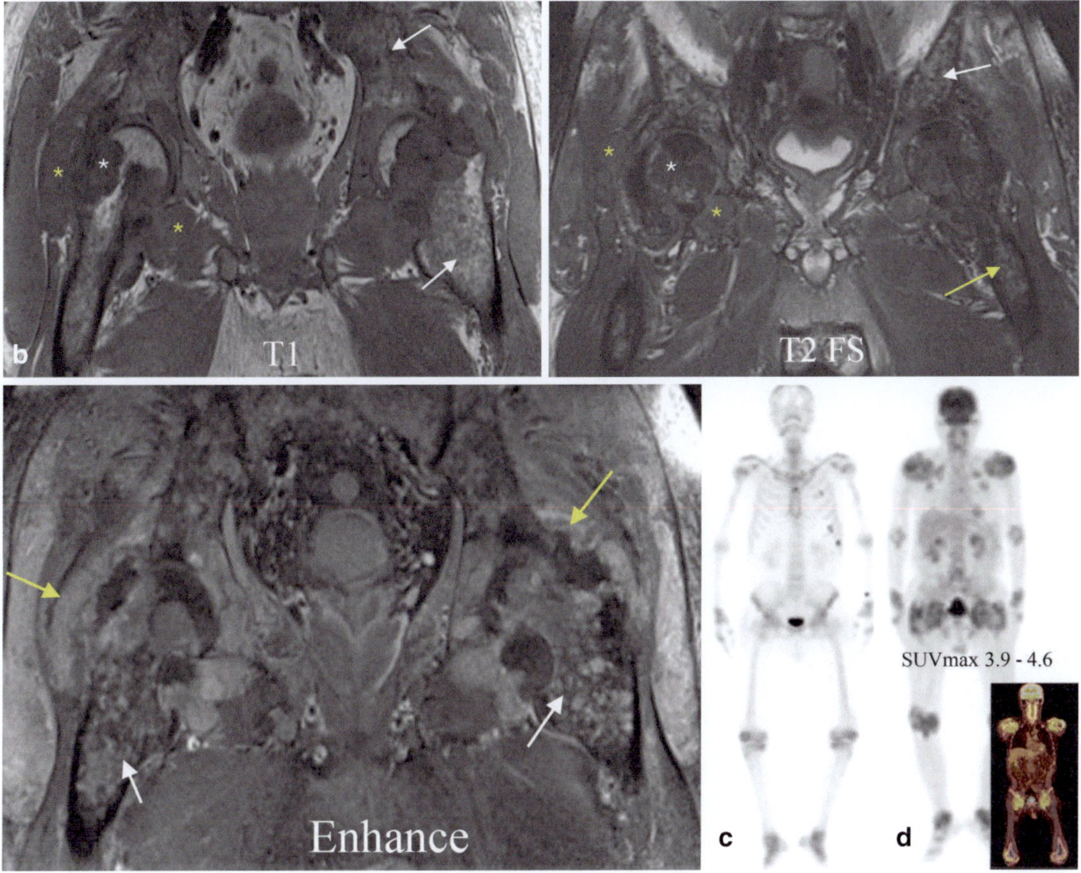

Fig. 6.1 (continued)

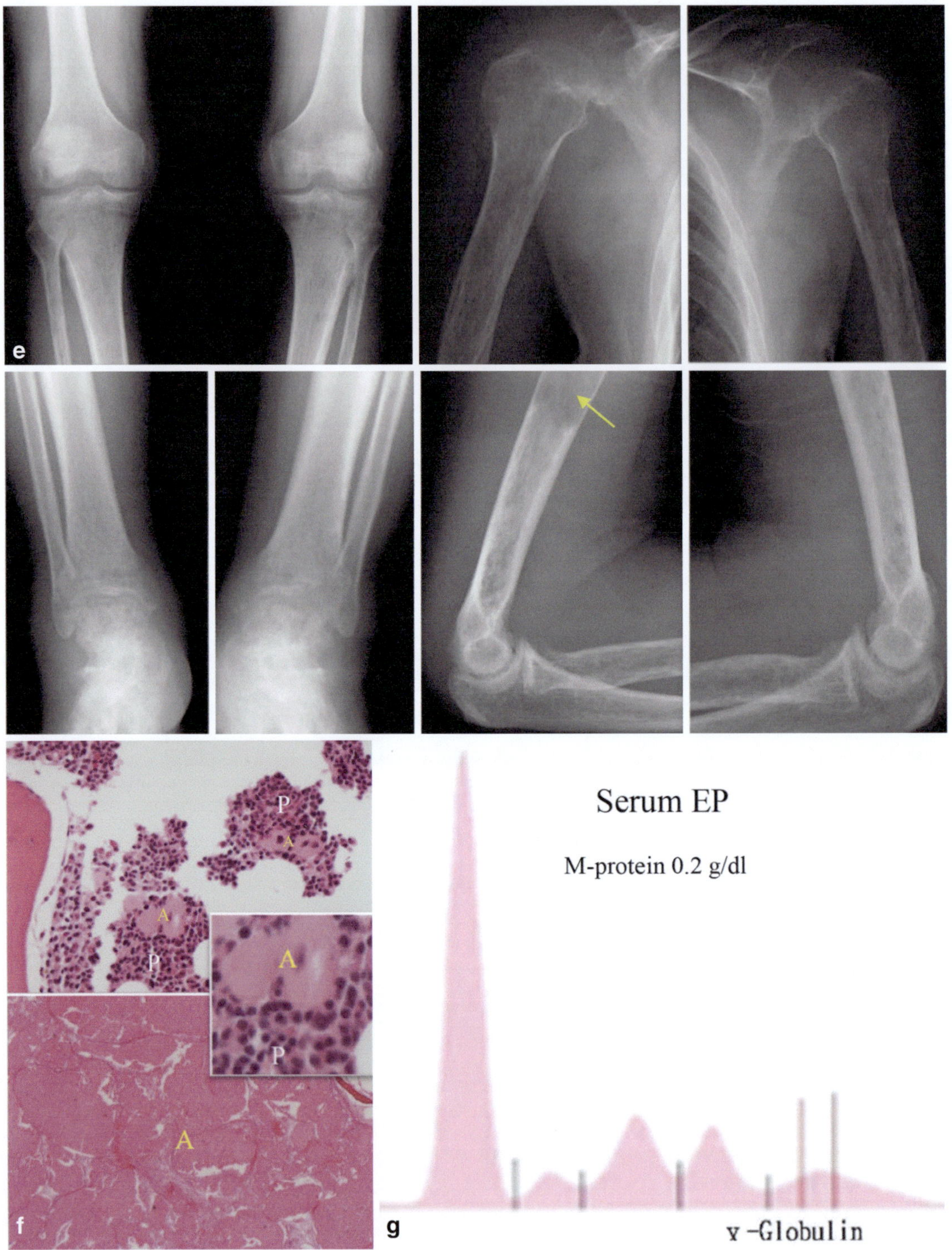

Fig. 6.1 (continued)

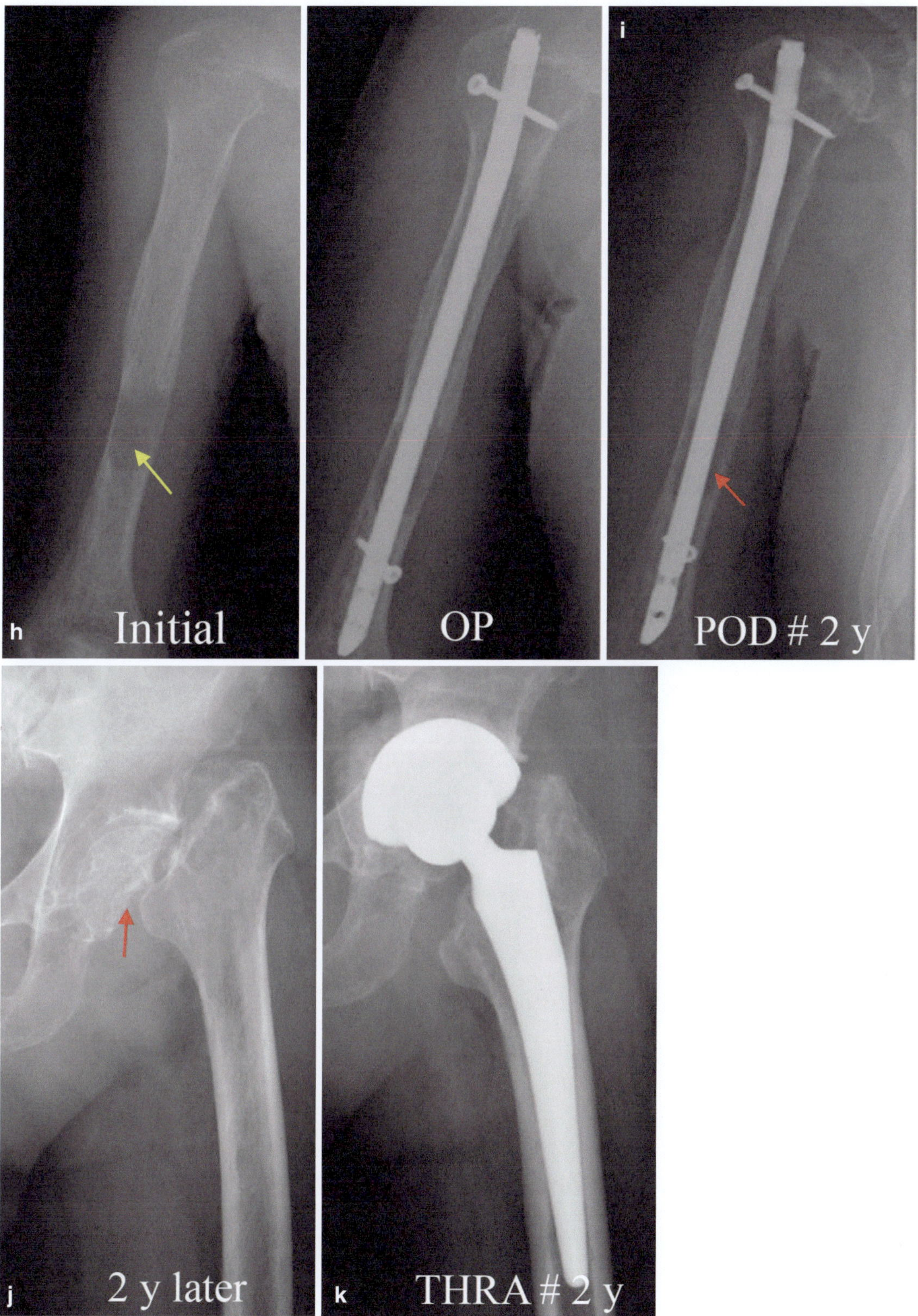

Fig. 6.1 (continued)

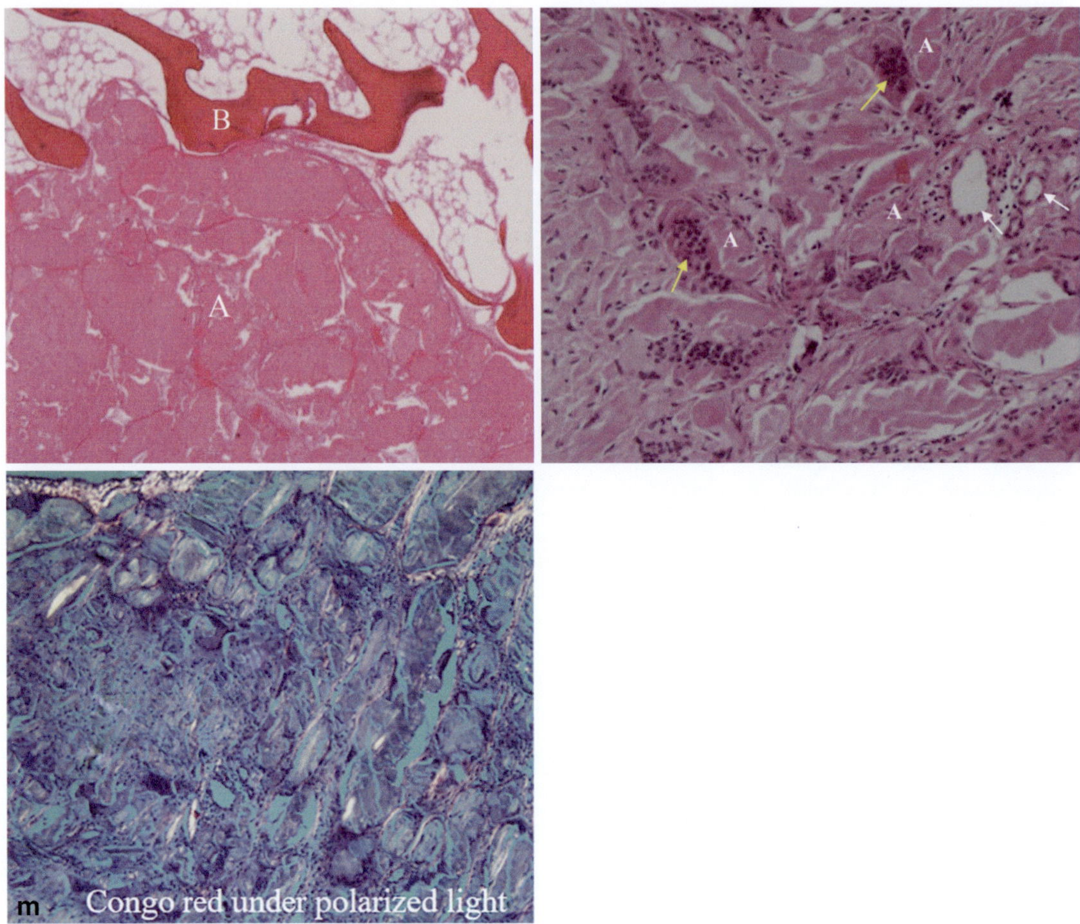

Fig. 6.1 (continued)

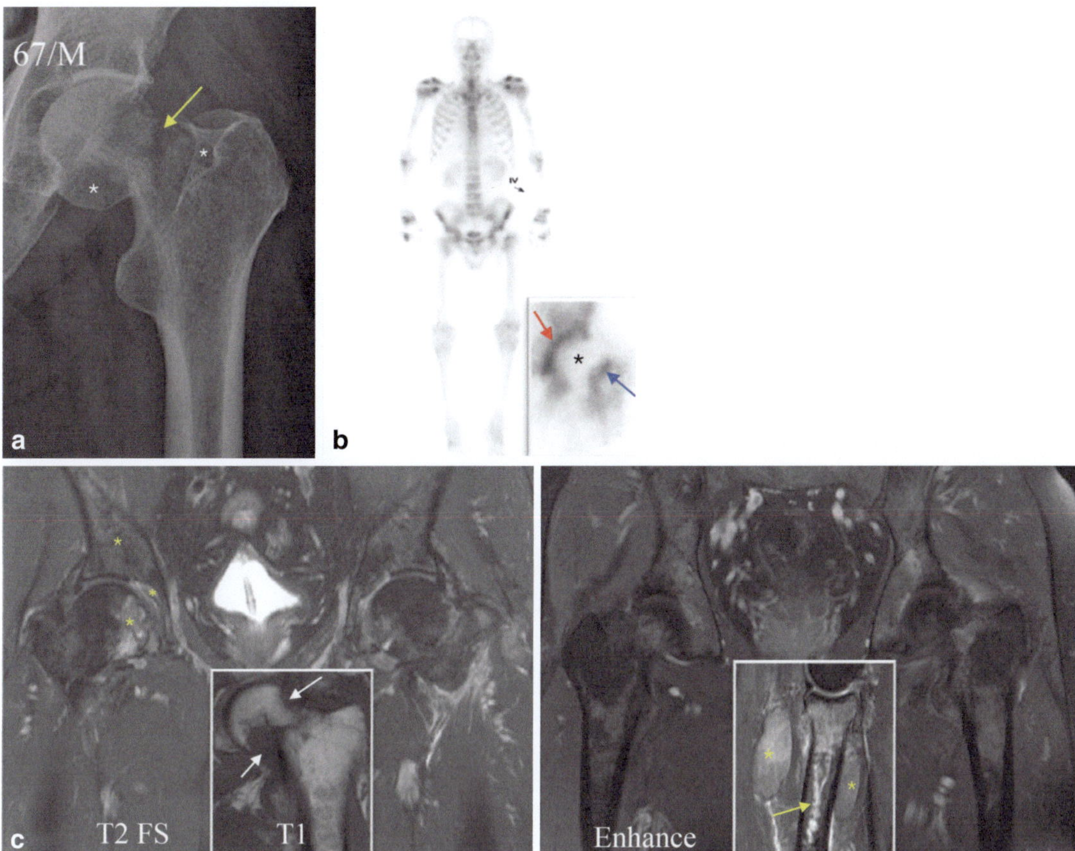

Fig. 6.2 ***AL amyloidosis*** (**a**) Radiograph taken for left hip pain of 2-week duration with a sudden aggravation in 67-year-old man shows hazy radiolucent lesions in the femoral head and neck area (asterisks) with pathologic neck fracture (arrow). In addition, he has also a right elbow mass and past history of carpal tunnel syndrome of both wrists with amyloid deposition, which were excised twice due to recurrence in another hospital years ago. (**b**) Bone scan reveals increased uptake in the shoulders, elbows, wrists, hands, and hips. Pinhole bone scan reveals a focal increased uptake (blue arrow) with central cold uptake area (asterisk) and in the femoral head and neck (inset). There is also reactive uptake in the acetabulum (red arrow). (**c**) MR images demonstrate multifocal ill-defined intramedullary lesions with low to intermediate SI on T1-weighted image (white arrows) and heterogeneous high SI (asterisks) on T2-weighted image in the both femoral heads, acetabulums, and hip joint spaces. The lesion is also seen in the trochanteric area of left femur and right iliopsoas/iliopectineal bursa in another cut. Additional MR images of right elbow mass notes a multi-lobulated soft tissue mass with similar SI as hip lesions as well as intraosseous bone lesion involving proximal radius (inset). The soft tissue mass (asterisks) as well as bony lesion (arrow) is heterogeneously enhanced. Amyloidosis with PCM or lymphoma was suspected. (**d**) Shoulder radiographs note symmetric moth-eaten destruction in the both lateral ends of clavicle, acromions and scapular bodies (circles), and small geographic destruction in the both scapular glenoid (arrows), reflecting increased uptake on bone scan (inset). Note numerous variable-sized tiny to small *"punch-out"* lesions in the both humeral shaft (blue arrow), but there is no uptake on bone scan (blue arrow). (**e**) Microscopic examination of specimen from excised femoral neck and elbow mass shows identical findings of dense aggregations of plasmatoid cell proliferation (P) and numerous pink eosinophilic globular structures representing amyloid deposit with giant cell reaction (arrows). The extracellular materials attained as reddish-orange color by Congo red stain (inset). (**f**) He was transferred to department of hematology for chemotherapy under diagnosis of amyloidosis with PCM confirmed by IEP/IFE, evaluation of the urine for M protein, and bone marrow biopsy. Follow-up radiograph after 30 months after hemiarthroplasty shows good maintenance with no evidence of infection and loosening. ***Amyloidosis associated with CRF*** (**g**). Radiographs taken for right hip pain after slip in another 54-year-old patient with CRF on long-term hemodialysis for 10 years reveals eccentric radiolucent geographic lesions surrounded by a thin rim of sclerosis in the both femoral neck and head (red arrow) with pathologic fracture in left femoral neck (yellow arrow). Hemiarthroplasty was done for femoral neck fracture. Gross specimen of resected femoral head notes cystic defect on the femoral head (inset). Microscopic examination of resected specimen showed typical findings of amyloidosis with no evidence of PCM

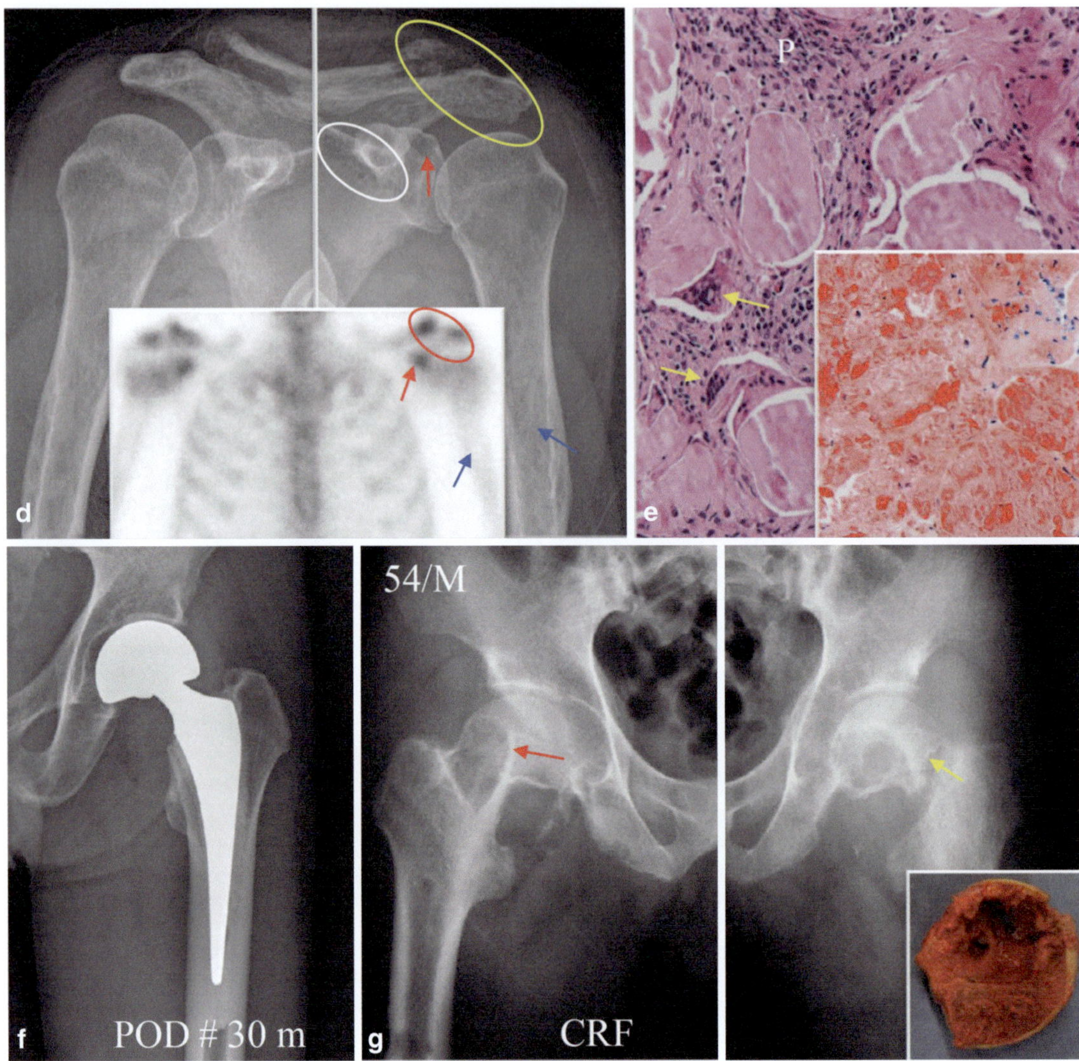

Fig. 6.2 (continued)

6.2 Classification

The amyloidosis can be subclassified into four forms depending on the abnormal protein produced: AL, AA, amyloid ß2-microglobulin, and transthyretin. (1) *AL (amyloid light chain) amyloidosis*, formerly called as primary amyloidosis, can be subdivided again into (a) AL and (b) AL with myeloma. The most common form involving skeleton is usually associated with PCM (Figs. 6.1 and 6.2). It could happen when plasma cells in the bone marrow make abnormal antibodies of light chain protein, which enter the bloodstream and produce amyloid deposition to damage multiple organs such as kidneys, heart, liver, spleen, gastrointestinal tract, muscle, nerves, and skin. (2) *AA amyloidosis*, previously known as secondary amyloidosis, stands for the fragment AA protein of serum amyloid A (SAA). It occurs when SAA level in the bloodstream remains high for a long period of time by high levels of inflammation as in uncontrolled chronic infectious or inflammatory process such as tuberculosis, rheumatoid arthritis, ankylosing spondylitis, Crohn's disease, or ulcerative colitis. It mostly affects kidneys, but it can also affect digestive tract, liver, and heart. (3) Later, *Aβ2M amyloidosis* has been described, which can be derived from amyloid ß2-microglobulin in patients with chronic renal failure (CRF) on long-term hemodialysis (Fig. 6.2g) or peritoneal dialysis [10–12]. This form is second most common after AL amyloidosis associated with PCM. In patients undergoing hemodialysis for more than 10 years, growing bone cysts with amyloid deposition were described in the carpus, humeral head, femur, and patella [13]. In a series with long-term follow-up, the frequency of symptoms was proportional to the duration of dialysis, and all patients on dialysis for over 20 years were affected [12]. (4) Transthyretin (prealbumin) is produced in rare form of familial or senile systemic amyloidosis.

6.3 Clinical Features and Diagnostic Analysis

A concurrent diagnosis of amyloidosis is made at presentation or sometime during the course of the myeloma in 7–15% of patients [14, 15]. M-protein was reported to be found in the serum or urine by immunoelectrophoresis (IEP)/immunofixation electrophoresis (IFE) in about 90% of the patients undertaken both tests at the time of the diagnosis [1]. In skeleton, amyloid may be deposited in capsule, synovium, articular cartilage, menisci [16, 17], and even in bone [12, 18]. Shoulder pain and carpal tunnel syndrome are most common initial symptoms, which are often bilateral. Patients can also develop osteolytic bone lesion (amyloidoma) and amyloid arthropathy as well particularly in hips, shoulders, and wrists. Those with a large subchondral lesion, particularly in femoral neck, have a high prevalence of pathologic fractures (Figs. 6.1 and 6.2). Amyloid myopathy commonly presents with proximal muscle weakness, and extensive deposition of amyloid material may result in pseudohypertrophy of the skeletal muscles. When affecting spines, cord compression or radicular symptoms due to nerve root compression may present. In systemic amyloidosis, fatigue, generalized weakness or malaise, and weight loss are the most common initial presentations. Cutaneous manifestations such as petechiae, ecchymosis, papules, plaques, nodules, bullous lesions, and nail dystrophy are common in systemic disease [19]. In a series of 83 patients with long-term hemodialysis patients at least 10 years, joint pain with stiffness by day, particularly shoulder, in the absence of radiological changes of arthritis was the most common symptom (41%), and 70% of affected patients complained of sleep disturbance [12]. The authors reported carpal tunnel syndrome was the most frequent musculoskeletal manifestation requiring surgical treatment. Symptoms recurred 2–3 years later, and repeated decompression was done in 6 of 16 patients (23%) who continued on hemodialysis after carpal tunnel release. Other manifestations included trigger finger, flexor tendon contracture, spontaneous tendon rupture, and pathological fracture through amyloid bone.

6.4 Radiologic Findings

Amyloid arthropathy may exhibit similar radiographic features of erosive and destructive osteoarthropathy, such as periarticular soft tissue swelling, mild periarticular osteoporosis, subchondral cyst surrounded by a thin rim of sclerosis, and normal sparing joint space. Radiographic changes in bone and joint appear in late stage of the disease and sometimes severe. Typically, the lesion presents geographic destruction by a localized deposition of amyloid in sufficient amount simulating bone cyst or other bone tumor in associated with diffuse multiple *"punched-out"* lesions, mimicking hematopoietic lesion such as PCM (Figs. 6.1 and 6.2). Calcification may occur within the amyloid mass, simulating chondrosarcoma [20]. When involving spines, the intervertebral discs are affected and are often associated with endplate erosions that can mimic spondylitis. **MR images** Amyloidoma involving the bone may present geographic lesion with cortical thinning and erosions simulating a bone tumor. Frequently, numerous "*punched-out*" lesions can present when accompanied by myeloma (Fig. 6.1). The amyloidoma lesions show low signals on T1-, and more variable but usually low to intermediate signals on T2-weighted images with gadolinium enhancement. The abnormal material covers the synovial membrane, fills subchondral defects, and extends to periarticular soft tissue. In addition, joint effusions are often present.

6.5 Histologic Findings

Microscopic examination typically displays numerous amorphous pinkish, globular structures within stromal tissue and around the vascular structure. Amyloid deposit can be varying in amount from subtle abundant. When the deposition is so extensive, it may obliterate plasmatoid cells of the myeloma, and multinucleated giant cells of foreign body type can be prominent being reactive to amyloid deposits (Figs. 6.1i, l and 6.2e). Amyloid tumor of bone is very rare, and the presence of amyloid in bone usually indicates myeloma. However, deposit of amyloid-like material has been increasingly reported in patients with CRF on long-term hemodialysis or peritoneal dialysis [10–12]. Amyloidosis is presented in about 10% of patients with myeloma [20]. The diagnosis requires histological confirmation by pink-red amyloid deposits with Congo red stain (Fig. 6.2e) and apple-green birefringence under polarized microscopic examination (Fig. 6.i). IHC staining including CD38 and CD 138 and Kappa and lambda chain are useful tools for a diagnosis of associated myeloma.

6.6 Management

Treatment depends on the type of amyloidosis. Treatments for AL amyloidosis include chemotherapy similar to that used to combat cancer and stem cell transplantation. Management of underlying disease can improve symptoms in AA amyloidosis. For patients with neurologic symptoms, emergency cord decompression is indicated. If involving femoral neck, pathologic fracture will ultimately occur in nearly all these patients, requiring internal fixation or prosthetic replacement. High incidence of nonunion after internal fixation was reported in more than half of the patients [3, 6] because of poor bone quality associated with amyloidosis and CRF on long-term hemodialysis, which may be related to inhibitory effect of amyloid ß2-microglobulin on bone mineralization by osteoblasts [21]. In addition, higher failure rate of prosthetic replacement (35%) due to postoperative infection and loosening was reported in CRF patients on long-term hemodialysis [22]. The authors emphasized that risk-to-benefit ratio of hip arthroplasty is high in patients on hemodialysis who should be informed of the higher risks of arthroplasty. In the femoral neck, prophylactic curettage and bone graft for amyloid bone cysts with 2.5 cm or larger size, destruction over 50% of the femoral cortex, pain on weight-bearing was reported to be successful with the grafts incorporated into the bone defects [23]. Amyloid bone cysts involving other bones in hemodialysis patients can be also successfully treated by curettage and bone graft. For carpal tunnel syndrome, carpal tunnel release is usually successful. However, Kurer et al. [12] reported a high recurrence rate of 23% and disappointing results for recurrent carpal tunnel syndrome and for flexor tendon fibrosis. The amyloid material may infiltrate the tendons and their sheaths as well as the finger or carpal joints [24, 25].

6.7 Clinical Course

Prognosis depends on the type of amyloidosis and the affected organ system. Some varieties of amyloidosis may lead to life-threatening organ failure. The progressively debilitating nature of amyloidosis is at least partly responsible for premature death in affected patients. The presence of congestive heart failure (CHF) was reported to be an important factor. Patients with CHF have a median survival of 4 months but 16 months for patients without CHF [1]. The authors reported death attributed to cardiac involvement in 48% of patients who had died, infection in 8%, and renal failure in 6%.

References

1. Kyle RA, Gertz MA. Primary systemic amyloidosis: clinical and laboratory features in 474 cases. Semin Hematol. 1995;32(1):45–59.
2. Gertz MA, Comenzo R, Falk RH, Fermand JP, Hazenberg BP, Hawkins PN, et al. Definition of organ involvement and treatment response in immunoglobulin light chain amyloidosis (AL): a consensus opinion from the 10th International symposium on amyloid and amyloidosis. Am J Hematol. 2005;79(4):319–28.
3. Pambuccian SE, Horyd ID, Cawte T, Huvos AG. Amyloidoma of bone, a plasma cell/plasmacytoid neoplasm: report of three cases and review of the literature. Am J Surg Pathol. 1997;21(2):179–86.
4. Lipper S, Kahn L. Amyloid tumor: a clinicopathologic study of four cases. Am J Surg Pathol. 1978;2(2):141–6.
5. Lai K, Chan K, Siu D, Wong C, Yeung D. Pathologic hip fractures secondary to amyloidoma: case report and review of the literature. Am J Med. 1984;77(5):937–43.
6. Schonland SO, Hansmann J, Mechtersheimer G, Goldschmidt H, Ho AD, Hegenbart U. Bone involvement in patients with systemic AL amyloidosis mimics lytic myeloma bone disease. Haematologica. 2008;93(6):955–6.
7. Mizuno J, Nakagawa H, Tsuji Y, Yamada T. Primary amyloidoma of the thoracic spine presenting with acute paraplegia. Surg Neurol. 2001;55(6):378–82.
8. Unal A, Sütlap P-N, Kýyýk M. Primary solitary amyloidoma of thoracic spine: a case report and review of the literature. Clin Neurol Neurosurg. 2003;105(3):167–9.
9. Hay N, Mahony J. Pathological hip fracture due to amyloidosis occurring after successful renal transplantation. A case report. Int J Artif Organs. 1994;17(2):74–5.
10. Casey TT, Stone WJ, Diraimondo CR, Brantley BD, Diraimondo CV, Gorevic PD, et al. Tumoral amyloidosis of bone of beta2-microglobulin origin in association with long-term hemodialysis: a new type of amyloid disease. Human Pathol. 1986;17(7):731–8.
11. Drüeke T, Touam M, Zingraff J. Dialysis-associated amyloidosis. Adv Ren Replace Ther. 1995;2(1):24–39.
12. Kurer M, Baillod R, Madgwick J. Musculoskeletal manifestations of amyloidosis. A review of 83 patients on haemodialysis for at least 10 years. J Bone Joint Surg (Br). 1991;73(2):271–6.
13. Gielen J, Van Holsbeeck M, Hauglustaine D, Verresen L, Verbeken E, Baert A, et al. Growing bone cysts in long-term hemodialysis. Skeletal Radiol. 1990;19(1):43–9.
14. Merlini G, Bellotti V. Molecular mechanisms of amyloidosis. N Engl J Med. 2003;349(6):583–96.
15. Kyle RA, Rajkumar SV. Epidemiology of the plasma-cell disorders. Best Pract Res Clin Haematol. 2007;20(4):637–64.
16. Bardin T, Kuntz D, Zingraff J, Voisin MC, Zelmar A, Lansaman J. Synovial amyloidosis in patients undergoing long-term hemodialysis. Arthritis Rheum. 1985;28(9):1052–8.
17. Hardouin P, Flipo R, Foissac-Gegoux P, Lecomte-Houcke M, Duquesnoy B, Delcambre B. Current aspects of osteoarticular pathology of hemodialyzed patients. Study of a population of 80 patients. Rev Rhum Mal Osteoartic. 1987;54(6):469–73.
18. McCarthy E. Amyloidosis in bone. In: Santini-Araujo E, Kalil R, Bertoni F, Park YK, editors. Tumors and tumor-like lesions of bone. London: Springer; 2015. https://doi.org/10.1007/978-1-4471-6578-1_70.
19. Piette WW. Myeloma, paraproteinemias, and the skin. Med Clin North Am. 1986;70(1):155–76.
20. Unni K, Inwards Y. Myeloma. In: Dahlin's bone tumors: general aspects and data on 10,165 cases. Philadelphia, PA: Lippincott Williams & Wilkins; 2010. p. 191–200.
21. Kataoka H, Gejyo F, Yamada S, Kunitomo T, Arakawa M. Inhibitory effects of β2-microglobulin on invitro calcification of osteoblastic cells. Biochem Biophysic Res Comm. 1986;141(1):360–6.
22. Naito M, Ogata K, Shiota E, Nakamoto M, Goya T. Hip arthroplasty in haemodialysis patients. J Bone Joint Surg (Br). 1994;76(3):428–31.
23. Naito M, Ogata K, Shiota E, Oyama M. Amyloid bone cysts of the femoral neck. Impending fractures treated by curettage and bone grafting. J Bone Joint Surg (Br). 1994;76(6):922–5.
24. Charra B, Calemard E, Laurent G. Chronic renal failure treatment duration and mode: their relevance to the late dialysis periarticular syndrome. Blood Purif. 1988;6(2):117–24.
25. Clanet M, Mansat M, Durroux R, Testut M, Guiraud B, Rascol A, et al. Carpal tunnel syndrome, amyloid tenosynovitis and periodic hemodialysis. Rev Neurol. 1981;137(10):613–24.

7 Solitary Plasmacytoma

7.1 Definition

Solitary plasmacytoma (SP) is a rare single localized tumor consisting of a mass of neoplastic proliferation of a single clone of plasma cells in a single bone or soft tissue without evidence of systemic disease attributing to plasma cell myeloma (PCM). It is categorized into two main types of solitary bone plasmacytoma (SBP) and solitary extramedullary plasmacytoma (SEP).

7.2 Age

The tumor usually occurs in the middle-aged and elderly people with median age at diagnosis of 55–65 years that is a decade younger than that of people with PCM [1–3]. It is very rare under the age of 30.

7.3 Incidence

SPB is uncommon representing about 5% of all of the plasma cell disorders [1, 2, 4, 5]. SEP is even less frequent, only occupying 2% of plasma cell disoders [5]. A population-based analysis in 1691 patients with SP on Surveillance, Epidemiology and End Results (SEER) database from 1998 to 2007 showed 60% had) SBP, 30% had SEP, and unspecified plasmacytoma was noted in the rest 10% of patients [3].

7.4 Location

SBP most commonly occurs in the bones of the axial skeleton including vertebra and skull. Thoracic vertebra is more frequently affected than cervical or lumbar vertebra. Other commonly involved bones are pelvis, ribs, sternum, clavicle, and scapula as well as long bones above knee and elbow including femur and humerus. SEP is generally found in mucous membrane, the head, and neck, particularly in the mucous membranes of the upper airways (nose, throat and sinuses) and less commonly seen in gastrointestinal tract, lymph nodes, bladder, or lung.

7.5 Clinical Features and Diagnostic Analysis

Although some patients can be found incidentally on imaging studies for other reasons (Fig. 7.1), most patients present localized bone pain or painful mass or swelling and occasionally pathologic fracture due to bone destruction by the infiltrating plasma cells (Figs. 7.2, 7.3). Nasal stuffiness can be presented when the lesion involved nasopharyngeal area (Fig. 7.3a). Root or spinal cord compression by the tumor mass can produce radiating pain or muscle weakness. Diagnostic analysis includes history, physical examination, complete blood count, bone marrow biopsy, serum/urine immunoelectrophoresis

W.-J. Bahk, *Diagnosis and Management of Primary Bone Tumors*,
https://doi.org/10.1007/978-981-99-5498-8_7

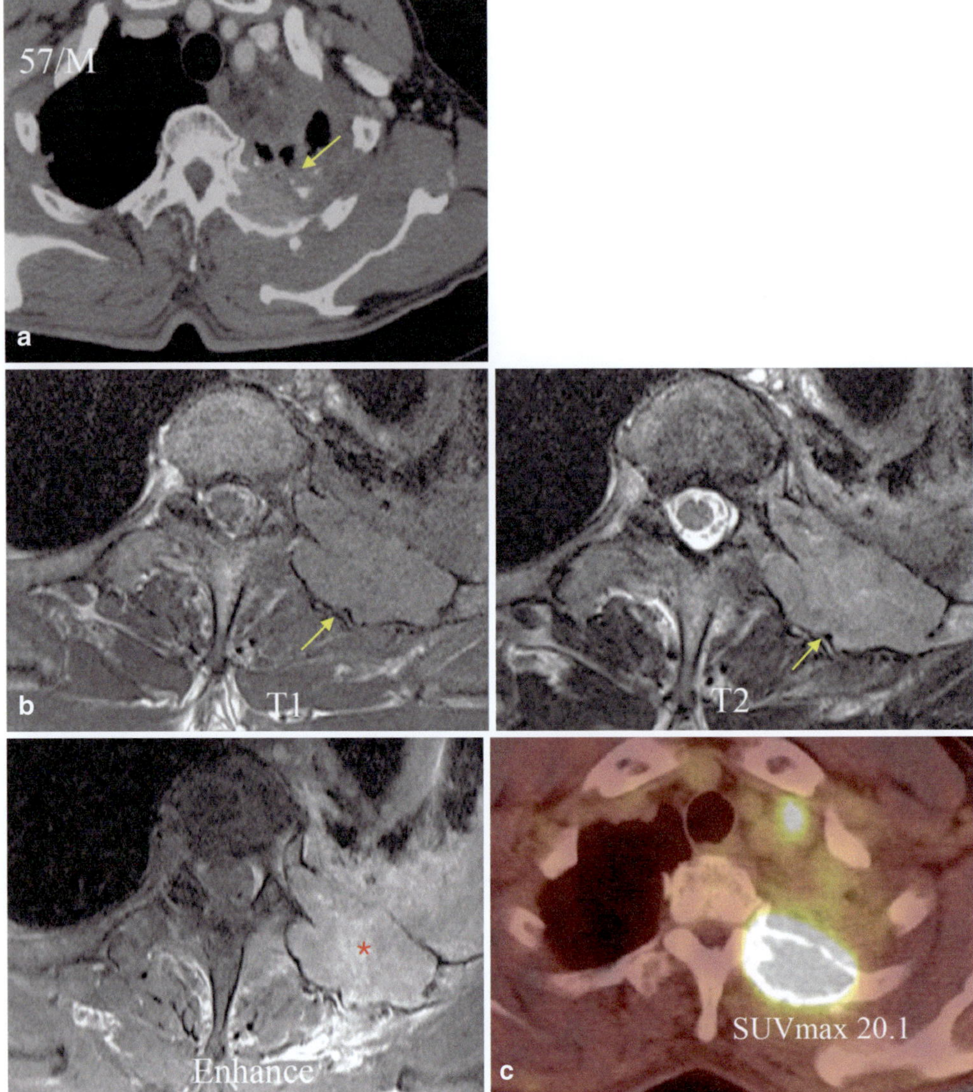

Fig. 7.1 ***Incidentally found SBP*** (**a**) Chest CT scan taken for hemoptysis in 57-year-old man incidentally shows an expansile, geographic destruction with soft tissue density in the transverse process of D3 vertebra and a part of posterior arc left third rib (yellow arrow). (**b**) MR images demonstrate a relatively well-defined medullary mass-like lesion forming a soft tissue mass with heterogeneous intermediate and high SI on T1-weighted image and intermediate to high SI on T2-weighted image. The soft tissue mass is surrounded by a thin dark signal of reactive rim (yellow arrows). The lesion is diffusely enhanced (red asterisk). (**c**) PET/CT scan reveals a hypermetabolic lesion (SUVmax 20.1) only in the area presented on the CT scan and MR images but in no other areas indicating a solitary lesion. (**d**) Serum IEP shows a faint band in the gamma globulin region with little concentration of M-protein (0.4 g/dL). (**e**) Microscopic examination of biopsy specimen notes neoplastic monoclonal proliferation of plasma cells, which replace the normal bone marrow. Bone marrow biopsy shows normocellular with 2% plasma cells. Based on the findings of single focus of bone lesion, microscopic finding of monoclonal proliferation of malignant plasma cells, but no evidence of myeloma on bone marrow biopsy, and no systemic manifestations of CRAB as well as little M-protein in serum, the final diagnosis of SBP was rendered, and radiotherapy was performed. (**f**) Bone scan at 3 years after irradiation reveals an ill-defined mild uptake only in the corresponding area (arrow) but no other bones. (**g**) The serum M-protein level has been continued to be little (0.2 g/dL) after irradiation. (**h**) Follow-up serum IEP at 9 years after radiotherapy shows no change of a faint band in the gamma globulin region but with little concentration of M-protein (0.2 g/dL). (**i**) Follow-up CT scan at 9 years after irradiation shows consolidation and stabilization of the lesion with thickening of cortex (red arrows) and internal sclerotic change. Follow-up bone scan also shows no newly developed abnormal uptake in other bones. He is doing well with no local recurrence and progression to systemic disease

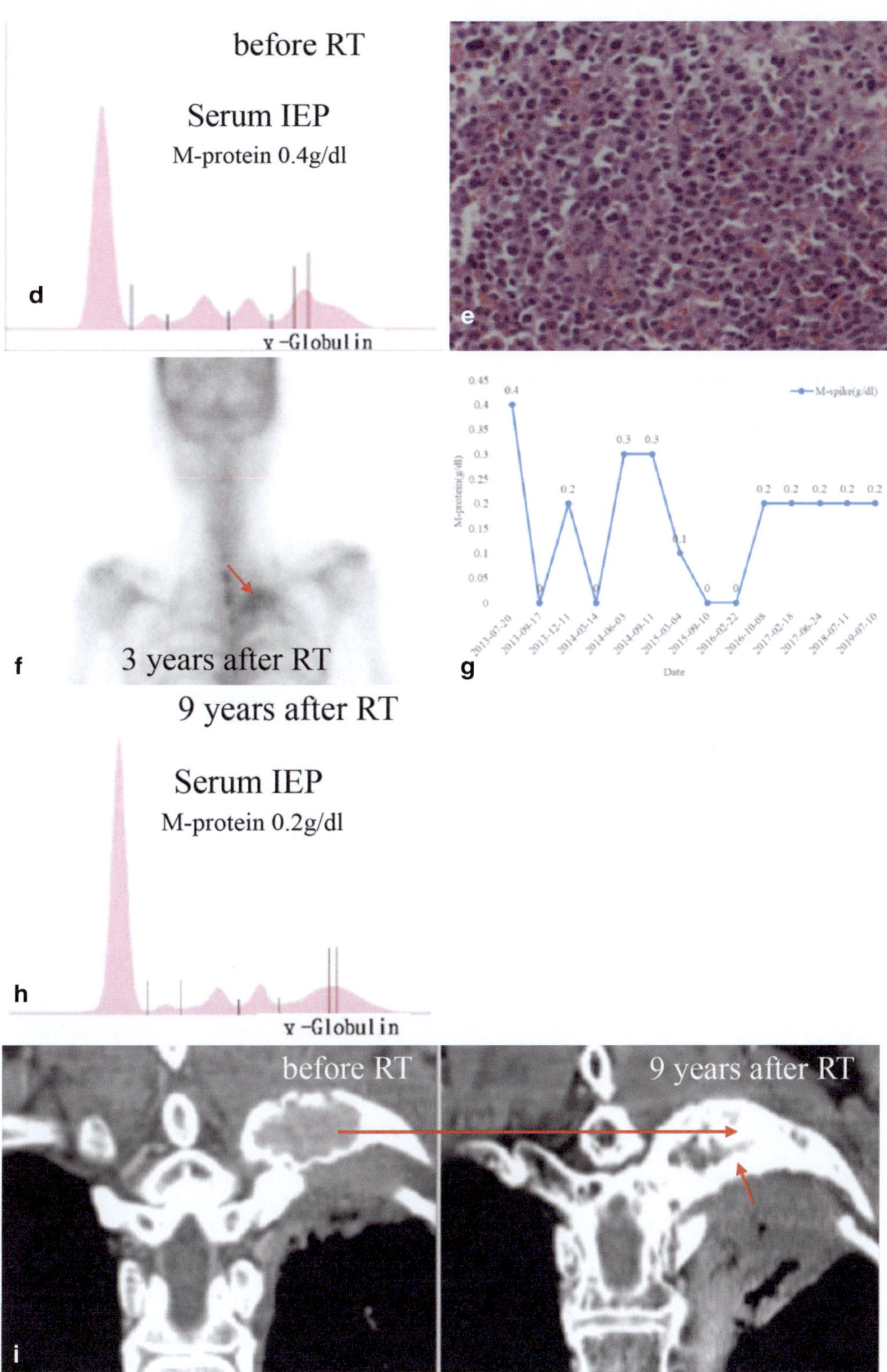

Fig. 7.1 (continued)

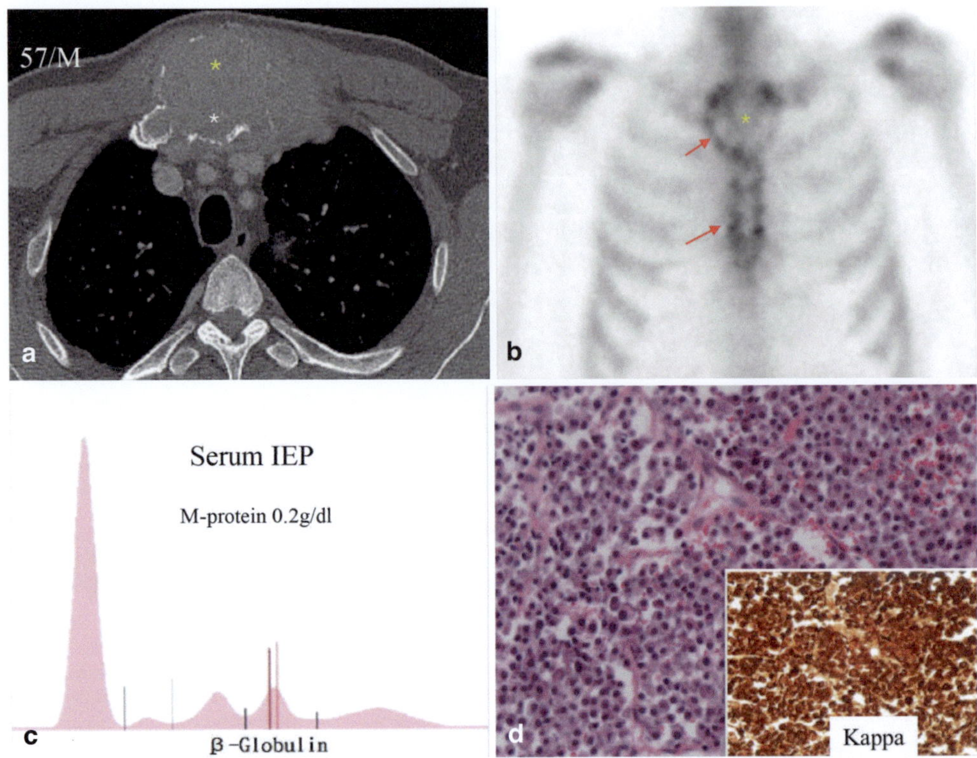

Fig. 7.2 ***SBP progressed to PCM*** (**a**) CT scan taken for sternal swelling of 18-month duration in 57-year-old man shows an expansile osteolytic destruction in the sternal manubrium and body (white asterisk) with cortical breakage and formation of large soft tissue mass (yellow asterisk). (**b**) Bone scan reveals heterogeneous marginal uptake (arrows) in the sternal manubrium and body with a photon defect area in the center (asterisk). No abnormal bony activity is seen in other bones at this time. (**c**) Serum IEP notes a faint band in the beta region suspecting a potential monoclonal gammopathy with a very low concentration of M-protein (0.2 g/dL), and IFE indicates a monoclonal gammopathy of IgE/kappa isotype. Urine IEP shows a prominent monoclonal band in the gamma region, and IFE indicates Bence-Jones proteinuria of kappa type. Bone marrow biopsy reveals clonal plasma cells less than 5% of all nucleated elements. (**d**) Microscopic examination shows neoplastic proliferation of dense monotonous plasmatoid tumor cells replacing bone marrow elements. ICH stain for kappa light chain is strongly positive (inset). PET CT noted a hypermetabolic lesion (SUVmax 17.2) in the sternal area but in no other areas indicating a solitary lesion (not shown here). A diagnosis of SBP of sternum is rendered when considering no other lesions in the bone or in the soft tissues on image studies, less than 5% of plasma cells on bone marrow biopsy, no signs of CRAB, and little serum M-protein (0.2 g/dL). Irradiation was performed over the sternal area. (**e**) Follow-up PET/CT scan at 2 months after irradiation demonstrates a stabilization of the lesion with a deceased size and surrounding reactive bone formation with significanly reduced SUVmax of 2.2 from 17.2 (white arrow). No other hyperactive lesion is seen in other bones or organs. (**f**) Follow-up chest CT scan at 5 years after irradiation shows restoration of the bone contour with thick surrounding new bone (arrow). (**g**) Follow-up bone scan taken for right arm pain at 9 months after irradiation reveals newly developed multiple bone lesions including right clavicle and humeral shaft as well as left clavicle and ribs, indicating multifocal dissemination of disease. (**h**) Radiographs show geographic and ill-defined moth-eaten destruction with no definite fracture in the humeral shaft (yellow arrow) and lateral ends of both clavicles (red circles). (**i**) Pathologic fracture is developed in the humerus shaft (arrow) by lifting of a heavy object while waiting for MRI evaluation. (**j**) MR images demonstrate marrow replacing mass-like lesion with angulation by a pathologic fracture. The SI is low on T1-weighted image and intermediate to high SI on T2-weighted image with heterogeneous enhancement. (**k**) Although serum M-protein level becomes zero, the disease progresses to multiple foci on follow-up bone scan. (**l**) Microscopic examination of curetted specimen shows different findings of variable-sized cells with more significant pleomorphism in size and shape when compared to initial pathologic findings (**d**). Bone marrow biopsy also shows significantly increased clonal plasma cells to more than 15% of all nucleated elements, which was initially less than 5%. A diagnosis of SBP progressed to PCM was rendered. (**m**) The lesion was managed by curettage and cementation with plate fixation followed by chemotherapy and autogenous BMT. (**n**) Follow-up radiograph at 4 years after surgery shows loosening of distal screws with mild angulation (arrow) but no evidence of local recurrence. And he is doing well without arm pain. However, there are newly developed lesions in other bones on follow-up PET/CT scan but no symptoms. He is alive with disease at 5 years after irradiation

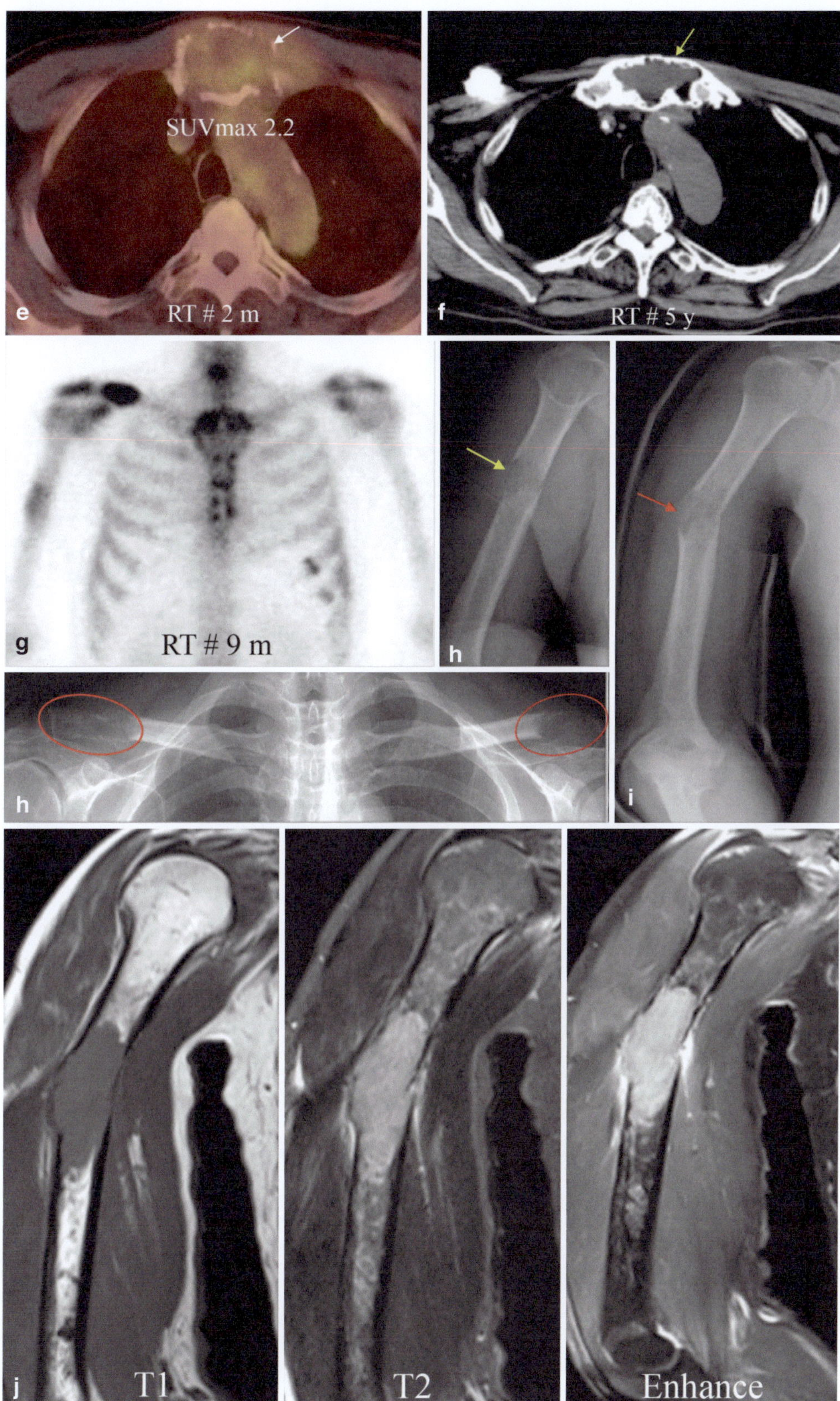

Fig. 7.2 (continued)

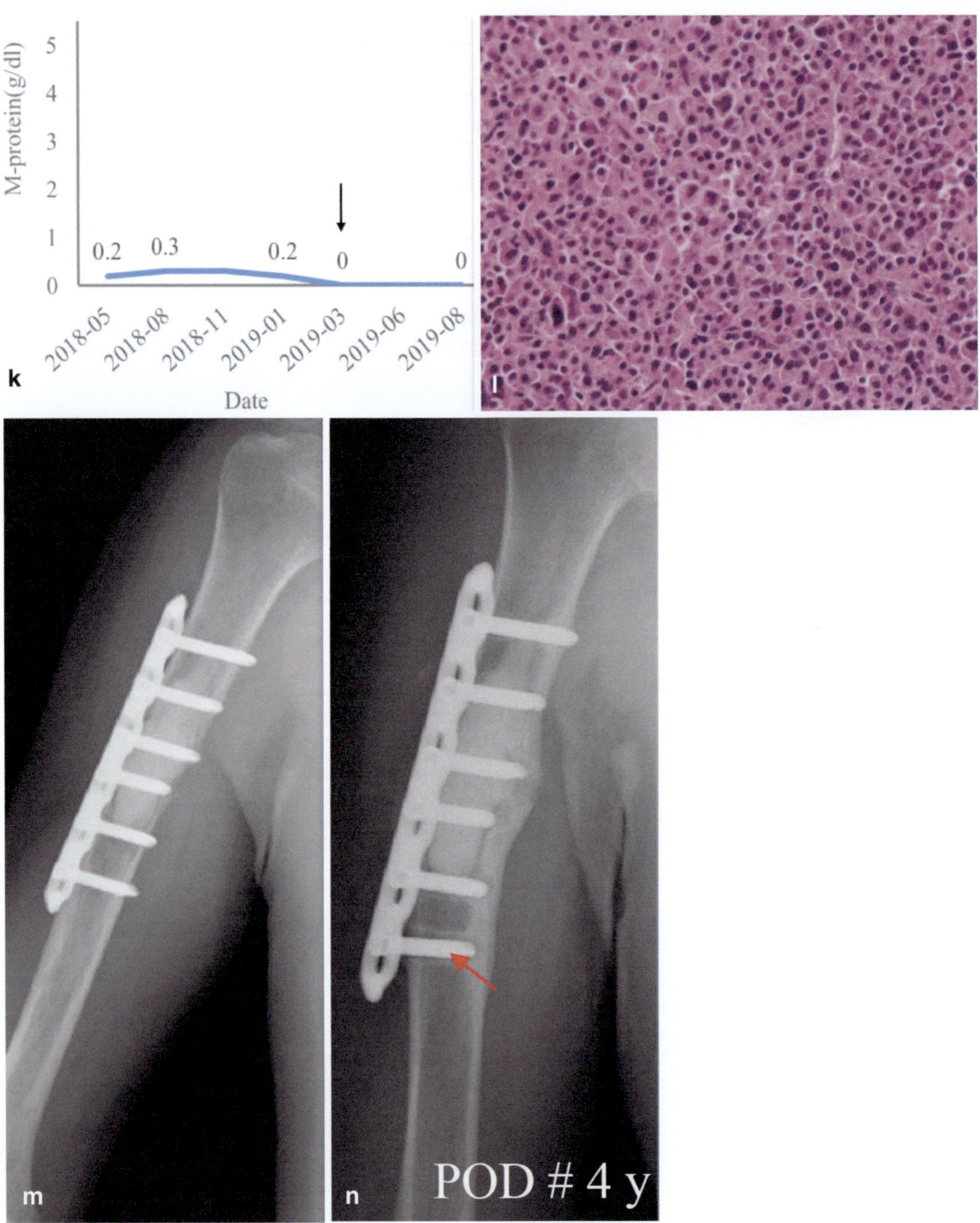

Fig. 7.2 (continued)

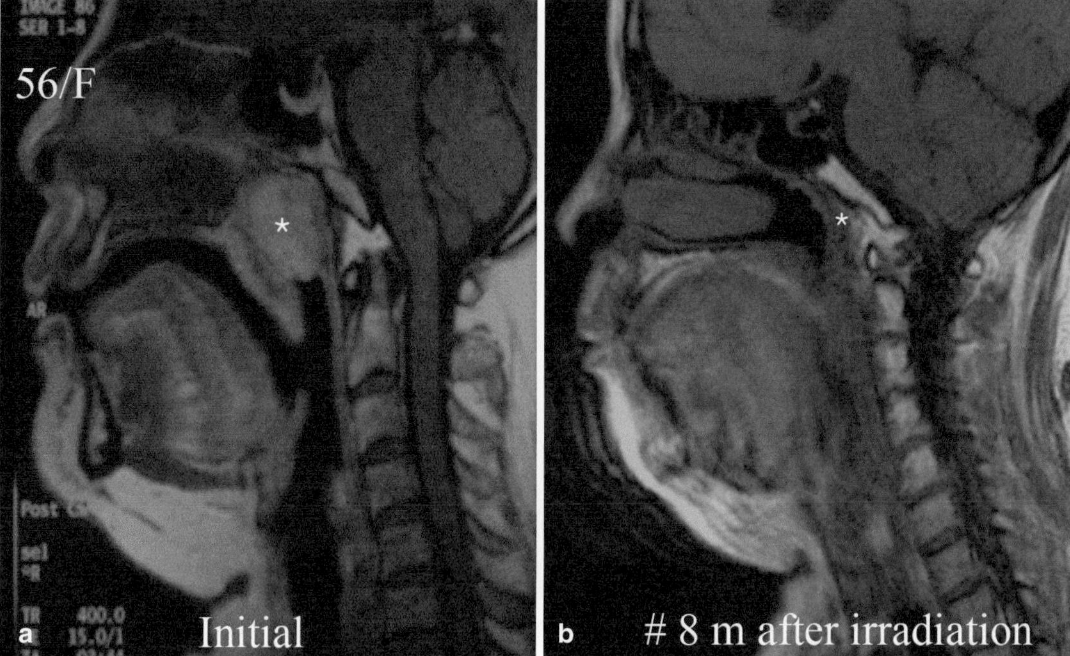

Fig. 7.3 ***EMP progreesed to PCM*** (**a**) MR image taken for nasal stuffiness of 6-month duration in 56-year-old woman at department of ENT shows a well-demarcated soft tissue mass but no bone involvement with good enhancement in the nasopharyngeal area (asterisk). Microscopic examination of biopsied specimen confirms a diagnosis of plasma cell neoplasm. However, serum and urine IEP reveal no diagnostic abnormality without M-protein detection. Bone marrow biopsy reveals no remarkable findings of disease involvement. There is normal skeletal survey and no end organ damage other than this solitary lesion. A diagnosis of SEP was rendered, and external irradiation was applied. (**b**) Follow-up MR image at 8 months after radiotherapy shows complete remission of the mass (asterisk). She has been doing very well without any symptoms. (**c**) Six years later, radiographs taken for newly developed finger pain reveal destruction of distal phalanx of right thumb and middle phalanx of left little finger (asterisks). (**d**) In addition, radiograph and CT scan taken for severe pain of right clavicle area by lifting of heavy object 2 days later while waiting for MRI evaluation of hand show a radiolucent lesion with pathologic fracture in the mid-shaft of right clavicle (yellow arrows). (**e**) MR images demonstrates a large bone marrow replacing lesion involving entire distal phalanx of left thumb with low SI on T1-weighted image and low to intermediate SI on T2-weighted image. The lesion is partially well enhanced (red arrow). (**f**) PET/CT scan shows multiple hypermetabolic bony lesions in the sternal body (SUVmax 12.5), right clavicle (SUVmax 6.29), thumbs, and tibias as well as spleen, splenic hilar lymph nodes, and gastric fundus. (**g**) Microscopic examination of specimen from resection of fractured clavicle shows a dense plasma cell proliferation with significant pleomorphism in size and shape. Serum IEP reveals a prominent monoclonal band in the gamma globulin region suggesting monoclonal gammopathy with concentration of serum M-protein (2.7 g/dL), and IFE indicates a monoclonal gammopathy of IgG/kappa isotype. Based on findings of involvement of multiple bones and other organs including spleen and multiple lymph node on PET/CT scan, histologic findings of poorly differentiated plasma cells proliferation as well as abnormal serum IEP and IFE, a diagnosis of PCM progressed from the SEP originally confined to the nasopharyngeal area has been rendered. She died of disease at 7 years after initial diagnosis of SBP and 10 months after progression to PCM

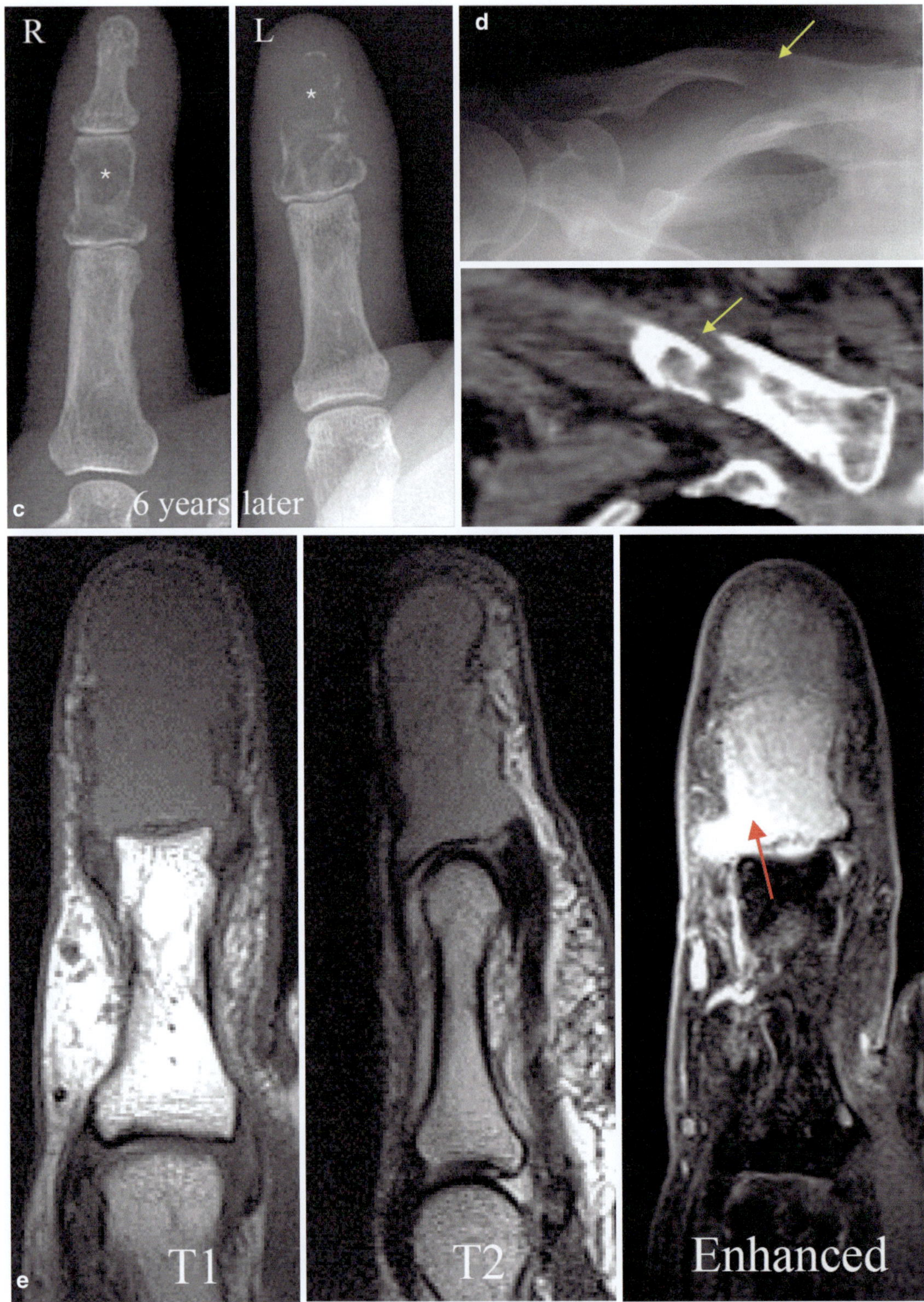

Fig. 7.3 (continued)

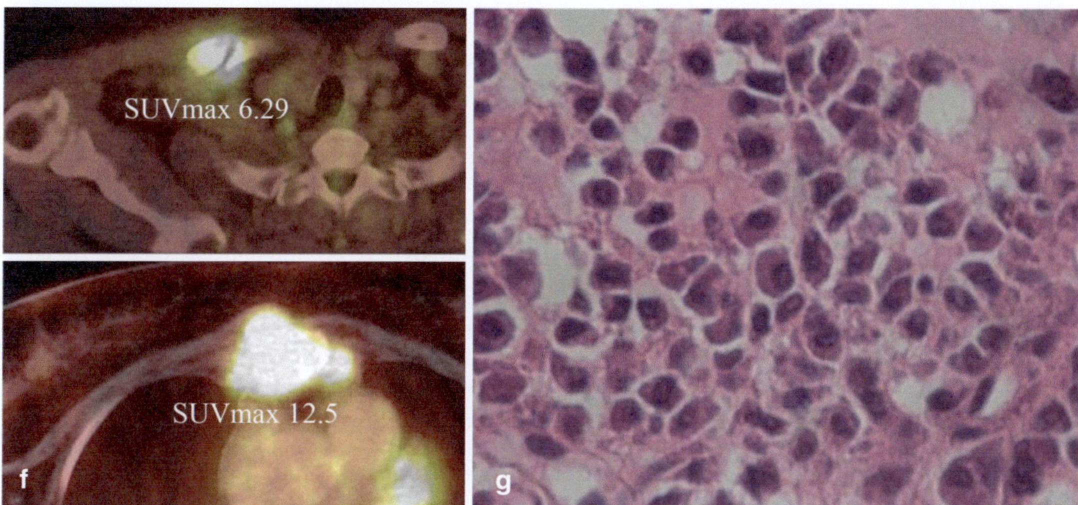

Fig. 7.3 (continued)

(IEP), evaluation of the urine for myeloma protein, and survey to exclude systemic manifestations of CRAB (increased calcium, renal insufficiency, anemia, or multiple bone lesions) due to myeloma. The diagnosis of SBP requires (a) a single area of bone destruction with no radiologic evidence of additional skeletal lesions confirmed by radiographs, MR images, PET/CT scan, and bone scan; (b) histologic finding of a localized proliferation of neoplastic monoclonal plasma cells; (c) no or little M-protein in serum/urine IEP; (d) lack of myeloma-related organ dysfunction (CRAB); and (e) bone marrow examination of morphologically normal or a very low clonal PC infiltration (less than 10%) [6, 7].

7.6 Radiologic Findings

SBP is typically well-defined, round to oval, *"punched-out"* lesion, predominantly osteolytic destruction as with PCM. There is absence of internal density and sclerotic reaction. The lesion is solitary and expansile with sharp or ill-defined margin. The cortex can be eroded, thinned, or destructed margin frequently with extraosseous soft tissue mass formation simulating metastatic cancer. It may exhibit a *"soap-bubble"* or *"trabeculated"* appearance with thick ridging around the periphery in advanced some cases. **Bone scan** frequently shows negative finding despite the extensive bone destruction. Thus, bone scan is not adequate for the workup in suspected or established disseminated myeloma. **PET/CT scan** is effective in detecting the distribution of the active myeloma both within bone and at extramedullary sites. It is useful to detect the solitary involvement of the disease with exclusion of the systemic distribution attributing to PCM (Fig. 7.1c). **CT scan** clearly demonstrates expansile lytic lesion with cortical thinning or destruction producing a soft tissue mass. CT scan also may can reveal thickening cortex as well as a rim of surrounding reactive sclerosis suggesting a less aggressive nature of SBP. **MR images** demonstrate an expansile mass-like lesion with low to intermediate SI on T1-weighted image and intermediate to high SI on T2-weighted image, and the lesion is usually heterogeneously enhanced (Figs. 7.1, 7.2 and 7.3). An interesting finding of curvilinear structures with low signal extending partially through the vertebral body on axial images, which suggest compensatory cortical thickening, has been described. The structures resemble the sulci seen in the brain and are named as a *"mini brain"* appearance, being thought to be pathognomonic for SBP in a vertebral body [8]. **Histologic findings** are identical to PCM and consist of sheets of monoclonal proliferation of malignant plasma cells, which replace the normal bone marrow. The lesions may contain mature, immature, plasmablastic, or even anaplastic plasma cells (Figs. 7.1, 7.2 and 7.3). Amyloid deposit can be also seen as pink amorphous material with scattered multinucleated giant cells in some cases.

7.7 Management

SP is a highly radiosensitive tumor, and radiation therapy (RT) is the first line of treatment in most patients with both types (SBP and SEP) providing a more an excellent local control rate compared to both surgery and chemotherapy as the only option for treatment [1, 7, 9, 10]. Surgical intervention is indicated for skeletal instability, impending, or pathologic fracture, rapidly progressive neurological symptoms due to spinal cord compression. Postoperative radiotherapy may be necessary to eradicate microscopic residual disease. Based on a large population study with SEER database, the authors concluded that combined therapy of RT and surgery is beneficial in axial plasmacytoma [3]. However, adjuvant chemotherapy has no beneficial effect on disease control or prevention of progression to PCM [11, 12].

7.8 Clinical Course

Three patterns of failure including local recurrence, development of new bone lesions in the absence of PCM, and development of PCM can be expected [13]. Although high rate of local control can be achieved with RT and/or surgery, progression to multifocal disseminated disease is still frequent, and 70–75% of patients who received RT have been reported to become PCM [3, 7]. Survival is closely related to the likelihood of developing PCM. Therefore, the parameters that influence progression to multifocal disease are likely to affect survival [14]. However, there is no clear evidence on the factors predicting the progression of SP into myeloma attributed to the low incidence of the disease and the lack of randomized controlled studies, although several parameters such as age over 60 years, size and number of involvements of the tumor, and persistence of M protein after treatment were reported to be indicating factors of a worse prognosis [3]. The progress rate to PCM is much lower in SEP than in SBP. A comprehensive review of large number of the patients with SEP in more than 400 publications between 1905 and 1997 reported that over 60% had no local recurrence or conversion to systemic involvement (PCM), about 20% had local recurrence, and some 15% had conversion to PCM [15]. However, SBP has been reported up to 70% of cases eventually progress to PCM usually within 3 years of initial diagnosis [9, 16–22]. Rarely, SBP may not progress to PCM for an extended period (15–35 years) [23]. Thus, every patient with SBP should be regularly monitored by lifelong follow-up with laboratory tests and imaging studies.

References

1. Dimopoulos MA, Kiamouris C, Moulopoulos LA. Solitary plasmacytoma of bone and extramedullary plasmacytoma. Hematol Oncol Clin North Am. 1999;13(6):1249–57.
2. Dimopoulos MA, Moulopoulos LA, Maniatis A, Alexanian R. Solitary plasmacytoma of bone and asymptomatic multiple myeloma. Blood. 2000;96(6):2037–44.
3. Thumallapally N, Meshref A, Mousa M, Terjanian T. Solitary plasmacytoma: population-based analysis of survival trends and effect of various treatment modalities in the USA. BMC Cancer. 2017;17(1):1–11.
4. Tong D, Griffin T, Laramore G, Kurtz J, Russell A, Groudine M, et al. Solitary plasmacytoma of bone and soft tissues. Radiology. 1980;135(1):195–8.
5. Liebross RH, Ha CS, Cox JD, Weber D, Delasalle K, Alexanian R. Clinical course of solitary extramedullary plasmacytoma. Radiother Oncol. 1999;52(3):245–9.
6. Rajkumar SV, Dimopoulos MA, Palumbo A, Blade J, Merlini G, Mateos M-V, et al. International myeloma working group updated criteria for the diagnosis of multiple myeloma. Lancet Oncol. 2014;15(12):e538–e48.
7. Soutar R, Lucraft H, Jackson G, Reece A, Bird J, Low E, Guidelines Working Group of the UK Myeloma Forum; British Committee for Standards

in Haematology; British Society for Haematology, et al. Guidelines on the diagnosis and management of solitary plasmacytoma of bone and solitary extramedullary plasmacytoma. Br J Haematol. 2004;124(6):717–26.
8. Major NM, Helms CA, Richardson WJ. The "mini brain" plasmacytoma in a vertebral body on MR imaging. Am J Roentgenol. 2000;175(1):261–3.
9. Knobel D, Zouhair A, Tsang RW, Poortmans P, Belkacémi Y, Bolla M, et al. Prognostic factors in solitary plasmacytoma of the bone: a multicenter rare cancer network study. BMC Cancer. 2006;6(1):1–9.
10. Hu K, Yahalom J. Radiotherapy in the management of plasma cell tumors. Oncology (Williston Park). 2000;14(1):101–8; 11; discussion 11.
11. Galieni P, Cavo M, Avvisati G, Pulsoni A, Falbo R, Bonelli M, et al. Solitary plasmacytoma of bone and extramedullary plasmacytoma: two different entities? Ann Oncol. 1995;6(7):687–91.
12. Shih L, Dunn P, Leung W, Chen W, Wang P. Localised plasmacytomas in Taiwan: comparison between extramedullary plasmacytoma and solitary plasmacytoma of bone. Br J Cancer. 1995;71(1):128–33.
13. Kyle RA. Monoclonal gammopathy of undetermined significance and solitary plasmacytoma: implications for progression to overt multiple myeloma. Hematol Oncol Clin North Am. 1997;11(1):71–87.
14. Mendenhall WM, Mendenhall CM, Mendenhall NP. Solitary plasmacytoma of bone and soft tissues. Am J Otolaryngol. 2003;24(6):395–9.
15. Alexiou C, Kau RJ, Dietzfelbinger H, Kremer M, Spieß JC, Schratzenstaller B, et al. Extramedullary plasmacytoma: tumor occurrence and therapeutic concepts. Cancer. 1999;85(11):2305–14.
16. Wiltshaw E. The natural history of extramedullary plasmacytoma and its relation to solitary myeloma of bone and myelomatosis. Medicine. 1976;55(3):217–38.
17. Wollersheim H, Holdrinet R, Haanen C. Clinical course and survival in 16 patients with localized plasmacytoma. Scand J Haematol. 1984;32(4):423–8.
18. Bolek TW, Marcus RB Jr, Mendenhall NP. Solitary plasmacytoma of bone and soft tissue. Int J Radiat Oncol Biol Phys. 1996;36(2):329–33.
19. Holland J, Trenkner DA, Wasserman TH, Fineberg B. Plasmacytoma. Treatment results and conversion to myeloma. Cancer. 1992;69(6):1513–7.
20. Kumar S, Fonseca R, Dispenzieri A, Lacy MQ, Lust JA, Wellik L, et al. Prognostic value of angiogenesis in solitary bone plasmacytoma. Blood. 2003;101(5):1715–7.
21. Frassica DA, Frassica FJ, Schray MF, Sim FH, Kyle RA. Solitary plasmacytoma of bone: Mayo Clinic experience. Int J Radiat Oncol Biol Phys. 1989;16(1):43–8.
22. Kilciksiz S, Celik OK, Pak Y, Demiral AN, Pehlivan M, Orhan O, et al. Clinical and prognostic features of plasmacytomas: a multicenter study of Turkish oncology group-sarcoma working party. Am J Hematol. 2008;83(9):702–7.
23. Dorfman HD, Czerniak B. Immunohematopoietic tumors. In: Dorfman HD, Czerniak B. editors. bone tumors. St. Louis: Mosby; 1998. p.644–679.

Lymphoma of Bone

8

(*Lympha* "Water, Fluid" + *Ōma* "Forming")

8.1 Definition

Lymphocytes are one of several different types of white blood cells made by bone marrow, which move to the lymphatic system such as spleen, tonsils, and lymph nodes. They include *natural killer cells,* also known as *NK cells* or *large granular lymphocytes* (cell-mediated, cytotoxic innate immunity to destroy viruses and some cancer cells), *T cells* (cell-mediated, cytotoxic adaptive immunity to destroy viruses and foreign cells with triggering the B cells to make antibodies), and *B cells* (humoral, antibody-driven adaptive immunity to make antibodies that fight bacteria and other infections). Lymphoma is a cancer that arises from lymphocytes and usually starts in the lymph nodes. However, primary lymphoma of bone (PLB) originates in bone and produces one or more masses within single or multiple bone marrow(s) without evidence of involvement of regional lymph nodes and extra-nodal sites. PLB is distinct from lymphoma that is started in the lymph nodes and then spread to the bones (bone metastases). Generalized disease may subsequently develop. Conventionally, an interval of 4–6 months between skeletal manifestation and the development of extra-skeletal lesion is necessary for the lesion to be a primary tumor in bone [1]. PLB is mostly *non-Hodgkin's lymphoma or diffuse large B-cell lymphoma* (DLBL) (Figs. 8.1, 8.2, and 8.3), rarely *NK/T cell lymphoma* (Fig. 8.4), *anaplastic large cell lymphoma* (ALCL) of T-cell or null cell lineage (Fig. 8.5), and *Hodgkin's lymphoma* (Fig. 8.6).

W.-J. Bahk, *Diagnosis and Management of Primary Bone Tumors*,
https://doi.org/10.1007/978-981-99-5498-8_8

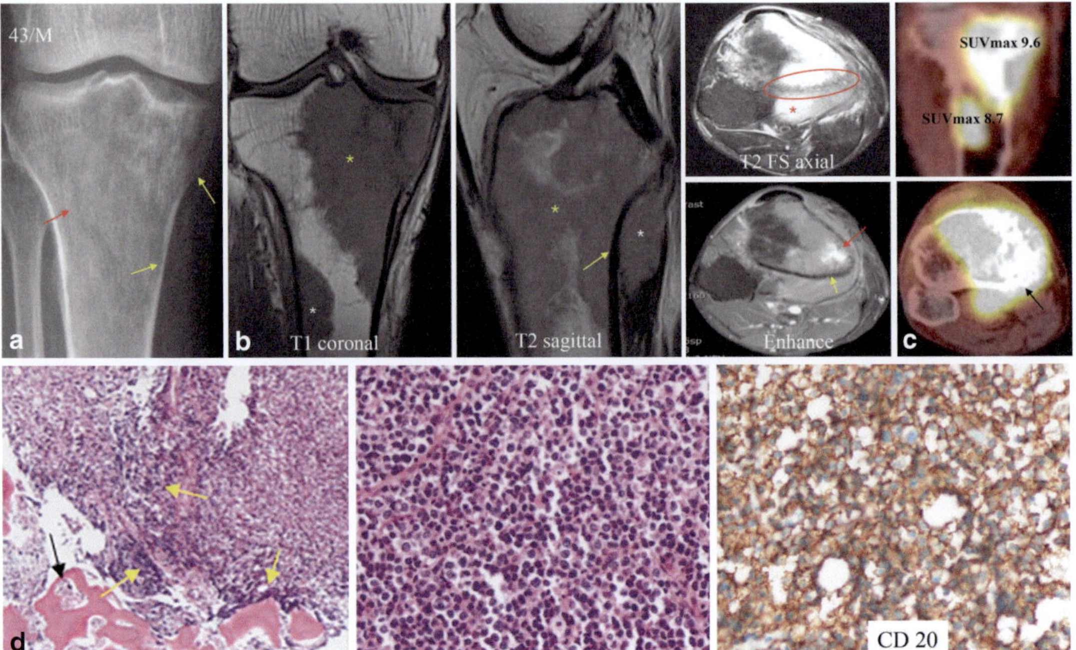

Fig. 8.1 ***Diffuse large B-cell lymphoma in a single bone***. (**a**) Radiograph taken for right knee pain of 2-month duration in 43-year-old man shows an ill-defined, osteolytic lesion mixed with sclerotic areas (mixed lytic and blastic lesion) affecting epi/metaphysis of proximal tibia (red arrow). The margin is infiltrative with wide zone of transition. There is cortical thinning with subtle to mild breach at the medial cortex (yellow arrows). (**b**) T1-weighted coronal MR image demonstrates a larger infiltrative medullary lesion (yellow asterisk) and another smaller satellite lesion with low SI (white asterisk) that is not clearly discernible on radiograph. T2-weighted sagittal image reveals a huge medullary replacing lesion with heterogeneous intermediated and focal high SI (yellow asterisk) and large soft tissue mass with intermediate SI (white asterisk) but no definite cortical destruction (arrow). Note numerous linear foci of high signal penetrating the posterior cortex with intact cortical architecture (red circle), so-called *"penetrating tunnels"* and a large soft tissue mass with intermediate and high SI (red asterisk) on fat saturated T2-weighted axial image as in Ewing's sarcoma. The lesion is partially enhanced (red arrow), and the tiny tunnels are also enhanced by the contrast media (yellow arrow). (**c**) PET/CT scan demonstrates an intense large FDG accumulation with extra-osseous extension at medial epi/metaphysis of proximal tibia (SUVmax 9.6) and another intense focal FDG accumulation at meta-diaphysis of proximal tibia (SUVmax 8.7). The lesion with an intense FDG uptake extends posteriorly to surrounding soft tissue through tiny cortical tunnels (black arrow). There is no evidence of abnormal FDG uptakes in other bones as well as regional lymph node or extra-nodal organs in the head, neck, chest, and abdomen, indicating a single bone lesion. (**d**) Microscopic examination. (Left) Low-power magnification shows a diffuse bone marrow replacement by small round blue cells. There are a few remained bony trabeculae in which tumor cells fill up the marrow space. Note crush artifacts (yellow arrows), which can be frequently seen in PLB. (Middle) Higher-power magnification reveals a not-cohesive diffuse sheet of tumor cells having round to oval nuclei of relatively uniformed size and shape with distinct cytoplasmic border. (Right) IHC stain for CD20, B-cell lymphocyte marker, is positive. Diffuse large B-cells lymphoma of tibia is finally rendered. He is doing well with complete remission of PLB at 3 years after chemotherapy in the Department of Hematoncology

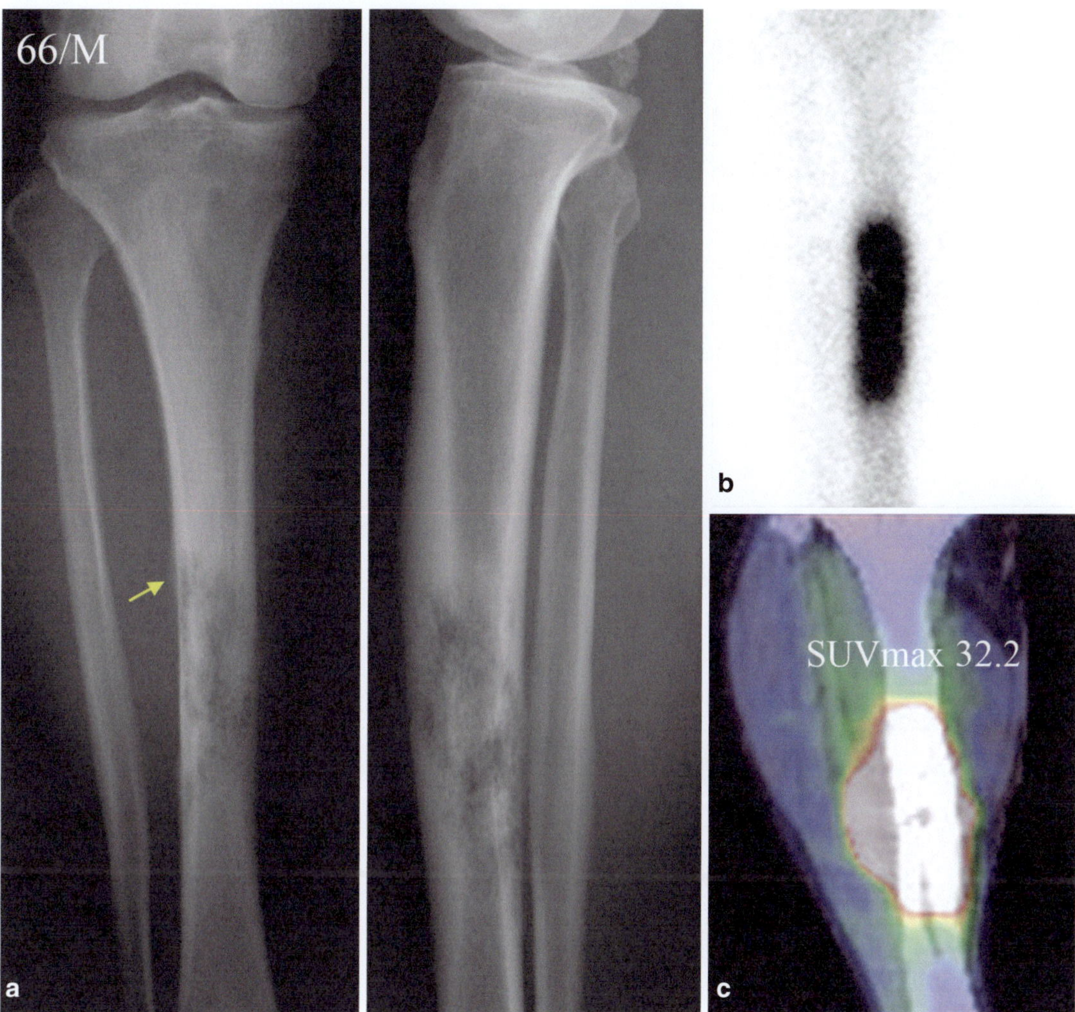

Fig. 8.2 ***Diffuse large B-cell lymphoma in a single bone***. (**a**) Radiographs taken for right leg pain of 3-month duration in 66-year-old man show an ill-defined moth-eaten to permeative destruction in both medulla and cortex of tibia mid-shaft with segmental faint periosteal reaction, so-called Codman's triangle (yellow arrow). (**b**) Bone scan reveals a segmental strong uptake in the mid-shaft of right tibia suggesting a possible osteomyelitis or an aggressive bone tumor. There is no such increased uptake in other bones. (**c**) PET/CT scan notes a hypermetabolic lesion (SUVmax 32.2) only in the mid-shaft of tibia and soft tissue adjacent to anterior tibial muscle. There is no evidence of abnormal FDG uptakes in other bones as well as regional lymph node or extra-nodal organs in the head, neck, chest, and abdomen indicating a single bony lesion. (**d**) MR images demonstrate an irregularly marginated bone marrow infiltrating and replacing lesion and soft tissue mass with low to intermediate SI on T1-weighted image and intermediate to high SI on T2-weighted image. Note focal intermediate to high signals within the intact cortex through which the bone lesion spreads into the surrounding soft tissue (arrows). (**e**) Follow-up radiographs at 4 years after chemotherapy under a pathologic diagnosis of diffuse large B-cell lymphoma shows a complete healing of the lesion with cortical thickness (arrows). However, he died of pneumonia 4 months later

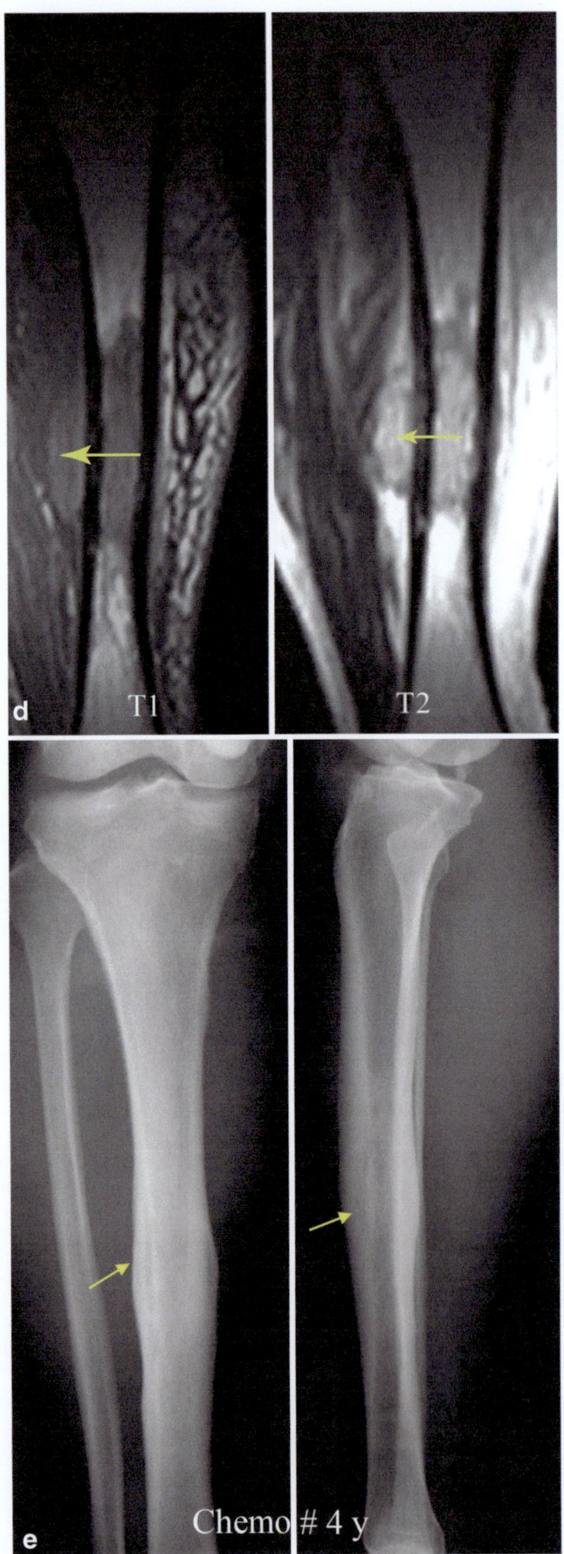

Fig. 8.2 (continued)

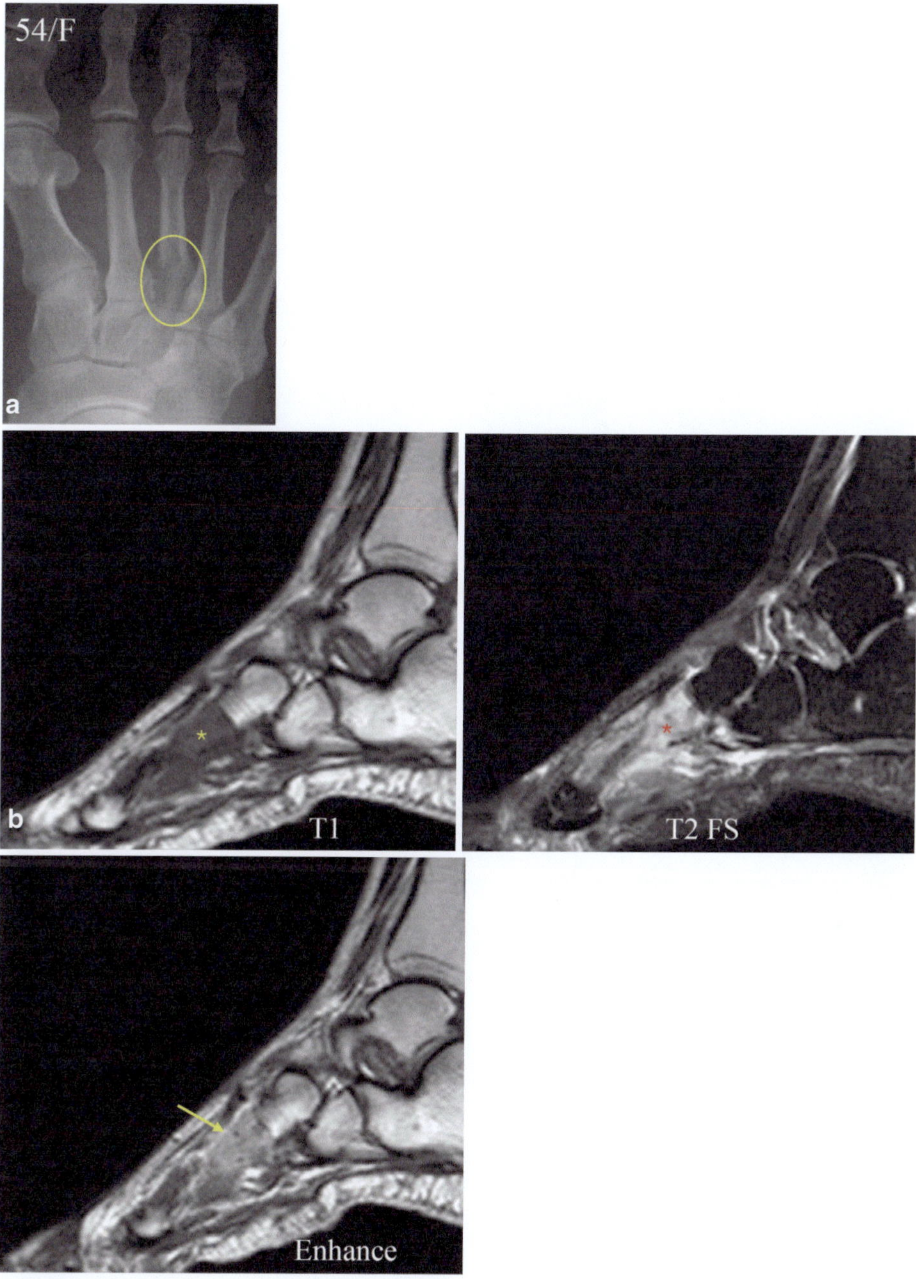

Fig. 8.3 ***Diffuse large B-cell lymphoma in multiple bones***. (**a**) Radiograph taken for left foot pain and swelling of 3-month duration in 54-year-old woman shows an ill-defined osteolytic lesion with moth-eaten destruction at base and proximal diaphysis of third metatarsal bone (yellow circle). (**b**) MR images reveal a bone marrow replacing lesion with cortical destruction and surrounding soft tissue extension. The SI is low on T1-weighted image and high on fat saturated T2-weighted image (asterisks). The lesion is partially enhanced (yellow arrow). (**c**) PET/CT scan demonstrates a focally increased FDG uptake in left mid-foot (yellow arrow) as well as both tibias and left distal femur (red arrows) but no uptakes in regional lymph node or extra-nodal organs in the head, neck, chest, and abdomen, suggesting multiple bone lesions. (**d**) The corresponding radiographs show an ill-defined multiple moth-eaten to permeative radiolucent lesions involving epi-metaphyseal area of right proximal tibia (red arrow) and meta-diaphyseal area of left proximal tibia (yellow arrows). (**e**) Follow-up radiograph at 18 months after chemotherapy under a pathologic diagnosis of diffuse, large B-cell lymphoma affecting multiple bones shows a partial consolidation of the foot lesion (yellow circle). However, she died of disease progression at 2 years after diagnosis

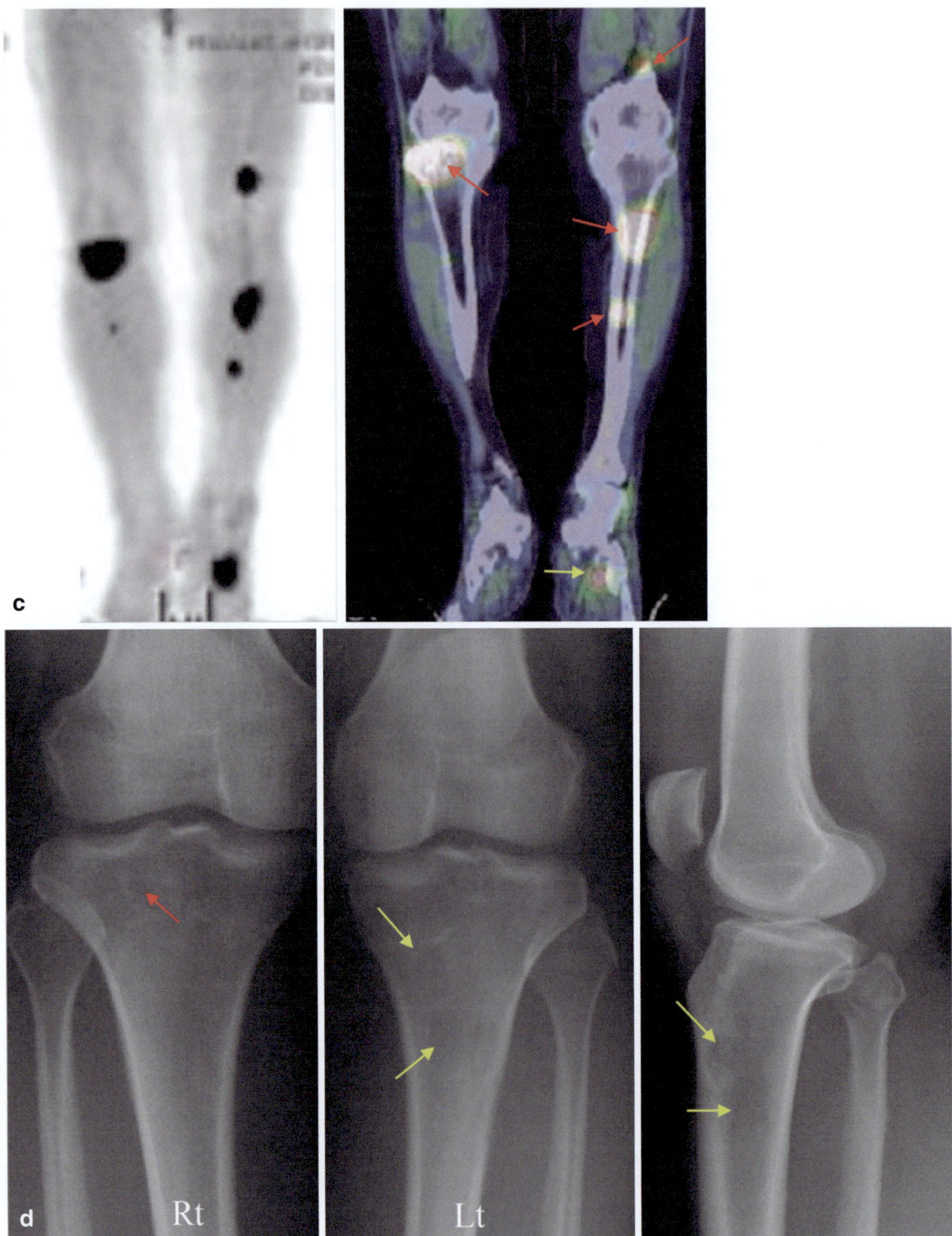

Fig. 8.3 (continued)

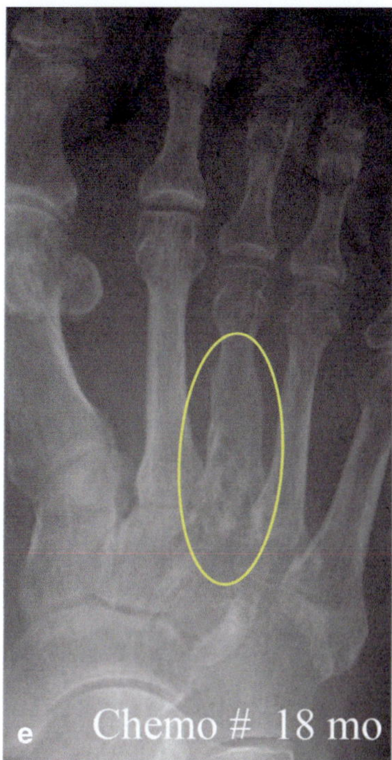

Fig. 8.3 (continued)

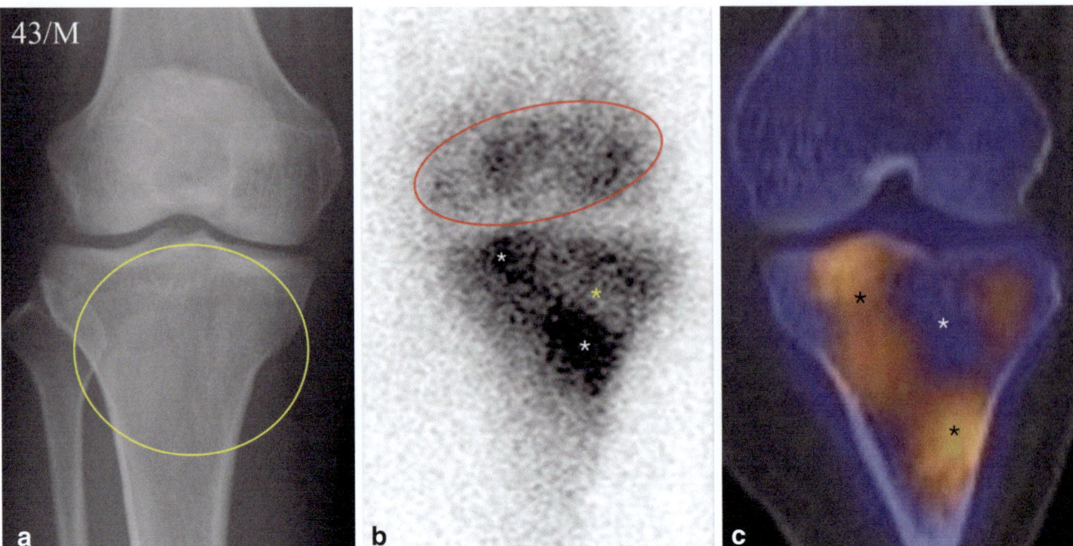

Fig. 8.4 ***NK/T cell lymphoma***. (**a**) Radiograph taken for intermittent pain of left knee for 7-month duration in 43-year-old lady shows near-normal to normal findings. (**b**) However, pinhole bone scan demonstrates an area of heterogeneous strong uptake (white asterisks) with internal decreased uptake area (yellow asterisk) in the epiphysis and metaphysis of proximal tibia. There is another mild uptake in the ipsilateral distal femur (red circle), suggesting a possible reactive uptake. (**c**) Bone SPECT demonstrates a same finding of increased uptake (black asterisks) with internal decreased uptake (white asterisk). However, there is no reactive uptake in the distal femur, which is seen on bone scan. (**d**) T2-wieghted fat saturation coronal view reveals an ill-defined, irregular, diffuse bone marrow changes with heterogeneous high SI with focal areas of low signal suggesting necrosis or fibrosis (red arrows) in the proximal tibia. However, there is no signal change in the distal femur, indicating the area with increased uptake on bone scan being reactive. Axial views show an ill-defined infiltrative bone marrow lesion with heterogeneous low to intermediate SI on T1-weighted image and high SI with anterior low signal suggesting necrosis (white asterisk) on T2-weighted image. Note pretibial extra-osseous extension (yellow asterisk) through numerous fine *"penetrating channels"* of high signals on both subsequences with intact cortical architecture (white arrows) as in Ewing's sarcoma. The lesion is centrally well enhanced (yellow arrow) and diffusely enhanced in the soft tissue mass and perilesional edema/inflammation (white arrows). Note migrating tumors through the fine channels are linearly enhanced (red arrows). (**e**) PET/CT image shows increased FDG uptake in the proximal tibia and pretibial subcutaneous soft tissue (SUVmax 6.8) and in left nasal cavity (SUVmax 4.8). (**f**) Microscopic examination of biopsy specimen from the tibia demonstrates diffuse infiltration of lymphoid cells in marked necrotic background, which is reflected as low signal on T2-weighted axial view. Higher microscopic examination reveals pleomorphic lymphoid cells in size and shape (inset). ICH for CD3 and CD 56, T-cell marker, are positive. Microscopic examination of biopsy specimen from the nasal cavity notes identical findings to those from the tibia. Epstein-Barr virus was found in a few cells by in situ hybridization. Bone marrow biopsy at iliac crest shows hypocellular bone marrow without abnormal findings. A final diagnosis of extra-nodal NK/T-cell lymphoma, nasal type, and associated with tibia involvement was made. She is doing well with complete remission at 3 years after autologous peripheral blood stem cell transplantation with chemotherapy

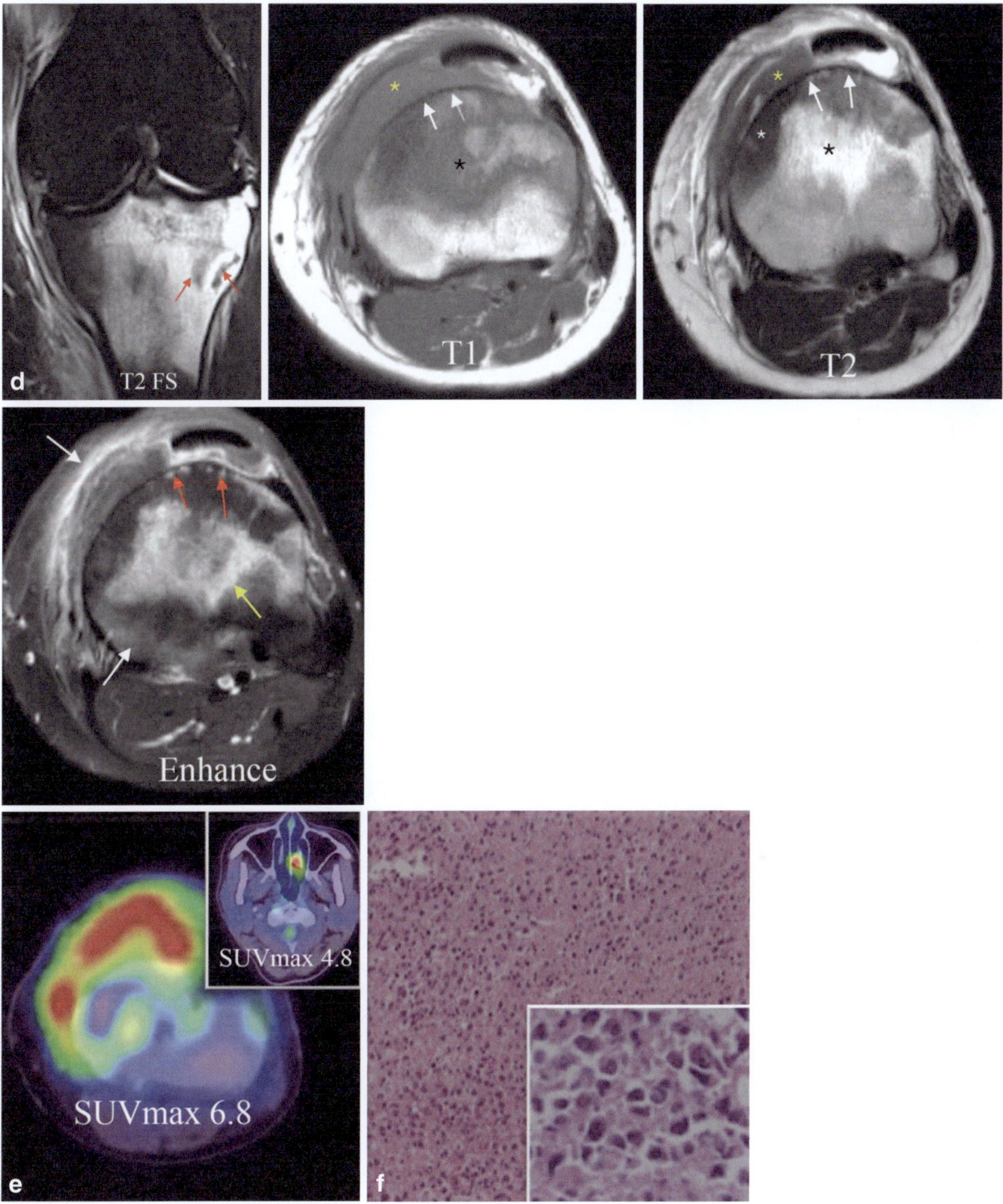

Fig. 8.4 (continued)

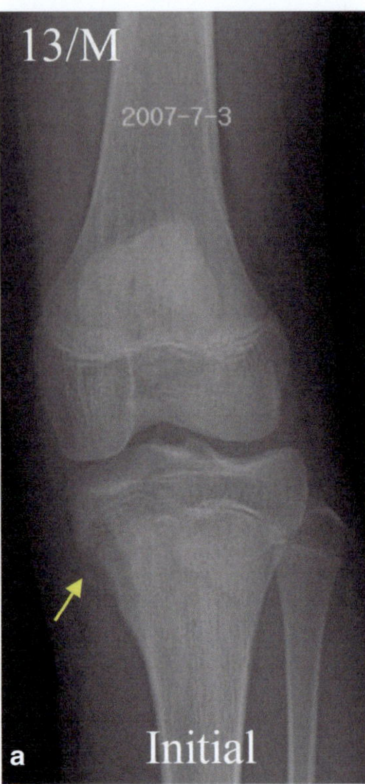

Fig. 8.5 ***Anaplastic large cell lymphoma.*** (**a**) Radiographs taken for left knee pain of 2-month duration in 13-year-old boy show an ill-defined osteolytic lesion with cortical destruction (yellow arrow) in medial aspect of metaphysis of proximal tibia. (**b**) Serial radiographs reveal chronologic progression of the lesion (arrows). Radiograph at 3-month follow-up notes a marked destruction with possible sequestrum (red arrow). (**c**) Serial MR images also demonstrate progression of the lesion with cortical breakage and soft tissue mass formation (red arrows). Three times of microscopic examinations of biopsy specimen demonstrate only findings of acute and chronic inflammation with lympho-plasmacytic and histiocytic infiltration but no clear evidence of lymphoma. (**d**) However, the last fourth incision biopsy confirms a diagnosis of anaplastic large cell lymphoma (ALCL). Microscopic examination: (Left) low-power magnification shows diffuse replacement of bone marrow space by infiltrative small tumor cells permeating and entrapping the lamellar bone spicules (L). (Middle) Medium-power magnification reveals large lymphocytic tumor cells with pleomorphism in size and shape. (Right) Higher-power magnification demonstrates bizarre cells with frequent mitoses. (**e**) IHC stains for ALK-1 and CD 30 are positive being essential for a diagnosis of ALCL

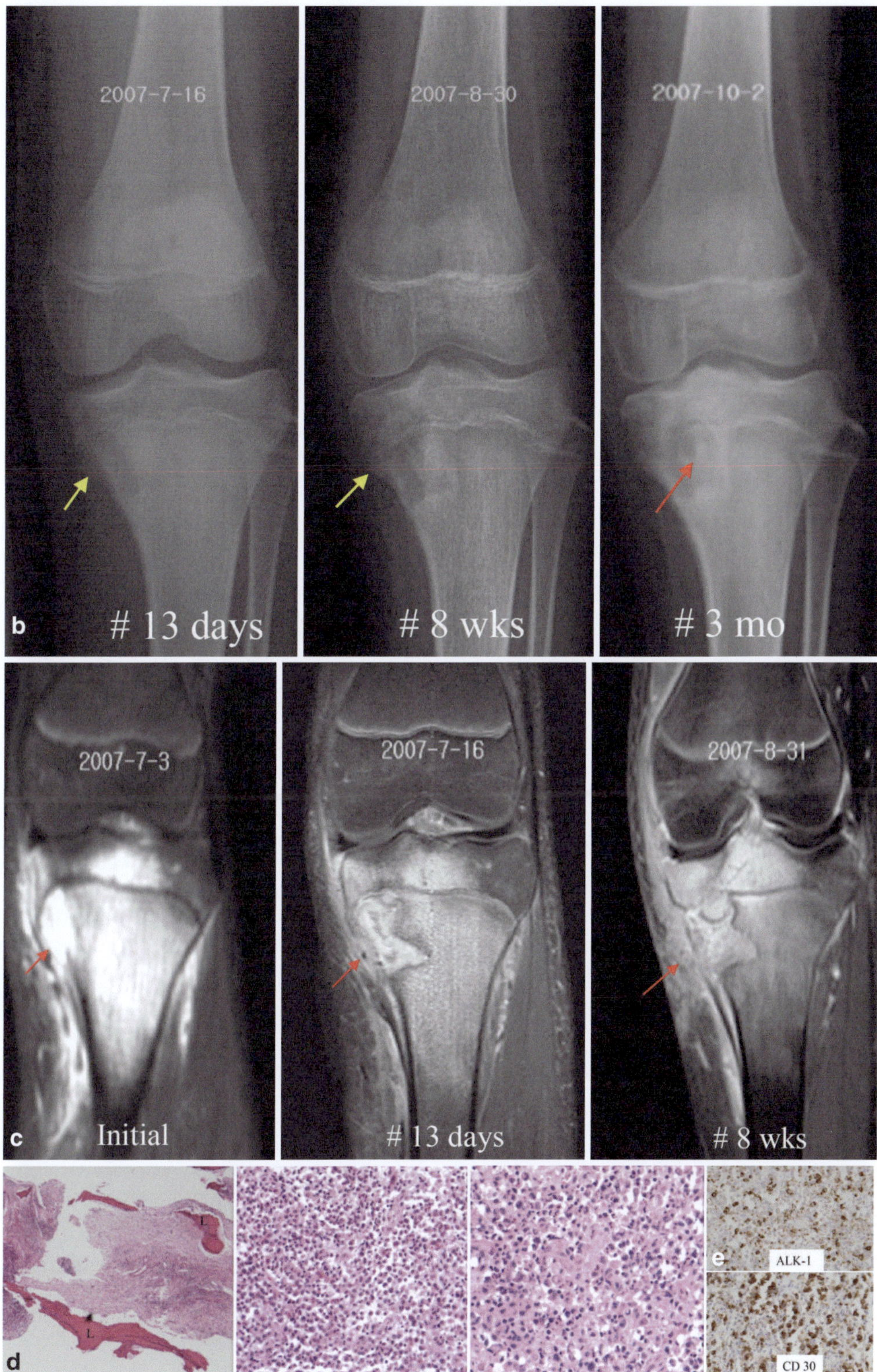

Fig. 8.5 (continued)

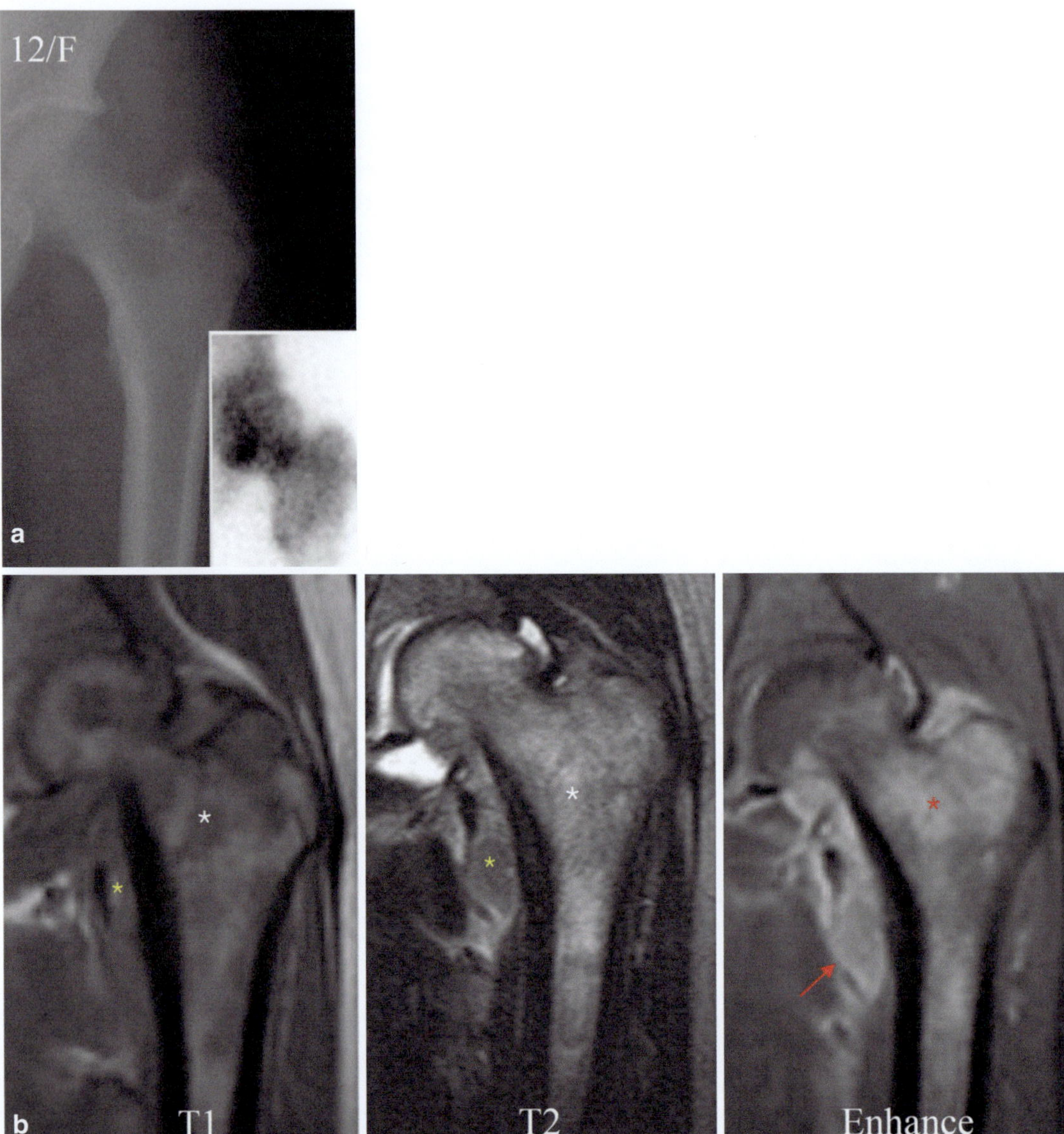

Fig. 8.6 ***Recurrent Hodgkin's lymphoma in bone and lymph node***. (**a**) Radiograph taken for left hip pain with limping gait of 2-month duration with constitutional systemic symptoms including generalized weakness, intermittent fever, and night sweat in 12-year-old girl shows normal bone appearance with no definite abnormal finding. She had a history of Hodgkin's lymphoma involving left clavicle but no regional lymph node or extra-nodal sites with remission by chemotherapy 3 year ago when she was 9 years old. The lesion was diagnosed as primary lymphoma of bone (PBT). Pinhole bone scan reveals, however, heterogeneously increased uptake only in the femoral head and neck as well as trochanteric area but no other bones (inset). (**b**) MR images demonstrate a diffuse, ill-defined marrow lesion (white asterisks) with heterogeneous low and intermediate SI on T1-weighted image and intermediate and high SI on T2-weighted image in the proximal femur. There are multiple enlarged lymph nodes around the inguinal area and along the left iliac vessels with the largest mass of 4 × 2.3 cm in diameter (yellow asterisks). The lesion is diffusely well enhanced especially at trochanteric region (red asterisk). The largest nodular mass is peripherally enhanced by the contrast media with focal internal enhancement (red arrow). (**c**) Microscopic examination of specimen from the bone and adjacent nodular mass notes atypical histiocytic reticulum cells with areas absent of chromatin, so-called perinuclear halo (black arrows), and bi-lobed Reed-Stenberg cell (yellow arrow) in cellular background rich in lymphocytes with a few other inflammatory cells, indicating recurrent Hodgkin's lymphoma spreading to proximal femur and lymph nodes around the hip joint. (**d**) Follow-up MR image at 5 years after auto PBSCT shows complete healing of the femoral lesion. She is donging well with uneventful findings of recurrent or metastatic foci on whole body MRI at 5 years' follow-up

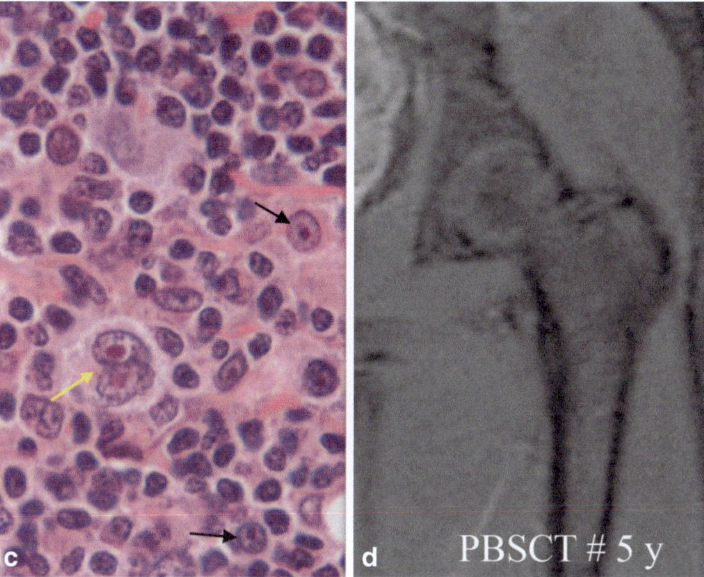

Fig. 8.6 (continued)

8.2 Synonym

Reticulum cell sarcoma (outdated)/ osteolymphoma.

8.3 Incidence

PLB is very rare, accounting for about 3–7% of all malignant bone tumors [2, 3], 0.2% of primary bone tumor [4], less than 5% of extranodal lymphomas [5, 6], and less than 2% of all lymphomas in adults [7]. Diffuse large B-cell lymphoma is the most common type, occupying about 65–80% of PLB in large series [8–10].

8.4 Age

PLB occurs in all age groups, usually in adults over 40 years with peak incidence of sixth and seventh decades of life and overall median age of 45 years [11]. More than half of the patients are older than age 60 years [9, 10]. It is very rare in children under 10 years and old patients over 80 years [4].

8.5 Location

Bones with red bone marrow are most frequently involved. They include flat bones such as pelvis, spine, and ribs as well as long bones. The spine, pelvis, and femur are the most common sites followed by humerus, tibia, rib, skull, and clavicle [4, 10]. A population-based study of 2558 patients registered in the SEER database from 1973 to 2016 reported that the most common site was vertebral column occupying 30% of all cases, followed by the long bones of lower limb and associated joints in 23% [8]. Occasionally, the lesions can be multifocal within one bone or multiple bones in some cases.

8.6 Clinical Features

Bone pain of variable intensity is the most common presentation even at rest in the majority. Local tenderness, swelling, or palpable mass often with local heat can be present. Pathological fracture can be occasionally the initial presentation particularly in the weight-bearing long bones. Half of the patients with vertebral involvement present neurologic symptoms by nerve compression [10]. Constitutional systemic symptoms such as fever, fatigue, night sweat, or weight loss can present, but rarer in contrast with Ewing's sarcoma. The patients with PLB are good in general health in comparison to those of secondary lymphoma which usually present severe constitutional symptoms [4]. Features of generalized systemic disease including lymphadenopathy, hepatosplenomegaly, or other organ involvement should not exist at presentation by definition.

8.7 Radiologic Findings

A false-negative rate is high (up to 50%) because of the requirement of advanced bone destruction affecting a minimum of 30–50% of the trabecular bone for lesion detection as for plasma cell myeloma (Refer Chaps. 1 and 5). Spectrums of radiologic findings are varying from a (near) normal bone to subtle appearing lesion (Figs. 8.4 and 8.6) or even to rapid and aggressive destructive process overlapping with other small cell tumors (Figs. 8.1, 8.2, and 8.3). Cases with near-normal to normal findings on radiograph may reveal significant abnormalities on radionuclide imaging, CT scan, or MR images as in other marrow infiltrating neoplasms. However, the most common feature is an ill-defined, variable-sized, purely osteolytic destruction eroding or breaching the cortices or mixed lytic and blastic lesion with or without moth-eaten to permeative pattern in mottled or patchy appearance. Frequently, the lesion is extensive, often occupying 25–50% of the affected host bone, and occasionally the entire bone [12]. A soft tissue mass formation with subtle or mild cortical disruption is a common feature (Figs. 8.1, 8.2, and 8.5) as in other round cell tumors such as Ewing's sarcoma and leukemia. Periosteal reaction is usually absent to faint or minimal (Fig. 8.2a), and *"onion-skin"* layers can be rarely present but is usually less evident than in Ewing's sarcoma if exists. *"Sequestrum"* (detached or dead bone spices from the involved segment) (Fig. 8.5b) has been reported in about 10% of PLB cases [13]. The sequestrum is most commonly seen in Brodie's abscess, osteomyelitis, and less commonly in a variety of bone tumors including eosinophilic granuloma, metastasis, osteoblastoma, aggressive fibrous tumors such as desmoplastic fibroma, fibrosarcoma, or undifferentiated pleomorphic sarcoma [14, 15]. Hodgkin's disease affects relatively frequently the bones, but it is very rarely detected on radiograph in only less than 3% of the patients [1] (Fig. 8.6a). Most frequently, patients with demonstrable bone lesions have the end stage of the disease with clinically apparent lymph node involvement [1].

Bone scan has been used traditionally in the evaluation of PLB [16–18]. The lesion is characterized by relatively discrete or localized strong uptake. One series reported a high rate of increased uptake in 98% of their patients, with a marked increase in 64% and mild to moderate uptake in 34%, but normal uptake was observed in only 2% [19]. It is useful to detect the case with subtle or absence of visible abnormalities on plain radiographs (Figs. 8.4 and 8.6), and in surveying the entire skeleton to detect additional foci because multiple involvement is a common feature in PLB.

PET/CT scan is a current state-of-the-art imaging in management of lymphoma. FDG uptake is increased in the lesion as well as in additional other bones or organs serving as a good tracer for identification of multifocal involvement (Fig. 8.3c). It can also clearly identify PLB lesions missed by plain radiographs or CT alone. FDG-PET/CT can reveal the post-chemotherapeutic response being predictive of outcome, which may identify a subgroup who benefits from radiotherapy and plays a major role in the various phases of lymphoma management [20].

8.8 MR Findings

T1-weighted pulse sequences are the best for demonstration of infiltrating marrow change with a homogeneous low SI (Fig. 8.1b). The lesion generally appears heterogeneously high to bright or sometimes low SI with fibrosis or necrosis on T2-weighted image, and is heterogeneously or partially enhanced by the contrast media. Typically, fat saturated T2-weighted axial image notes an associated extensive soft tissue extension through the numerous tiny channels (Figs. 8.1 and 8.4) or focal small breaches (Fig. 8.2) of high signal with a well-preserved cortical architecture, which are also enhanced well, as in other small round-cell tumors of bone such as Ewing's sarcoma or leukemia (Fig. 8.7).

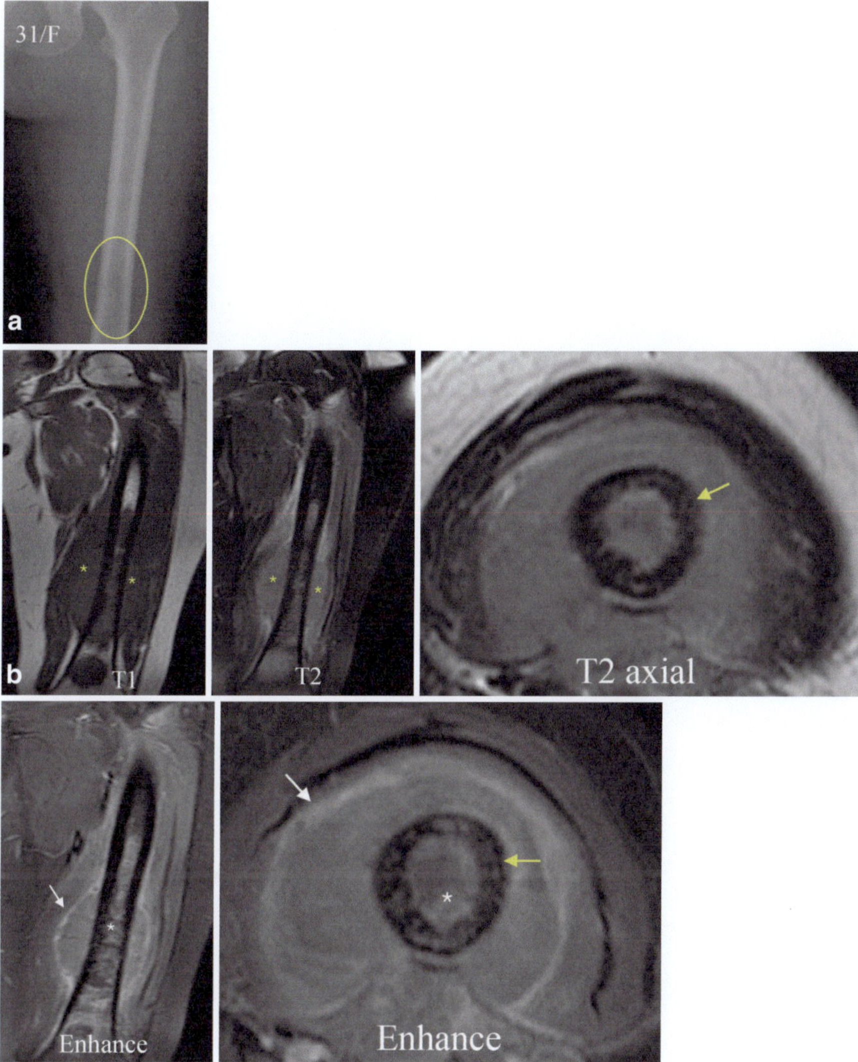

Fig. 8.7 ***Acute lymphoblastic leukemia*.** (**a**) Radiograph taken for right knee and leg pain for 2-week duration in 31-year-old lady shows no definite abnormality of the femur. She has a history of acute lymphocytic leukemia (ALL) managed with chemotherapy and allo PBSCT 1 year ago. (**b**) MR images reveal, however, an ill-defined multifocal marrow signal changes and a large para-osseous mass encircling the femur without severe cortical destruction having low SI on T-weighted image and intermediate to high on fat saturated T2-weighted image. Axial view exhibits more clearly visible numerous *"penetrating channels"* within the cortex with no definite cortical breakage though which the tumor cells invading surrounding soft tissue (yellow arrows) as in other small round-cell tumors of bone such as lymphoma (Figs. 8.1 and 8.4) and Ewing's sarcoma. The medullary lesion is partially enhanced (yellow arrow), and the soft tissue mass is peripherally enhanced (white arrow). The tiny tunnels are also enhanced by the contrast media (yellow arrow). (**c**) Radiograph taken for newly developed pain of right iliac bone area 2 weeks later shows an ill-defined moth-eaten destruction of a part of iliac wing (yellow circle). (**d**) MR images demonstrate bone marrow replacing lesion with a well-defined huge soft tissue mass through cortical breakage (yellow arrows). The SI is low to intermediate SI on T1-weighted image and heterogeneously high SI on T2-weighted image. The lesion is heterogeneously enhanced by the contrast media. Microscopic examination in association with IHC stains confirms leukemic infiltration of ALL. (**e**) Radiograph taken for newly developed pain of right shoulder 1 month later shows moth-eaten to permeative destruction involving proximal humerus (yellow circle). (**f**) MR images show an ill-defined bone marrow signal change and cortical disruption extending into axillary recess to form soft tissue mass (yellow asterisks) with low to intermediate SI on T1-weighted image and heterogeneously high SI on T2-weighted image. The lesion is heterogeneously enhanced with a focal non-enhancing area that reflects a focally increased to intermediate signal area on T1-weighted image (white asterisk), suggesting a possible necrosis. Palliative radiotherapy was performed for each bony lesion, but she died of disease progression at 19 months after initial diagnosis of ALL

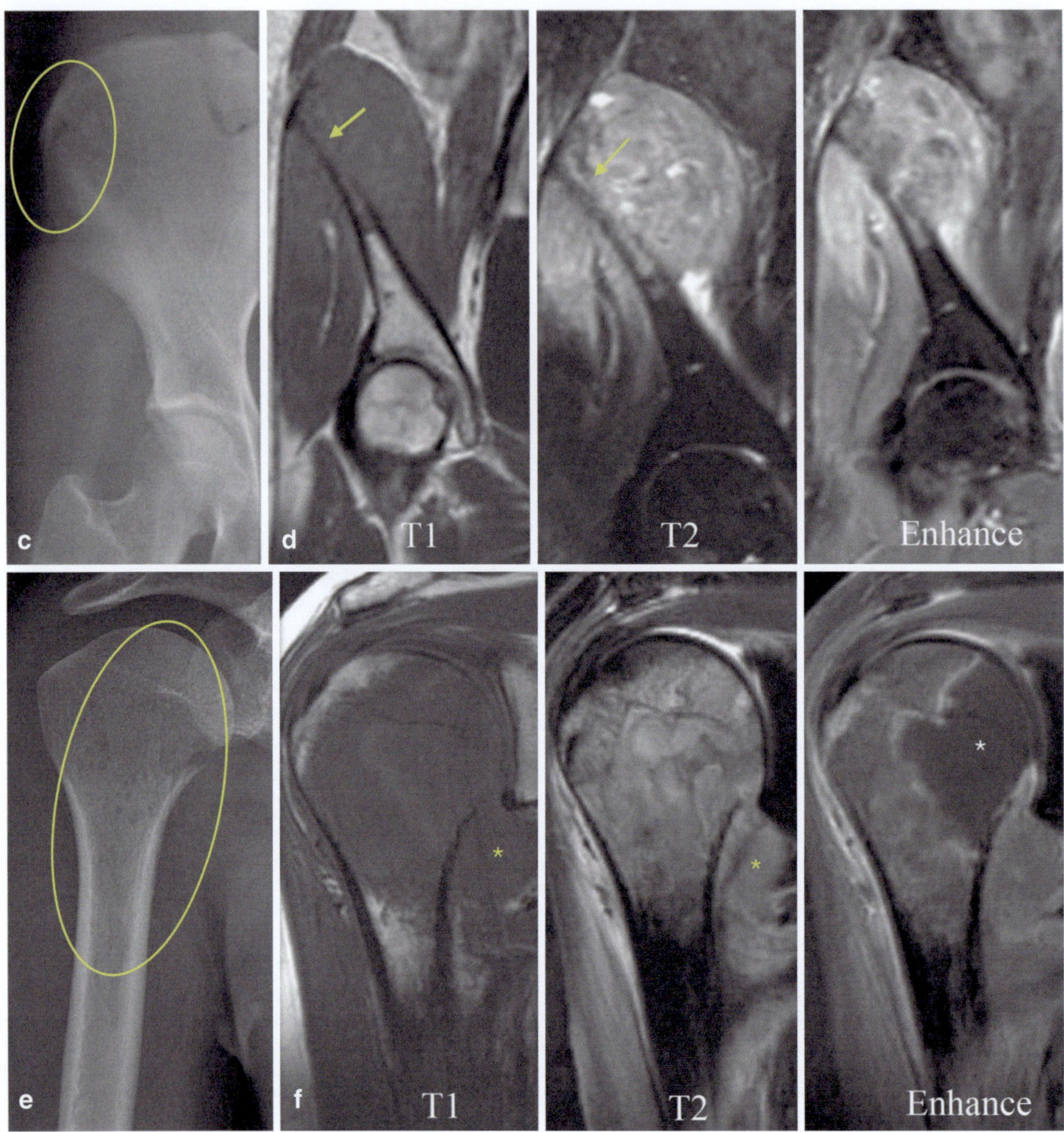

Fig. 8.7 (continued)

The phenomenon is probably represented by a theory that certain soluble cytokine mediators produced by tumor cells may activate osteoclastic resorption and form the fine "*penetrating channels*" within the relatively intact cortical architecture, through which the lymphoma cells can escape from the medullary space to the adjacent soft tissue forming a large soft-tissue mass without extensive cortical destruction [21]. If extensive bone marrow infiltration is associated with extensive soft tissue extension through the *"penetrating channels"* or focal small breaches without marked cortical destruction in a patient over 40 years, a diagnosis of PLB should be firstly considered.

8.9 Histologic Findings

The most frequent histologic type is DLBL (Figs. 8.1, 8.2, and 8.3). It is characterized by diffuse sheets of solid proliferation of large, atypical, quite round, lymphocytic cells filling the marrow space in diffuse growth pattern to permeate the lamellar bone and Harversian channels. The growth pattern is typified by central destruction with peripheral preservation of medullary bones and fat components, sometimes with prominent fibrosis. The bone trabeculae may be normal or irregularly thickened with reactive change. The sheets consist of predominantly large cells or polymorphous mixed with small and large cells. The individual cells are usually clear with more distinct cytoplasmic border, and spaces between the cells are not-cohesive, separable, and more evident when compared to those of Ewing's sarcoma in which the cells are closely packed in true sarcomatous cohesive sheets with indistinct border. The tumor cells have large cleaved or multi-lobulated nuclei, fine chromatin, and inconspicuous to prominent nucleoli. The tumor cells can be often associated with reactive, non-neoplastic smaller lymphocytes. Crush artifact is frequently seen particularly in trephine or core biopsy materials, which can make the diagnosis more obscure especially when the reactive smaller lymphocytes or reactive bone spicules are admixed. Another characteristic feature is the near complete obliteration of the normal fatty marrow except at the peripheral infiltrating edge of the lesion [7]. Other subtypes are very rare. *NK/T cell lymphoma* is characterized by a diffuse lymphocytic infiltrate with numerous, evenly dispersed, ill defined, small clusters of epithelioid histiocytes, angiodestruction, marked necrosis, and association with Epstein-Barr virus (Fig. 8.4). ALCL is characterized by diffuse sheets of solid proliferation of anaplastic and pleomorphic large lymphocytic cells filling the marrow space in diffuse growth pattern and permeating the lamellar bone (Fig. 8.5). Secondary bone involvement of Hodgkin's lymphoma is relatively common but the primary type is extremely rare. *Hodgkin's lymphoma* is typified by atypical histiocytic reticulum cells with areas absent of chromatin and the hallmark bi-lobed "*Reed-Stenberg cells*" in a cellular background rich in lymphocytes with a few other inflammatory cells such as plasma cells and eosinophils (Fig. 8.6).

8.10 Special Stains

IHC stains are mandatory to exclude other hematopoietic round-cell tumors. The positive stains for a diagnosis of PLB include leukocyte common antigen (LCA), CD20 as a pan B-cell marker, UCHL-1 or CD3 as a T-cell marker, both ALK-1 and CD 30 for ALCL.

8.11 Management

Chemotherapy with or without radiotherapy is the cornerstones of treatment for all lymphomas. Patients with DLBL reported to have a favorable prognosis when treated with primary anthracycline-based chemotherapy whether followed by radiotherapy or not [22]. However, whether chemotherapy in combination with radiotherapy is superior to chemotherapy alone remains still controversial [8]. The optimal treatment strategies, including agents with novel mechanisms of action and radiation doses and fields, need to be verified by future studies and clinical trials. Bone marrow transplantation (BMT) or peripheral blood stem cell transplantation (PBSCT) would be considered if chemotherapy and radiotherapy do not lead to remission or the lesion comes back after initial treatment (Fig. 8.6). Surgical management including internal fixation for impending or pathologic fracture and wide en-bloc resection with reconstruction for significantly destructive lesion or recurrent tumors can be indicated.

8.12 Clinical Course

Multivariate analysis in 1559 patients with PLB identified from 1973 through 2005 in the SEER database revealed that younger age and localized disease were the only identifiable prognostic indicator for survival [9]. In a population-based study of 2558 patients with PLB registered in the Surveillance, Epidemiology, and End Results (SEER) database from 1973 to 2016, the 5-year progression-free and overall survival rates of DLBC lymphoma patients have been reported to be 80% and 93%, respectively, superior to other subtypes [8]. The authors also reported the 3-, 5-, 10-, and 20-year overall survival rates were about 71%, 66%, 54%, and 40%, respectively. A better prognosis has been reported in PLB than in systemic lymphoma with bone involvement. In other series, while the disease-free 5-year survival for patients with PLB was 81%, for patients with systemic lymphoma with bone involvement, it was only 44%. For patients younger than 60 years old and those older than 60 years, the survival rates were 90% and 62%, respectively. The authors concluded that age was the only prognostic factor for survival [11].

References

1. Ewton A. Hematopoietic tumors. In: Dorfman HD, Czerniak B, editors. Dorfman and Czerniak's bone tumors (eBook). 2nd ed. Elsevier; 2016. p. 817–902.
2. Limb D, Dreghorn C, Murphy J, Mannion R. Primary lymphoma of bone. Int Orthop. 1994;18(3):180–3.
3. Cleven AHG, Ferry JA. Primary non-Hodgkin lymphoma of bone. In: The WHO Classification of Tumors Editorial Board, editor. Soft Tissue and bone tumours. 5th ed. Lyon: WHO; 2020. p. 489–91.
4. Mirra JM. Lymphoma and leukemia. In: Mirra JM, editor. Bone tumors: clinical, radiologic, and pathologic correlation. 2nd ed. Philadelphia, PA: Lea & Febiger; 1989. p. 1148–73.
5. Freeman C, Berg JW, Cutler SJ. Occurrence and prognosis of extranodal lymphomas. Cancer. 1972;29(1):252–60.
6. Rosenberg SA, Diamond HD, Jaslowitz B, Craver LF. Lymphosarcoma: a review of 1269 cases. Medicine. 1961;40(1):31–84.
7. Dubey P, Ha CS, Besa PC, Fuller L, Cabanillas F, Murray J, et al. Localized primary malignant lymphoma of bone. Inter J Radiat Oncol biol phys. 1997;37(5):1087–93.
8. Li X, Xu-Monette ZY, Yi S, Dabaja BS, Manyam GC, Westin J, et al. Primary bone lymphoma exhibits a favorable prognosis and distinct gene expression signatures resembling diffuse large B-cell lymphoma derived from centrocytes in the germinal center. Am J Surg Pathol. 2017;41(10):1309–21.
9. Jawad MU, Schneiderbauer MM, Min ES, Cheung MC, Koniaris LG, Scully SP. Primary lymphoma of bone in adult patients. Cancer. 2010;116(4):871–9.
10. Ramadan K, Shenkier T, Sehn L, Gascoyne R, Connors J. A clinicopathological retrospective study of 131 patients with primary bone lymphoma: a population-based study of successively treated cohorts from the British Columbia Cancer Agency. Ann Oncol. 2007;18(1):129–35.
11. Demircay E, Hornicek FJ, Mankin HJ, Degroot H. Malignant lymphoma of bone: a review of 119 patients. Clin Orthop. 2013;471(8):2684–90.
12. Unni K, Inwards Y. Malignant lymphoma of bone. In: Dahlin's bone tumors: general aspects and data on 10,165 cases. Philadelphia, PA: Lippincott Williams & Wilkins; 2010. p. 201–10.
13. Mulligan M, Kransdorf M. Sequestra in primary lymphoma of bone: prevalence and radiologic features. Am J Roentgenol. 1993;160(6):1245–8.
14. Resnick D, Niwayama G. Osteomyelitis, septic arthritis and soft tissue infection: the mechanisms and situations. In: Resnick D, editor. Diagnosis of bone and joint disorders. 2nd ed. Philadelphia, PA: Saunders; 1988. p. 2525–754.
15. Helms CA, Jeffrey RB, Wing VW. Computed tomography and plain film appearance of a bony sequestration: significance and differential diagnosis. Skel Radiol. 1987;16(2):117–20.
16. Orzel J, Sawaf N, Richardson M. Lymphoma of the skeleton: scintigraphic evaluation. Am J Roentgenol. 1988;150(5):1095–9.
17. Schechter JP, Jones SE, Woolfenden JM, Lilien DL, O'Mara RE. Bone scanning in lymphoma. Cancer. 1976;38(3):1142–8.
18. Ferrant A, Rodhain J, Michaux J-L, Piret L, Maldague B, Sokal G. Detection of skeletal involvement in Hodgkin's disease: a comparison of radiography, bone scanning, and bone marrow biopsy in 38 patients. Cancer. 1975;35(5):1346–53.
19. Mulligan M, McRae G, Murphey M. Imaging features of primary lymphoma of bone. Am J Roentgenol. 1999;173(6):1691–7.
20. El-Galaly TC, Villa D, Gormsen LC, Baech J, Lo A, Cheah CY. FDG-PET/CT in the management of lymphomas: current status and future directions. J Int Med. 2018;284(4):358–76.
21. Hicks DG, O'Keefe RJ, Rosier RN, Sickel JZ, Judkins AR, Gokan T, et al. Primary lymphoma of bone. Correlation of magnetic resonance imaging features with cytokine production by tumor cells. Cancer. 1995;75(4):973–80.
22. Bruno Ventre M, Ferreri AJ, Gospodarowicz M, Govi S, Messina C, Porter D, et al. Clinical features, management, and prognosis of an international series of 161 patients with limited-stage diffuse large B-cell lymphoma of the bone (the IELSG-14 study). Oncologist. 2014;19(3):291–8.

Part III

Notochordal Tumors

9 Benign Notochordal Cell Tumor

(***Noton*** "back" + ***chordaē*** "cord" + ***cella*** *"compartment"* + ***tumere*** "to swell")

9.1 Definition

Benign notochordal cell tumor (BNCT) is a distinctive, slow-growing, benign intraosseous tumor derived from notochordal cells.

9.2 Synonyms

Giant notochordal rest/notochordal hamartoma/ecchordosis physaliphora.

9.3 Incidence

BNCTs have been reported to be surprisingly common with an incidence of up to 20% in cadaveric specimens [1], although the prevalence of BNCT detected on images including CT scan and MRI was reported to be only 0.76% [2]. Some of BNCTs are so small in size (a few millimeters) that may not cause any symptoms or show up on images.

9.4 Age

Patient ages widely ranged from 7 to 82 with a mean age of 63 years in autopsy patients [1].

9.5 Location

BNCTs may occur anywhere from the skull base to the sacrum being identical to that of chordoma. The sacro-coccygeal region and skull base are the most frequent sites, followed by cervical and lumbar vertebrae.

9.6 Clinical Presentations

The lesions are usually asymptomatic and found incidentally on images taken for unrelated reasons. However, a small number of patients present with chronic neck or back pain with or without tingling sense of extremities and coccygodynia.

9.7 Radiologic Findings

BNCT can manifests as ill-defined irregular area of vague to mild sclerosis within a vertebral body or clivus, often mimicking intra-osseous hemangioma. Rarely, the lesion may be diffusely sclerotic presenting as an ivory vertebra. However, radiograph often fails to identify any abnormal findings (Figs. 9.1a, 9.2a). **CT scan** may reveal irregular sclerotic lesion(s) usually

W.-J. Bahk, *Diagnosis and Management of Primary Bone Tumors*,
https://doi.org/10.1007/978-981-99-5498-8_9

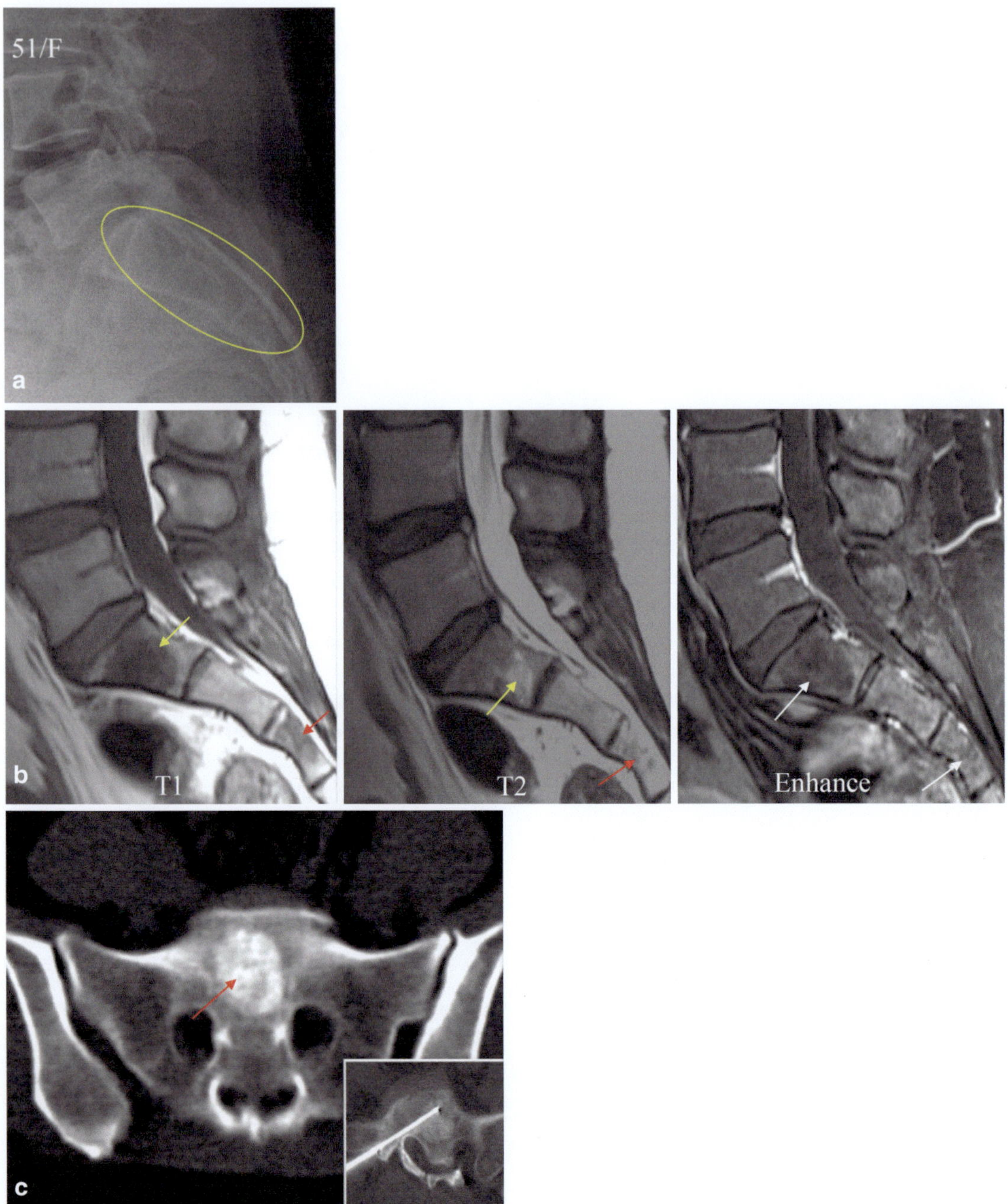

Fig. 9.1 (**a**) Radiograph taken for tingling sense of lower leg in 51-year-old female shows no definite abnormal findings of third lumbar spines (yellow circle). (**b**) However, MR images reveal an irregular intramedullary lesions (arrows) confined to the first and third sacral body with low SI on T1-weighted image and intermediate to high SI on T2-weighted image. The lesion is not enhanced by contrast media (white arrows). (**c**) CT scan demonstrates an irregular sclerotic, round to oval, mass-like lesion in the sacral body. CT-guided biopsy was done (inset). (**d**) Microscopic examination. (Left) Low-power magnification shows sheets of abundant adipocyte-like cells with clear cytoplasm and hematopoietic cells between under-decalcified host bony trabeculae (T). (Right) Higher-power magnification reveals variable-sized adipocyte-like cells with well-defined cell boundaries. Most tumor cells have clear to pale pink cytoplasm. The vacuolated cells have centrally or peripherally located round to oval nuclei with small dense nucleoli mimicking fat cells (black arrows). Less vacuolated tumor cells have pinkish eosinophilic cytoplasm (red arrows). There are no mitoses or myxoid matrix

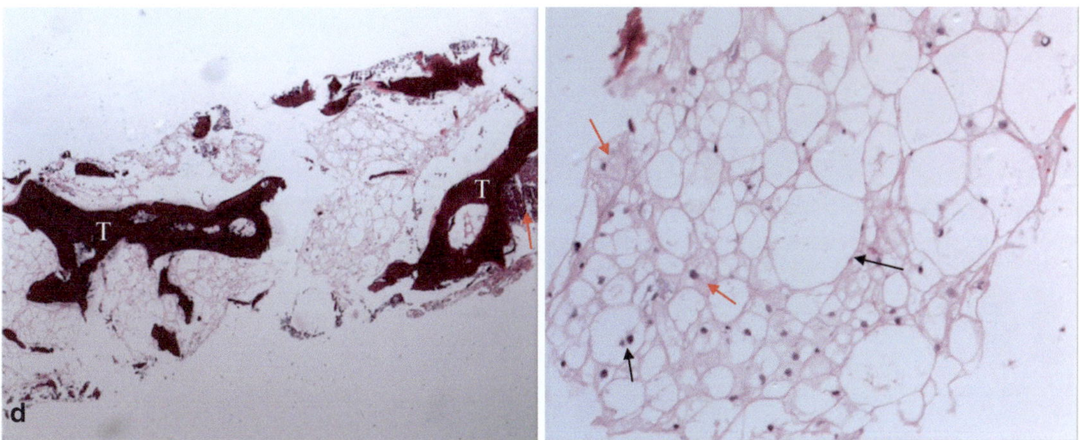

Fig. 9.1 (continued)

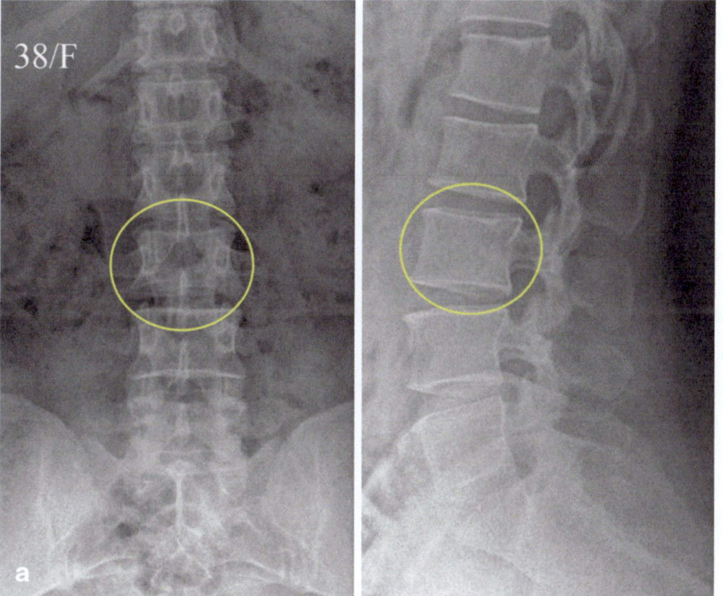

Fig. 9.2 (**a**) Radiograph taken for a routine physical checkup in 38-year-old healthy female shows no definite abnormal findings of third lumbar spines (yellow circles). (**b**) However, MR images reveal an ill-defined irregular osseous lesion confined to the spine body (arrows) with homogeneous low SI on T1-weighted image and heterogeneous intermediate and high SI on T2-weighted image. There is intralesional punctuated foci of high signal on T1-weighted image (yellow arrows), possibly representing fat lobules. Biopsy was not performed

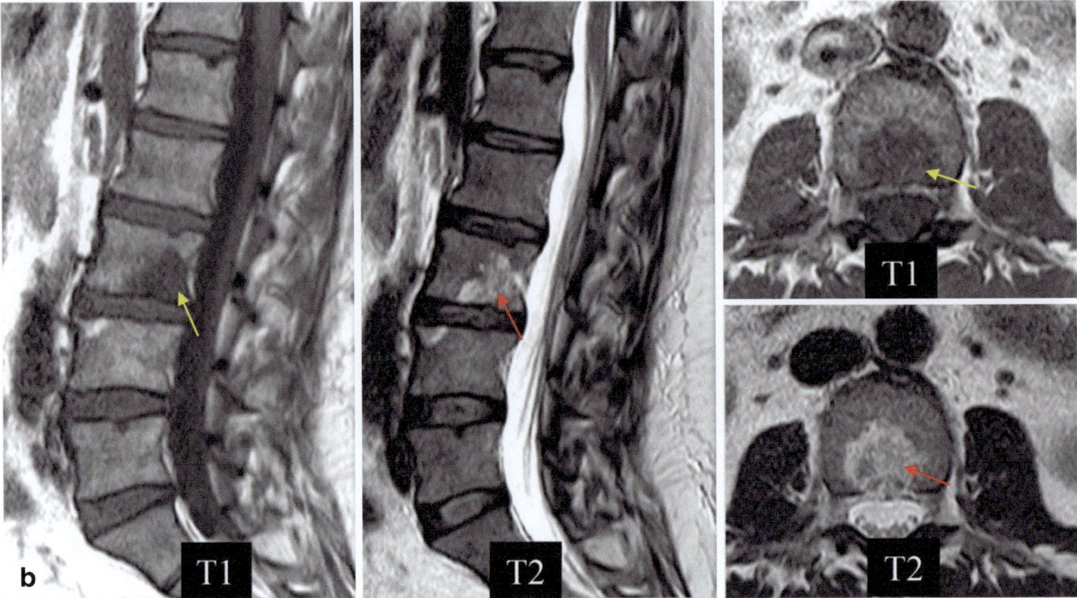

Fig. 9.2 (continued)

confined to the vertebral body without definite cortical destruction (Fig. 9.1c) but rarely can extend into the adjacent soft tissue through cortical defect. **Bone scan** generally shows no abnormal uptake. **MR images** demonstrate irregular osseous lesion(s) usually confined to the vertebral body with low SI on T1-weighted image and intermediate to high SI on T2-weighted image (Figs. 9.1b, 9.2b). The lesion is not enhanced by contrast material (Fig. 9.1b). Intralesional punctuated foci of high signal may be occasionally observed on T1-weighted image representing fat lobules due to entrapped bone marrow (Fig. 9.2b). Rarely, the lesion may present a small extra-osseous component. Thus, a possibility of chordoma arising in BNCT should be excluded if size of the soft tissue mass is moderate or large, particularly when any lytic areas are associated.

9.8 Histologic Findings

BNCT is sharply demarcated and surrounded by reactive new bone trabeculae and entraps hematopoietic marrow. The lesion consists of solid sheets of adipocyte-like *vacuolated cells* with clear cytoplasm intermingled with less vacuolated eosinophilic *pale pink* cells of varying degrees (Fig. 9.1d). The vacuolated cells have centrally or peripherally located, bland to mildly atypical, round to oval nuclei with small dense nucleoli mimicking fat cells. The less vacuolated eosinophilic cells contain round, intracytoplasmic hyaline globules of varying size. The nuclei are usually bland but can be mildly pleomorphic. Cystic spaces filled with colloid-like eosinophilic material can be present in some cases. There are no mitoses or myxoid matrix, which can distinguish BNCT from chordoma. Islands of hematopoietic bone marrow are often observed within the lesions.

9.9 Management

The current preferred choice of treatment is periodic follow-up with imaging studies to exclude incipient chordoma or rare progression into chordoma for asymptomatic lesions. Surgical treatment is indicated only for large lesions and biopsy may be necessary for differential diagnosis.

9.10 Clinical Course

Most BNCTs are quiescent, but the lesions may enlarge very slowly over many years. Mirra and Brien [3] described no enlargement of a giant BNCT lesion after 9 years of natural course, and Iorgulescu et al. [4] also reported no radiographic and symptomatic progression in eight patients during follow-up from about 9 to 71 months with an average of 22 months. Several other authors reported sporadic cases of chordoma arising from an intraosseous BNCT [5–9]. However, the relationship between chordoma and BNCT still remains to be elucidated.

References

1. Yamaguchi T, Suzuki S, Ishiiwa H, Ueda Y. Intraosseous benign notochordal cell tumours: overlooked precursors of classic chordomas? Histopathology. 2004;44(6):597–602.
2. Golden LD, Small JE. Benign notochordal lesions of the posterior clivus: retrospective review of prevalence and imaging characteristics. J Neuroimaging. 2014;24(3):245–9.
3. Mirra JM, Brien EW. Giant notochordal hamartoma of intraosseous origin: a newly reported benign entity to be distinguished from chordoma. Report of two cases. Skeletal Radiol. 2001;30(12):698–709.
4. Iorgulescu JB, Laufer I, Hameed M, Boland P, Yamada Y, Lis E, et al. Benign notochordal cell tumors of the spine: natural history of 8 patients with histologically confirmed lesions. Neurosurgery. 2013;73(3):411–6.
5. Kyriakos M. Benign notochordal lesions of the axial skeleton: a review and current appraisal. Skelet Radiol. 2011;40(9):1141–52.
6. Peris-Celda M, Salgado-Lopez L, Inwards CY, Raghunathan A, Carr CM, Janus JR, et al. Benign notochordal cell tumor of the clivus with chordoma component: report of 2 cases. J Neurosurg. 2019;133(5):1355–9.
7. Nishiguchi T, Mochizuki K, Tsujio T, Nishita T, Inoue Y. Lumbar vertebral chordoma arising from an intraosseous benign notochordal cell tumour: radiological findings and histopathological description with a good clinical outcome. Br J Radiol. 2010;83(987):e49–54.
8. Yamaguchi T, Watanabe-Ishiiwa H, Suzuki S, Igarashi Y, Ueda Y. Incipient chordoma: a report of two cases of early-stage chordoma arising from benign notochordal cell tumors. Mod Pathol. 2005;18(7):1005–10.
9. Yamaguchi T, Yamato M, Saotome K. First histologically confirmed case of a classic chordoma arising in a precursor benign notochordal lesion: differential diagnosis of benign and malignant notochordal lesions. Skelet Radiol. 2002;31(7):413–8.

10 Chordoma

(***chordaē*** "cord" + ***ōma*** "forming")

10.1 Definition

Chordoma is a slow-growing, low- to intermediate-grade malignant tumor with notochordal differentiation thought to originate from embryonic rest of primitive notochord. Three recognized subtypes include *conventional chordoma* (the most common), *chondroid chordoma* (the best prognosis), and *dedifferentiated chordoma* (the least common and worst prognosis).

10.2 Incidence

The incidence is relatively rare accounting for 1–4% of primary bone tumors [1–4]. But it is the most common primary malignant tumor affecting spines in adults.

10.3 Age

No age group can be exempt, but most patients are adults between 30 and 70 years of age with a peak of 40–50 years. Those in the spheno-occipital region usually occur in younger patients between 20 and 40 years of age, whereas sacrococcygeal chordomas are typically seen in a slightly older age group over 50 years.

10.4 Location

Chordoma is almost exclusively located in axial skeleton from the base of the skull to coccyx. About 80–90% of cases occur in the sacrococcygeal and spheno-occipital regions, and remaining cases arise in the mobile cervical and lumbar spine. Over 50% of chordomas occur in the sacrococcygeal region, being the most common primary malignant sacral tumor [3, 5]. Thoracic spine is very rarely affected. In the sacrum, chordoma usually involved caudal sacrum below S3 in comparison to other tumors including giant cell tumor, chondrosarcoma, or osteosarcoma, which frequently occur in the more cephalad sacrum.

10.5 Clinical Presentations

Insidious pain of several months to years duration is the most frequent presentation. Other symptoms depend on the location of the lesion due to mass effect on adjacent structures (brainstem, cranial nerves, nasopharynx, spinal cord). Diplopia, headaches, and cranial nerve palsies can be associated when skull base is affected. Pharyngeal mass is frequent presentation of cervical chordoma. Pain and neurologic symptoms are related

W.-J. Bahk, *Diagnosis and Management of Primary Bone Tumors*,
https://doi.org/10.1007/978-981-99-5498-8_10

to the lesion involving mobile spines. Pain, constipation, incontinence, bladder dysfunction, and erectile dysfunction can be presented by sacral lesion.

10.6 Radiologic Findings

Typical findings are axial sacral or clival location as well as central lobular to geographic destruction with soft tissue mass and scattered, discrete intralesional calcification (Fig. 10.1a). However, sacral chordoma is often difficult to recognize due to overlying shadows of bowel gas and stool on plain radiographs, particularly if the quality of radiograph is poor. Thus, careful observation of a symmetricity or obliteration of outline of the sacral foramen as well as expansion of the sacrum is mandatory first step. Even careful observation may not permit to recognize the lesion on anteroposterior view with gas or stool, but the bone destruction lesion and soft tissue mass can be more clearly seen on lateral view without the obstacles (Fig. 10.2a). **CT scan** clearly reveals destructive lytic lesion, sometimes with marginal sclerosis and expansile soft tissue mass that is often disproportionately large relative to the bony destruction with or without calcification. **MR images** demonstrate a lobulated or septate lesion with low to intermediate SI sometimes with scattered small foci of very high signal suggesting hemorrhage or a mucus pool on T1-weighted image and high to extremely bright SI similar to the nucleus pulposus probably reflecting the high fluid content of vacuolated cells on T2-weighted image with focal dark signal of calcification on both sequences (Figs. 10.1b, 10.2c). In an analysis of MR features of chordoma in skull base, histologic examination revealed small sites of hemorrhage and mucinous collections in the lesions that may account for the high signal characteristics [6]. A degree of bone involvement as well as extent of soft tissue extension can be clearly evaluated. The huge soft tissue mass located anterior to sacrum may displace and compress the rectum or bladder producing related dysfuction. The lesion may no enhancement to mild or intense, homogeneous or heterogeneous enhancement sometimes in a honeycomb appearance, with linear areas of non-enhancement [7]. **Bone scan** notes variably increased uptake frequently with central void area suggesting a possible necrosis (Fig. 10.2b). **FDG PET/CT scan** is useful in the staging, response, and surveillance of rare tumor chordoma and efficiently detect metastatic disease, occult residual/recurrent local disease, and guide management in chordoma. It shows a large destructive bony lesion with soft tissue mass located anteriorly in the sacrococcygeal region and heterogeneously increased FDG uptake within the lesion (Figs. 10.1, 10.2).

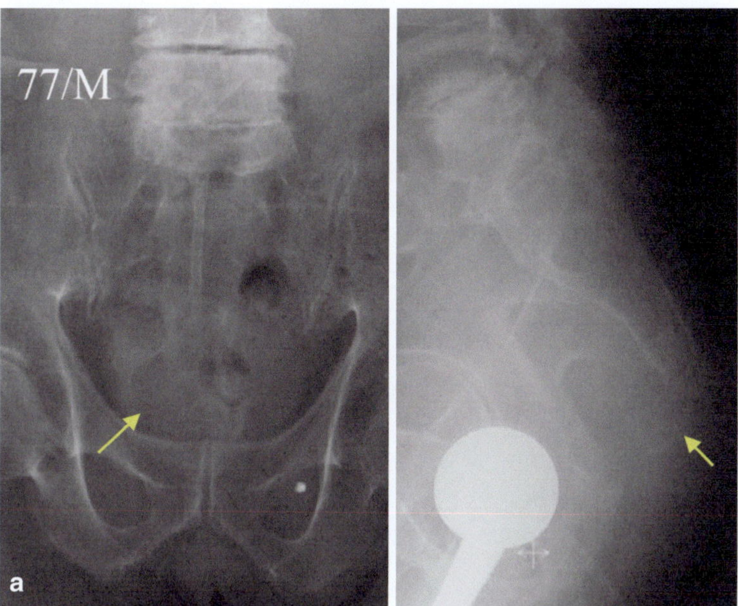

Fig. 10.1 (**a**) Radiograph taken for coccygodynia of 2-year duration in 77-year-old man shows an ill-defined geographic destruction in the sacro-coccygeal bone (yellow arrows). (**b**) MR images reveal a lobulated medullary mass-like lesion (white asterisks) and cortical destruction with a ventral huge soft tissue mass (yellow asterisks) in the sacrum from S3 to coccyx. The SI is low with scattered small foci of very high signal suggesting hemorrhage or a mucus pool on T1-weighted image and heterogeneous intermediate and very high SI with low and focal dark signals, which may also be associated with mucous, hemorrhage, and calcification on T2-weighted image. Both lesions in the bone and soft tissue are heterogeneously enhanced with a honeycomb appearance. (**c**) PET/CT scan demonstrates a heterogeneous hypermetabolic lesion (SUVmax 5.9) in the sacro-coccygeal area. (**d**) Wide resection from S3 to coccyx with negative margin followed by adjuvant radiotherapy was performed under a histologic diagnosis of conventional chordoma. (**e**) Follow-up MR images at 20 months after surgery note a well-defined small mass lesion confined to S1 body and posterior cortical perforation with focal soft tissue extension, which is heterogeneously enhanced suggesting a local recurrence. (**f**) PET/CT scan shows a small hypermetabolic mass (SUVmax 5.4) in the S1 body indicating a local recurrence. (**g**) Extended curettage and cementation (black arrow) was performed because the patient did not want radical surgery. Microscopic examination confirmed a local recurrence of chordoma. (**h**) Follow-up PET/CT scan at 2 years after second operation reveals increased metabolic activity around the cement suggesting a possible second local recurrence (yellow arrows). In addition, newly developed multiple tiny nodules are found in both lungs and T10 vertebra possibly suggesting distant metastases. The patient does not want any further management. (**i**) Follow-up MR image at 3 years after second operation notes irregular nodular lesion around the bone cement in the sacrum probably suggesting remnant or recurred tumor, which has been remained with little change for 1 year. He is still alive with disease at 5 years after initial surgery and radiotherapy

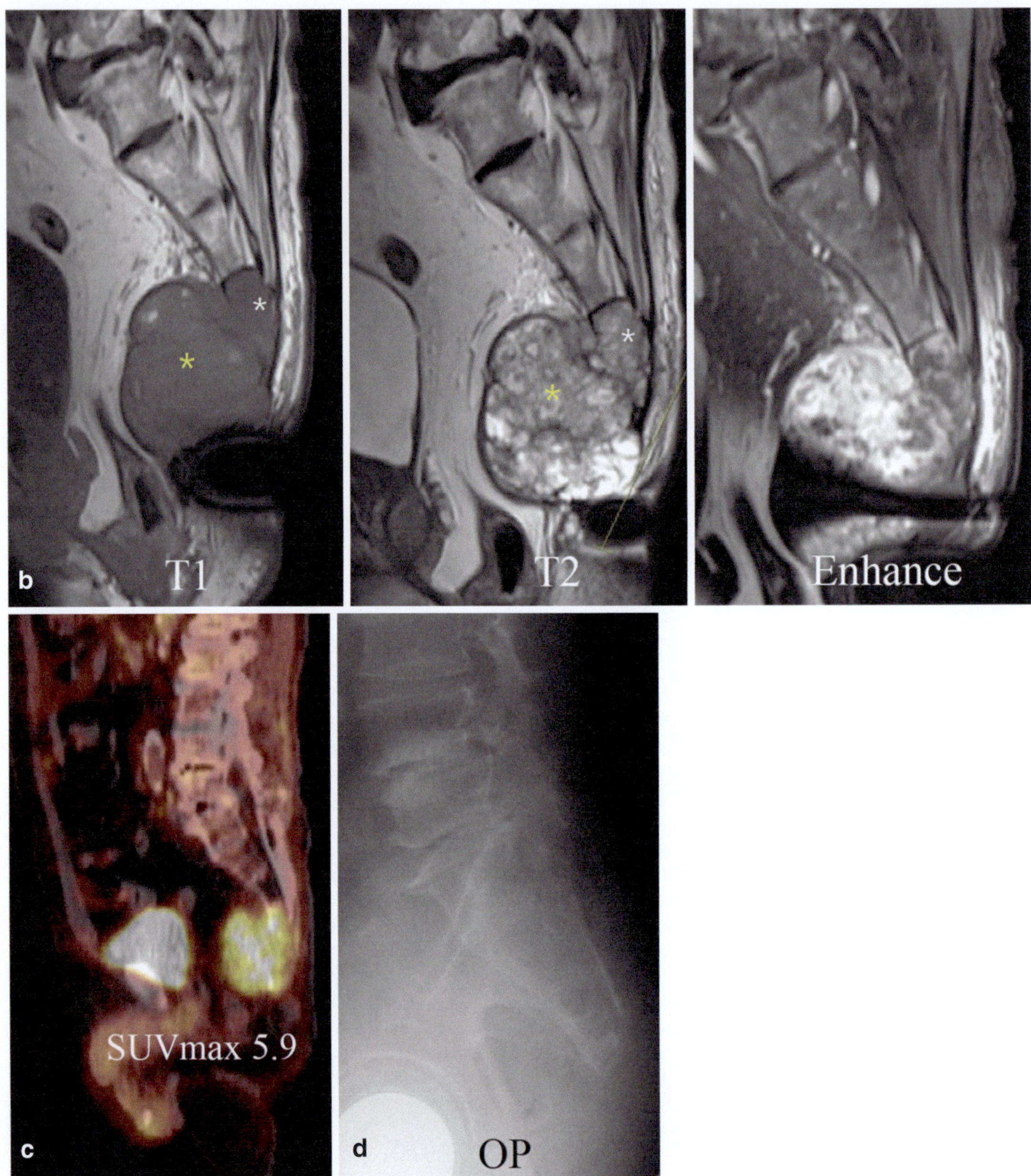

Fig. 10.1 (continued)

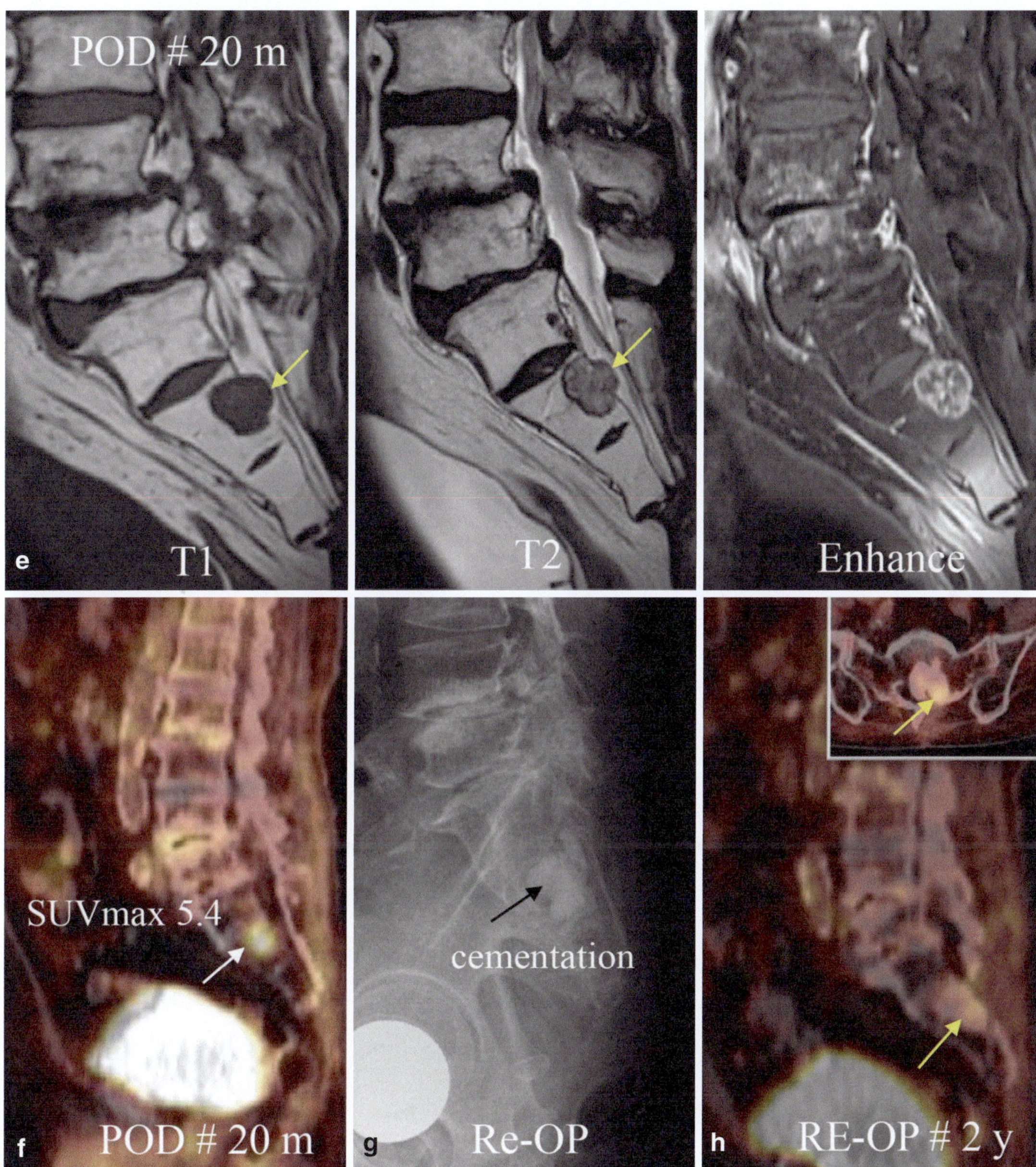

Fig. 10.1 (continued)

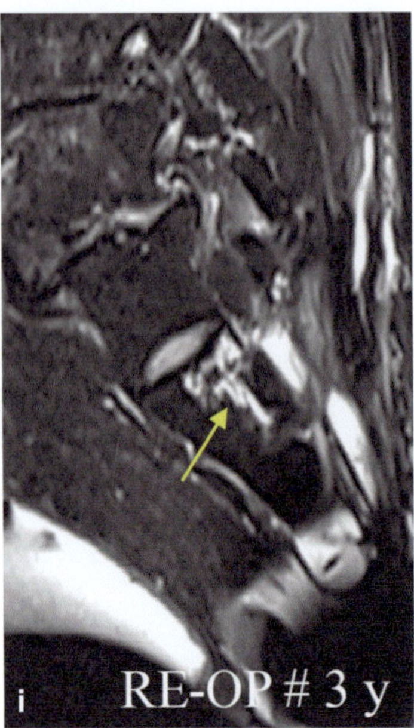

Fig. 10.1 (continued)

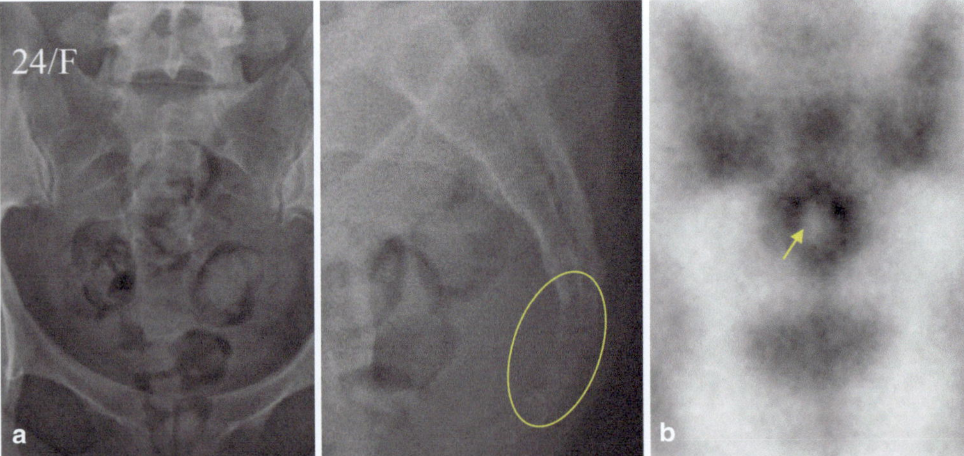

Fig. 10.2 (**a**) Anteroposterior radiograph taken for coccygodynia of 2-week duration in 24-year-old young lady does not allow to evaluate the sacral lesion due to overlapping shadows of bowel gas and stool. However, later view with no gas or stool around the bone reveals an ill-defined hazy geographic destruction in the sacro-coccygeal bone (circle). (**b**) Bone scan reveals thick ring of hot activity with central void area suggesting necrosis in the lower sacrum (arrow). (**c**) MR images demonstrate a lobulated medullary lesion with low SI on T1-weighted image and heterogeneous bright SI with focal dark signal of calcification on T2-weighted image from S4 sacrum to coccyx in association with a huge soft tissue mass (asterisks) in the ventral aspect of sacro-coccygeal junction, which is heterogeneously enhanced. (**d**) PET/CT scan notes a heterogeneous hypermetabolic lesion (SUVmax 5.1) in the sacro-coccygeal area. (**e**) Resection of from S3 to coccyx with limited negative margin followed by adjuvant radiotherapy was performed under a histologic confirmation of conventional chordoma. (**f**) Follow-up MR images at 53 months after initial surgery show newly developed mass in subcutaneous area (black asterisk) as well as muscle area in the resection bed (yellow asterisk). (**g**) PET/CT scan reveals hypermetabolic lesion in the subcutaneous area (SUVmax 4.2) and resected bed area (SUVmax 5.0), suggesting a local recurrence. Wide resection of the lesions was performed again, and microscopic examination conformed a local recurrence of the chordoma. (**h**) Follow-up MR image at 5 years after initial surgery and adjuvant radiotherapy notes postoperative change by second surgery with no evidence of local recurrence. (**i**) However, follow-up MR image at 72 months after initial managemnt demonstrates recurrent huge mass at ischiorectal fossa, which encases rectum and anteriorly displaces bladder and cervix. She does not want further surgery

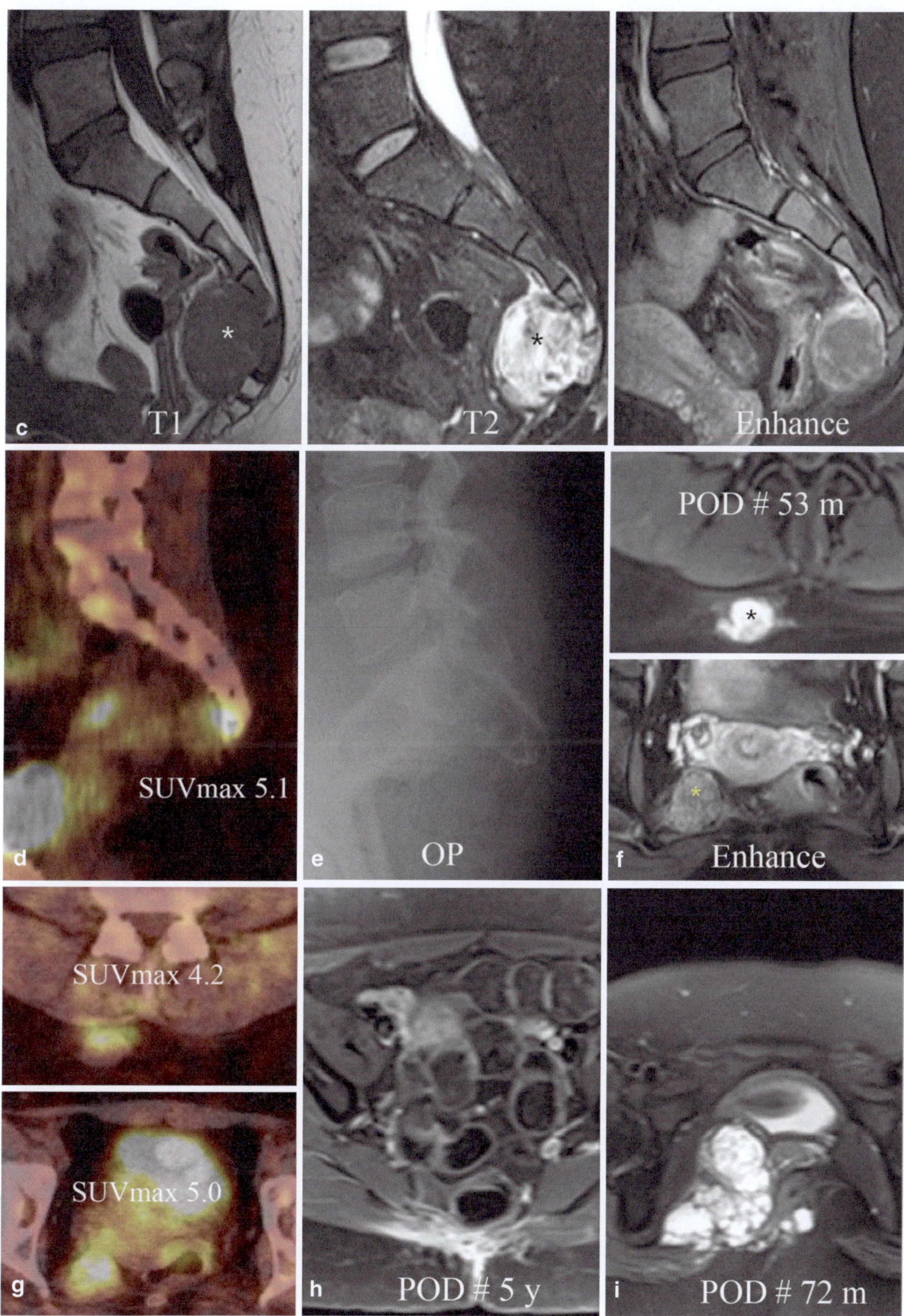

Fig. 10.2 (continued)

10.7 Histologic Findings

Macroscopically, a chordoma present as friable, encapsulated, glistening, multi-lobulated mucoid to gelatinous mass. Microscopic examination shows distinct lobules typically separated by nonneoplastic, reactive fibrous bands (Fig. 10.3a). Typically, the tumor cells show a syncytial arrangement in the form of interconnecting cords or nests within focal pools of a prominent mucinous material (Fig. 10.3b). This syncytial arrangement is very useful to differentiate chordoma from liposarcoma. The tumor cells are characteristically composed of hallmark cells with foamy to vacuolated cytoplasm, so-called *"physaliferous (basket-like) cells"* and other cells with homogeneously deep pink cytoplasm, so-called *"pink cells,"* reminiscent of early embryonic notochord. Some cells appear as intermediate shape between the *"physaliferous cell"* and *"pink cell"* (Fig. 10.3c). The ratio of both cells is varying from case to case and even from fields to fields in a same case. On rare pink cell variant, the *"pink cells"* are prominent, but *"physaliferous cells"* are sparse to total absence, which may be easily mistaken for metastatic carcinoma [2]. Cytoplasmic vacuolization is almost invariably present with varying size. Frequently, the vacuoles are large enough to displace the nucleus peripherally leading *"signet-ring"* like appearance (Fig. 10.3b). Extensive vacuolization can make clear cell appearance mimicking adipocytes (Fig. 10.3d), and minimal vacuolization with dense eosinophilic cytoplasm may simulate epithelial neoplasm. The nuclei are usually large and round to oval with a prominent nucleolus. Most lesions show clearly recognizable pleomorphism with occasional large atypical nuclei and rare giant bizarre nuclei mimicking high-grade sarcoma. Mitotic activity is usually minimal, and atypical mitoses are not present in most cases. Areas of necrosis and hemorrhage are frequently seen. Rarely, chondroid or true hyaline to myxoid cartilage ranging from small foci to large areas resembling low-grade chondrosarcoma can be observed, so-called *"chondroid chordoma"* (Fig. 10.3e). If cartilaginous differentiation is prominent, it may be difficult to distinguish from chondrosarcoma. If even tiny foci of cartilage are included, cartilaginous differentiation is not that rare phenomenon [1]. *"Dedifferentiated chordoma"* is characterized by biphasic appearance containing high-grade sarcoma component, usually undifferentiated pleomorphic sarcoma, juxtaposed to the conventional chordoma (Fig. 10.3f).

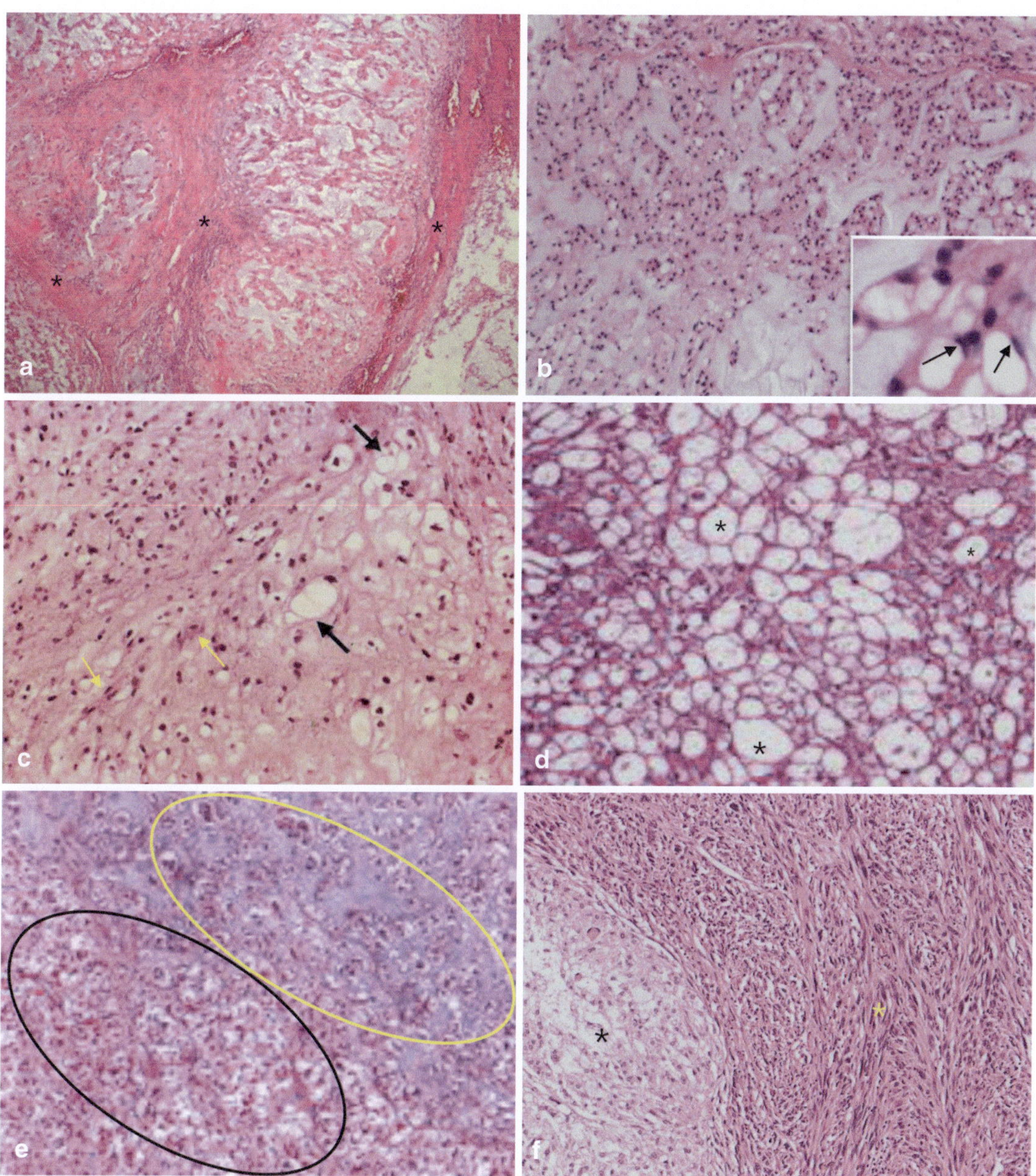

Fig. 10.3 (**a**) Low-power magnification shows distinct lobules typically separated by non-neoplastic, reactive fibrous bands (asterisks). (**b**) Mixture of foamy to vacuolated *"physalipherous"* cells and pink cells is arranged in syncytial cord in richly mucoid stroma in some fields. Frequently, the vacuoles are large enough to displace the nucleus peripherally leading *"signet-ring"* appearance simulating those in mucinous gastric carcinoma (black arrows in inset). (**c**) Higher-power magnification clearly shows the hallmark cells with foamy to vacuolated cytoplasm, so-called *"physalipherous cells"* (black arrows) and other cells with homogeneously deep pink cytoplasm, so-called *"pink cells"* (yellow arrows). Some cells are intermediate shaped between the two cells. (**d**) Some *"physalipherous"* cells have large single cytoplasmic vacuole that causes them mimicking adipocytes (asterisks). (**e**) *Chondroid chordoma* contains areas of conventional chordoma (black circle) and abruptly abutting chondroid area (yellow circle) resembling low-grade chondrosarcoma. (**f**) *Dedifferentiated chordoma* contains an area of conventional chordoma (black asterisk) juxtaposed to area with an appearance of a pleomorphic spindle cell sarcoma (yellow asterisk)

10.8 Special Stains

Intercellular myxoid stroma is stained with PAS, mucicarmine, and alcian blue. Chordoma cells typically co-express S100, epithelial markers such as keratin and EMA. An affinity for cytokeratin is useful to differentiate chordoma from chondrosarcoma particularly when the biopsy specimen is inadequate because the latter is negative for the stain.

10.9 Management and Prognosis

Wide resection with negative margin is the only curative treatment. Multidisciplinary approach is required to improve the local control of the disease. Adjuvant radiotherapy can be considered for patients with en bloc resection with positive margin or debulking, although chordoma is radioresistant to irradiation. High-dose irradiation, particularly with protons and carbon ions, is a therapeutic alternative in patients with inoperable or recurrent tumor. Currently, there is no approved medical treatment for chordoma. Clinical trials exploring additional therapeutic modalities are ongoing [8]. **Prognosis** can be influenced by histologic subtype, location, size, respectability, age of the patients, and distant metastasis. Local recurrence rate is high due to locally aggressive nature and location which is not adequate for wide resection. Sacral locations show the best prognosis because they may allow wide resection with negative margin. However, wide resection with adequate margin is difficult to achieve in the mobile spines. Rate of distant metastasis to lung, bone, and lymph node has been reported very widely from 5 to 43% [9–12]. In an analysis of 808 patients with primary chordoma (The Surveillance, Epidemiology, and End Results (SEER) Registry) database between 1973 and 2014, overall survival and disease-specific survival was about 80 and 89% at 3 years, 68 and 81% at 5 years, and 39 and 60% at 10 years. The median overall survival and disease-specific survival was 7.8 years and 13.8 years, respectively. The overall rate of distant metastasis was 7.7%. Additionally, spinal chordoma patients with an elderly age (age ≥ 60), performed with nonsurgical therapy, and with distant metastasis were associated with worse prognosis and poor overall survival [13].

References

1. Czerniak B. Chordoma and related lesions. In: Dorfman HD, Czerniak B, editors. Dorfman and Czerniak's bone tumors. 2nd ed. Philadelphia, PA: Elsevier; 2016. p. 1174–216.
2. Mirra JM. Chordoma. In: Mirra JM, editor. Bone tumors: clinical, radiologic, and pathologic correlation. 2nd ed. Philadelphia, PA: Lea & Febiger; 1989. p. 648–72.
3. Murphey MD, Smith W, Smith S, Kransdorf M, Temple H. From the archives of the AFIP. Primary tumors of the spine: radiologic pathologic correlation. Radiographics. 1996;16(5):1131–58.
4. Das P, Soni P, Jones J, Habboub G, Barnholtz-Sloan JS, Recinos PF, et al. Descriptive epidemiology of chordomas in the United States. J Neuro-Oncol. 2020;148(1):173–8.
5. Diel J, Ortiz O, Losada RA, Price DB, Hayt MW, Katz DS. The sacrum: pathologic spectrum, multimodality imaging, and subspecialty approach. Radiographics. 2001;21(1):83–104.
6. Meyers SP, Hirsch W, Curtin HD, Barnes L, Sekhar LN, Sen C. Chordomas of the skull base: MR features. Am J Neuroradiol. 1992;13(6):1627–36.
7. Pamir MN, Ozduman K. Analysis of radiological features relative to histopathology in 42 skull-base chordomas and chondrosarcomas. Eur J Radiol. 2006;58(3):461–470.
8. Scheipl S, Igrec J, Leithner A, Smolle M, Haybäck J, Liegl B. Chordome: Gibt es eine molekulargenetische Grundlage für diagnostik und therapie? (Chordoma: is there a molecular basis for diagnosis and treatment?) Pathologe. 2020;41(2):153–62.
9. Vergara G, Belinchón B, Valcárcel F, Veiras M, Zapata I, de la Torre A. Metastatic disease from chordoma. Clin Transl Oncol. 2008;10(8):517–21.
10. McPherson CM, Suki D, McCutcheon IE, Gokaslan ZL, Rhines LD, Mendel E. Metastatic disease from spinal chordoma: a 10-year experience. J Neurosurg Spine. 2006;5(4):277–80.
11. Delank K-S, Kriegsmann J, Drees P, Eckardt A, Eysel P. Metastasizing chordoma of the lumbar spine. Eur Spine J. 2002;11(2):167–71.
12. Sopta J, Tulic G, Mijucic V, Mamontov P, Mandic N. Solitary lymph node metastasis without local recurrence of primary chordoma. Eur Spine J. 2009;18(2):191–5.
13. Pan Y, Lu L, Chen J, Zhong Y, Dai Z. Analysis of prognostic factors for survival in patients with primary spinal chordoma using the SEER registry from 1973 to 2014. J Orthop Surg Res. 2018;13(1):1–8.

Part IV

Cysts and Cyst-Like Lesions

11 Aneurysmal Bone Cyst

(***aneurysma*** "widening" + **kystis** "sac")

11.1 Definition

Aneurysmal bone cyst (ABC) is a benign but locally destructive expansile lesion of bone characterized by multilocular blood-filled cystic spaces surrounded by walls predominantly consisting of fibrous tissue. ABC can be divided into primary, de novo ABC without a definite precursor lesion and secondary ABC with various pre-existing lesions.

11.2 Possible Pathogenesis

A possibility of a hemorrhagic "blowout" working on pre-existing lesion has been suggested by Jaffe [1] who introduced the term ABC with Lichtenstein [2]. They separated ABC as a distinct lesion from giant cell tumor. Later, it has been postulated that locally disturbed blood circulation by arteriovenous anomaly might be operating on a precursor lesion [3]. Recent cytogenetic studies showing recurrent cytogenetic abnormality of chromosomal translocation suggested that at least some primary ABCs are true neoplasms and not reactive tumor- simulating lesions [4–7]. More recently, Oliveira et al. [8] proposed that primary and secondary ABCs have a different pathogenesis by observation of ubiquitin-specific protease (USP6) or CDH11 rearrangements in about 70% of primary ABC but not in secondary ABC, suggesting that the latter is not a neoplasm. Thus, they concluded that secondary ABC would likely represent a common end point of differentiation in non-ABC bone tumors.

11.3 Clinical Importance

ABC can be easily mistaken for sarcoma such as telangiectatic osteosarcoma radiographically due to severe bone destruction and expansion or blowout with rapid growth pattern and histologically due to significantly high cellularity with plump and ominous nuclei particularly at incipient phase. Another clinical importance is that ABC can be frequently associated various locally aggressive benign or even malignant pre-existing lesions. In a series of 215 ABCs [9], about half of the cases (114 cases; 53.0%) are secondary in nature and associated with both benign and malignant lesions including giant cell tumor (GCT), chondroblastoma (CB), fibrous dysplasia (FD), osteosarcoma (OSA), non-ossifying fibroma, osteoblastoma, and simple bone cyst (SBC) in decreasing order. GCT, CB, and FD occupied about 70% (79 of 114 cases) of secondary ABC. Approximately half of secondary ABCs (52 of 114 cases; 45.6%) were linked with locally aggressive giant cell tumor (39 cases) and malignant tumor of osteosarcoma (13 cases).

W.-J. Bahk, *Diagnosis and Management of Primary Bone Tumors*,
https://doi.org/10.1007/978-981-99-5498-8_11

Scrutinized and careful histologic examination should be warranted to find such aggressive pre-existing tumors for appropriate management. Another clinical importance is that very rare case may have cytological aberration that may be severe and bizarre enough to simulate malignant tumor but no equivocal atypical mitosis and frank anaplasia showing absolutely benign clinical course, so-called *"peudoanaplastic"* ABC which should be differentiated from the true malignant tumors [10].

11.4 Incidence

Primary ABC is relatively uncommon, accounting for about 1% of biopsy-proven primary bone tumor and approximately 2–2.5% when secondary ABC component is included [11].

11.5 Age

ABC affects all age groups ranged from 1 to 83 years, but about half [9] and up to 80–85% of the patients [11, 12] occur in skeletally immature patients younger than 20 years of age. It is very rare age under 5 years and over 50 years. Secondary ABC occurs often in much older patient depending on the pre-existing lesions.

11.6 Location

ABC can affect any bones but usually affects medullary portion and much less commonly the cortex and periosteum. The lesion occurs most commonly in the metaphysis of long bones, especially femur, tibia, and humerus as well as posterior element of spine and craniofacial bone. Diaphysis of the long bones is less frequently involved. Small bones of hand and foot and flat bones such as pelvis, scapula, rib, or patella are next frequently involved sites.

11.7 Clinical Features

Most common symptoms are pain and swelling. Swelling can be severe and rapidly developed due to blowout nature of the lesion. Rarely, pathologic fracture can be associated (Fig. 11.2a, 11.6e). The skin temperature over the affected bone may be increased. Movement in adjacent joints may be restricted. Nerve root or spinal cord compression symptoms can be associated when involving vertebrae.

11.8 Radiologic Findings

Radiologic findings are protean and can vary depending on the phase of the lesion [11] (Fig. 11.1). (1) *Incipient/Early Phase*. Two types of presentation are existed in this phase. The lesions can exhibit a diffusely moth-eaten to permeative destruction mimicking rapidly progressing malignant tumor. Other cases may be presented as a well-circumscribed benign-looking lytic lesion. (2) *Mid-phase* ("blowout" due to explosive growth). Features are usually indicative of ABC in this phase (Figs. 11.2, 11.3, 11.4 and 11.5). Most lesions are purely lytic without mineralized matrix. Rapid growing of the lesion can expand the affected bone and destruct the cortex with pushing out of the periosteum. The lesions show eccentric or concentric expansion with internal linear trabeculations due to endosteal ridges produced by tumoral resorption of cortex, so-called *"bubbly appearance."* Some cases present significant cortical destruction with a soft tissue mass imitating a malignant tumor. A thin reactive shell of periosteal new bone is extended from the Codman's triangle area fusing together and begins to encircle the lesion in a "balloon-like" fashion. With shaft of long bone protruding into the expanded area with buttress of periosteal reaction, overall appearance becomes *"finger-in-a balloon"* appearance, which is highly indicative of ABC

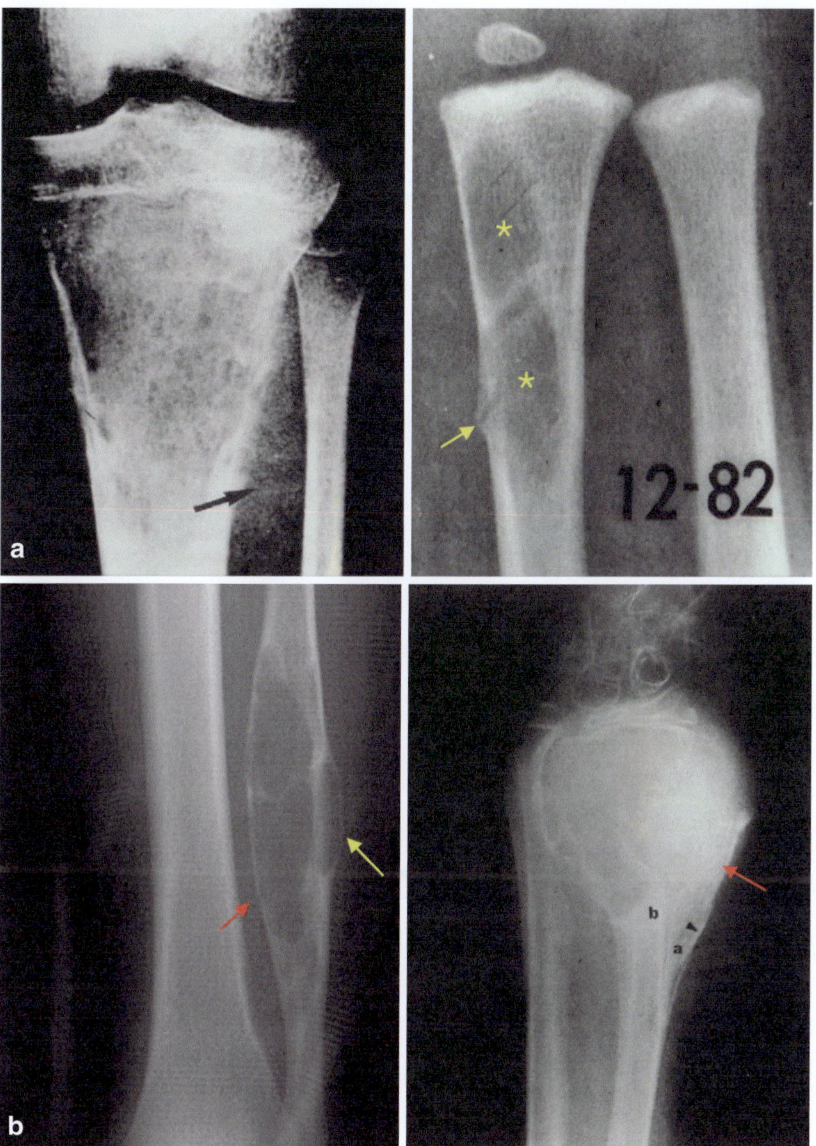

Fig. 11.1 (**a**) *Incipient or early phase* This phase may show either benign- or malignant-looking presentation. (Left) Radiograph taken for left knee pain in adolescent male reveals an ill-defined moth-eaten to permeative destruction with a naked soft tissue mass (black arrow) in the proximal tibia suggesting a locally aggressive or even malignant bone tumor. However, biopsy confirmed a diagnosis of ABC. (Right) Radiograph taken for wrist pain after minor injury in young boy shows a benign-looking multi-lobulated round to oval osteolytic lesion (yellow asterisks) surrounded by a suspicious hazy rim of sclerosis involving meta-diaphysis of distal ulna with buckling and crack indicating incomplete fracture (yellow arrow). (**b**) *Mid-phase* Findings are suggestive of ABC. (Left) Radiograph taken for leg pain in young boy shows a well-demarcated, multi-lobulated geographic destruction with internal linear septa involving distal fibula. The lesion is moderately expansive, and the cortices are markedly thinned but not perforated (yellow arrow). Cortical crack is suspected (red arrow). (Right) Radiograph taken for wrist pain with rapid swelling in young boy reveals a significantly concentric expansion of the distal radius. Note "balloon-like" expansion with a thin cuff of periosteal new bone (arrowhead) extending from the former Codman's triangle (a) and newly forming shell of periosteal new bone (red arrow). The overall shape of inwardly intruding shaft of the radius (b) within the expanded radius is like a *"finger-in-a balloon,"* highly indicative if not pathognomonic of ABC. (**c**) *Late-phase of equilibrium and stabilization* The lesion progressively ossifies and becomes stabilized with coarse trabeculations and a thin complete rim of new bone formation (red arrow). Note a trace of old "finger-in-a balloon" sign (black arrow) indicating stabilization of ABC. Thus, the lesion is no more considered as malignancy

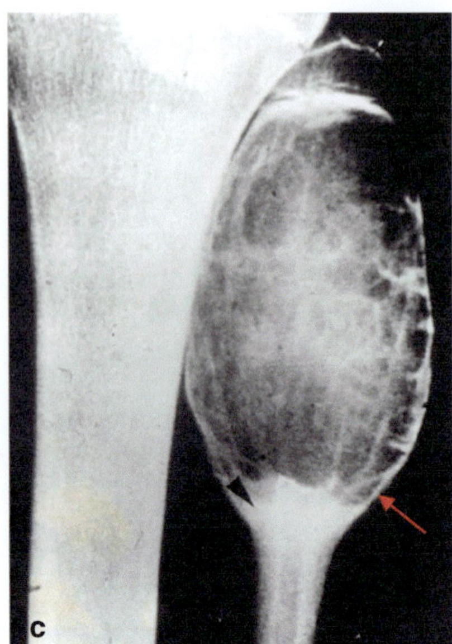

Fig. 11.1 (continued)

although not pathognomonic sign. (3) *Late phase* (equilibrium and stabilization). Finally, the procedure reaches equilibrium, and the lesion becomes stabilized. The lesion progressively ossifies with coarse tabulations, and the ballooning very slowly decreases with complete rim of new bone formation. Thus, the lesion is no more considered as malignancy. **Bone scan** usually reveals peripherally increased uptake related to reactive sclerotic new bone with little activity (photon defect) in the center of cystic lesion, so-called *"doughnut"* sign. But it may show diffuse homogeneous increased uptake when trabeculae of new bone within fibrous tissue septa are formed throughout the lesion. **MR images** demonstrate an expansile, multi-lobulated cystic lesion of varying size with low SI on T1-weighted image and heterogeneously high SI with varying degree of low and intermediate signal T2-wieghted image surrounded by a thin dark signal of periosteal new bone on both images. Frequently, the presence of a solid component with different signal suggests that the ABC may be secondary to pre-existing lesions. Perilesional bone marrow and/or neighboring soft tissues is often associated. The *"fluid-fluid levels"* of different densities representing precipitation of red blood cells at the bottom and serum on the top with different densities atop one another are characteristically demonstrated (Figs. 11.9, 11.10, 11.11, 11.12, 11.13, and 11.14). However, it can be also seen in SBC with pathologic fracture and telangiectatic OSA; thus, it is by no means unique to ABC. The signal of different densities is variably manifested depending on the age of the blood and the type of hemoglobin (oxy-, deoxy-, or met-). Contrast images exhibit peripheral and septal enhancement but no diffuse internal enhancement. Focal solid areas with enhancement may represent either solid portion of thickened ABC wall (Figs. 11.2b, 11.6b and 11.13c) or component of pre-existing another tumor from which secondary ABC develops (Fig. 11.10c, 11.11b, 11.12b).

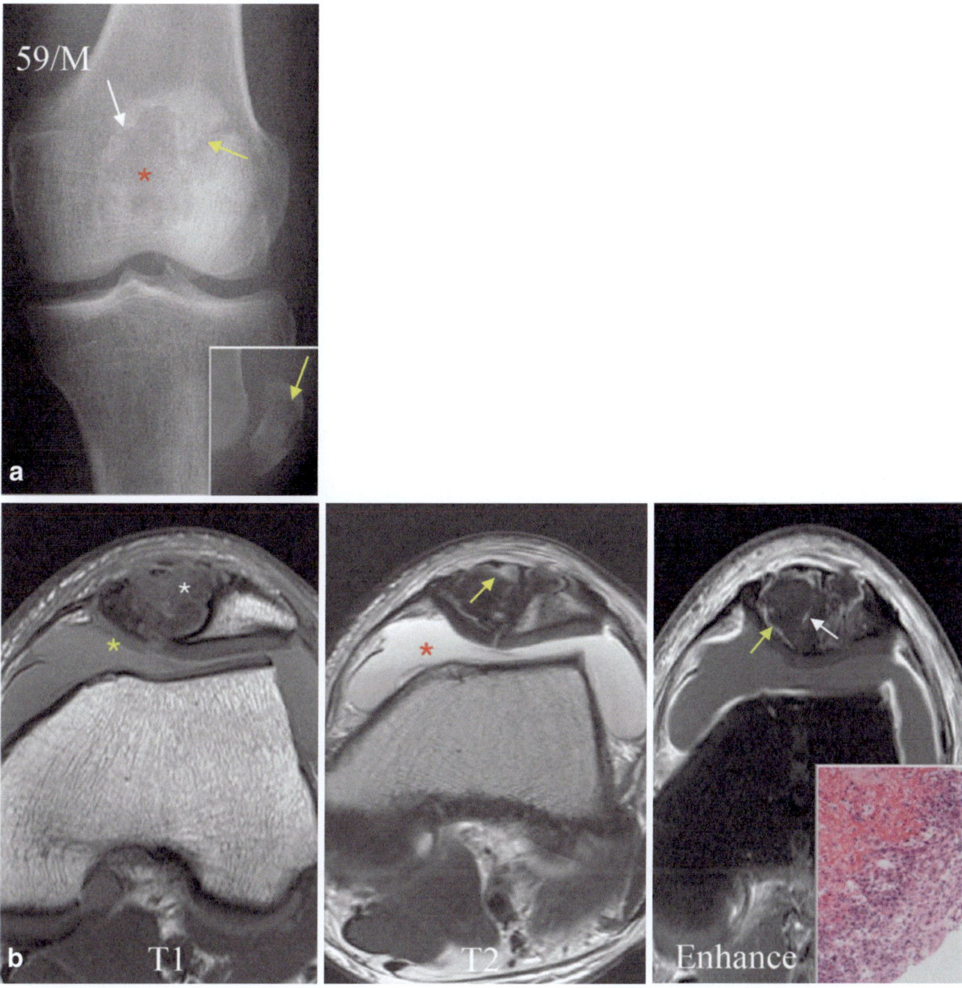

Fig. 11.2 (**a**) Radiograph taken for left knee pain of 3-year duration, which is aggravated after slip in 59-year-old man show a relatively well-defined lytic lesion (asterisk) surrounded by an irregular thin rim of sclerosis (white arrow) with a fracture line (yellow arrows) in the patella. (**b**) MR images reveal a multi-lobular cystic lesion (white asterisk) with low and intermediate SI on T1-weighted image and mixed signal of mainly low and small high signal making a "fluid-fluid" level (yellow arrow) on T2-weighted images. There is extensive hemorrhage (red and yellow asterisk) in the patella-femoral joint due to a pathologic fracture. The lesion is peripherally enhanced (yellow arrow) with focal tiny internal enhancement (white arrow), which may represent a sold portion of thickened ABC wall (inset). (**c**) Before frozen biopsy, aspiration from the patella lesion showed pure dark fresh blood rather than blood-tinged clear yellow fluid. Then, frozen biopsy confirmed a diagnosis of primary ABC with several sold portion of thickened ABC walls but no of evidence of pre-existing tumor. (**d**) Follow-up radiograph at 6 months after thorough curettage, allo-chip bone graft and fixation using tension band wiring demonstrates consolidation of the lesion with fracture union. (**e**) Radiograph taken for right knee pain of 4-month duration in 23-year-old young lady shows an eccentric geographic radiolucent lesion (asterisk) with no clear rim of sclerosis in the proximal tibia. Note cortical destruction and soft tissue extension suggesting aggressive lesion on lateral view (arrow in inset). (**f**) Bone scan reveals strong uptake with internal photon defect (asterisk). (**g**) SPECT/CT images also note an intense focal uptake with little activity in the center of lesion (yellow asterisks). Cortical loss is seen with soft tissue extension with intense uptake (arrow in inset). (**h**) MR images demonstrate an eccentric geographic destruction with anterior cortical destruction and soft tissue extension. There are multiple "fluid-fluid" levels of different densities on T2-weighted image. The lesion is peripherally enhanced (yellow arrows) with enhancing solid portion (red arrow). However, pre-existing other solid tumor is not histologically observed, and a final diagnosis of primary ABC is rendered. (**i**) Extended curettage using high-speed bur and allo-chip bone graft was performed. (**j**) Radiograph at 4 years after surgery notes some resorption of graft bone (red asterisk), but no definite evidence of local recurrence. She is also doing very well without any symptoms

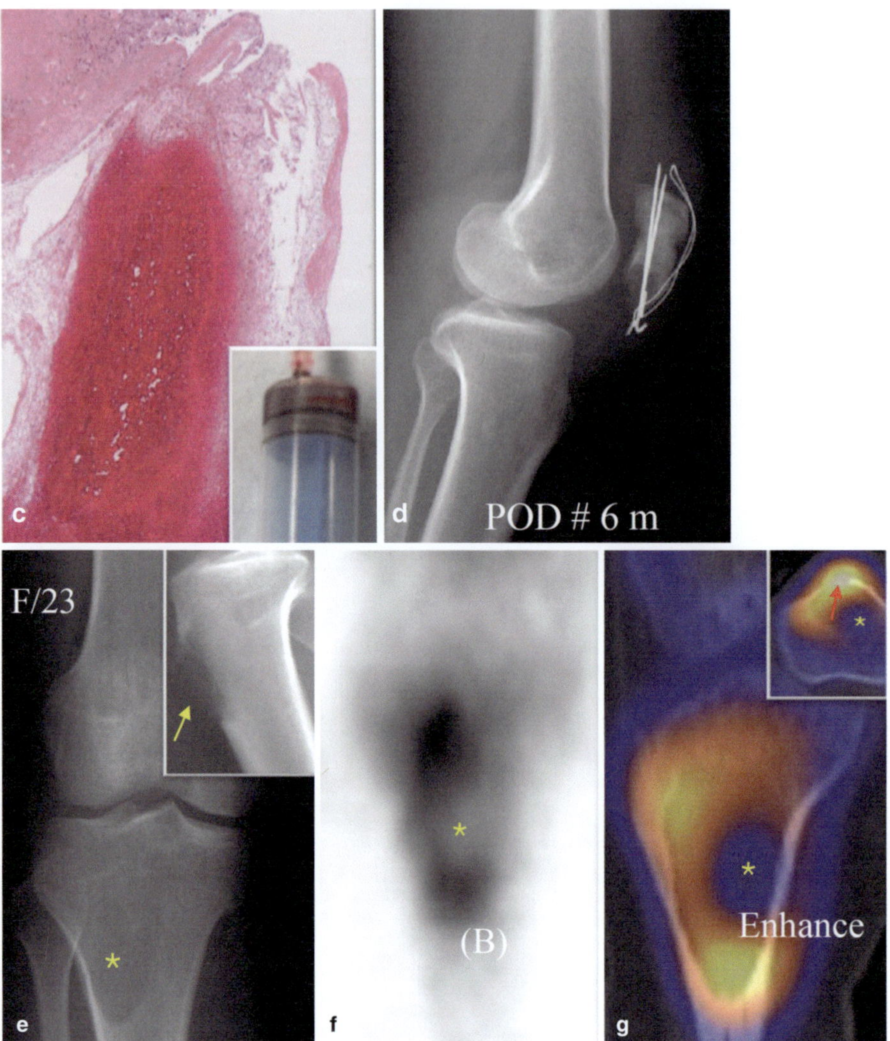

Fig. 11.2 (continued)

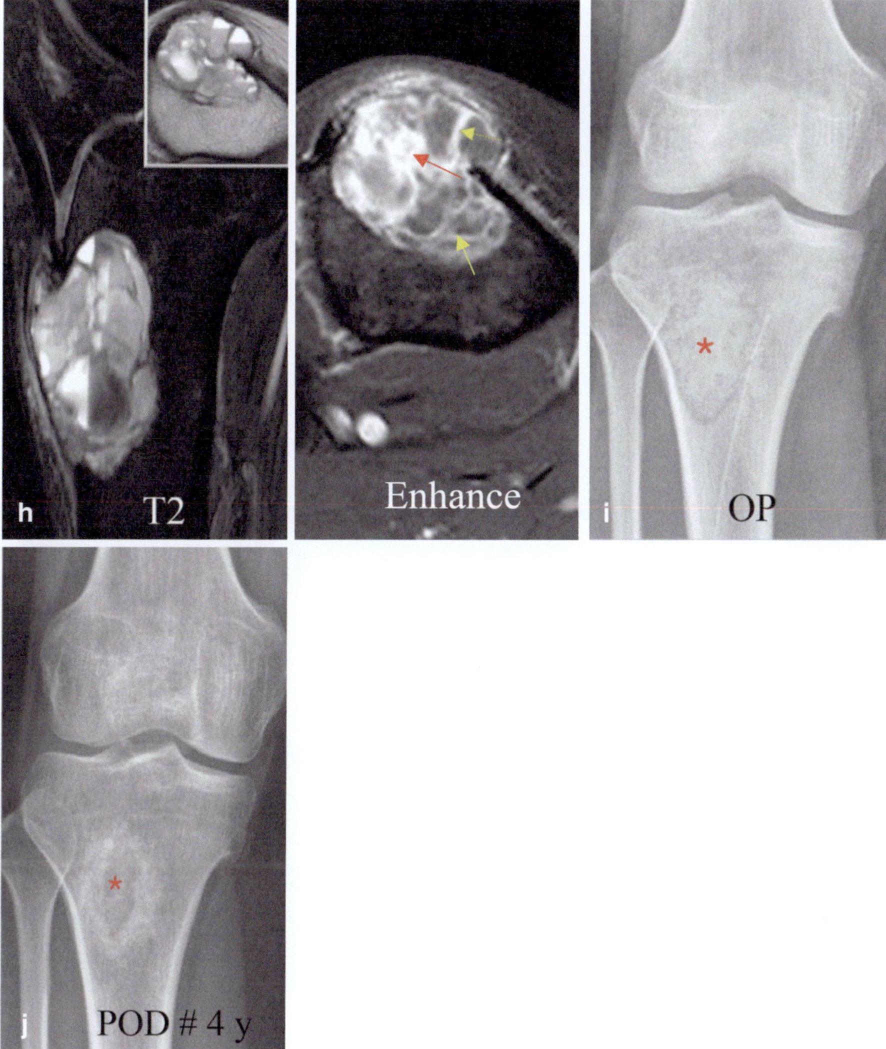

Fig. 11.2 (continued)

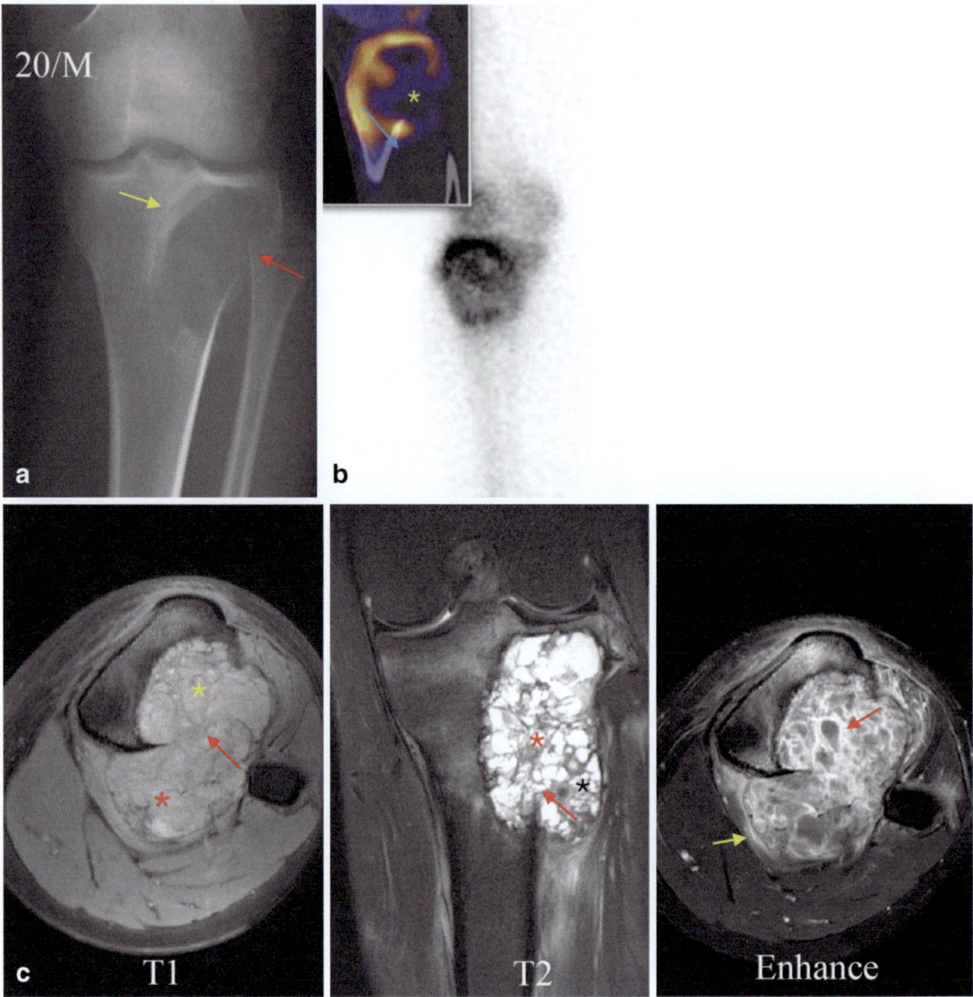

Fig. 11.3 (**a**) Radiograph taken for left knee pain of 3-month duration in 20-year-old young man shows an eccentric lytic geographic destruction surrounded by a rind of surrounding sclerosis (yellow arrow) with cortical breakage (red arrow) involving epi-metaphysis of proximal tibia. (**b**) Bone scan reveals an inhomogeneous strong uptake along the periphery of the lesion with a weaker uptake or photon defect in the center of the lesion. On SPECT/CT image, inhomogeneous uptake at the periphery of the lesion with internal photon defect is also seen with cortical destruction in left proximal tibia (asterisk in inset). (**c**) MR images demonstrate an eccentric multi-lobulated medullary lesion (yellow asterisk) with cortical destruction (red arrows) forming a large soft tissue mass (red asterisks). The SI is intermediate or iso to muscle on T1-weighted image and heterogeneous high SI with numerous "fluid-fluid" levels of various densities in the bony lesion (black asterisk) as well as soft tissue mass lesion (black asterisk) on T2-weighted image. On contrast image, both lesions show peripheral (yellow arrow) and septal (red arrow) enhancement. (**d**) Incision biopsy followed by cement packing to reduce postoperative bleeding was performed (red arrow). (**e**) Microscopic examination. (Left) Lower-magnification reveals multi-lobulated cystic thickened wall architecture with blood-filled cystic spaces of variable size separated by significantly thickened fibrous septa. There are moderate to high number of bland spindle cells, inflammatory cells, numerous capillary channels, and extravasated red blood cells with primitive slivers of osteoid to woven bone rimmed by osteoblasts (black arrows), which are highly suggestive of benignancy. Some of blood vessels are dilated resembling small aneurysmal spaces containing blood cells (black asterisks). (Right) There are several multinucleated osteoclast-like giant cells sprinkled on the markedly thickened wall (yellow arrows). (**f**) Extended curettage using high-speed bur and chemical cauterization with anhydrous ethanol followed by bone cementing and plate fixation was performed. (**g**) Follow-up radiograph at 3 years after surgery notes no evidence of local recurrence

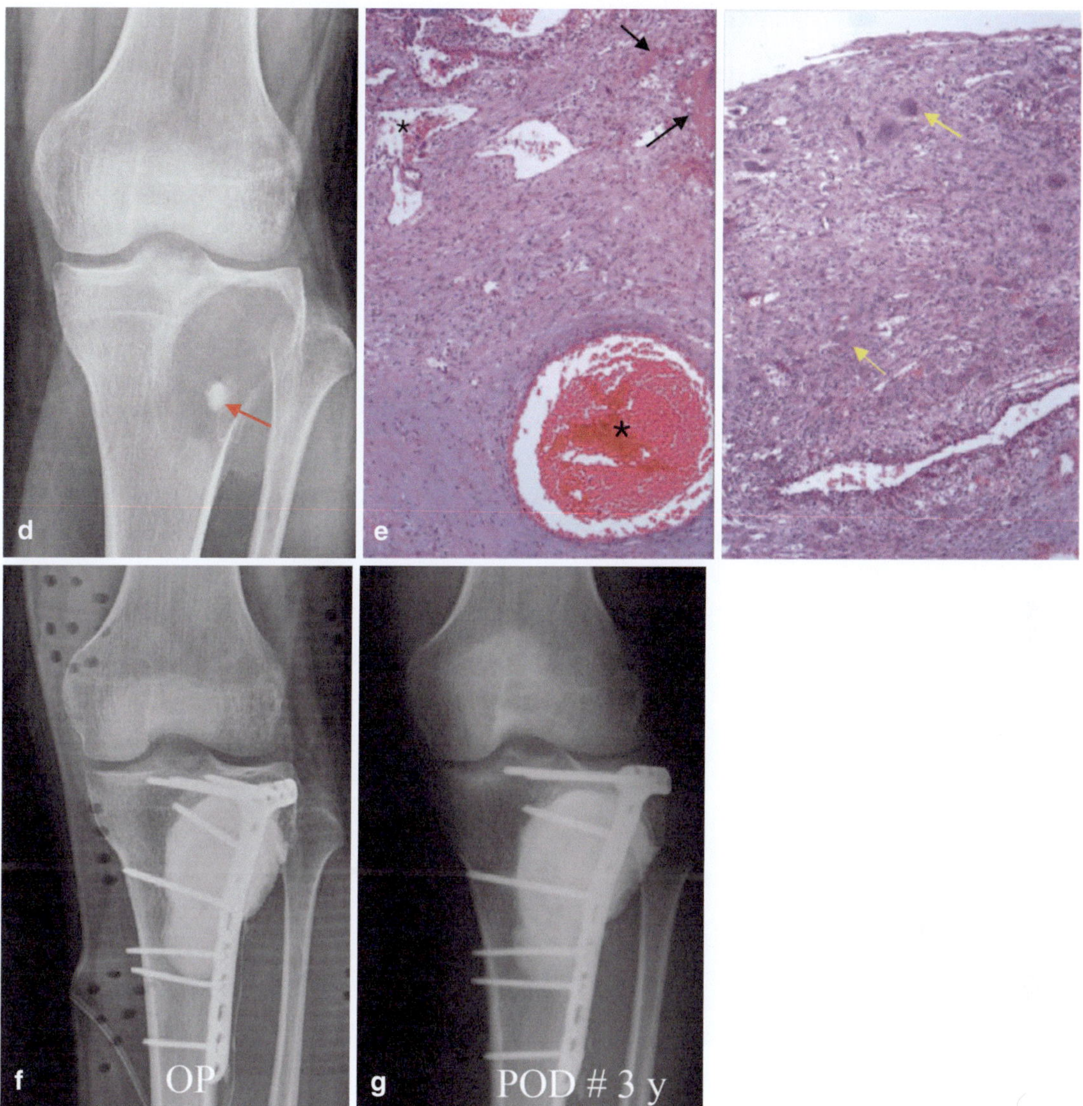

Fig. 11.3 (continued)

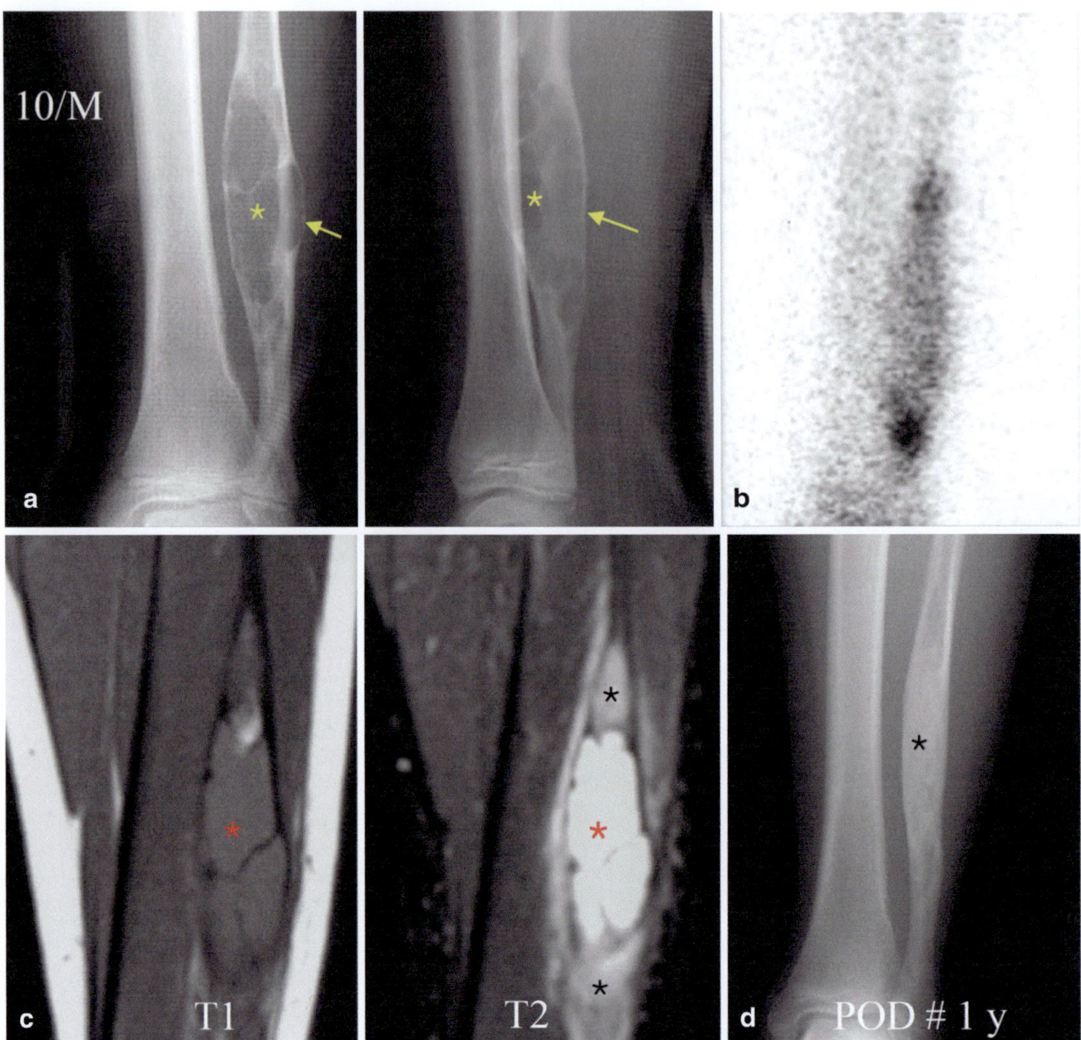

Fig. 11.4 (**a**) Radiograph taken for left distal leg pain after blunt trauma in 10-year-old boy shows a multi-lobulated expansile cystic lesion (asterisks) with a marked cortical thinning but no perforation (arrows) mainly affecting diaphysis of distal fibula. (**b**) Bone scan reveals a peripherally increased uptake with internal milder uptake in the diaphysis of distal fibula. (**c**) MR images demonstrate a multi-lobulated expanded intramedullary lesion (red asterisks) with low SI on T1-weighted image and high SI on T2-weighted image. There is peri-tumoral bone edema (black asterisks). (**d**) Radiograph at 1 year after extended curettage and allo-chip bone graft notes good consolidation with remodeling but no evidence of local recurrence (asterisk). (**e**) Radiograph taken for right ankle pain of 1-year duration in 20-year-old young man shows an ill-defined round to oval osteolytic lesion at superior-lateral aspect of talus (circle). (**f**) Bone scan reveals a heterogeneously increased uptake with a focal internal photon defect (asterisk). (**g**) MR images demonstrate a well-defined multi-lobulated cystic lesion with low SI on T1-weighted image and heterogeneous high SI with "fluid-fluid" levels on fat saturated T2-weighted image. The lesion is well defined by a dark signal of reactive sclerotic bone on both sequences (yellow arrows). Contrast images exhibit peripheral (white arrow) and septal (yellow arrow) enhancement but no internal enhancement indicating primary ABC. Microscopic examination of curette specimen also fail to find other pre-existing bone tumor. (**h**) Follow-up radiograph and CT scan (inset) at 2 years after thorough curettage and allo-chip bone graft notes consolidation with no evidence of recurrence (red circle)

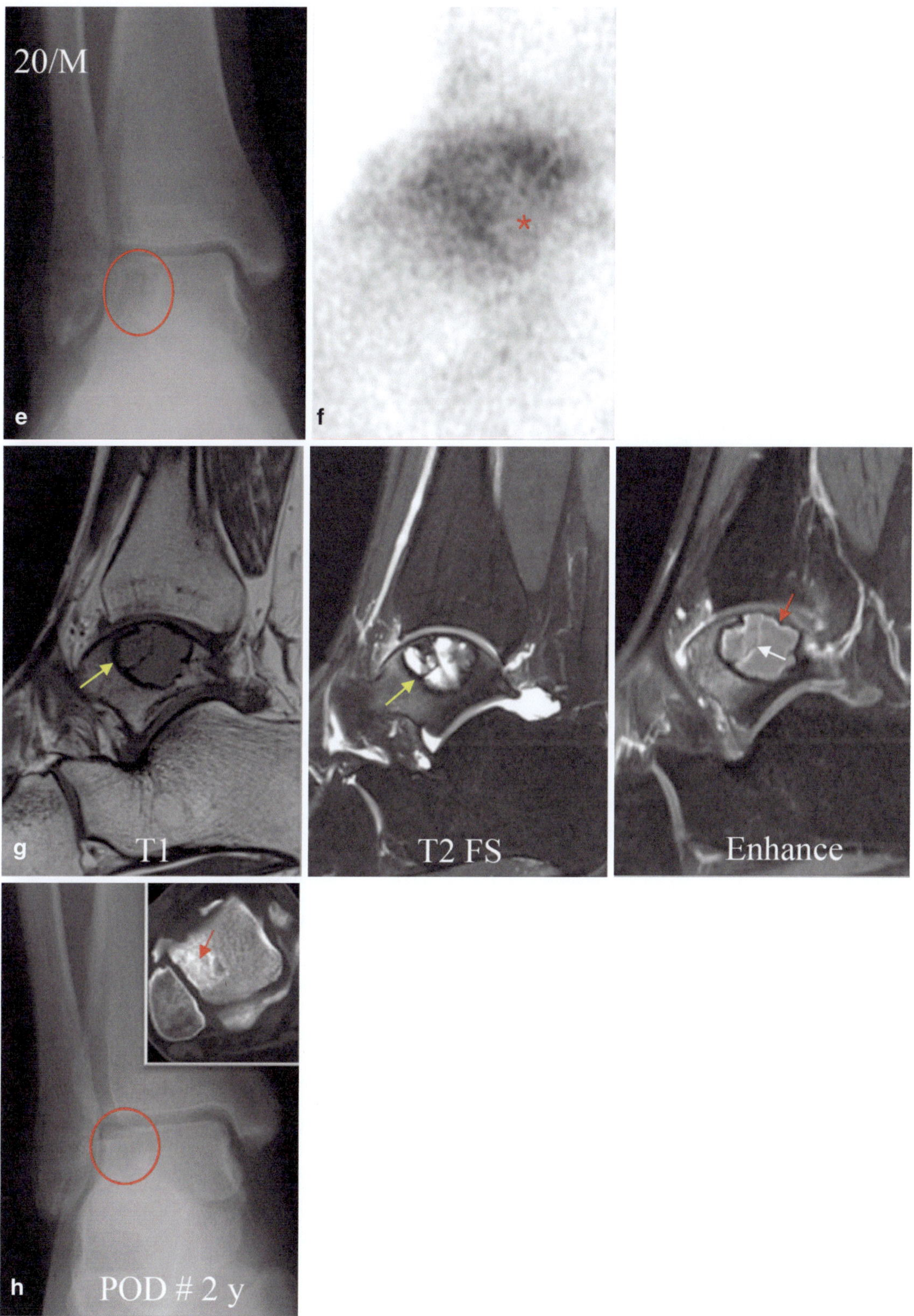

Fig. 11.4 (continued)

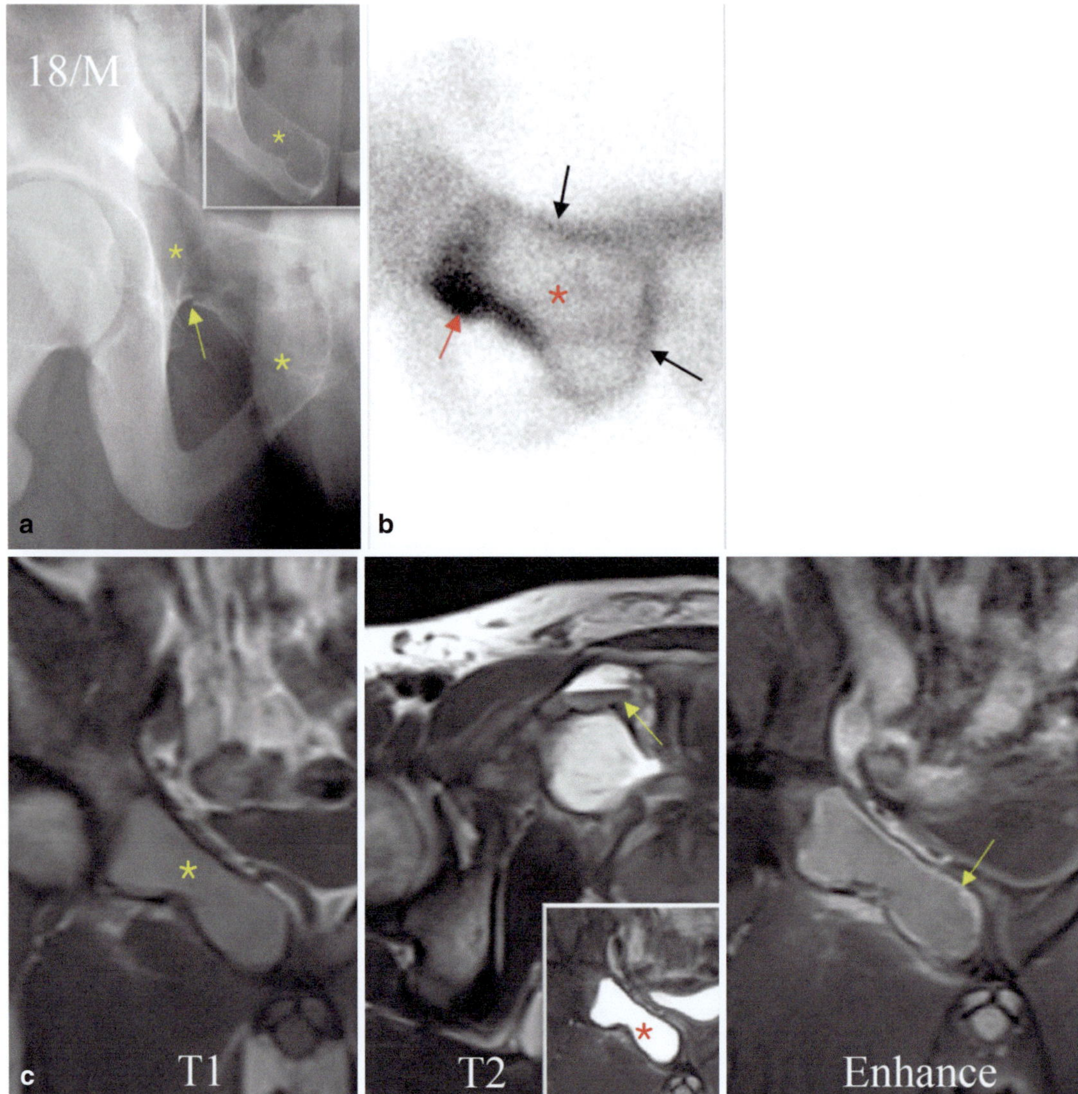

Fig. 11.5 (**a**) Radiograph taken for right inguinal intermittent pain of 2-year duration in 18-year-old adolescent shows an ill-defined expansile radiolucent lesion (asterisks) with a cortical breakage (yellow arrow) in the right pubic rami to tubercle and part of inferior rami. (**b**) Pinhole bone scan reveals heterogeneously increased activity along the rim of the lesion with a focal strong uptake indicating pathologic cortical breakage and internal void area (asterisk). (**c**) MR images demonstrate a well-defined cystic lesion (asterisks) with intermediate SI on T1-weighted image and high SI with multiple thin septations and a "fluid-fluid" level (yellow arrow). The lesion is peripherally enhanced (yellow arrow) with no internal solid enhancement. (**d**) Follow-up radiograph at 1 year after extended curettage and allo-chip bone graft was performed under presumptive diagnosis of primary ABC notes consolidation of the lesion (asterisk). The diagnosis was confirmed by microscopic examination of curetted specimen. (**e**) Radiograph taken for left inguinal pain for 4-month duration in 17-year-old adolscent shows an expansile radiolucent lesion (asterisk) with a well-defined hazy ballooning (arrows) in the left pubic bone. (**f**) CT scan reveals an expansile osteolytic lesion (asterisk) with an interrupted rim of surrounding sclerosis (arrow). (**g**) MR images demonstrate a multi-lobulated ballooning cystic lesion with low SI (yellow arrow) on T1-weighted image and heterogeneous intermediate and high SI on T2-weighted image. The lesion is peripherally enhanced (yellow arrow) with internal focal tiny enhancement. However, microscopic examination confirmed primary ABC without any pre-existing lesions. (**h**) Radiograph at 3 years after thorough curettage and allo-chip bone graft notes healing of the lesion with no evidence of local recurrence (asterisk)

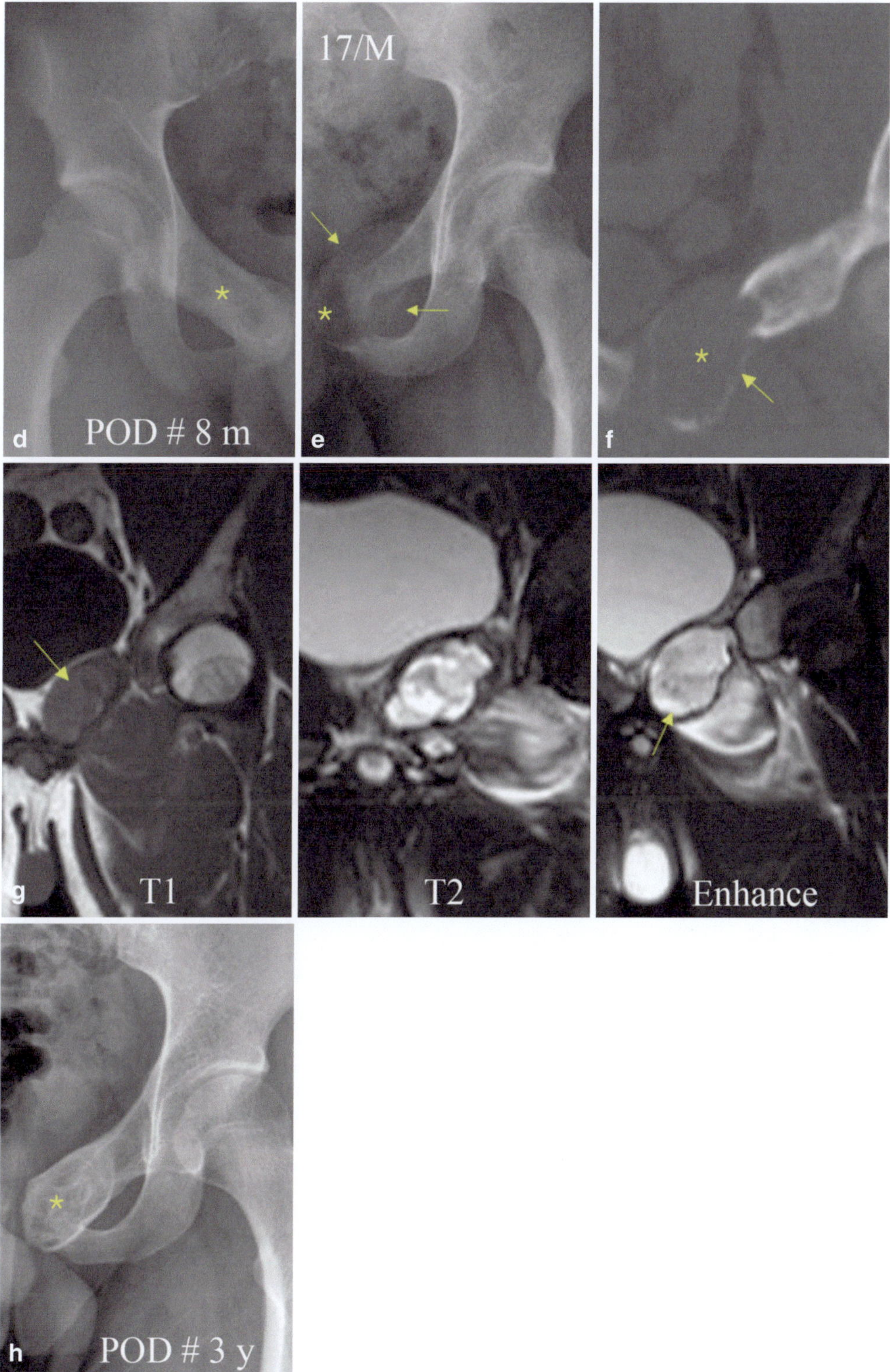

Fig. 11.5 (continued)

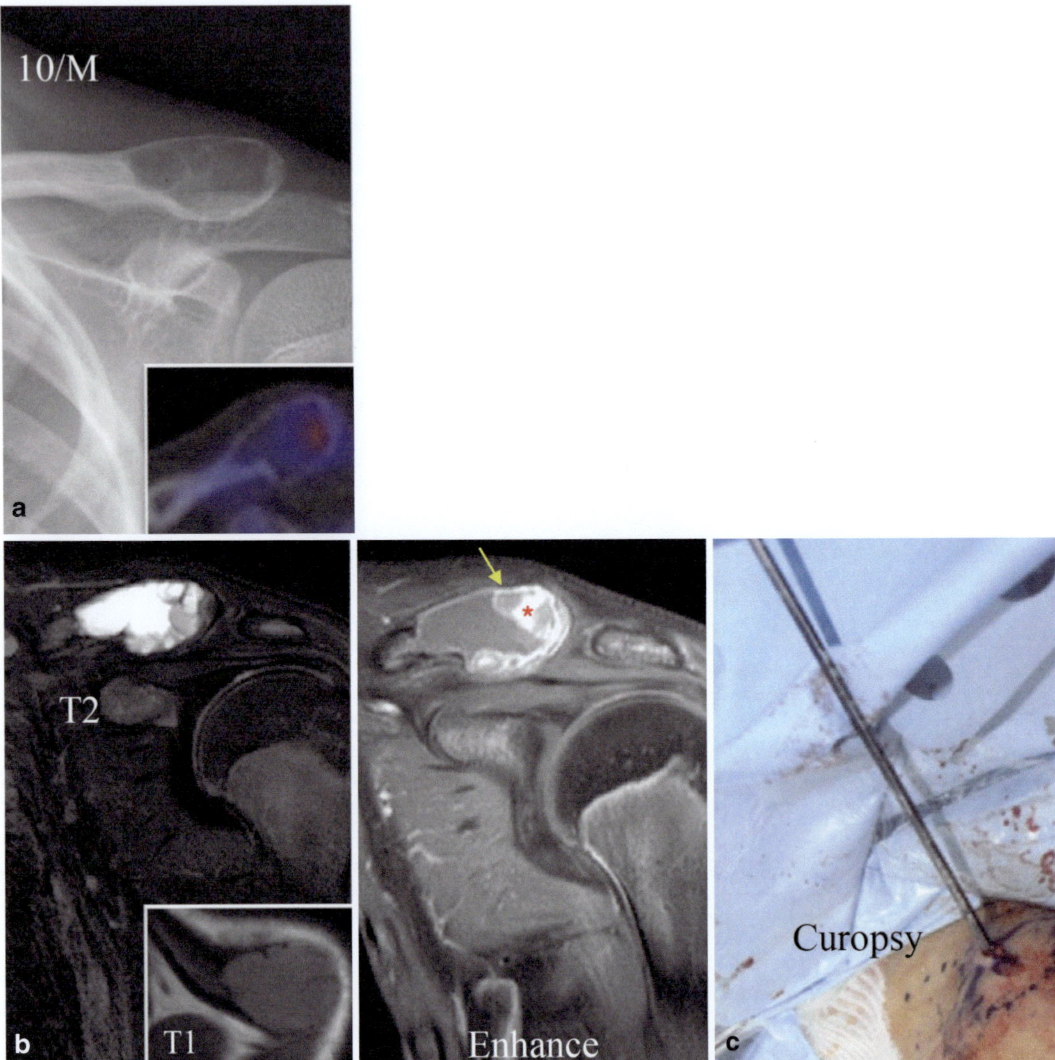

Fig. 11.6 (**a**) Radiograph taken for painful swelling in left shoulder area of 1-year duration in 10-year-old boy shows a well-demarcated multi-lobulated radiolucent lesion with mild expansion affecting the lateral end of the clavicle. SPECT/CT image reveals a mild heterogeneous uptake in the expansile osteolytic lesion without a clear cortical destruction (inset). (**b**) MR images demonstrate a multi-chambered cystic lesion with low SI on T1-weighted image (inset) and heterogeneous high SI with fluid-fluid levels on T2-weighted image. The lesion peripherally well enhanced (yellow arrow), and the thick septa or internal focal solid area (asterisk) is also well enhanced. The enhanced solid area is thought to be a thickened solid part of ABC wall because there is no histologic evidence of other underlying tumor. (**c**) With a diagnosis of primary ABC by frozen sections obtained through a small incision, curettage using pituitary rongeur *("curopsy")* were performed. (**d**) Follow-up radiograph at 18 months after surgery shows a partial consolidation of the lesion (arrow). The patient is free of pain. (**e**) Radiograph taken left forearm pain after fall in 66-year-old woman shows a multi-lobulated expansile radiolucent lesion with cortical thinning (yellow arrow) and displaced pathologic fracture (red arrow) in the distal shaft of the radius. (**f**) Pinhole bone scan reveals irregular strong uptake distally around the fracture site (white asterisk) and milder uptake proximally (yellow asterisk). (**g**) MR images demonstrate an ill-defined lobulated cystic lesion (asterisks) with low to intermediate SI on T1-weighted image and heterogeneous high SI on T2-weighted image. There are associated extensive hemorrhage and edema around the fracture site. The lesion is peripherally well enhanced (red arrow) with focal enhancing area (yellow arrow). Incision biopsy confirms a diagnosis of primary ABC with no underlying lesion. (**h**) Extended curettage using high-speed bur followed by allo-chip bone graft and plate fixation was done. (**i**) Follow-up radiograph at 1 year after surgery shows union of fracture with mild shortening resulting in ulna plus variant of the wrist (red arrow). The lesion itself is remodeled with no evidence of local recurrence

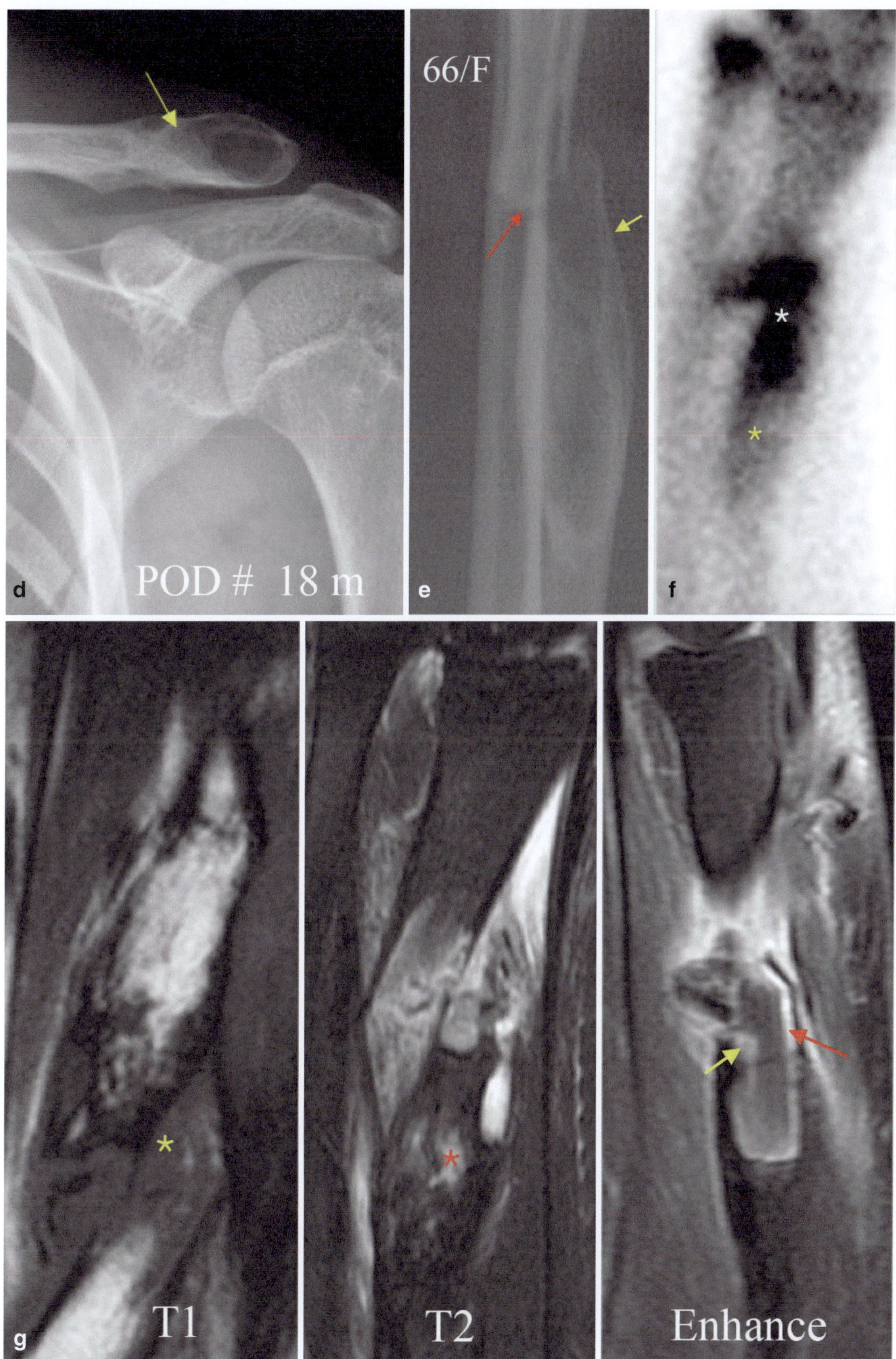

Fig. 11.6 (continued)

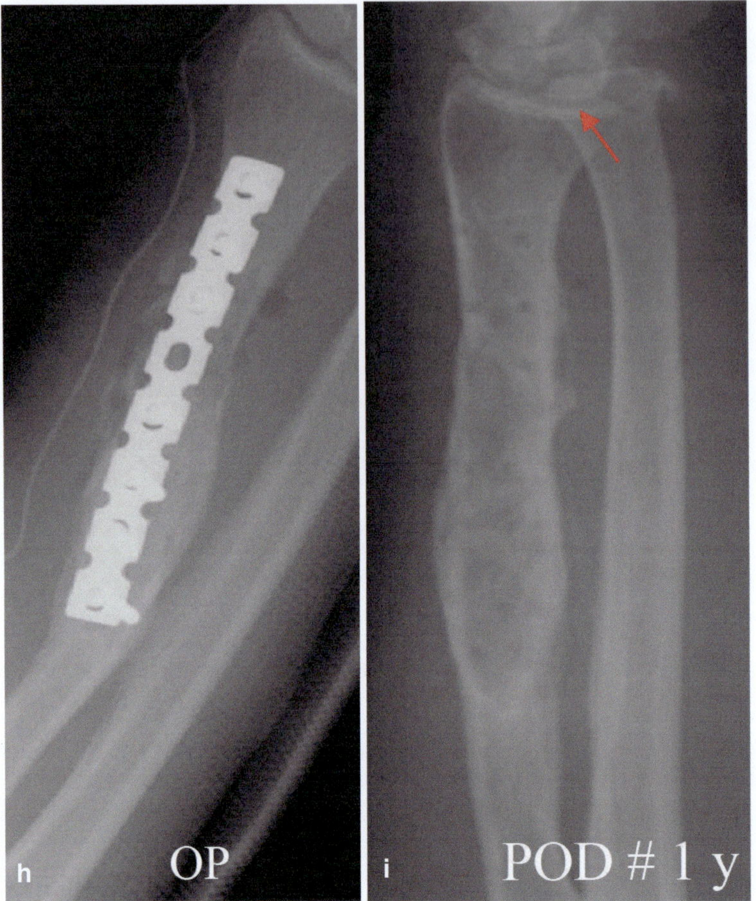

Fig. 11.6 (continued)

11.9 Histologic Findings

A fine needle aspiration cytology is usually non-diagnostic. However, aspiration before making window for curettage during surgery is often dominated by dark red blood rather than blood-tinged serous fluid, which is simple and useful finding in differentiation ABC from SBC (Fig. 11.2c). For histologic confirmation, biopsy sample includes lining tissue of the cystic lesion by incision biopsy. (1) *Constant findings.* To recognize multi-lobulated cystic wall-like structure on low-power view is the first step in histologic diagnosis of ABC (Fig. 11.7a). However, only a minor number of cases show as simple as this because most specimens are obtained by surgical curettage that can disrupt and distort the wall structures and blood-filled channels (Fig. 11.7b). A thickness of cystic walls is variable from fairly thin to significantly thickened with solid portion, which may be focally enhanced by a contrast medium on MR image. Rarely, blood can be seen in the dilated vascular lumen (Fig. 11.7c), but it is usually washed out when the specimen is placed in formalin. Medium-power view shows a moderate to high cellularity of plump or bizarre-looking nuclei, numerous sprinkled multinucleated giant cells, and focal deposition of primitive osteoid within the wall (Fig. 11.7d). Higher-power magnification reveals that the loose fibrous tissue within the cystic walls consists of moderate to high number of bland fibroblast-like cells, numerous capillary channels, extravasated red blood cells, inflammatory cells, or hemosiderin pigment deposition. Some blood vessels may be dilated resembling small aneurysmal spaces. There is specialized endothelium with basement membrane and intercellular junctions in the blood vessels. However, aneurysmal spaces are typically lined by bundles of collagen, fibrin, and cell debris devoid of specialized endothelial lining cells, but occasional elongated cells resembling fibroblasts can be present on the surface of the cyst [13]. On the contrary, SBC consists of a thin layer of loose fibrous tissue lined with a single layer of flattened to mildly plump cells resembling endothelial or synovial lining cells. Some blood vessels were dilated resembling small aneurysmal spaces and contains endothelial cells [13]. (2) *Variable findings*. Cases in the rapid growth phase may show severely thickened septa with fairly significant fibroblastic cellular exuberance due to maximal reparative stimulation (Fig. 11.7e). Osteoid or reactive woven bone trabeculae rimmed by osteoblasts often present in the form of long thin strands oriented along long axes of septa (Fig. 11.7f). However, random orientation is not unusual. Curetted specimen may reveal multiple fragmentations of host lamellar bone. Various numbers of multinucleated osteoclast-like giant cells are scattered throughout the septa (Fig. 11.7d–f). Peculiar, mineralized matrices can be observed in a clump. Earlier, they are chondroid-like pinkish material with microcalcification within spindle cells in the process of degeneration and necrosis stimulating pericellular calcium deposition. The deposited matrices gradually grew larger and become confluent. With time, the substance typically turns dark blue or purple in color and lacy or reticulated in texture, so-called *"blue reticulated chondroid"* (Fig. 11.7g, h). The peculiar material is not pathognomonic but valuable to differentiate ABC from telangiectatic OSA if present and has been reported to be found in about one fourth of the ABCs [9]. Mitotic activity is easily identified, but necrosis is rare. Extremely rare case with significant cytologic aberration showing extremely bizarre nuclei but no equivocal atypical mitosis and anaplasia, so-called *"pseudoanaplastic"* ABC, has been described [10]. In such a difficulty case with exceedingly rarely marked bizarre cytologic changes, clinico-radiologic-pathologic correlation should be made for a correct diagnosis with maximum accuracy to prevent overtreatment with overdiagnosis of sarcoma [10]. About half of the ABCs are associated with GCT, CB, FD, OSA, SBC, or others (Figs. 11.8, 11.9, 11.10, 11.11, 11.12, 11.13, and 11.14.

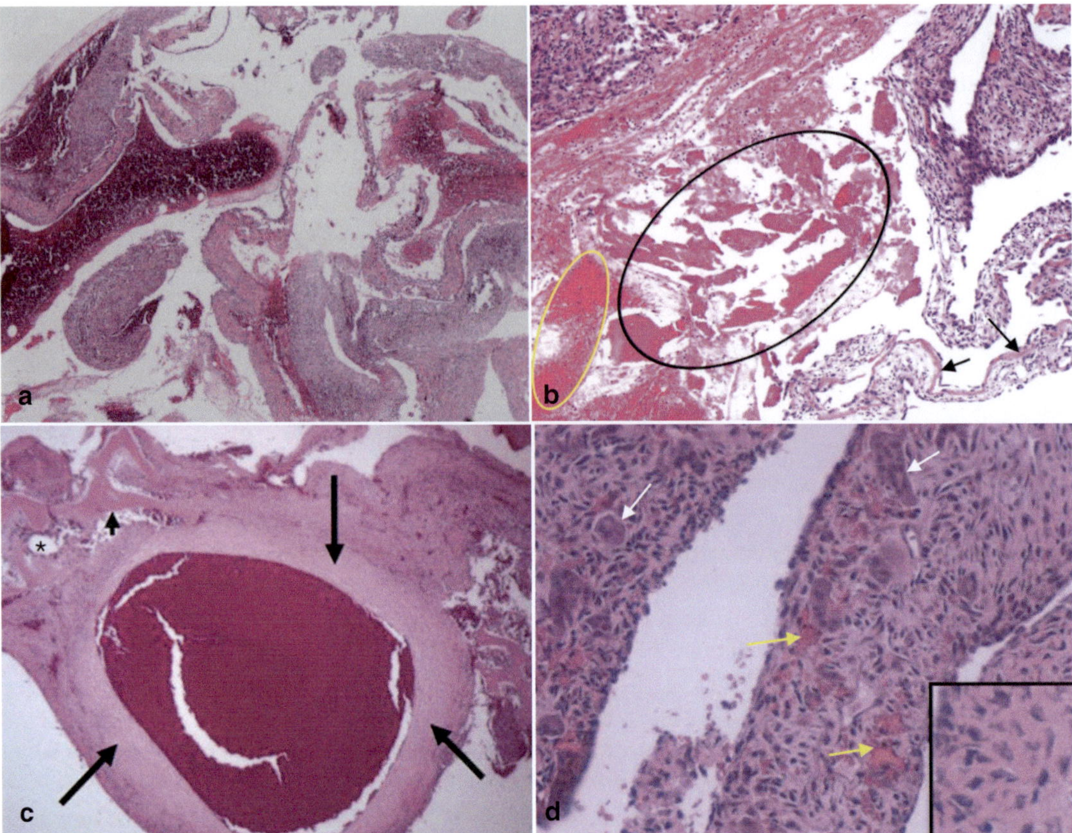

Fig. 11.7 ***Microscopic features***. (**a**) On low-power magnification, multi-lobulated cyst-like walls of variable thickness from fairly thin to significantly thick with blood-filled spaces are constant feature of conventional ABC. To recognize the walls is the first step in histologic diagnosis of ABC. However, only a minor number of cases show as simple as this case because most specimens are obtained by surgical curettage that can distort the wall structures. (**b**) The typical walls are usually torn apart with multiple fragmentations of lamellar bone (black circle) and severe hemorrhage (yellow circle) between cystic wall structures by surgical curettage. Reactive woven bone is deposited frequently in paralleling to axis of the wall (black arrows). (**c**) Note that blood remains in a dilated channel containing cyst-like space surrounded by moderately thick wall-like structure (long black arrows). Outer edge of the wall-like structure is covered by thin rim of reactive woven bone spicules (short black arrow). But blood is frequently washed out when the specimen is placed in formalin. There is a small cyst-like space in which blood is washed out (asterisk). (**d**) Medium-power magnification reveals moderate to high cellularity of plump or bizarre-looking nuclei (inset), numerous sprinkled multinucleated giant cells (white arrows) and focal deposition of primitive osteoid (yellow arrows) within the wall. (**e**) Some cases, particularly in rapid growth phase, reveal fairly thick wall with moderate to severe proliferation of uniform plump spindle fibroblast-like cells in the severely thickened septa due to maximal reparative stimulation. There are also abundant capillary channels and extravasated red blood cells in the septa. Typically, aneurysmal spaces are lined by bundles of collagen, fibrin, and cell debris devoid of specialized endothelial lining cells (arrow), but occasional elongated cells resembling fibroblasts can be present on the surface of the cyst. (**f**) Another characteristic finding is a spotty, winding, snakelike ribbons of osteoid (black arrows) with incipient row of osteoblasts (white arrows) strongly suggesting benignancy despite occasional bizarre, pleomorphic cells (yellow arrows). However, there is no definite anaplasia or unequivocal atypical mitoses. (**g**) Peculiar mineralized matrices can be observed in a clump. Earlier, they were chondroid looking pinkish material with microcalcification within spindle cells (dotted circles) stimulating pericellular calcification. The deposited matrices gradually grew larger and became confluent. (**h**) With time, the substance typically turned dark blue or purple in color and lacy or reticulated in texture (arrows), so-called *"blue reticulated chondroid,"* which is not pathognomonic but valuable to differentiate ABC from telangiectatic OSA if present

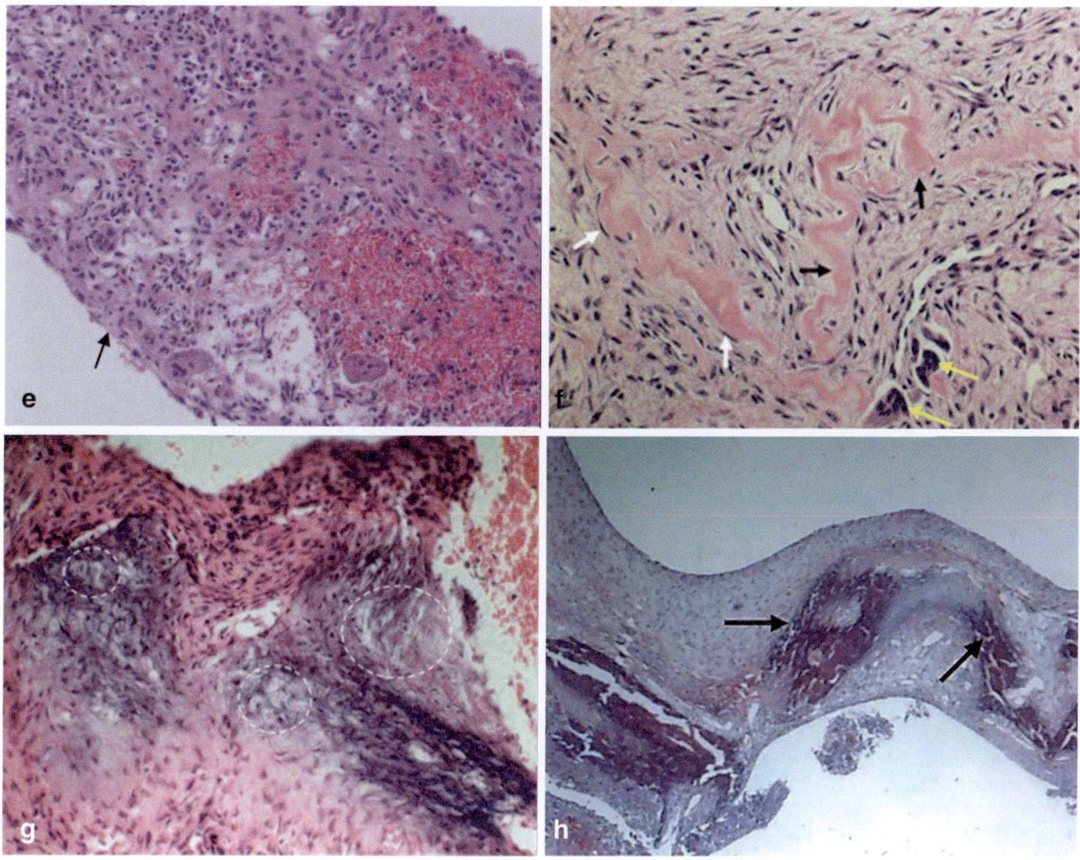

Fig. 11.7 (continued)

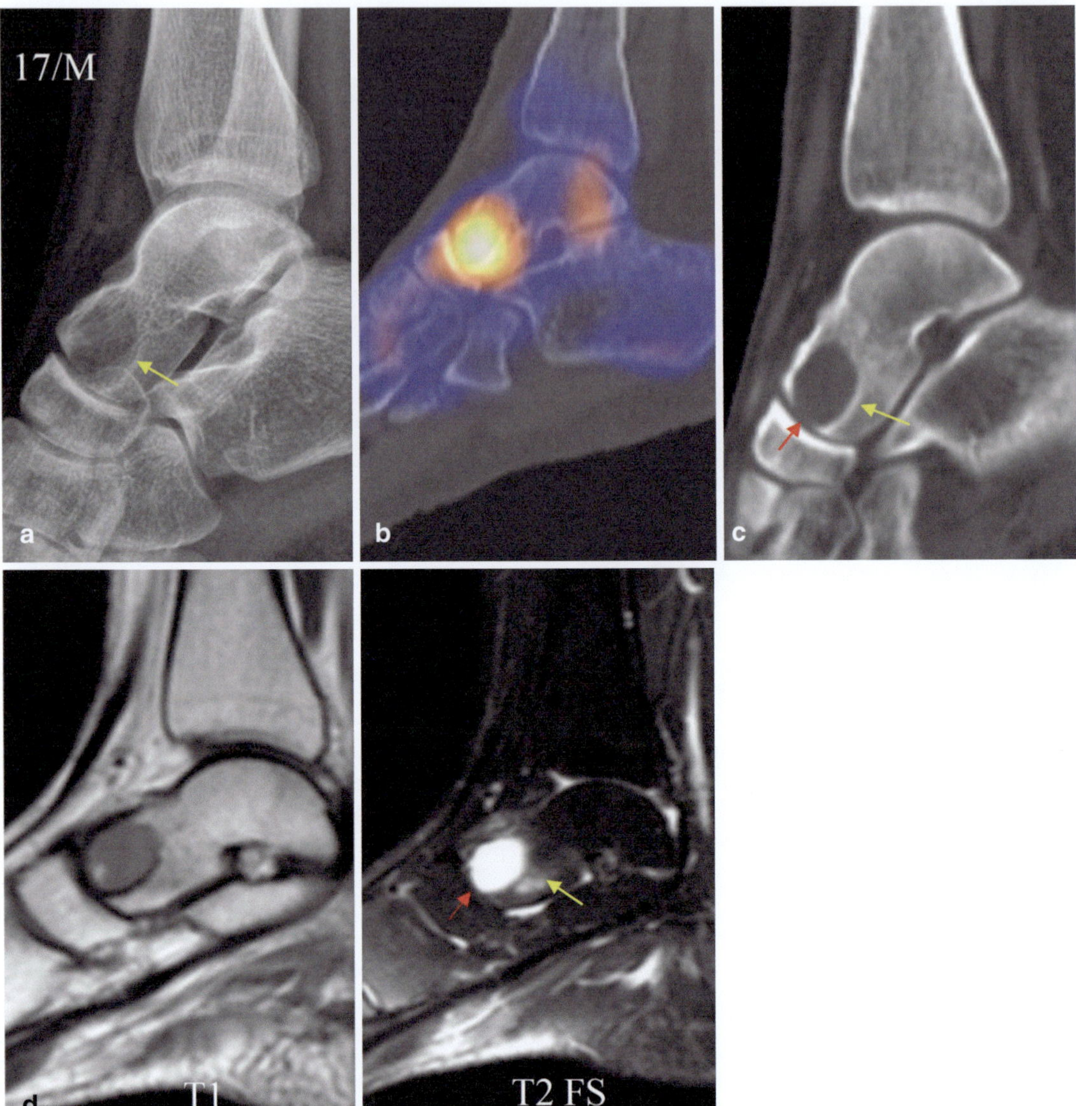

Fig. 11.8 ***Secondary ABC with GCT***. (**a**) Radiograph taken for right ankle pain of 2 months' duration in 17-years-old boy shows a well-defined oval radiolucent lesion surrounded by a thin rind of sclerosis (arrow) affecting anterior aspect of talus. (**b**) Bone SPECT reveals a heterogeneous strong uptake at anterior portion of talus. (**c**) CT scan notes a well-defined lytic lesion with internal non-enhancing low density surrounded by a thin sclerotic rim (yellow arrow). A cortical breakage is seen in the talonavicular joint (red arrow). (**d**) MR images demonstrate a well-defined cystic lesion with low SI with focal high signal on T1-weighted image and bright SI on fat saturated T2-weighted image. Cortical breakage is also seen in the talonavicular joint (red arrow), and surrounding bone marrow edema is associated (yellow arrow). (**e**) Microscopic examination shows two different components of solid component of conventional GCT and cystic component of ABC, indicating secondary ABC associated with GCT. (**f**) Thorough curettage and all-chip bone graft (asterisk) was performed. (**g**) Follow-up radiograph at 4 years after surgery reveals consolidation of the lesion with no evidence of local recurrence (asterisk)

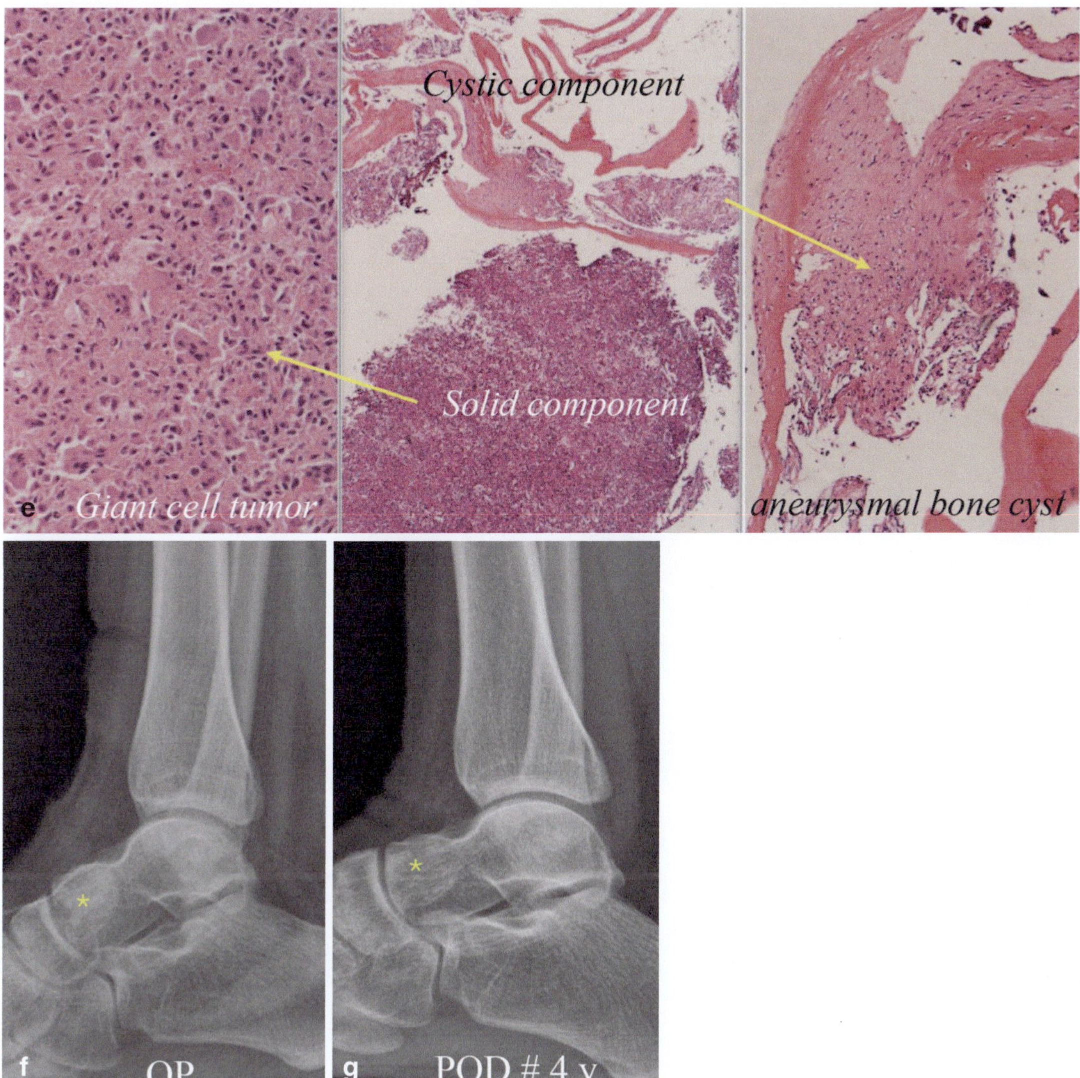

Fig. 11.8 (continued)

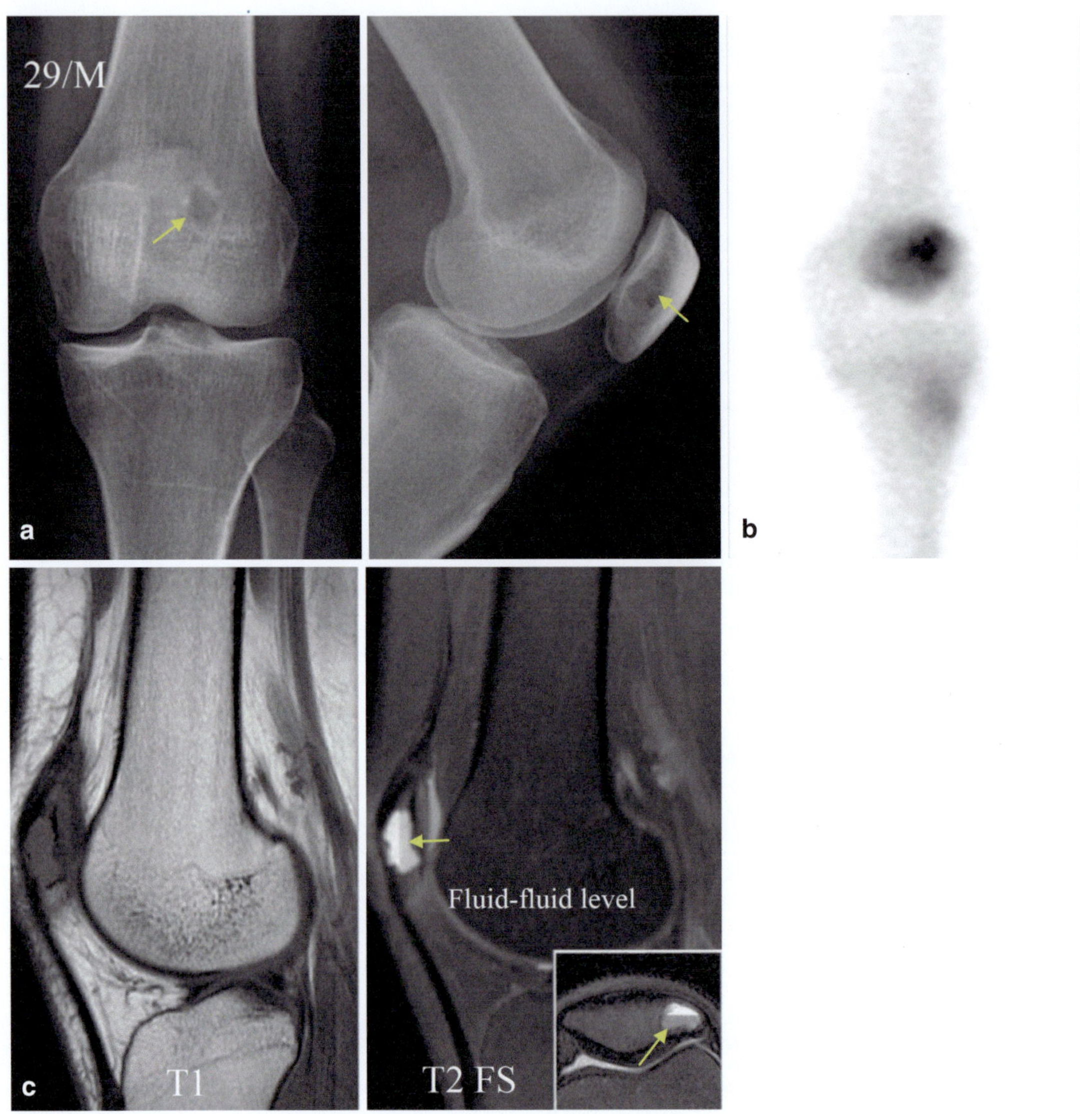

Fig. 11.9 ***Secondary ABC with CB***. (**a**) Radiograph taken for left knee pain for 3 months' duration in 29-years-old man shows a relatively well-defined small round to oval radiolucent lesion (arrows) in the patella. (**b**) Bone scan reveals heterogeneously strong uptake. (**c**) MR images demonstrate a well-circumscribed small oval cystic lesion with low SI on T1-weighted image and heterogeneous high SI showing a *"fluid-fluid"* level of different density (arrows) on fat saturated T2-weighted image. (**d**) Microscopic examination notes two different solid and cystic components. (Left and middle) Solid component is noted polygonal mononuclear chondroblasts and multinucleated giant cells with eosinophilic chondroid matrix indicating CB. (Right) Cystic component shows a multilobulated cyst-like wall architecture of varying degree of thickness consisting of bland fibroblast-like cells, woven bone formation, hemosiderin pigments, and scattered multinucleated cells indicating secondary ABC. (**e**) Thorough curettage and allo-chip bone graft was performed (asterisk). (**f**) Follow-up radiograph at 3 years after surgery reveals complete healing of the lesion with no evidence of recurrence (asterisk)

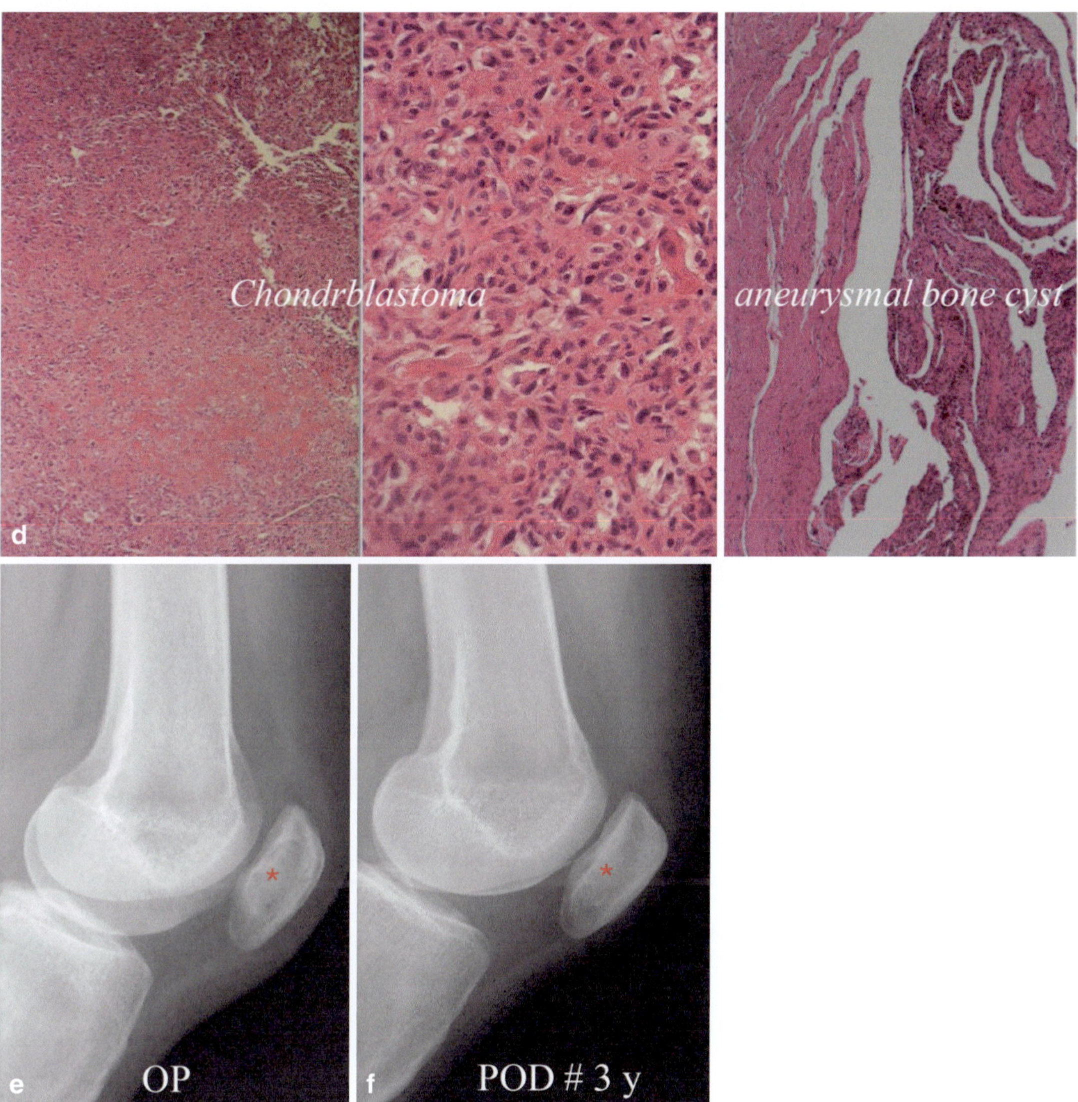

Fig. 11.9 (continued)

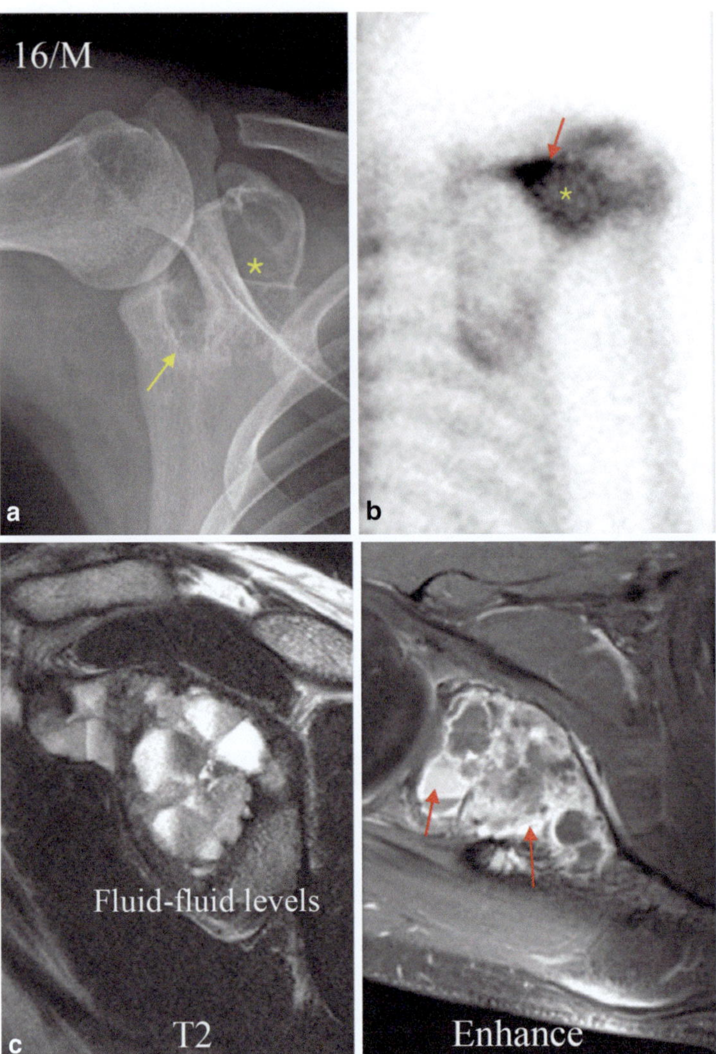

Fig. 11.10 ***Secondary ABC with CB***. (**a**) Radiograph taken for right shoulder discomfort of 3-month duration in 16-year-old boy shows a multi-lobulated geographic destruction (asterisk) surrounded by a thin sclerotic rim (arrow) in the scapular neck and glenoid. (**b**) Bone scan reveals heterogeneously increased uptake at the periphery of the lesion (red arrow) with central lesser degree of uptake (asterisk). (**c**) MR image demonstrate a locally aggressive looking medullary lesion with multiple "*fluid-fluid*" levels on T2-weighted images. The lesion is enhanced in peripheral and septal pattern indicating cystic lesion. Note other pattern of focal solid enhancement suggesting a probable solid component (arrows). (**d**) Microscopic examination. Low-power magnification notes two different components of multi-lobulated thickened cyst-like and several solid components (Middle). Higher-power magnification reveals thickened cyst wall consisting moderate to high cellular bland fibroblast-like spindle cells and extravasated red blood cells with scattered multinucleated giant cells indicating ABC (Left) and other area consisting of polygonal mononuclear chondroblasts with eosinophilic chondroid to cartilage matrix indicating CB (Right). (**e**) Patient and his parents do not want further surgery because of no severe pain to bother him. Follow-up radiograph at 6 months after biopsy and cement packing shows no definite interval change. And then, he was lost for follow-up

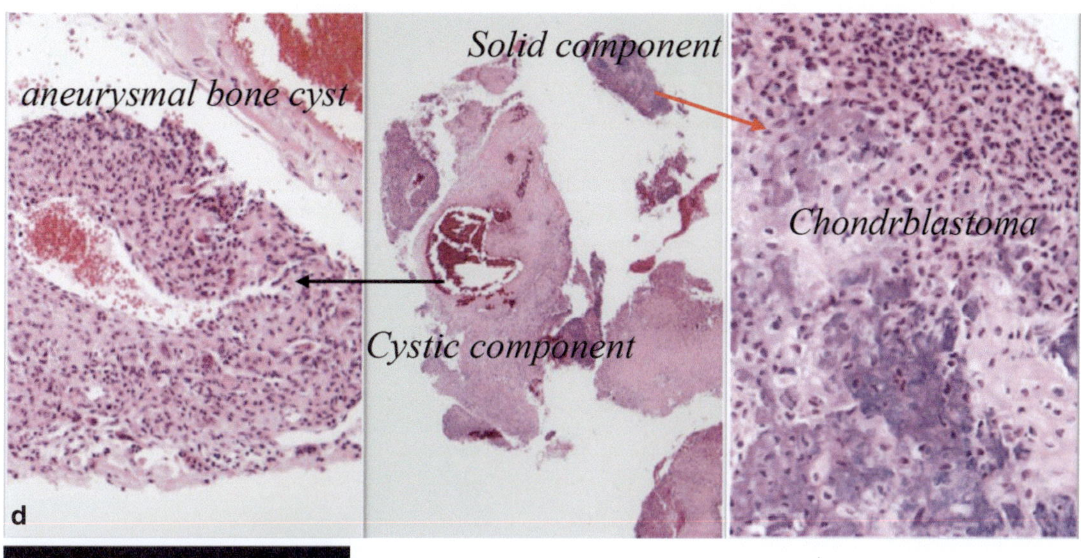

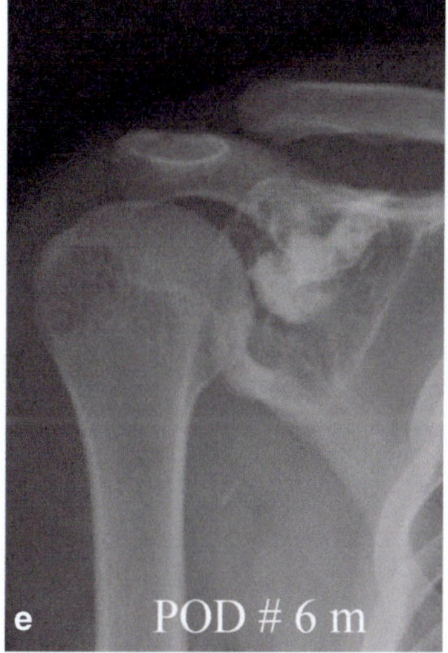

Fig. 11.10 (continued)

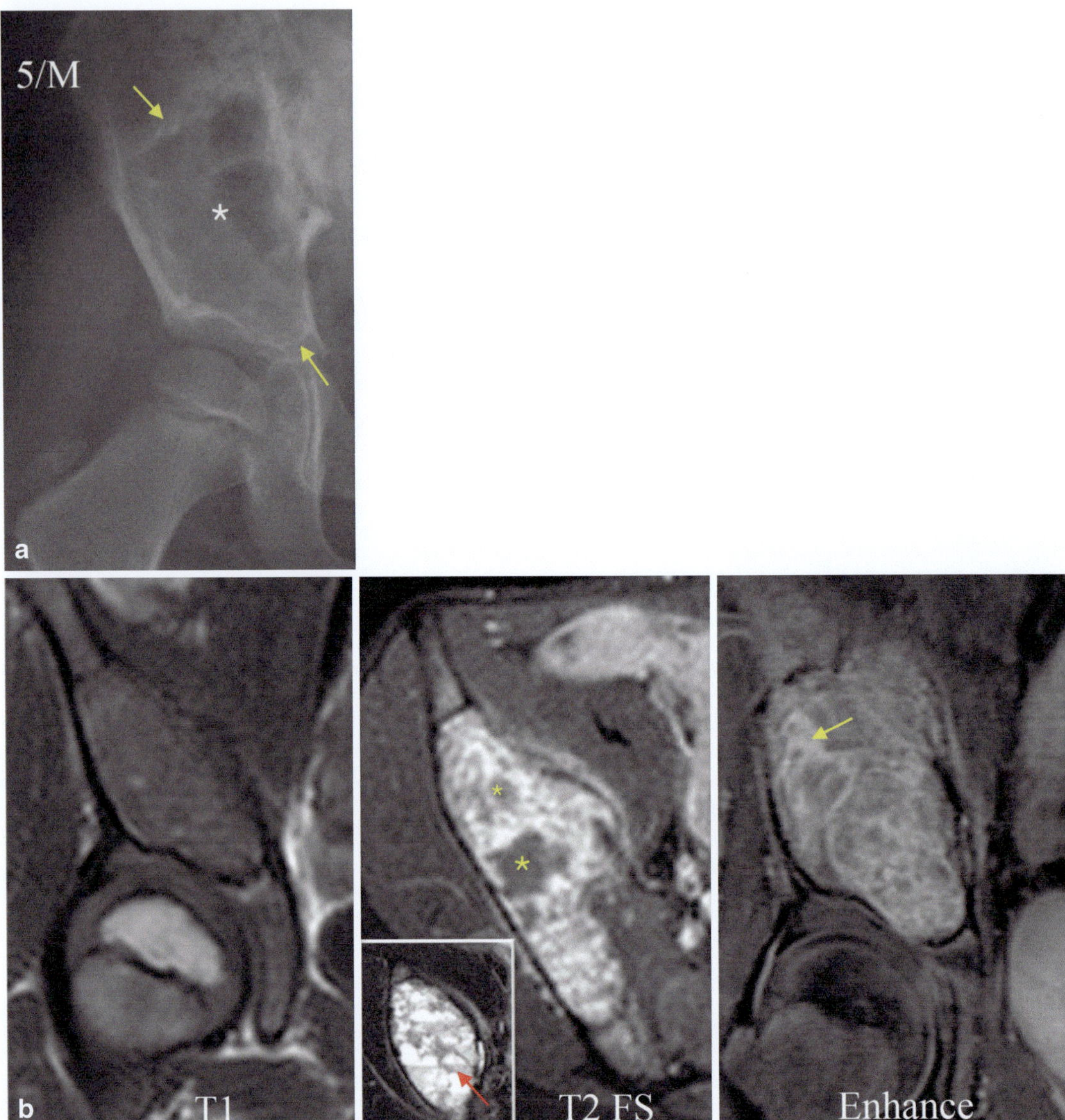

Fig. 11.11 ***Secondary ABC with FD.*** (**a**) Radiograph taken for pain of right pelvic area of several months duration in 5-year-old boy shows a multi-chambered expansive lytic lesion with a thin rim of surround sclerosis (arrows) in the acetabulum and iliac wing. (**b**) MR images demonstrate a large expansile destructive lesion with low SI with tiny focal areas of high signal on T1-weighted image and heterogeneous high SI with focal areas of low signal (asterisks) on fat saturated T2-weighted image, suggesting mostly cystic lesion with focal solid areas. Note multiple *"fluid-fluid"* levels (inset). The lesion is enhanced in peripheral and septal pattern with internal solid areas of focal enhancement (yellow arrow). However, aspiration and steroid injection were done without biopsy at private clinic. (**c**) Follow-up radiograph at 5 months after injection notes that the lytic becomes slightly hazier (asterisk). Incision biopsy has been performed because of continuous pain and follow-up MR features of slight enlargement. (**d**) Microscopic examination demonstrates two different solid and cystic components. (Left) Solid component shows bland spindle cells in fibrous-appearing tissue and dysplastic bone trabeculae indicating FD. (Right) Cystic area reveals multi-lobulated cyst-like wall architecture having thickened fibrous septa consisting of numerous dilated vascular channels with extravasated red blood cells, bland fibroblast-like cells, woven bone formation, as well as sprinkled multinucleated giant cells, indicating secondary ABC. (**e**) Follow-up radiograph at 10 years after extended curettage and allo-chip bone grafting reveals consolidation of the lesion with evidence of local recurrence (asterisk)

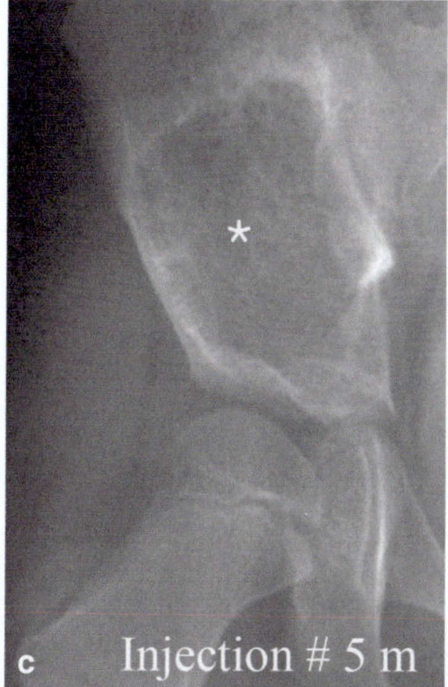

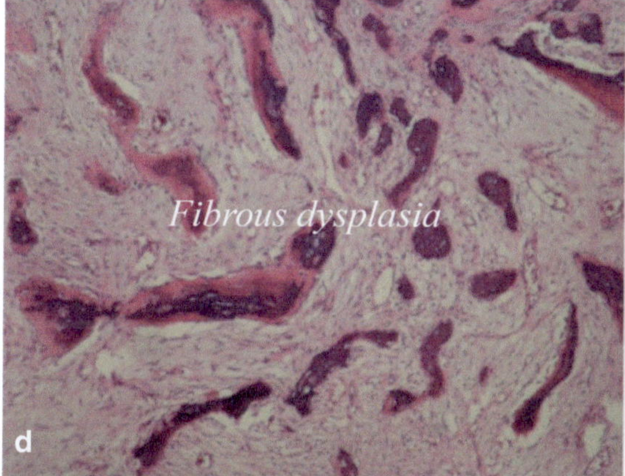

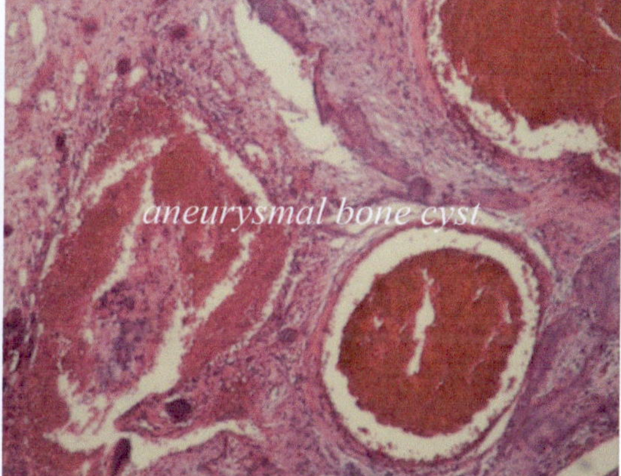

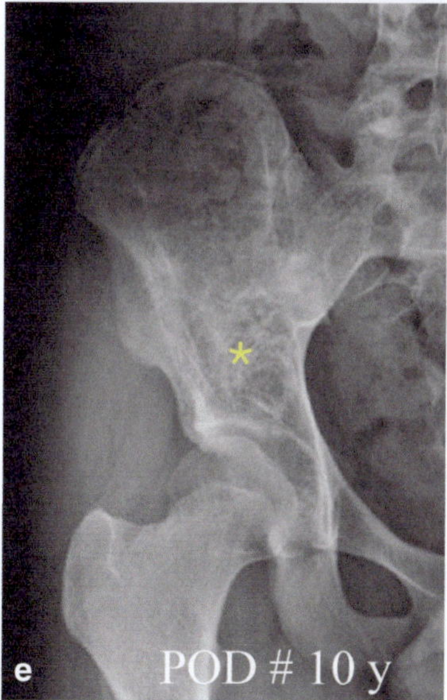

Fig. 11.11 (continued)

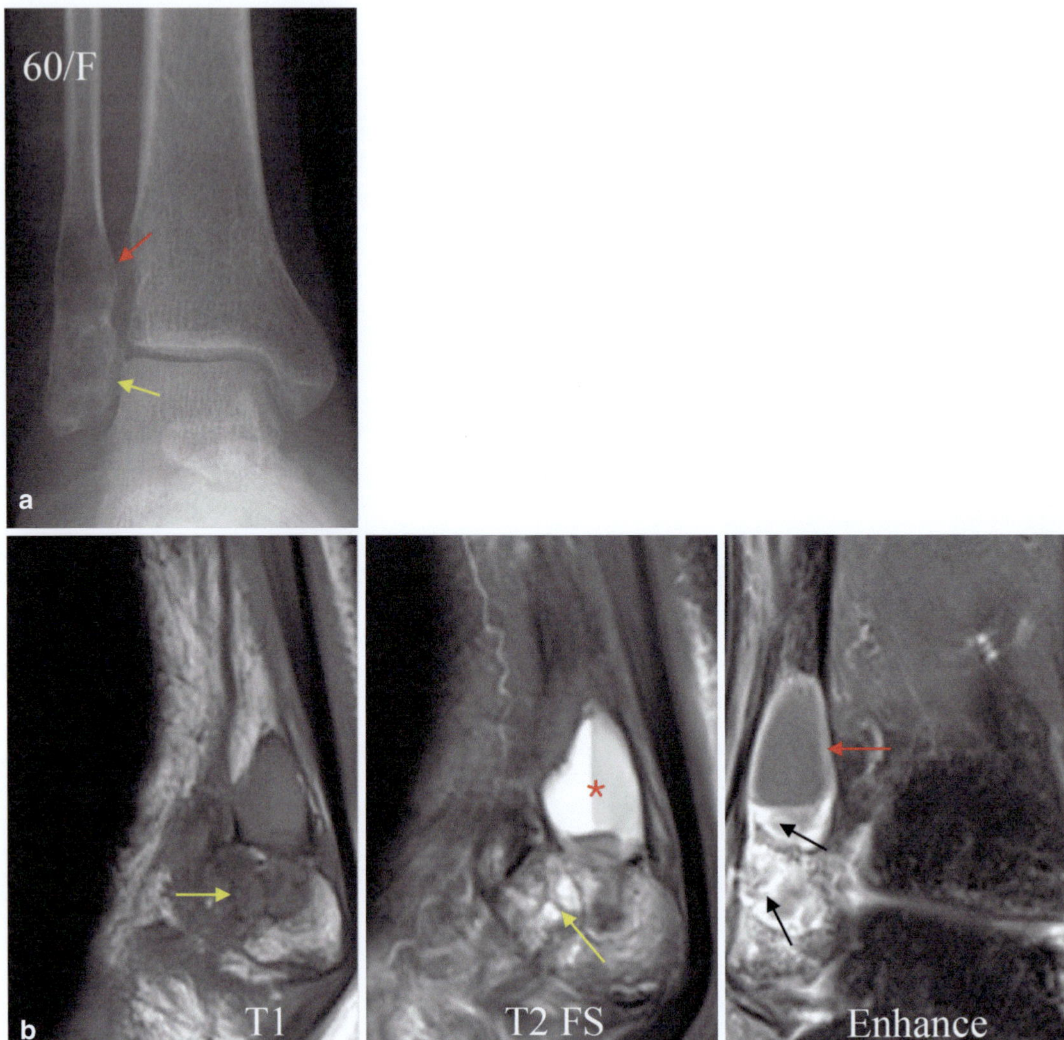

Fig. 11.12 ***Secondary ABC with FD***. (**a**) Radiograph taken for painful swelling of right ankle of 3-month duration in 60-year-old woman shows a multi-lobulated radiolucent lesion with mild expansion cortical thinning proximally in the diaphysis (red arrow), and another area of osteoblastic and osteolytic lesion with focal cortical disruption distally in the epi-metaphysis of distal fibula (yellow arrow). (**b**) MR images reveal a well-demarcated cystic lesion proximally with low SI on T1-weighted image and heterogeneous high SI with a *"fluid-fluid"* level (asterisk) on fat saturated T2-weighted image. There is poorly demarcated another lesion distally with low SI on T1-weighted image and heterogeneous intermediate and high SI on T2-weighted fat saturation image (yellow arrows). There is perilesional soft tissue edema and fluid or hemorrhage collection in tibiofibular and tibiotalar joint. The proximal lesion is peripherally enhanced indicating cystic component (red arrow), and the distal lesion is internally heterogeneously enhanced suggesting sloid component (black arrows). (**c**) Incision biopsy followed by cement packing was performed. (**d**) Follow-up radiograph at 1 year after thorough curettage, cement packing, and plate fixation notes good maintenance with no evidence of local recurrence. (**e**) Low-power microscopic examination shows two different components of variable-sized cystic walls and another solid structure consisting of fibrous-appearing tissue and bone trabeculae. (**f**) Higher-power magnification of cystic component reveals the loose fibrous tissue consisting of scanty to moderate number of bland fibroblast-like cells, inflammatory cells, and extravasated red blood cells but no clearly visible lining cells. You can see markedly thickened wall with massive hemorrhagic foci in the particular wall (asterisk). (**g**) Higher-power magnification of solid component notes proliferation of bland spindle cells in fibrous-appearing tissue with woven bone trabeculae indicating FD

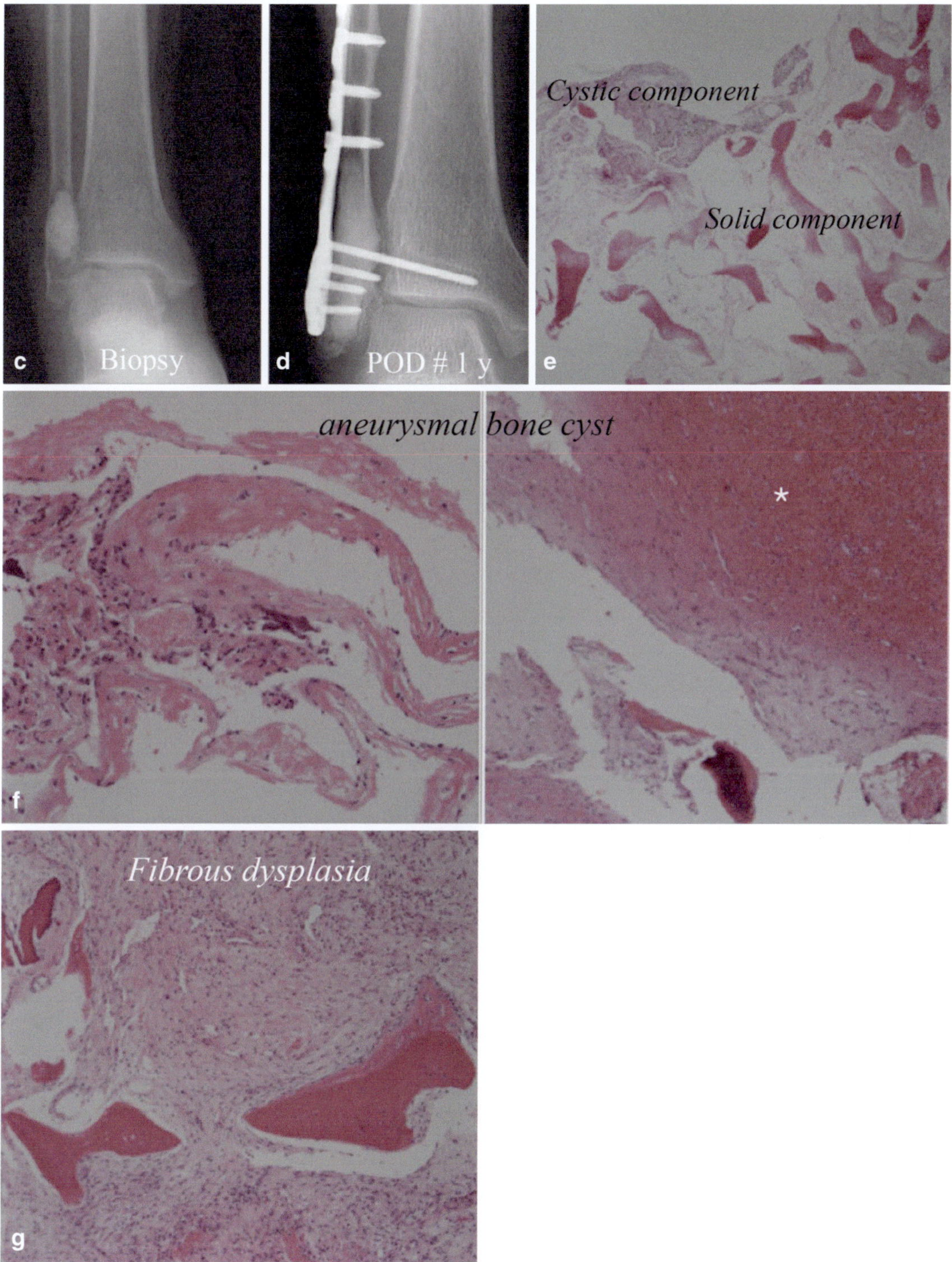

Fig. 11.12 (continued)

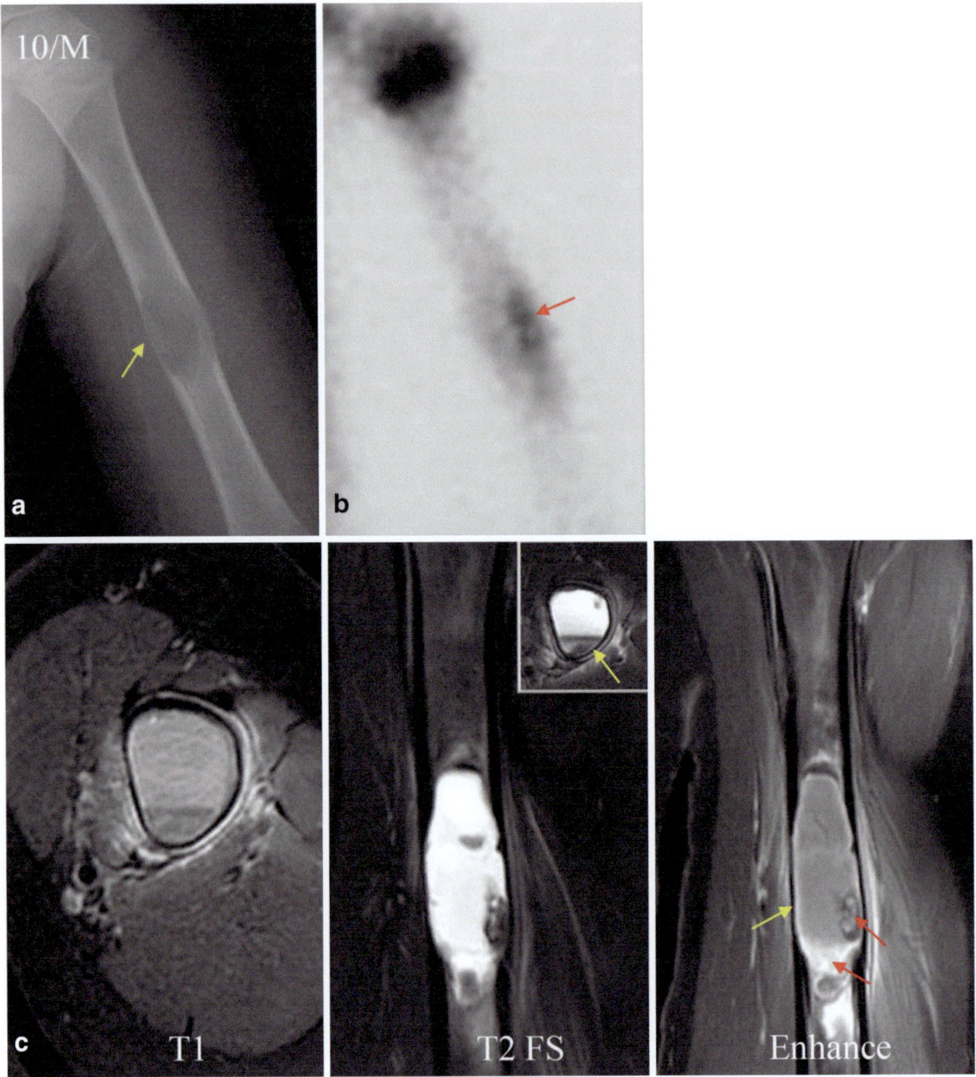

Fig. 11.13 ***Secondary ABC with SBC***. (**a**) Radiograph taken for left arm pain of 1-month duration in 10-year-old boy shows a well-demarcated radiolucent lesion with mild expansion and cortical thinning (arrow) in the mid-shaft of humerus. (**b**) Bone scan reveals a focal moderately increased uptake (arrow). (**c**) MR images reveal a well-defined cystic lesion with low to intermediate SI on T1-weighted image and high SI with focal dark signals on fat saturated T2-weighted image. Note a *"fluid-fluid"* level of different densities (inset). The lesion is peripherally enhanced (yellow arrow) with focal internal enhancement (red arrow) which may represent thickened portion of ABC or pre-existing lesion. (**d**) Simple curetted with allo-chip bone graft was done under radiologic impression of SBC in private clinic. (**e**) However, microscopic examination demonstrates two different types of cystic walls. (Left) Low-power magnification shows a single continuous folded membrane consisting of a thin layer of loose fibrous tissue lined with a single layer of flattened to mildly plump cells resembling endothelial cells (arrows). (Right) Higher-power magnification of a thick wall reveals abundant unique acellular pinkish *"cementum-like"* matrix (white arrow) and cholesterol clefts (yellow arrow) indicating SBC. (**f**) Another field notes a multi-lobulated cyst-like wall architecture consisting of loose fibrous tissue with blood-filled cystic spaces of variable size separated by fibrous septa but no clearly visible lining cells suggesting secondary ABC. (**g**) Follow-up radiograph taken for left arm pain at 16 months after simple curettage shows a markedly enlarged lesion with mild expansion and cortical thinning (red arrow) suggesting a local recurrence. (**h**) Enhanced MR images reveal a significant enlargement of the lesion with mild expansion and cortical thinning with a peripheral thin enhancement (yellow arrow). (**i**) Follow-up radiograph at 3 years after extended curettage, allo-graft impaction graft and fixation using flexible nails to prevent perioperative pathologic fracture notes good consolidation of the lesion with no local recurrence

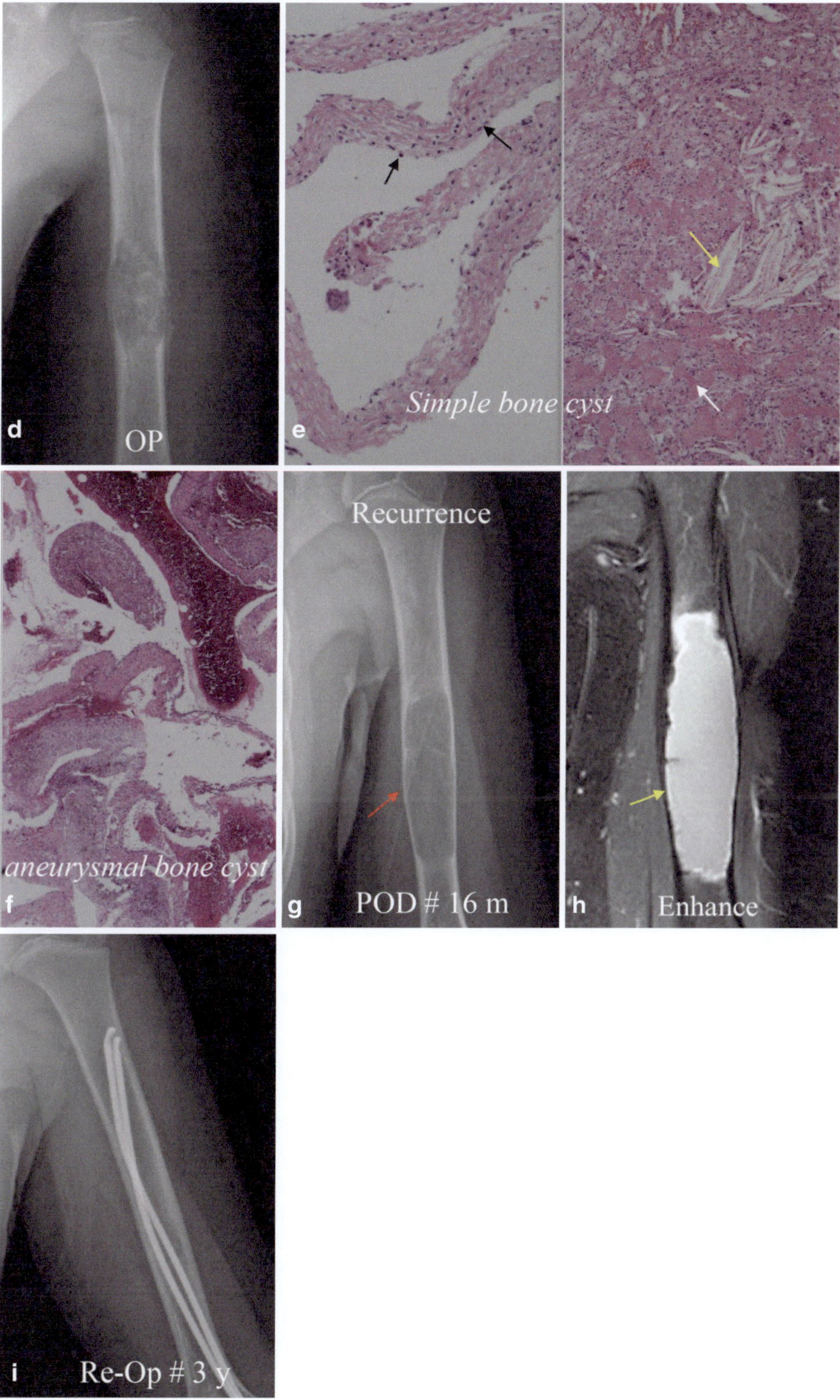

Fig. 11.13 (continued)

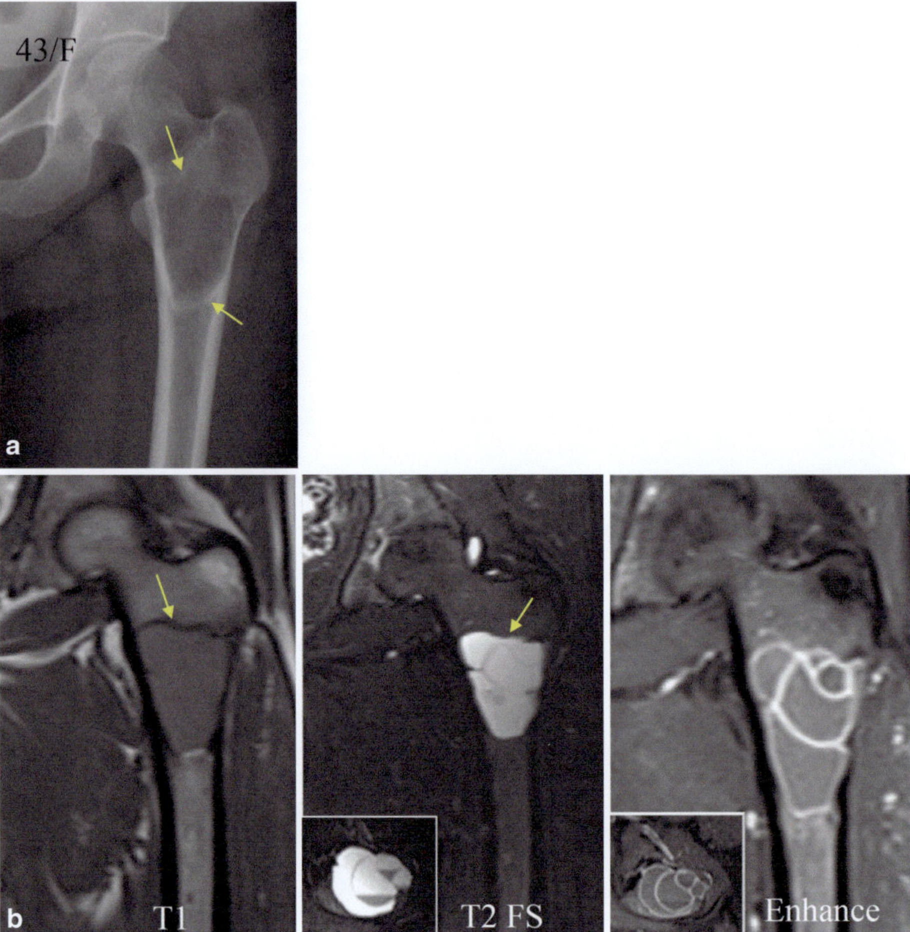

Fig. 11.14 ***Secondary ABC with OSA***. (**a**) Radiograph taken for left hip pain of 5-month duration in 43-year-old lady shows a relatively well-defined radiolucent lesion with a thin rim of surrounding sclerosis distally and proximally (arrows) in the trochanteric area of the femur. (**b**) MR images reveal a well-demarcated multi-lobulated cystic lesion with low SI on T1-weighted image and high SI on fat saturated T2-weighted image with multiple *"fluid-fluid levels"* (inset). The lesion is surrounded by a thin rim of dark signal on both sequences and characteristically enhanced in peripheral and septal pattern with no internal enhancement suggesting a solid lesion. (**c**) Microscopic examination of biopsy specimen demonstrates multi-lobulated cystic walls with moderate to high cellularity of fibroblast-like cells showing moderate atypia but no equivalent anaplasia or pleomorphism. A diagnosis of primary ABC was rendered. (**d**) Extended curettage using high-speed burr and allo-chip bone graft with plate fixation to prevent postoperative fracture was performed. (**e**) Follow-up radiograph at 5 months after surgery shows radiolucent change (arrows) around the consolidated grafted chip bones (yellow asterisk) suggesting a possible local recurrence. (**f**) Follow-up radiograph at 1 year after surgery reveals progression of the disease (red arrow) with resorption of some grafted bones (asterisk). (**g**) Incision biopsy was performed to exclude malignancy. Microscopic examination notes area of bizarre pleomorphic spindle cells with atypical mitoses. The tumor cells produce osteoid and primitive woven bones and permeate the host lamellar bone indicating OSA (Left). There is another area with bland looking, multi-lobulated cyst-like wall architecture with extensive hemorrhage fibrous septa suggesting secondary ABC (Right). It is hard to consider the case a malignant change from pre-existing ABC because the interval between initially surgery and development is too short (5 months)

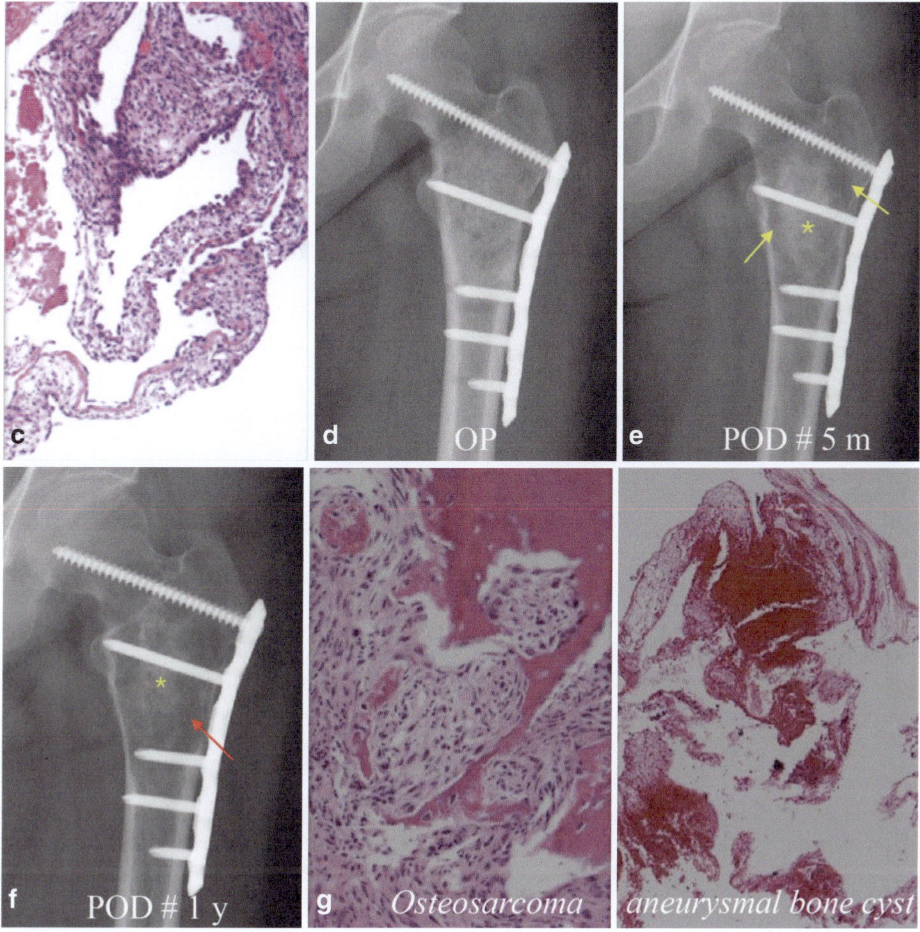

Fig. 11.14 (continued)

11.10 Management

Standard management is thorough curettage and bone grafting or cementing for the resultant defect. Bone cementing is usually not employed for the lesion in metaphysis of a growing child because of a possible thermal effect to growth plate. Due to variable recurrence rates with high rate up to 59% after best efforts with curettage [3], various adjuvant therapies including the use of cement, high-speed burr, argon beam cauterization (burning the tumor bed), phenol (a chemical), or cryotherapy (liquid nitrogen) have evolved to reduce the recurrence. Gibbs et al. [14] and Dorfmans et al. [15] reported local control rates up to 80–90% by augmented curettage using high-speed burr. Marcove et al. [16] reported a recurrence rate of 17.6% with curettage and cryosurgery and reduced rate of 4% by second cryosurgery. However, postoperative fracture, soft tissue or skin necrosis, or wound infection can be complicated when a surgeon is not familiar with the procedure. Polymethylmethacrylate cement can provide immediate stability, thermal effect to the tumor cells during hardening, and early detection of local recurrence with radiolucent line around the inserted cement. However, it can injure the articular cartilage and growth plate by the heat, is biologically inert with no chance of bone incorporation, has no growth potential, provides increasing the risk of future pathologic fracture due to stress shielding, and may act as a possible foreign nidus for infection. Ozaki et al. [17] reported lower recurrence rate of 17% with curettage and cementing compared to higher rate of 37% after curettage and bone grafting. En bloc resection with or without reconstruction may be necessary for a huge, significantly destructive or frequently recurrent lesion in expandable bones and small bones such as fibula and rib. Percutaneous treatment with fibrosing agents or selective arterial embolization is rarely indicated in localization to vertebra, pelvis, and proximal femur with expectation of a favorable result without surgical treatment. Radiation therapy is reserved for inoperable tumors involving bones of skull base. More recently, "curopsy," a percutaneous limited curettage at the time of biopsy (Fig. 11.6c), has been introduce with a successful consolidation in 80% of the patient [18]. A percutaneous core needle or small open biopsy obtains lining membranes from various parts of the lesion for a histologic diagnosis, and simultaneous curettage by pituitary rongeur or curette destroys the internal cyst architecture to induce healing of the lesion. Bisphosphonate has been introduced for treatment of symptomatic inoperable benign bone tumors including ABC with near universal pain relief by varying degrees of lesion ossification [19]. More recently, denosumab is proposed as a potentially effective neoadjuvant therapy for osteoporosis, skeletal metastasis, or GCT. It has been introduced to use for ABC [20], and several authors reported pain reduction with tumor regression in sacral and spinal lesions [21–23] .

11.11 Clinical Course

ABC is a locally aggressive benign lesion with high recurrence rate that renders its treatment challenging. The prognosis of secondary ABC may depend on the biology of the pre-existing lesion. If ABC superimposed on GCT or OSA, it would be worse. The reported recurrence rates after surgical treatment are varying with range from 10 to 59%. Higher rate is expected after simple curettage without adjuvant therapy. The presence of open growth plates and younger age is related with higher risk for recurrence with a statistical significance [14]. Malignant transformation occurs almost exclusively in the context of prior radiation exposure. However, sporadically rare cases of malignant transformation of ABC have been reported without history of irradiation [24–26].

References

1. Jaffe HL. Aneurysmal bone cyst. Bull Hosp Joint Dis. 1950;11:3–13.
2. Lichtenstein L. Aneurysmal bone cyst. A pathological entity commonly mistaken for giant-cell tumor and occasionally for hemangioma and osteogenic sarcoma. Cancer. 1950;3(2):279–89.
3. Biesecker J, Marcove R, Huvos A, Mike V. Aneurysmal bone cysts. A clinicopathologic study of 66 cases. Cancer. 1970;26(3):615–25.
4. Baruffi M, Neto JB, Barbieri C, Casartelli C. Aneurysmal bone cyst with chromosomal changes involving 7q and 16p. Cancer Genet Cytogenet. 2001;129(2):177–80.
5. Herens C, Thiry A, Dresse MF, Born J, Flagothier C, Vanstraelen G, et al. Translocation (16; 17)(q22; p13) is a recurrent anomaly of aneurysmal bone cysts. Cancer Genet Cytogenet. 2001;127(1):83–4.
6. Leithner A, Machacek F, Haas OA, Lang S, Ritschl P, Radl R, et al. Aneurysmal bone cyst: a hereditary disease? J Pediatr Orthop B. 2004;13(3):214–7.
7. Panoutsakopoulos G, Pandis N, Kyriazoglou I, Gustafson P, Mertens F, Mandahl N. Recurrent t (16; 17)(q22; p13) in aneurysmal bone cysts. Genes Chromosomes Cancer. 1999;26(3):265–6.
8. Oliveira AM, Perez-Atayde AR, Inwards CY, Medeiros F, Derr V, Hsi B-L, et al. USP6 and CDH11 oncogenes identify the neoplastic cell in primary aneurysmal bone cysts and are absent in so-called secondary aneurysmal bone cysts. Am J Pathol. 2004;165(5):1773–80.
9. Bahk WJ, Mirra JM. Differential diagnostic value of "blue reticulated chondroid-like material" in aneurysmal bone cysts: a classic histopathologic analysis of 215 cases. Am J Clin Pathol. 2015;143(6):823–9.
10. Bahk WJ, Mirra JM. Pseudoanaplastic tumors of bone. Skelet Radiol. 2004;33(11):641–8.
11. Mirra JM. Aneurysmal bone cyst. In: Mirra JM, editor. Bone tumors: clinical, radiologic, and pathologic

correlation. 2nd ed. Philadelphia, PA: Lea & Febiger; 1989. p. 1267–312.

12. Czerniak B. Cystic lesions. In: Dorfman HD, Czerniak B, editors. Dorfman and Czerniak's bone tumors. 2nd ed. Philadelphia, PA: Elsevier; 2016. p. 1055–99.
13. Aho H, Aho A, Pelliniemi L, Ekfors T, Foidart J. Endothelium in aneurysmal bone cyst. Histopathology. 1985;9(4):381–7.
14. Gibbs CP Jr, Hefele MC, Peabody TD, Montag AG, Aithal V, Simon MA. Aneurysmal bone cyst of the extremities. Factors related to local recurrence after curettage with a high-speed burr. J Bone Joint Surg Am. 1999;81(12):1671–8.
15. Dormans JP, Hanna BG, Johnston DR, Khurana JS. Surgical treatment and recurrence rate of aneurysmal bone cysts in children. Clin Orthop Relat Res. 2004;421:205–11.
16. Marcove RC, Sheth DS, Takemoto S, Healey JH. The treatment of aneurysmal bone cyst. Clin Orthop Relat Res. 1995;311:157–63.
17. Ozaki T, Hillmann A, Lindner N, Winkelmann W. Cementation of primary aneurysmal bone cysts. Clin Orthop Relat Res. 1997;337:240–8.
18. Reddy KI, Sinnaeve F, Gaston CL, Grimer RJ, Carter SR. Aneurysmal bone cysts: do simple treatments work? Clin Orthop Relat Res. 2014;472:1901–10.
19. Cornelis F, Truchetet M, Amoretti N, Verdier D, Fournier C, Pillet O, et al. Bisphosphonate therapy for unresectable symptomatic benign bone tumors: a long-term prospective study of tolerance and efficacy. Bone. 2014;58:11–6.
20. Lange T, Stehling C, Fröhlich B, Klingenhöfer M, Kunkel P, Schneppenheim R, et al. Denosumab: a potential new and innovative treatment option for aneurysmal bone cysts. Eur Spine J. 2013;22(6):1417–22.
21. Dubory A, Missenard G, Domont J. Interest of denosumab for the treatment of giant-cells tumors and aneurysmal bone cysts of the spine. About nine cases. Spine. 2016;41(11):E654–E60.
22. Pelle DW, Ringler JW, Peacock JD, Kampfschulte K, Scholten DJ II, Davis MM, et al. Targeting receptor-activator of nuclear kappaB ligand in aneurysmal bone cysts: verification of target and therapeutic response. Transl Res. 2014;164(2):139–48.
23. Skubitz KM, Peltola JC, Santos ER, Cheng EY. Response of aneurysmal bone cyst to denosumab. Spine. 2015;40(22):E1201–E4.
24. Kyriakos M, Hardy D. Malignant transformation of aneurysmal bone cyst, with an analysis of the literature. Cancer. 1991;68(8):1770–80.
25. Brindley GW, Greene JF Jr, Frankel LS. Malignant transformation of aneurysmal bone cysts. Clin Orthop Relat Res. 2005;438:282–7.
26. Kansagra AP, Wan JJ, Devulapalli KK, Horvai AE, O'Donnell RJ, Link TM. Malignant transformation of an aneurysmal bone cyst to fibroblastic osteosarcoma. Am J Orthop. 2016;45(6):E367–E72.

12 Simple/Unicameral Bone Cyst

(***unus*** "one" + ***cameras*** "cavity" + ***kystis*** "sac")

12.1 Definition

Simple or unicameral bone cyst (SBC/UBC) is usually a unilocular, fibrous-walled cystic cavity lined by a single row of mesothelial-like epithelium filled with serous or serosanguineous fluid. It is only primary, true cyst of bone by the pathologic definition of an abnormal closed cavity lined by epithelium or less likely endothelium. A cavity that is not lined by epithelium is commonly referred to pseudocyst.

12.2 Synonym

Solitary bone cyst.

12.3 Incidence

The true incidence is not known because most patients are asymptomatic and discovered incidentally on image studies for unrelated problems or even do not seek a medial attention. However, SBC is thought to be the second most frequent next to exostosis, accounting for about 3% of primary bone tumor [1].

12.4 Age

The lesion usually detected in childhood to adolescence less than 20 years old with a peak age between 5 and 15 years of age with open growth plate. Less than 15% of patients are older than 20 years [1].

12.5 Location

The cases occur most frequently in proximal humerus (60%) and next frequently in the proximal femur (30%). Metaphyseal area adjacent to growth plate is usually affected in most cases. As the lesion grows, it slowly migrates toward the diaphysis and may eventually be incorporated into the diaphyseal area (Figs. 12.1 and 12.3). Rarely, it can be found in metaphysis of other remaining long bones (Fig. 12.5a, f), or iliac bones, and occasionally, calcaneus in older patients, so-called *"calcaneal cyst"* (Fig. 12.6).

W.-J. Bahk, *Diagnosis and Management of Primary Bone Tumors*,
https://doi.org/10.1007/978-981-99-5498-8_12

Fig. 12.1 (**a**) Radiograph taken for left shoulder pain after slip in 11-year-old girl incidentally shows a large well-defined radiolucent lesion with trabeculated appearance due to endosteal bony ridges from the metaphysis abutting the growth plate to the diaphysis of proximal humerus. Note moderate expansion with cortical thinning (yellow arrow) and foal cortical breakage (red arrow). (**b**) MR images reveal a well-defined, expansile, centrally located cystic lesion with low SI in T1-weighted image and high SI on T2-weighted image. The cortex is markedly thinned and broken with a fracture line (red arrows). (**c**) Dual-trocar technique of aspiration and instillation was performed. Cystography with contrast medium after confirmation of clear yellowish fluid through the first trocar indicating SBC rather than ABC notes a complete opacification (asterisk) suggesting no septations. The dye is drained through the second trocar followed by cleansing with saline. And then one trocar was removed, and steroid (methylprednisolone) was injected by remained trocar. Bone marrow cells obtained from the iliac crest were additionally injected. (**d**) Follow-up radiograph at 3 months after the procedure notes a significant sclerotic change with thickening of the cortex (arrow). (**e**) Follow-up radiograph at 11 years after the procedure shows no evidence of local recurrence with normalized cortex (arrow). (**f**) Radiograph taken for right upper arm pain of 1-month duration in 12-year-old girl shows a relatively well-defined purely lytic lesion with mild thinning and scalloping of the cortices from the metaphysis apart from the growth plate to the diaphysis of proximal humerus (between red lines). (**g**) MR images reveal a well-defined, lobulated cystic lesion that is slightly apart from the growth plate (double-headed arrows) with low SI in T1-weighted image and high SI on T2-weighted image with focal intermediate and high signal on both sequences (red asterisks). (**h**) Cystography demonstrates areas of opacification (white asterisks) and another areas of non-opacification (red asterisks) suggesting septations. The same procedure as in previous patient was performed. (**i**) Follow-up radiograph at 3 months after the procedure notes, however, a mild sclerotic change but no milder cortical thickening (arrow) in contrast to Fig. D. (**j**) Another same procedure was repeated, and follow-up radiograph at 6 years after the second procedure shows no evidence of local recurrence with normalized cortex (arrow)

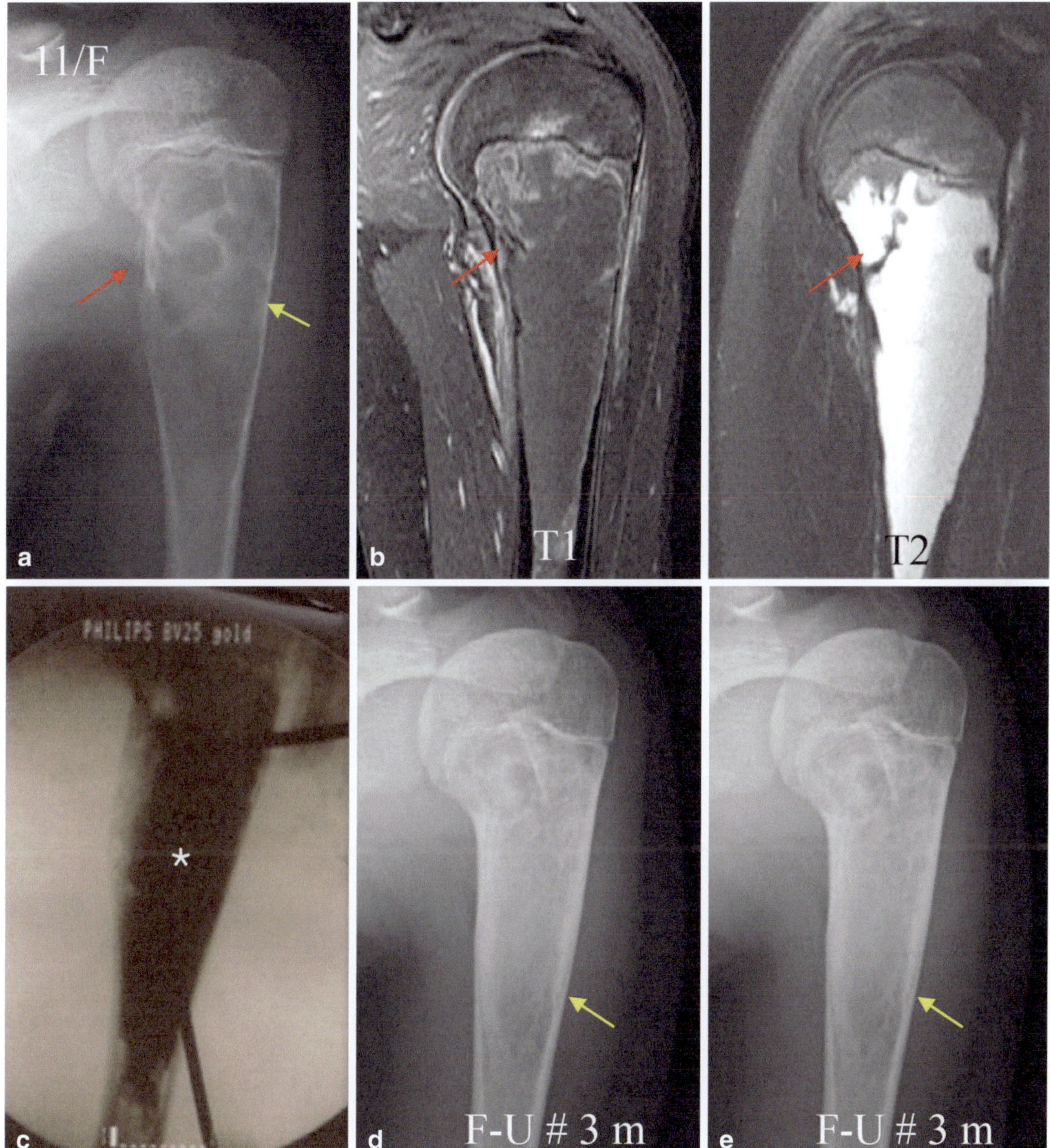
11/F
a
T1
b
T2
PHILIPS BV25 gold
*
c
F-U # 3 m
d
F-U # 3 m
e

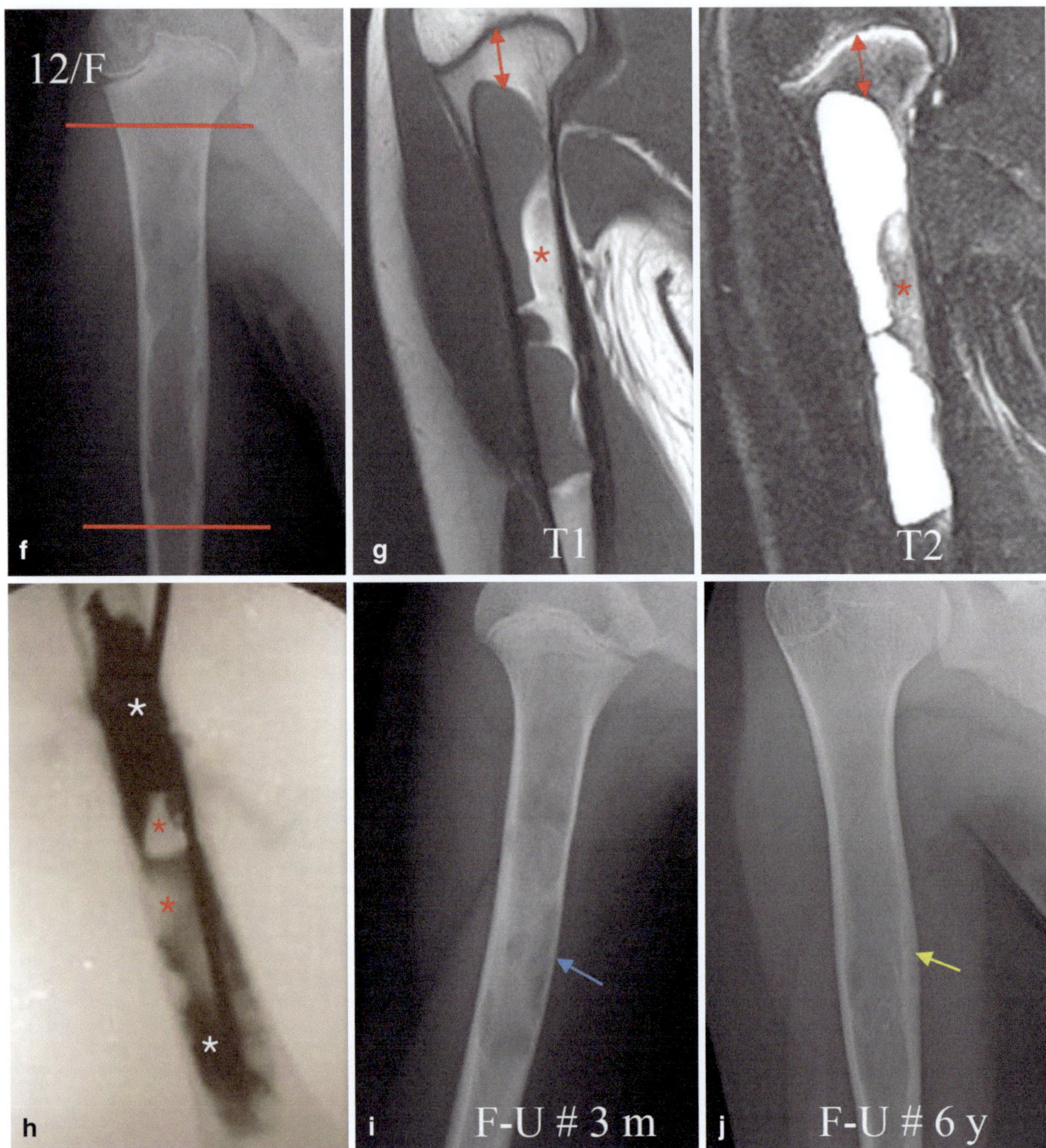

Fig. 12.1 (continued)

12.6 Clinical Features

SBC is mostly asymptomatic and discovered incidentally on radiographs or CT scans performed for unrelated problems (Figs. 12.1a and 12.2a). Pain or swelling is frequently associated with pathologic fracture by trivial injury event or slip (Figs. 12.3f, 12.4a). The lesion grows during skeletal growth (active cyst) and becomes inactive or latent after skeletal maturity (inactive cyst). The lesion is considered to be "*active*" when it develops in patients under 10–12 years of age, and cyst arises adjacent to growth plate and occupies most of metaphysis. *The active cyst* has a single cavity with very thin cortical shell, or continues to enlarge during observation that is prone to cause a pathologic fracture.

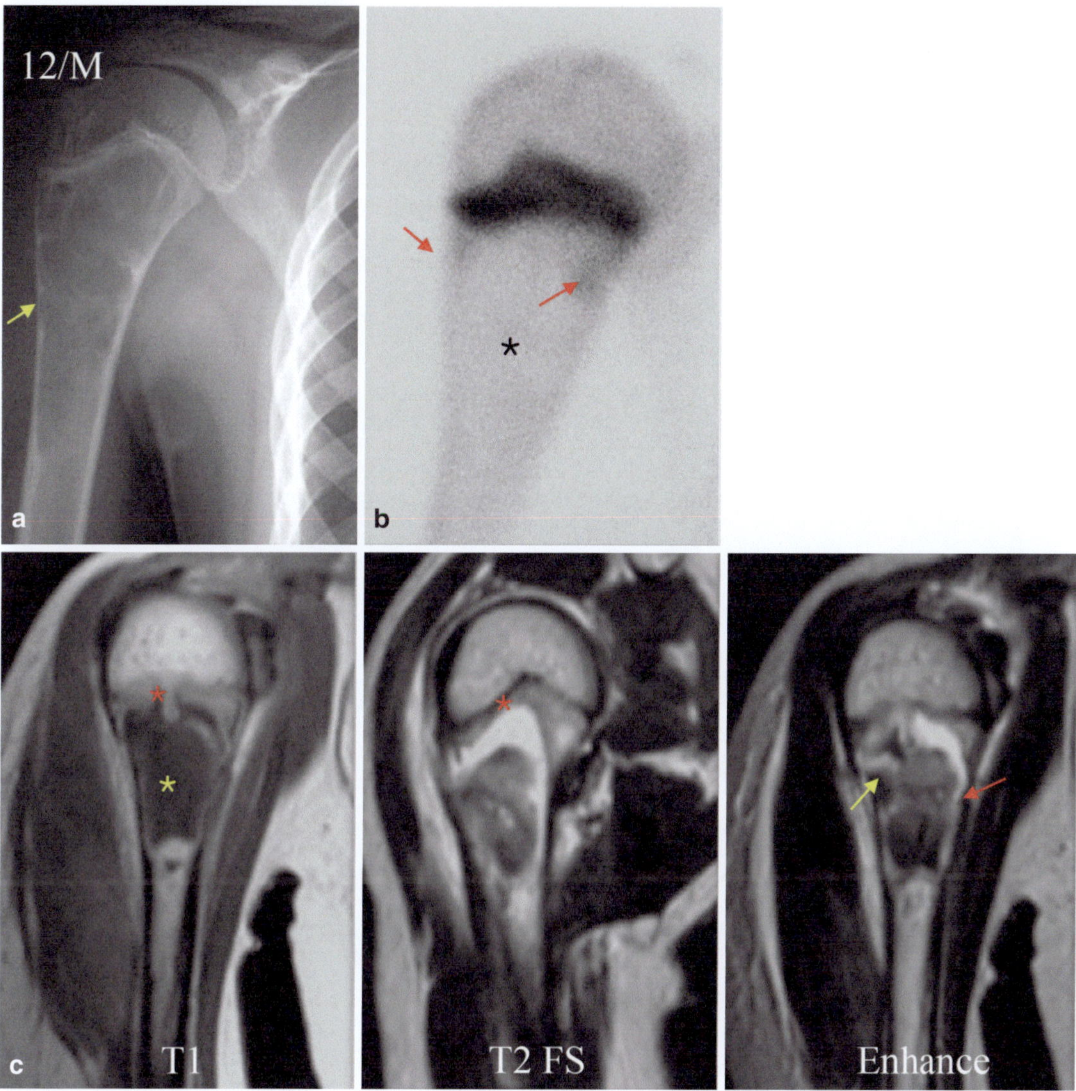

Fig. 12.2 (**a**) Radiograph taken for right shoulder pain after slip in 12-year-old boy incidentally shows a centrally located, multi-lobulated, purely lytic lesion with mild expansion and cortical thinning (arrow) in the meta-diaphysis of the proximal humerus. Proximal part of the lesion is abutting the growth plate. (**b**) Pinhole bone scan reveals a large photon defect (asterisk) with focal areas of very mild uptake (arrows). (**c**) MR images demonstrate a relatively well-defined centrally located cystic lesion abutting the growth plate (red asterisks) with low SI on T1-weighted image and heterogeneous low and high SI on T2-weighted image. The lesion is peripherally well enhanced (red arrow) with focal septal enhancement (yellow arrow). Curettage with allo-chip bone graft was performed in consideration of a large size of the lesion and his activity. (**d**) Follow-up radiograph at 6 years after surgery notes consolidation of the most lesion. But there is still focally remained radiolucent area with endosteal scalloping (asterisk). The patient does not present any symptoms. ***The oldest patient in our series*** (**e**) Radiograph taken for left shoulder pain of 2-week duration in 24-yeard-old young man shows a well-defined multi-lobulated purely lytic lesion mainly affecting metaphysis of the proximal humerus. (**f**) Pinhole bone scan reveals a hazy peripheral uptake (arrows) with internal photon defect (asterisk). (**g**) MR images demonstrate a well-demarcated unichambered cystic lesion with low and intermediate SI on T1-weighted image and intermediate and high SI on T2-weighted image. There is a *"fluid-fluid"* level of different densities (yellow arrows), which may be associated with focal cortical breakage and hemorrhage. The lesion is only peripherally enhanced (red arrows). (**h**) Curettage and allo-chip bone graft was performed, and he was lost for follow-up. The histologic diagnosis was SBC

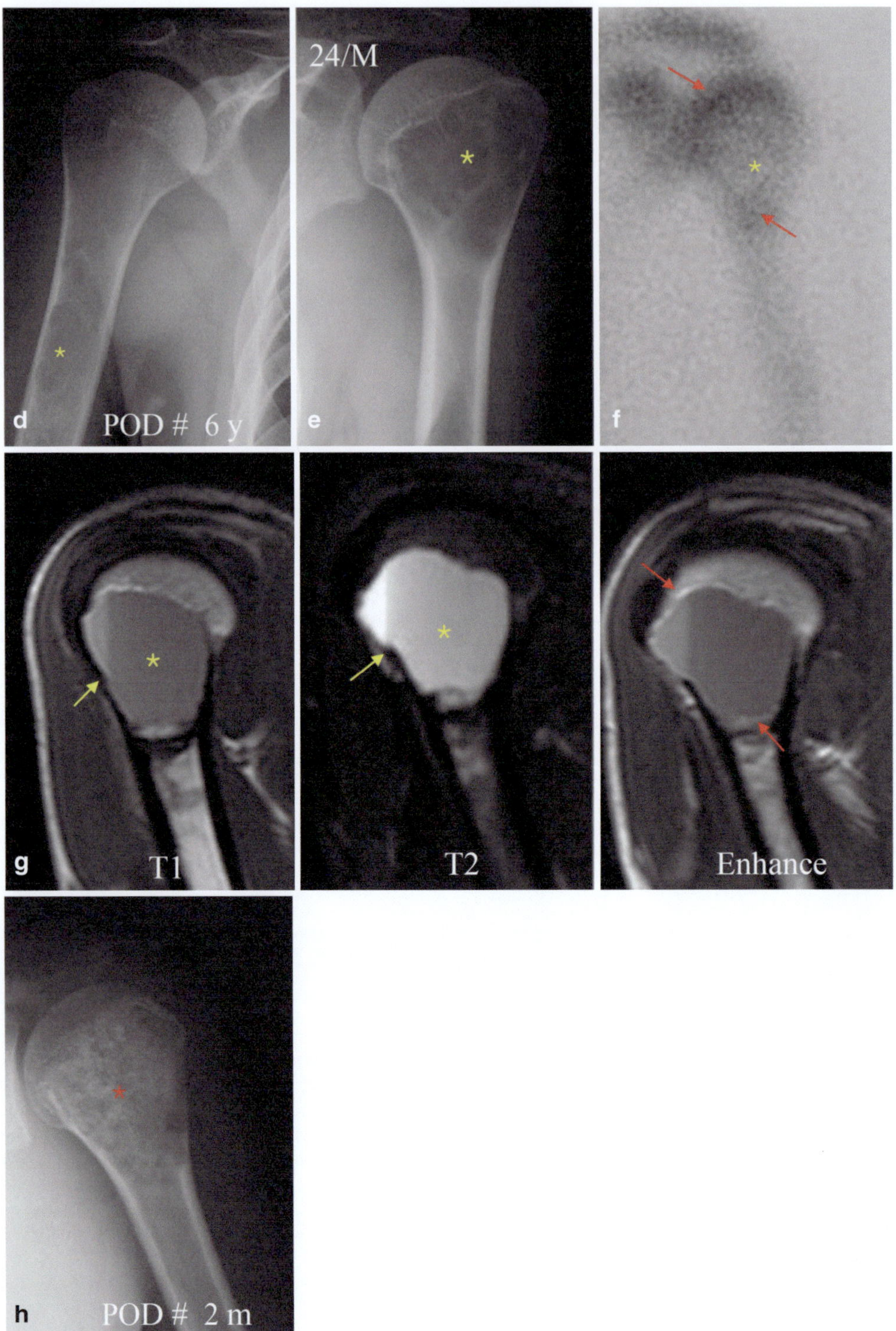

Fig. 12.2 (continued)

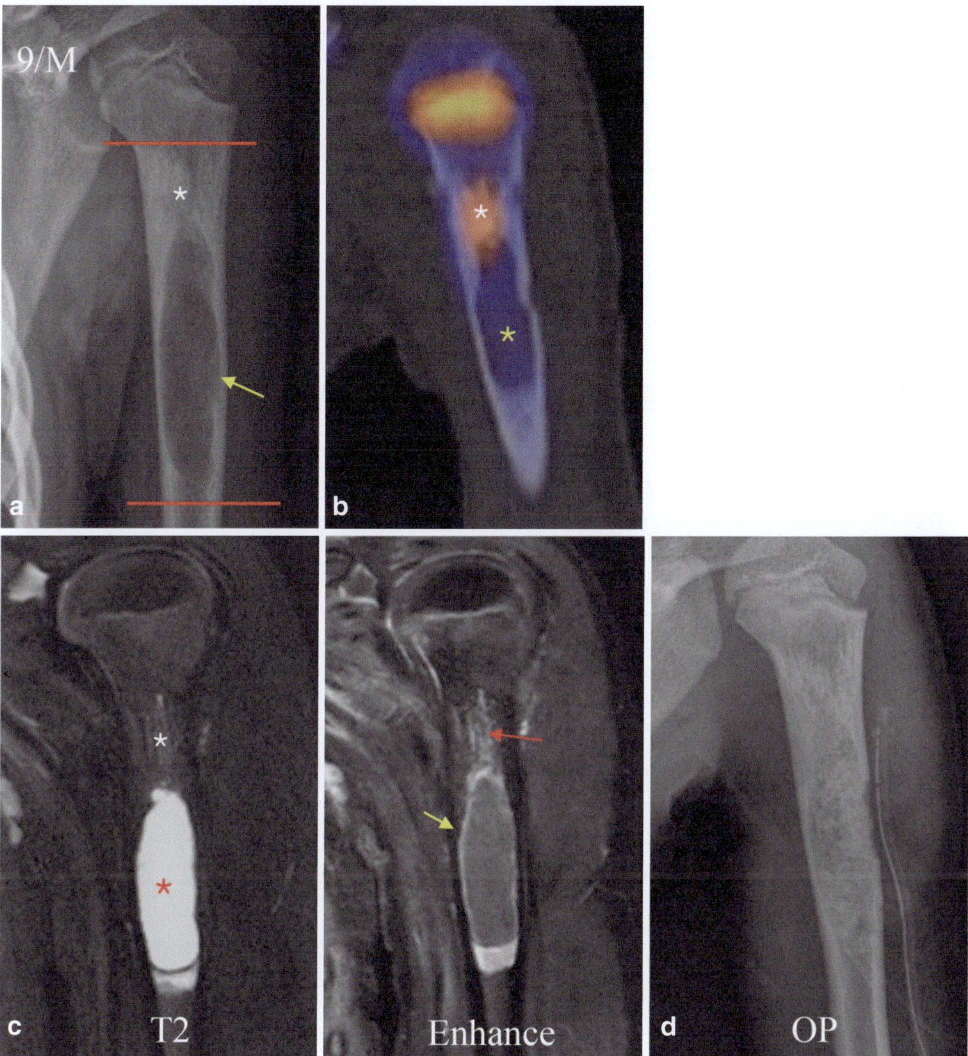

Fig. 12.3 ***Diaphyseal migration*** (**a**) Radiograph taken for left upper arm pain of 1-month duration in 9-year-old boy shows a well-defined purely radiolucent lesion with mild expansion, endosteal scalloping, and cortical thinning (arrow) in the diaphysis of proximal humerus (between red lines). Note a sclerotic healing lesion (asterisk) proximal to the main radiolucent lesion. (**b**) Bone SPECT/CT reveals increased uptake (white asterisk) in the meta-diaphyseal junctional area of the proximal humerus, which corresponds to the sclerotic healing lesion on the radiograph and MR image. However, there is no increased uptake in the more distally located main cystic lesion (yellow asterisk). (**c**) MR images demonstrate a well-defined cystic lesion (red asterisk) in the diaphysis associated with healing sclerotic lesion (white asterisk) in the meta-diaphysis area. The main cystic lesion is peripherally enhanced (yellow arrow), and the proximal sclerotic lesion is heterogeneously enhanced (red arrow). (**d**) Curettage and allo-chip bone graft was done for the diaphyseally located cystic lesion. (**e**) Follow-up radiograph at 2 years after surgery notes consolidation of the lesion (red asterisk) with cortical thickening (red arrow). (**f**) Another radiograph taken for right shoulder pain after slip in 5-year-old boy reveals a similar lesion in the proximal diaphysis with pathologic fracture (white arrow). Note several fallen pieces of fractured or fragmented cortex, so-called *"fallen fragment"* sign (yellow arrow). (**g**) Bone scan shows a moderately inceased heterogeneous uptake in the proximal sclerotic area (white asterisk) but no uptake in the diaphyseally located cystic lesion (red asterisk) as in bone SPET/CT (**b**) of former patient. (**h**) MR images reveal a cystic lesion with low SI and linear dark signal of fallen cortex (inset) on T1-weighted image and high SI with internal dark and intermediate signal (yellow arrow) suggesting fractured fragments with associated hemorrhage on fat saturated T2-weighted image. The lesion is peripherally enhanced (yellow arrow) and surrounding hemorrhage is well enhanced (red arrow). (**i**) Curettage with allo-chip bone graft and fixation of the fracture by Khai-nails was performed. (**j**) Follow-up radiograph at 5 years after surgery notes consolidation of the lesion (yellow asterisk) with cortical thickening

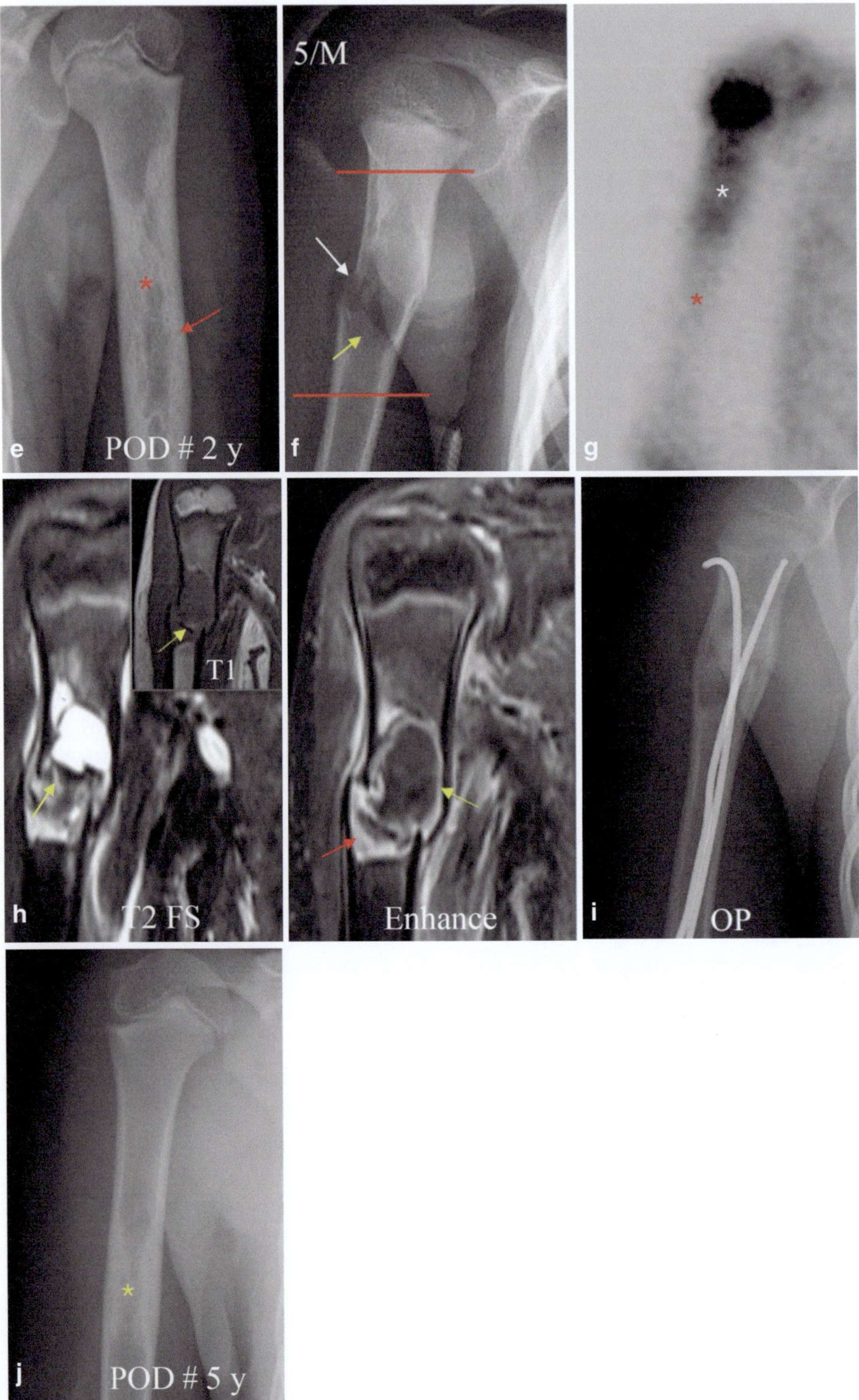

Fig. 12.3 (continued)

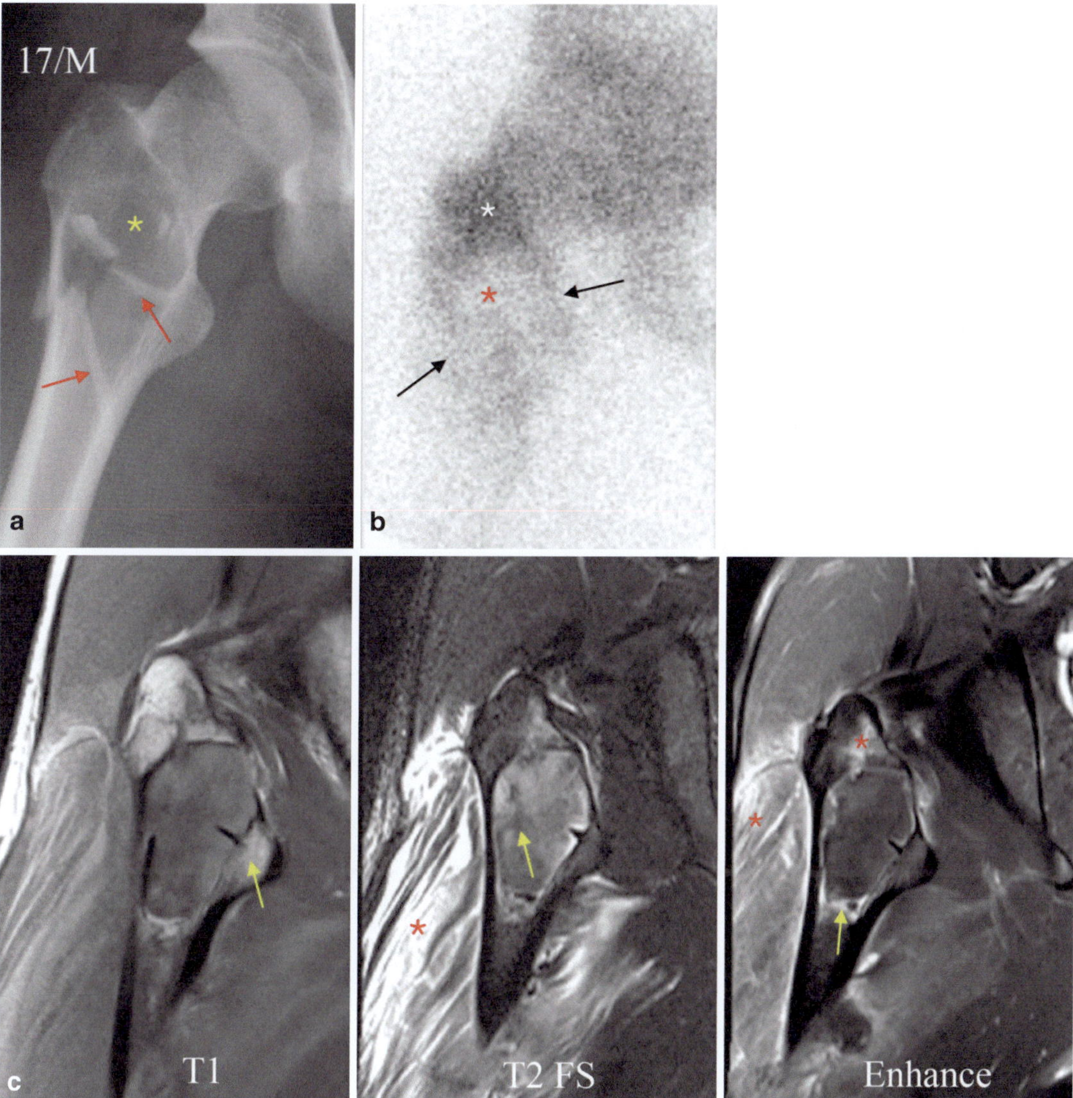

Fig. 12.4 ***Pathologic fracture*** (**a**) Radiograph taken for right hip pain by slip down shows a pathologic fracture with underlying radiolucent lesion (asterisk) in the trochanteric area. There are fallen pieces of fractured cortical fragment floating in the fluid, so-called *"fallen fragment"* sign (red arrows). (**b**) Pinhole scan reveals a focal photon defect in the lucent cystic lesion (red asterisk) with mild increased uptake along the periphery of the lesion (black arrows) and moderately increased focal uptake in the greater trochanter (white asterisk). (**c**) MR images demonstrate a large well-defined uni-chambered cystic lesion with low and intermediate SI on T1-weighted image and heterogeneous intermediate and high SI on fat saturated T2-weighted image. There are associated high signal on T1-weighted image and low signal on fat saturated T2-weighted image (yellow arrows). In addition, bright signal are diffusely seen in the adjacent muscle and subcutaneous tissue (red asterisk) representing extensive hemorrhage and edema by pathologic fracture. The lesion is only peripherally enhanced (yellow arrow). Enhancement also is noted in the muscles and subcutaneous fat tissues as well as marrow (asterisks). (**d**) Open biopsy at fracture gap followed by closed reduction, curettage with allo-chip bone graft, and PFNA nailing was performed. (**e**) Microscopic examination. (Left) Low-power magnification shows thickened cystic wall components (inset). Medium-power magnification reveals the thickened wall is composed of fibroblasts, wavy wisps of collagen fibers, reactive osteoid or woven bone, foamy histiocytes, massive hemorrhage, and cholesterol clefts in some areas (black asterisks). (Right) Additional area of explosive growth of mesenchymal cells, fibrinoid necrosis, acute and chronic inflammatory cell infiltration, and primitive osteoid (white asterisks) with cartilage (yellow asterisks), which is equivalent to a callus of 7–10 days' estimated age, is recognized. Practically, biopsy was performed 7 days after fracture event. (**f**) Follow-up radiograph at 11 years after surgery reveals complete healing of SBC lesion with no recurrence

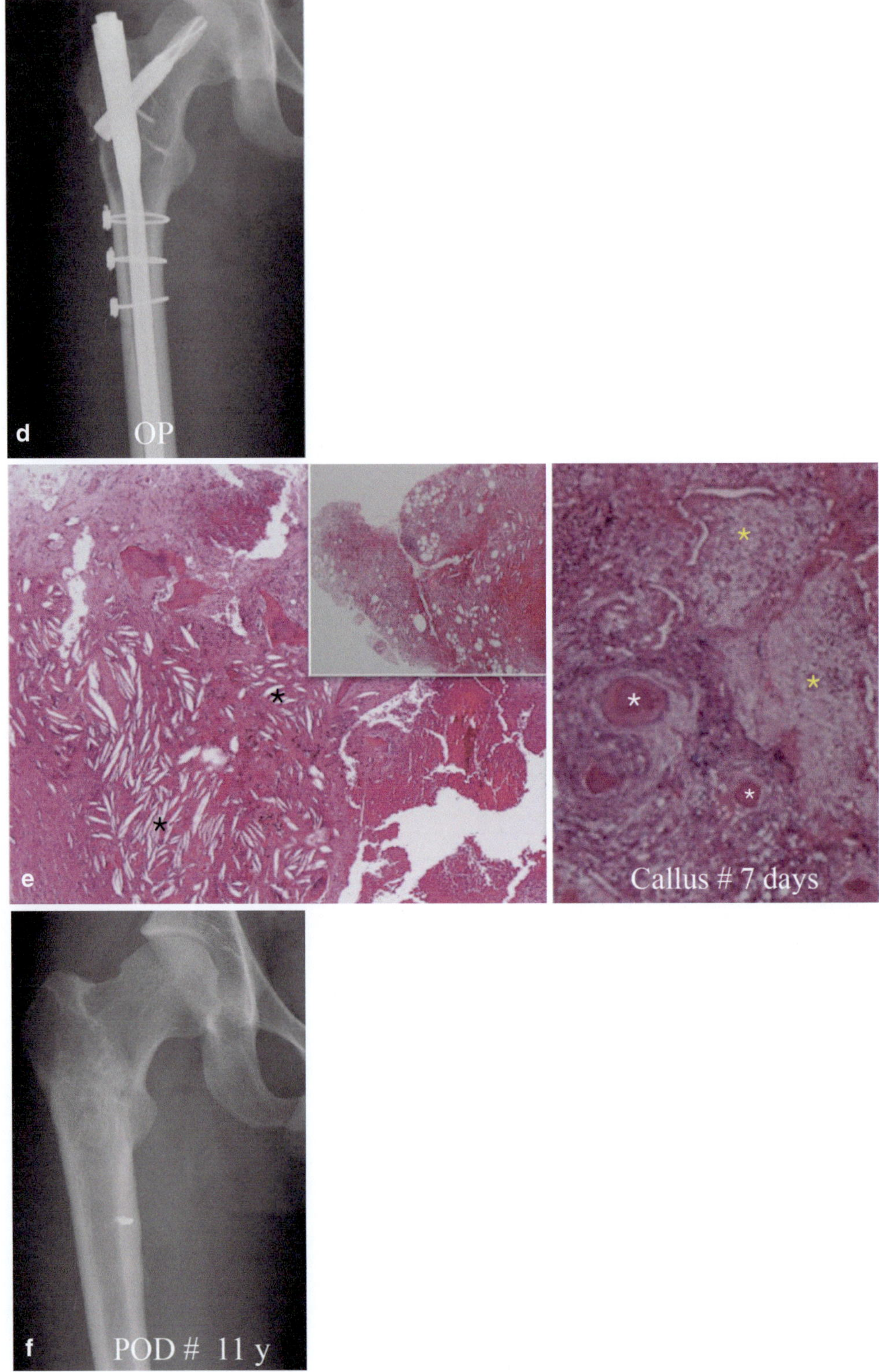

Fig. 12.4 (continued)

However, it is considered to be *inactive* when patient is over 12 years of age, the lesion ceases to expand and migrate to a diaphyseal location far from the growth plate (more than 1–2 cm). *The inactive cyst* has a multilocular cavity with thicker bony wall and evidence of healing/ossification, which less likely to result in a pathologic fracture.

12.7 Radiologic Findings

Radiologic findings are highly characteristic, although not pathognomonic, which present as a well-defined purely lytic lesion with or without trabeculation, generally originating in the metaphysis of long bone that abuts open growth plate (Figs. 12.1, 12.2). However, the lesion may migrate away from the growth plate to be centered in the diaphysis as the bone grows (Figs. 12.1 and 12.3). SBC is usually composed of one contiguous cystic space, but it may present a trabeculated appearance due to prominent endosteal bony ridges. Rarely, it is truly multi-lobulated in late inactive stage. The lesion usually shows a sharp border with variable thinning of the cortex and symmetric bone expansion. A rim of sclerosis is rarely observed despite the benign nature of the cyst probably because the lesion is "expanding" at a faster rate than that of a surrounding sclerotic reactive bone formation. The width of cyst is usually not greater than width of epiphyseal plate. Piece(s) or sliver(s) of cortical bone or linear fragments of fractured cortical bone may drop down to the bottom of the cyst by gravity and float in the fluid, producing a pathognomonic *"fallen fragment"* sign (Figs. 12.3f and 12.4a). **Bone scan** Active lesion shows peripherally increased uptake with internal foci of photon defect (cold spot) in the center. There is no increased uptake in inactive lesion. **MR findings** MR signals are characteristic for fluid content with homogenous low on T1-weighted image and high SI on T2-weighted images but no solid internal component. If solid areas existed in the lesion, the cystic lesion is not a primary but secondary degenerative cystic change of pre-existing lesion. There are usually no fluid-fluid levels. However, a simple fluid level can be seen if hemorrhage is associated with or without fracture (Fig. 12.2). Repeated fracture can make trabeculations producing a multi-lobulated appearance with fluid level(s). The lesion is peripherally enhanced with or without septal enhancement. Nodular-like enhancement may suggest associated fracture with hemorrhage or hematoma.

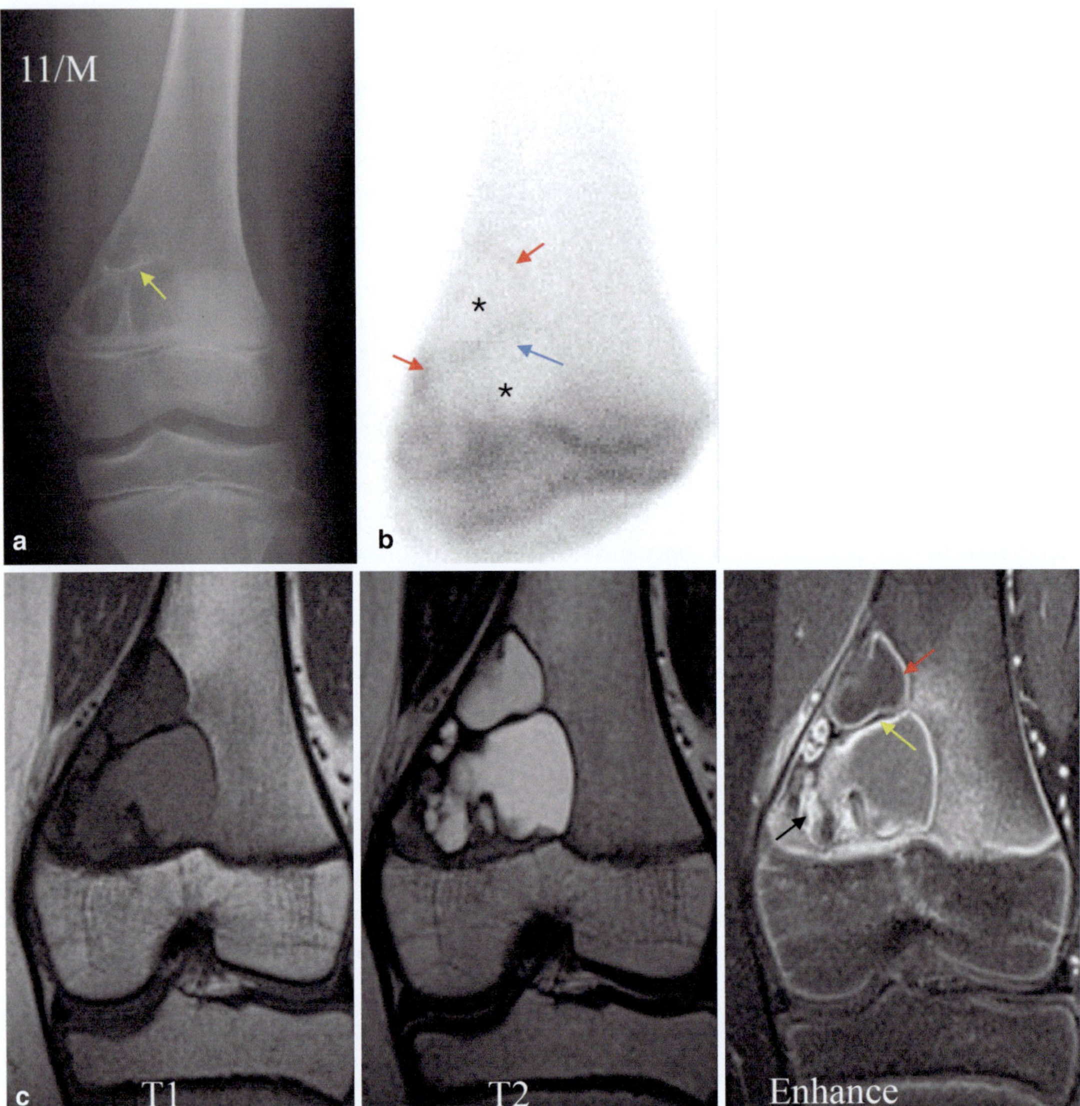

Fig. 12.5 ***Rare location of distal femur*** (**a**) Radiographs taken for left knee pain of 3-month duration in 11-year-old boy shows an eccentric, multi-lobular, radiolucent lytic with thin trabeculations (arrow), mild expansion, and cortical thinning involving metaphysis of medial aspect of the distal femur. (**b**) Pinhole bone scan reveals mild to moderately increased uptake along the wall (red arrows) and internal septa (blue arrow) with central photon defects (asterisks). (**c**) MR images reveals a well-demarcated, eccentric, multi-lobulated cystic lesion with low SI on T1-weighted image and high SI on T2-weighted images with dark signals of septa and surrounding rims of sclerotic bone. The lesion is well enhanced along the wall (red arrow) and internal septa (yellow arrow) with focal thick enhancement (black arrow) probably suggesting markedly thickened walls. (**d**) Microscopic examination notes thickened cystic wall composed of fibroblasts and wavy wisps of collagen fibers as well as cholesterol cleft and abundant cementum-like material significantly thickening the wall (inset). (**e**) Follow-up radiograph at 5 years after curettage and allo-chip bone graft shows consolidation of the lesion. ***Rare location of distal fibula with secondary ABC*** (**f**) Radiograph taken for right ankle pain in 12-year-old boy shows a well-defined radiolucent lesion with mild expansion and cortical thinning in the distal fibula. MR images reveal a clear fluid signal within the lesion indicating UBC (not available here). Dual-needle technique was performed for management. Aspiration of clear yellow fluid indicating SBC followed by saline irrigation and drain through the first needle was performed, and then steroid was injected through the second needle after removal of the first needle. (**g**) Follow-up radiograph taken after several weeks reveals a progression of expansion and cortical thinning (white arrow). (**h**) Another follow-up radiograph taken a few more weeks later demonstrates a further progression and expansion of the lesion with a possible cortical breakage (yellow arrow). Microscopic examination confirmed secondary ABC arising from SBC (Courtesy from Prof. JM Mirra)

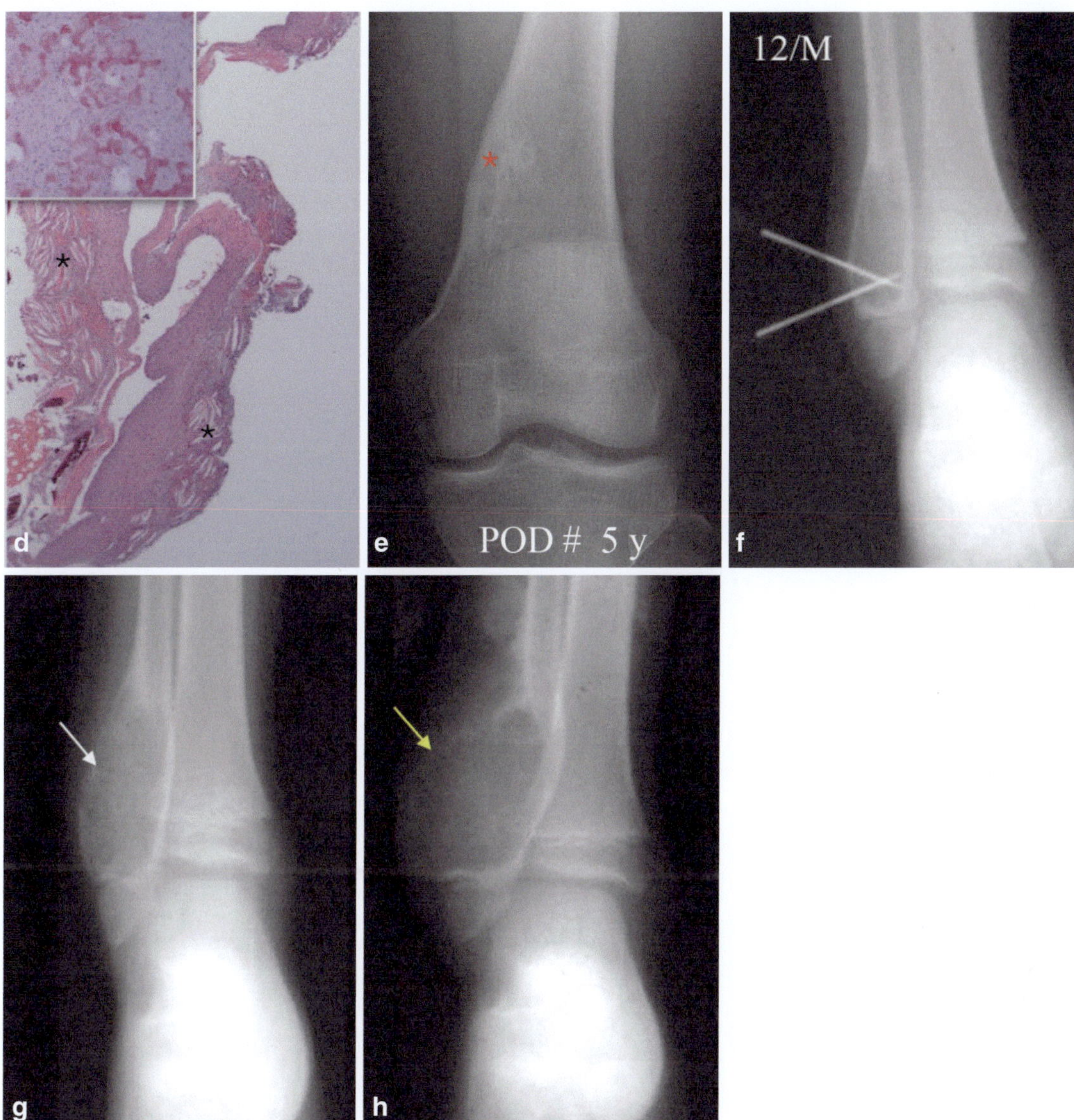

Fig. 12.5 (continued)

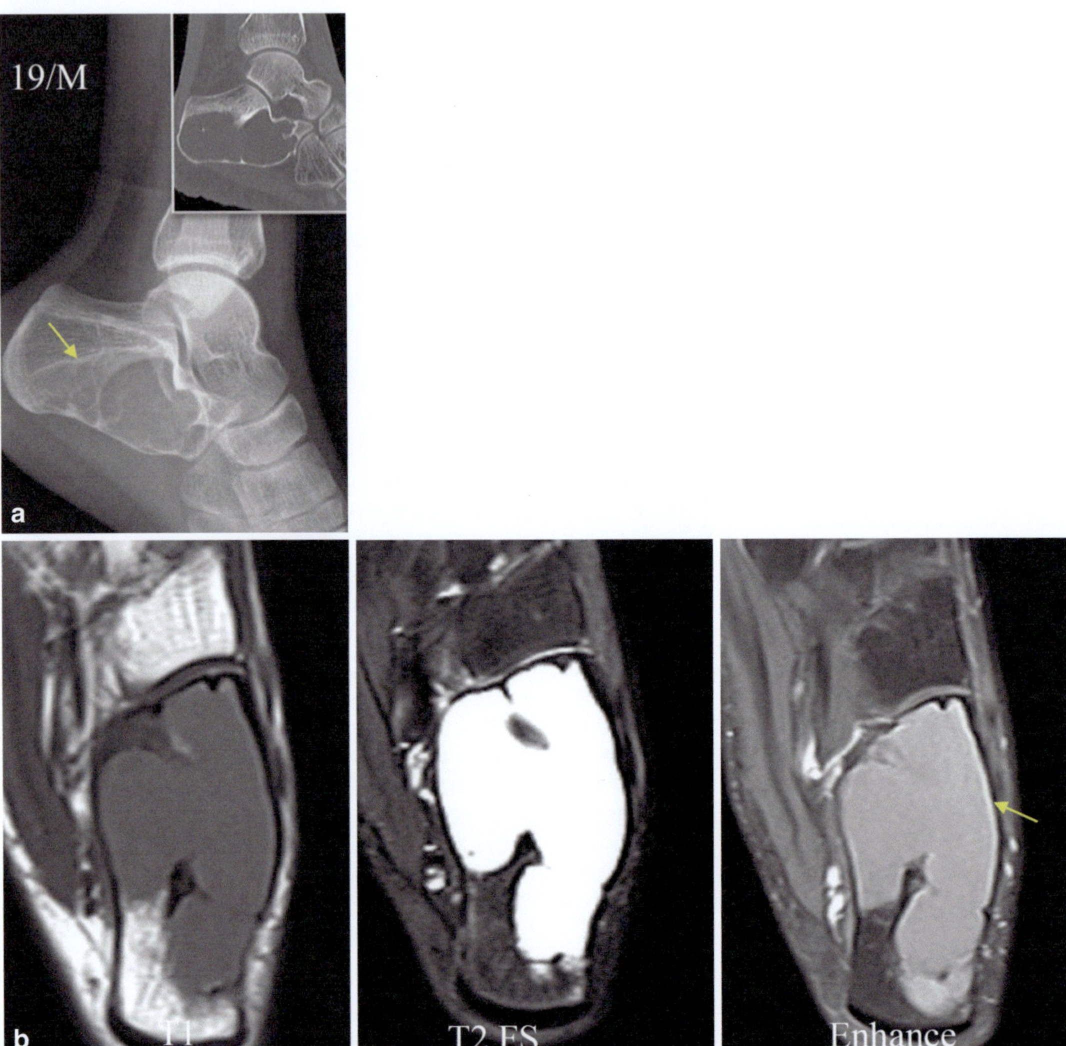

Fig. 12.6 *Calcaneal cyst* (**a**) Radiographs taken for left heel pain in 19-year-old young man shows a multilobulated, trapezoidal, radiolucent lesion surrounded by a sclerotic border (arrow) occupying over one-third of the calcaneus. CT scan more clearly notes such features (inset). (**b**) MR images demonstrate a well-defined unilocular cystic lesion with low SI on T-weighted image and bright SI on fat saturated T2-weighted image. The lesion is only peripherally enhanced (arrow). (**c**) Microscopic examination reveals a markedly thickened cystic wall with abundant cholesterol clefts (yellow asterisks) within the wall consisting prominent fibrous tissues and irregular bone spicules (yellow arrows) as well as marrow fat (black asterisk). (**d**) Follow-up radiograph at 1 year after curettage and allo-chip bone graft notes consolidation of the lesion without local recurrence. (**e**) Radiograph taken for left heel pain during military drill in 24-year-old soldier shows an oval to trapezoidal radiolucent lesion surrounded by a sclerotic border (arrow) in the calcaneus. (**f**) Non-enhanced MR images reveals a well-defined lesion with mostly low SI on T1-weighted image and high SI on T2-weighted image suggesting fluid containing cyst (larger asterisks). In addition, there is intermediate to high signal along the periphery of the lesion on both sequences, which may indicate fat component (smaller red asterisks) probably in the process of healing. There are thin dark signals of reactive sclerosis at outer most area (red arrows). (**g**) Microscopic examination. (Left) Low magnification demonstrates two different structures of cystic tissue (white asterisk) and fatty tissue (black asterisk). The calcaneal cyst shows epithelial-like lining with more abundant fibrous tissue (inset) and cholesterol clefts than SBC of long bones. (Right) Higher magnification clearly notes transition or conversion of thickened cystic wall with heavy cholesterol cleft to fatty tissue with bone spicules. Some areas show prominent fat cells (inset). (**h**) Follow-up radiograph at 1 year after curettage and allo-chip bone graft notes consolidation of the lesion, and he has no pain during military drill

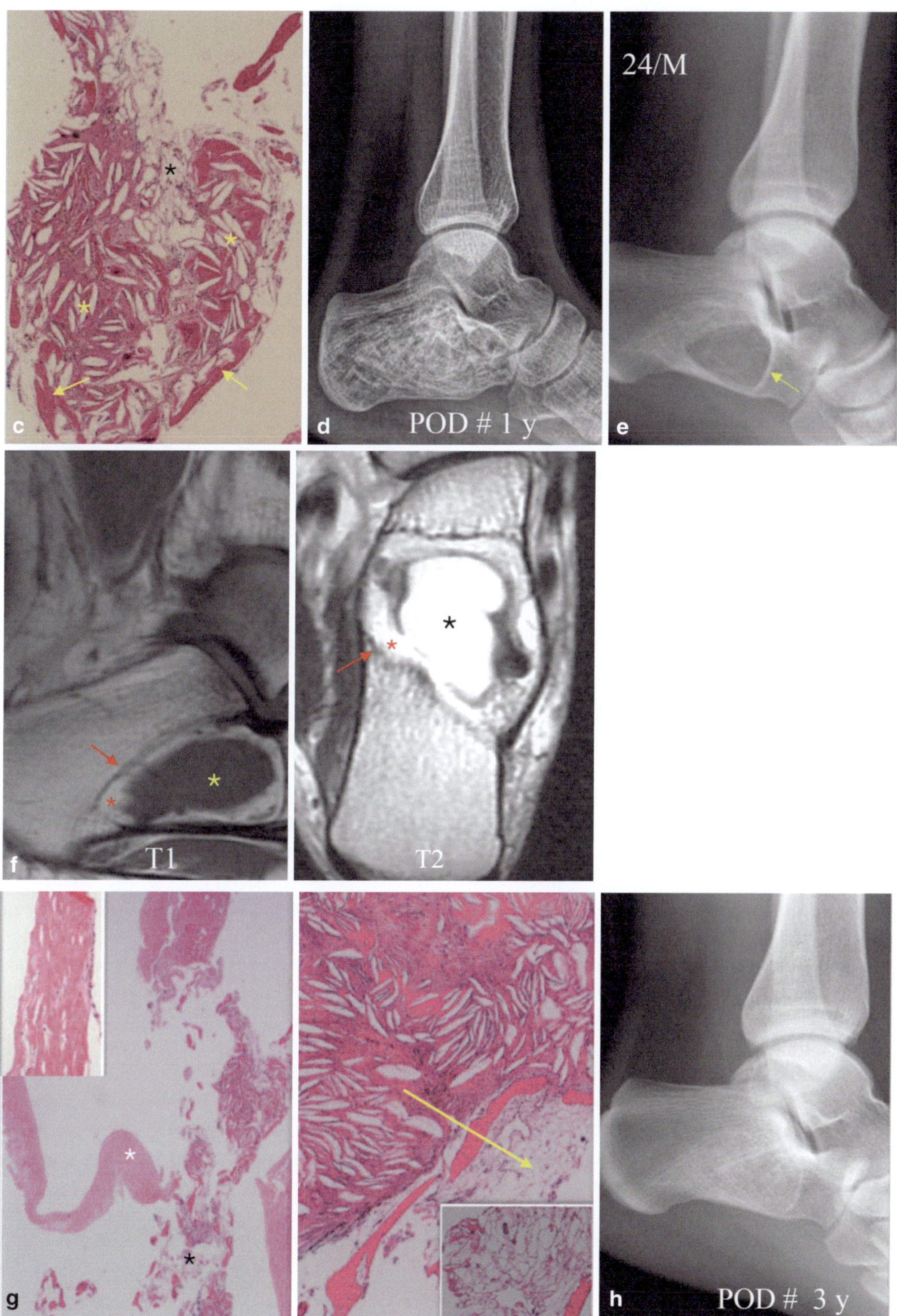

Fig. 12.6 (continued)

12.8 Histologic Findings

SBC is usually unicameral and filled with clear yellow serious or often serosanguineous blood tinged fluid, while aneurysmal bone cyst (ABC) is a multi-loculated cystic architecture with a dark, red pure blood. It can be easily differentiated by a simple needle aspiration before surgical procedure. The key histologic finding is a wall-like structure composed of thin membrane with fibroblasts, collagen fibers, and fibrin. The cystic wall consists of a thin layer of loose fibrous tissue lined with a single layer of flattened to mildly plump cells resembling mesothelial-like or synovial-like lining cells (Fig. 12.7a) or less likely endothelial-like cells. The cystic wall of SBC is a single continuous membrane, analogous to that lining the internal surface of a fowl's egg. However, ABC is typically lined by bundles of collagen, fibrin, and cell debris devoid of specialized endothelial lining cells, but occasional elongated cells resembling fibroblasts can be present on the surface of the cyst (see histologic findings in ABC chapter). But it can be confused with the wall of ABC if the membrane of SBC is curetted off the bone and twisted into undulating folds as well as the lining cells are torn apart by surgeon's procedure [1]. The wall components beneath the lining cells are composed of fibroblasts, wavy wisps of collagen fibers, usually thin slivers of reactive osteoid or woven bone, scattered multinucleated giant cells, foamy histiocytes, hemosiderin pigments, or sometimes cholesterol cleft (Figs. 12.4e and 12.7b). When calcaneus is affected, almost all cases are more prominent in cholesterol cleft and fibrosis (Figs. 12.6c and 12.7c). Cementum-like material (calcified eosinophilic fibrinous material) can be observed within significantly thickened walls in rare cases (Fig. 12.7d). Electron microscopic studies of cementum-like material by Mirra et al. [2] demonstrated collagen fibers and numerous matrix vesicles, which form the initial sites of calcification. They concluded that so-called *"cementoma"* of long bone is not a distinct entity, but a form of SBC with acellular form of bone mimicking tooth cementum. In addition, they also first reported the lining cells had features identical to those of synovial cells and suggested that SBC may represent a congenital "rest" of synovial tissue displaced into the thin, cortical metaphyseal region of bones at the synovial-capsular-bone reflection. The thesis may explain the reason for a significant preponderance of proximal femur (hip joint) and humerus (shoulder joint), which have the largest area of capsular-metaphyseal bone reflection. Fracture callus at different estimated age is observed in case with pathologic fracture (Fig. 12.7e, f), which should be aware for a correct diagnosis. Particularly, early callus aged 1–2 weeks can make a confusion in diagnosis. Rarely, secondary ABC can be associated with SBC (Fig. 11.12 in Chap. 11).

12.9 Management

The options should be individualized for each patient based on the clinical and radiologic features such as size of the cyst, the strength of the bone, patient's activity level, pathologic fracture, and symptoms. ***Observation*** Asymptomatic small lesion can be observed with regular radiographs to keep track of any changes in the cyst until the cyst resolves. The cyst may be healed and resolved spontaneously in less than 10% patients with pathologic fracture occurring through the cyst [3]. ***Aspiration and Injection*** The procedure is only effective in active lesion in younger patients and usually consists of penetrating the cyst with two needles or trocars. After aspiration of the fluid, cleansing with saline and removing one needle or trocar, substances such as steroid or autologous bone marrow is injected by a remained needle to decrease the chance of the cyst coming back (Fig.12.1). However, several procedures are required in many patients. ***Surgical treatment*** is considered particularly for painful lesion, growing larger during observation or large enough to weaken the bone with high risk of fracture with mild force, lesion in a location that may more easily cause fracture such as hip, or associated pathologic fracture (Figs. 12.2, 12.3, and 12.4). A standard option is curettage of lining membrane followed by allo/autobone graft or hydroxyapatite bone substitute with or without internal fixation. Only decompression of cystic cavity without bone graft by multiple drill holes, cannulated screw, K-wires or flexible intramedullary nails, hydroxyapatite cannulated pin insertion has been reported to be effective. More recently, minimally invasive endoscopic curettage has been introduced with relatively higher success rate with minor complications [4–6]. Each management method has advantages and disadvantages. Observation method requires a longer duration for consolidation of the lesion and prolonged restriction of activity to prevent pathologic fracture. Steroid or bone marrow injection is non-surgical, but it has to be repeated in every 2 months, and usually 2-5 times of injection are required [7]. Curettage and bone graft is aggressive option sometimes with postoperative complications. Pathologic fracture can be man-

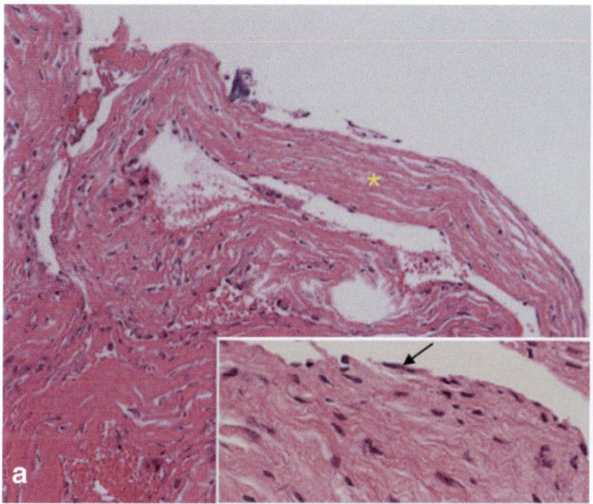

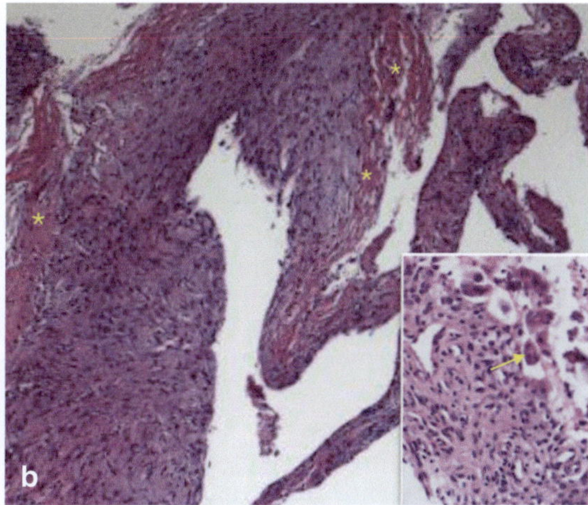

Fig. 12.7 ***Microscopic features*** (**a**) Key histologic finding is a wall-like structure (asterisk) composed of thin membrane with fibroblasts, collagen fibers, and fibrin lined with single layer of mesothelial-like or synovial-like lining cells (black arrow in inset). The membrane usually assumes a folded shape with multiple lobulations by curettage, which may be mistaken for ABC. However, the latter notes no definite lining cells. (**b**) The wall components beneath the lining cells include fibroblasts, wavy wisps of collagen fibers, foamy histiocytes, deposition of reactive osteoid or woven bone (yellow asterisks), hemosiderin pigments, and scattered multinucleated giant cells (inset). (**c**) Some cystic walls are significantly thickened with large masses of cholesterol deposition and heavy fibrosis, particularly in calcaneal cyst as this case. (**d**) A unique uncalcified globular acellular to hypocellular substance similar to the cementum of the teeth, so-called *"cementum-like material"* (asterisks) can be found in associated with fibrin, which make the wall significantly thickened in rare cases. (**e**) Additionally, fracture callus of various ages should be recognized if existed for correct diagnosis. There are areas of explosive growth of mesenchymal cells, which are quite ominous (yellow asterisks) in association with primitive woven bone spicules (white asterisks) and chondroid to immature cartilage (black asterisks), mimicking osteosarcoma. However, a fracture callus can be easily differentiated when considering image findings of cyst with pathologic fracture. Estimated age is about the end of first week to early second week (7–10 days). In this particular case, the specimen was obtained 8 days after fracture. (**f**) The callus in another case presents more matured woven bone spicules (yellow asterisk) embedded within the bland spindle stroma with prominent injury vessels and higher cellularity (black asterisk), suggesting a fracture callus of early second week's estimated age. Clinically, the specimen was obtained 10 days after fracture event

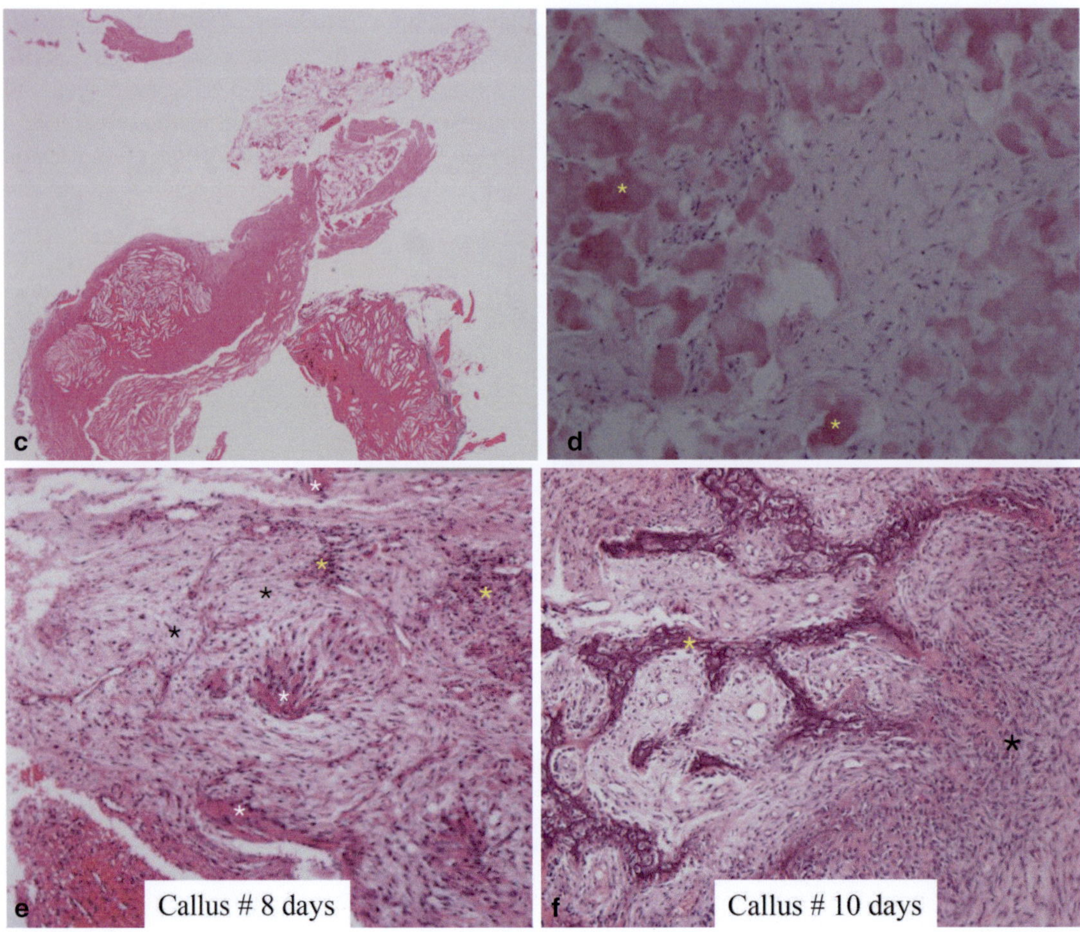

Fig. 12.7 (continued)

aged by splinting or internal fixation depending on the age, size and location of the lesion as well as the patients' activity levels. Conservative splinting for proximal humerus and internal fixation for proximal femur can be considered.

12.10 Clinical Course

SBC develops in the metaphysis of the long bones abutting open growth plate, then migrates toward the diaphysis, and finally ends up filled and ossified with growth. SBC is rarely found in adults suggesting a possible spontaneous resolution with aging. The cysts constantly become inactive around pubertal age. After then, the thinned cortex is slowly reinforced, and the fracture risk becomes almost nil. However, some kinds of management are necessary in many patients to reduce the risk of pathologic fracture or to treat fracture itself before such spontaneous healing. Regardless management methods, most authors reported local recurrence rate between 10 and 30%. It thus seems to be reasonable to try the minimally aggressive procedure first and then more aggressive surgical treatment when recurred. In general, the earlier the cyst is treated in a child, the higher the chance of recurrence is expected. The recurrence rate is much higher in active cysts and significantly lower in latent cysts. Exceptionally rarely, secondary ABC could arise from SBC by puncture (Fig. 12.6). A possible relationship between SBC and intraosseous lipoma has been described particularly in the calcaneus cyst [8]. SBCs can heal with fatty conversion of the cystic cavity with complete filling or with partly cystic remnants in calcaneal cyst (Fig. 12.6f) [9]. The exact opposite finding of cystic change in intraosseous lipoma has also been described [10–12]. Extraordinarily, malignant change without a history of previous irradiation has been reported [13–16].

References

1. Mirra JM. Simple bone cyst. In: Mirra JM, editor. Bone tumors: clinical, radiologic, and pathologic correlation. 2nd ed. Philadelphia, PA: Lea & Febiger; 1989. p. 1235–61.
2. Mirra JM, Bernard GW, Bullough PG, Johnston W, Mink G. Cementum-like bone production in solitary bone cysts.(so-called" cementoma" of long bones). Report of three cases. Electron microscopic observations supporting a synovial origin to the simple bone cyst. Clin Orthop Relat Res. 1978;135:295–307.
3. Green NM, Pagkalos J, Jeys LM, Stevenson JD, Gregory JJ. Humeral simple bone cysts: observational versus interventional management. J Pediatr Orthop. 2019;39(6):e472–e7.
4. Yildirim C, Akmaz I, Sahin O, Keklikci K. Simple calcaneal bone cysts: a pilot study comparing open versus endoscopic curettage and grafting. J Bone Joint Surg Br. 2011;93(12):1626–31.
5. Nishimura A, Matsumine A, Kato K, Aasanuma K, Nakamura T, Fukuda A, et al. Endoscopic versus open surgery for calcaneal bone cysts: a preliminary report. J Foot Ankle Surg. 2016;55(4):782–7.
6. Aiba H, Kobayashi M, Waguri-Nagaya Y, Goto H, Mizutani J, Yamada S, et al. Treatment of simple bone cysts using endoscopic curettage: a case series analysis. J Orthop Surg Res. 2018;13(1):1–9.
7. Campanacci M. Simple bone cyst. In: Bone and soft tissue tumors. Cham: Springer; 1999. p. 791–811.
8. Malghem J, Lecouvet F, Vande BB. Calcaneal cysts and lipomas: a common pathogenesis? Skelet Radiol. 2017;46(12):1635–42.
9. Tins BJ, Berkowitz YJ, Konala P, Davies M, Cassar-Pullicino VN, Lalam R, et al. Intraosseous lipomas originating from simple bone cysts. Skelet Radiol. 2021;50(4):801–6.
10. Chung CB, Murphey M, Cho G, Schweitzer M, Hodler J, Haghihi P, et al. Osseous lesions of the pelvis and long tubular bones containing both fat and fluid-like signal intensity: an analysis of 28 patients. Eur J Radiol. 2005;53(1):103–9.
11. Milgram JW. Intraosseous lipomas: radiologic and pathologic manifestations. Radiology. 1988;167(1):155–60.
12. Milgram JW. Intraosseous lipomas. A clinicopathologic study of 66 cases. Clin Orthop Relat Res. 1988;(231):277–302.
13. Picci P, Sieberova G, Alberghini M, Balladelli A, Vanel D, Hogendoorn PC, et al. Late sarcoma development after curettage and bone grafting of benign bone tumors. Euro J Radiol. 2011;77(1):19–25.
14. Johnson LC, Vetter H, Putschar WG. Sarcomas arising in bone cysts. Virchows Arch Pathol Anat Physiol Klin Med. 1962;335(4):428–51.
15. Grabias S, Mankin HJ. Chondrosarcoma arising in histologically proved unicameral bone cyst: a case report. J Bone Joint Surg Am. 1974;56(7):1501–9.
16. Li Y-J, Zhang Y, Yin X-X, Zhang W-L, Tu C-Q. Osteosarcoma at the site of a previously treated simple bone cyst. Transl Cancer Res. 2016;5(6):877–88. https://doi.org/10.21037/tcr.2016.11.02.

13 Ganglion Cyst

(***ganglion*** "knot" + ***kystis*** "sac")

13.1 Definition

Intraosseous ganglion cyst (IGC) is a rare non-neoplastic pseudocyst histologically identical to its soft tissue counterpart, which contains mucinous fluid but no epithelial or synovial lining. Subchondral cyst associated with adjacent degenerative arthritis is not included in this category. That, particularly near hip joint surface, can be further been confused with the peri-articular cysts by the degenerative joint disease, in which articular disruption with joint communication frequently exist

13.2 A Possible Mechanism

A theory of mechanical stress and repeated minor trauma near the surface of the bone producing intramedullary vascular disturbance with consequent foci of aseptic bone necrosis was suggested [1]. To some extent, IGC is similar to the so-called subchondral cyst in degenerative joint, and the mechanism producing both conditions may be similar, in fact [2].

13.3 Incidence

The true incidence is unknown because most lesions are asymptomatic and discovered incidentally. There is no doubt that the incidence of IGC should be much more frequent than reported in earlier publications [1]. It is, however, very rare accounting for only 0.1% of biopsy-proven primary bone tumor of bone [3].

13.4 Age

It is typically identified in the skeletally mature individuals over 20 years old with a peak incidence between the fourth and fifth decades of life on the data from the major reports [4–6]. In the largest series, about 80% of 88 patients were reported to occur in adults between 20 and 29 years of age [1].

13.5 Location

IGC usually develops in subchondral area of bones around the hip, knee, ankle, wrist, and shoulder [2, 3].

13.6 Clinical Presentation

Many patients are clinically symptom free. Chronic, insidious, or intermittent mild pain of long durations is often associated. The pain can be aggravated by use of the affected region or physical activity

W.-J. Bahk, *Diagnosis and Management of Primary Bone Tumors*,
https://doi.org/10.1007/978-981-99-5498-8_13

13.7 Radiologic Findings

The lesion is typically an eccentric, sharply defined, purely radiolucent with a rim of sclerosis constantly in the epiphysis of the long bone, carpal or tarsal bones, or flat bones adjacent to the joint particularly hip, know, shoulder, or ankle (Figs. 13.1, 13.2 and 13.3). Occasionally, it can be multi-lobulated or partially septate due to bone ridges. Many cases reveal complete or incomplete cortical shell. The cyst is usually apart from the joint surface, and the adjacent joint space and articular surface appear to be normal with no evidence of degenerative changes. **CT scan** clearly presents a well-defined osteolytic lesion in a subchondral region with a sclerotic rim. By tomography, Menges et al. reported that a connection with the adjacent joint in 57% (13/23) in his cases and stated that IGC should be included in the differential diagnosis of cystic epiphyseal bone lesions [6]. **MR images** reveal a well-circumscribed round to ovoid cystic lesion with low SI on T1-weighted image and high to bright SI on T2-weighted image. A surrounding rim of sclerosis usually presents as low signal on both sequences. The cyst is separated from the joint surface by a layer of bone with or without a connection to the joint space (Figs. 13.1 and 13.2). The lesion shows no central enhancement but a thin peripheral enhancement by a contrast media. **Bone scan** demonstrates a peripherally increased uptake with a central photon defect area as in other cyst lesions (Fig. 13.1g). **Histologic findings** are identical to ganglion of soft tissue (Figs. 13.1, 13.2 and 13.3). The lesion is com-

Fig. 13.1 (**a**) Radiograph taken for left ankle pain of 2-month duration in 26-year-old young lady shows a well-defined, eccentrically located, small, round to ovoid radiolucent lesion surrounded by a thin rim of sclerosis (arrow) in the talus with normal joint space. (**b**) MR images reveals a small, round to oval, subcortical cystic lesion in the posterolateral aspect of the talus with low SI on T1-weighted image and high SI on T2-weighted image. The lesion is surrounded by a dark signal of surrounding reactive sclerosis (white arrows). On both sequences. The tibiotalar and subtalar joint is normal looking. The bony lesion is peripherally enhanced and associated a focal breach of the posterior cortex with adjacent bone marrow (yellow arrow) and soft tissue edema (red arrow) which are diffusely enhanced. (**c**) Curettage without bone graft was performed through the small window at posterolateral aspect of talus. A true connection between the lesion and joint space was not found in operative field, but adhesion with surrounding soft tissue was observed. Note a curetted material of a thin, fibrous capsule containing a clear gelatinous fluid (inset). (**d**) Microscopic examination notes multi-lobulated cystic walls of variable thickness composed of flattened fibrous elements without lining cells. The cyst contains abundant pools of mucinous fluid indicating IGC. (**e**) Follow-up radiograph at 1 year after surgery shows a hazy small lucent hole but the is free of pain. (**f**) Radiograph taken for discomfort of right shoulder after traffic accident in 58-year-old woman incidentally shows a well-defined radiolucent lesion with a thin complete rim of sclerosis affecting the scapular neck and glenoid (arrow). (**g**) Bone scan reveals a moderately increased peripheral uptake with an internal photon defect area (asterisk). (**h**) MR images demonstrate a well-defined cystic lesion with low SI on T1-weighted image and bright SI on fat saturated T2-weighted image with a thin dark signal of surround sclerosis on both sequences. The cyst is separated from the joint surface by a thin layer of bone without a connection to the joint space (white arrows). The lesion is only peripherally enhanced (yellow arrow) with no internal enhancement. (**i**) A needle aspiration under C-arm image intensifier was performed. A sticky, clear, blood-tinged, mucoid to gelatinous fluid being identical to that of soft tissue ganglion rather than yellow serious fluid of UBC or blood of ABC was aspirated (inset). Curettage was not performed because the lesion is incidentally found without pain before the traffic accident. (**j**) Follow-up radiograph taken at 3 years after aspiration notes the lesion seems to become smaller with a hazy inferior portion (arrow)

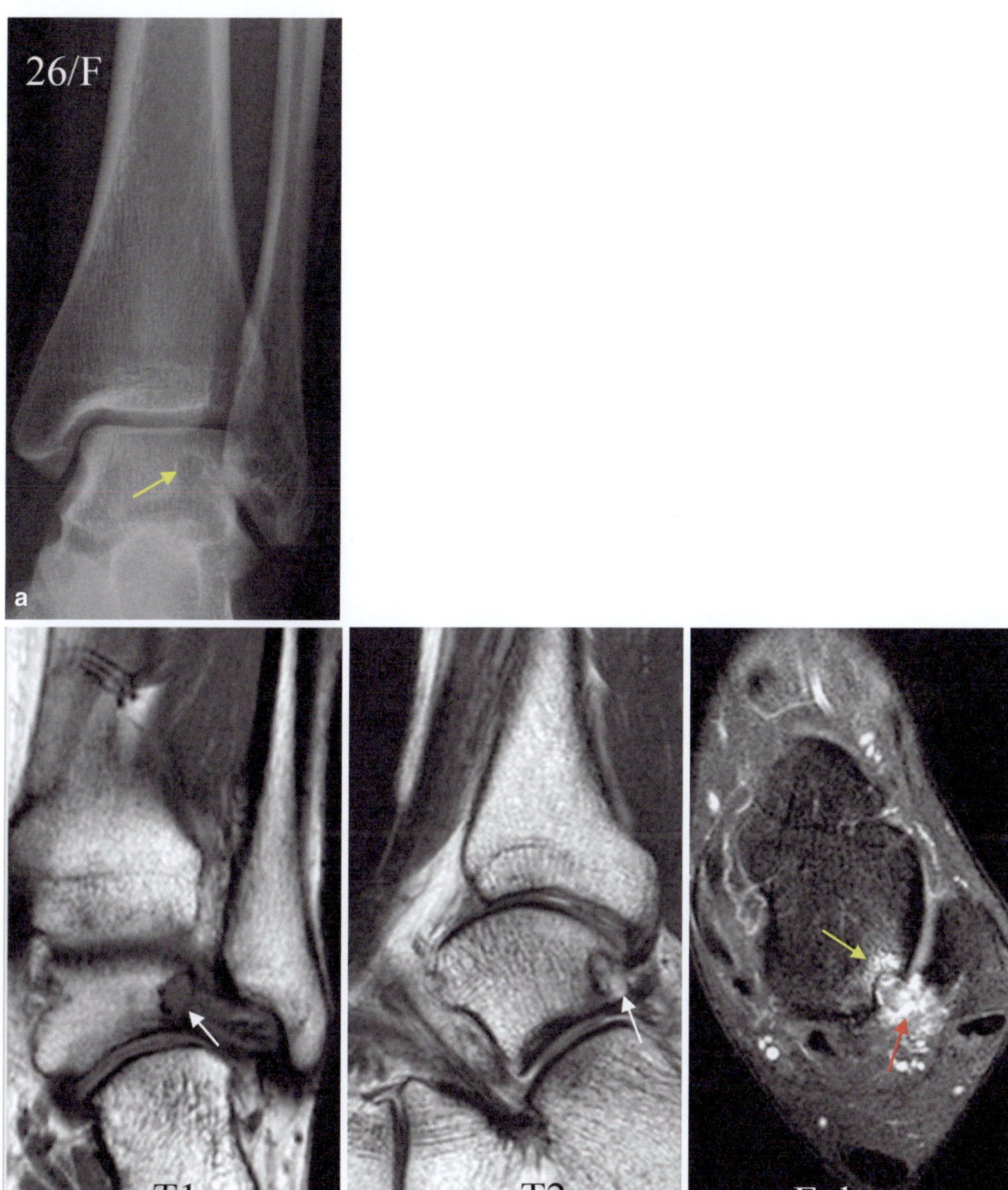
26/F
a
b
T1
T2
Enhance

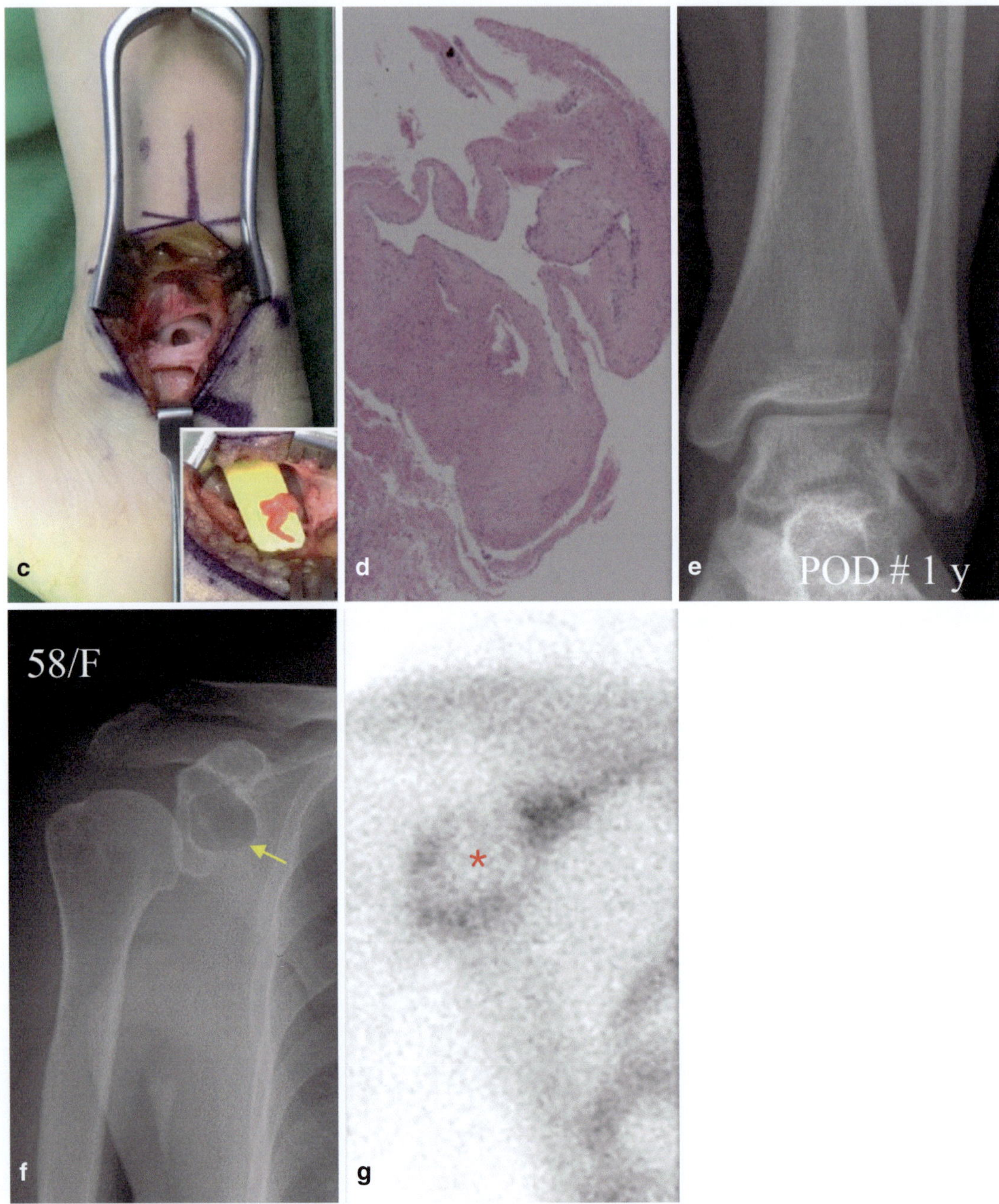

Fig. 13.1 (continued)

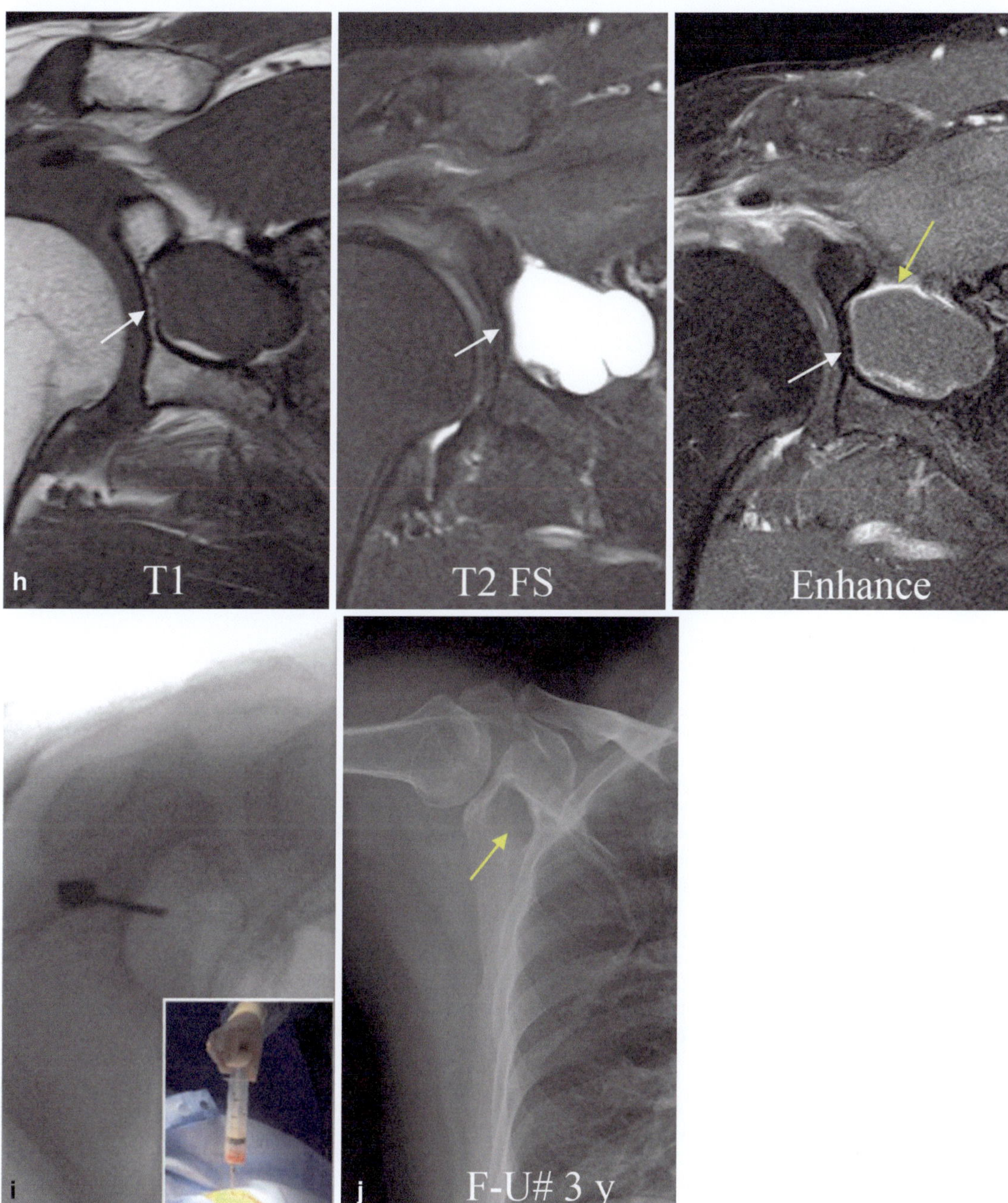

Fig. 13.1 (continued)

posed of multi-lobulated, thick fibrous cystic walls with mucinous pools. The cystic wall is composed of hypocellular loose fibrous connective tissue with no lining cells, which would be indicative of a true cyst. Focal myxoid change can be seen with scattered inflammatory cells and foamy macrophages. Varying size of pools of amorphous gelatinous or mucinous matrix can be seen with occasional inflammatory and red blood cells in some areas.

Fig. 13.2 (**a**) Radiograph taken for right knee pain of 10-month duration in 92-year-old man shows two separated eccentric well-defined multi-lobulated radiolucent lesions surrounded by a thin rim of sclerosis in the medial and lateral condyles of distal femur (asterisks) as well as significant narrowing of both joint spaces (arrows) indicating degenerative arthritis. (**b**) MR images reveal two separated well-defined cystic lesions at medial and lateral collateral ligament attachment sites (asterisks) with low SI on T1-weighted image and intermediate and high SI on T2-weighted image surrounded by a thin dark signal of sclerosis on both sequences. Despite the marked arthritic changes of the adjacent knee joint, the cysts are certainly separated from the joint surface by a thick layer of cancellous bone and do not connect to the joint space (double-headed arrows). The cyst is believed to be incidentally found IGCs rather than degenerative subchondral cysts. (**c**) Total knee replacement was performed with curettage of the cyst followed by cementing of the defect (asterisk). The cyst is surrounded by a thin fibrous membrane containing mucinous or gelatinous fluid. (**d**) Microscopic examination notes multi-lobulated, thick fibrous cystic walls with mucinous pools representing IGCs. (**e**) Follow-up radiograph at 1 year after surgery shows good maintenance with no evidence of recurrence of the IGC (asterisk). (**f**) Radiograph taken for right hip pain of 1-month duration in 42-year-old lady shows a hazy multi-lobulated radiolucent lesion surrounded by a thin rim of sclerosis (yellow arrow) with mild irregularity and sclerosis of the hip joint. (**g**) CT scan reveals the cyst is separated from the joint surface by a layer of bone without a connection to the joint space (red arrow), suggesting IGC rather than degenerative subchondral cyst. (**h**) Radiograph for left ankle pain in 45-year-old man notes in a well-defined eccentric radiolucent lesion in medial malleolus of tibia (circle). (**i**) Microscopic examination demonstrates multi-lobulated thin fibrous cystic walls with a markedly thickened wall by abundant mucinous pools (asterisks), indicating IGC

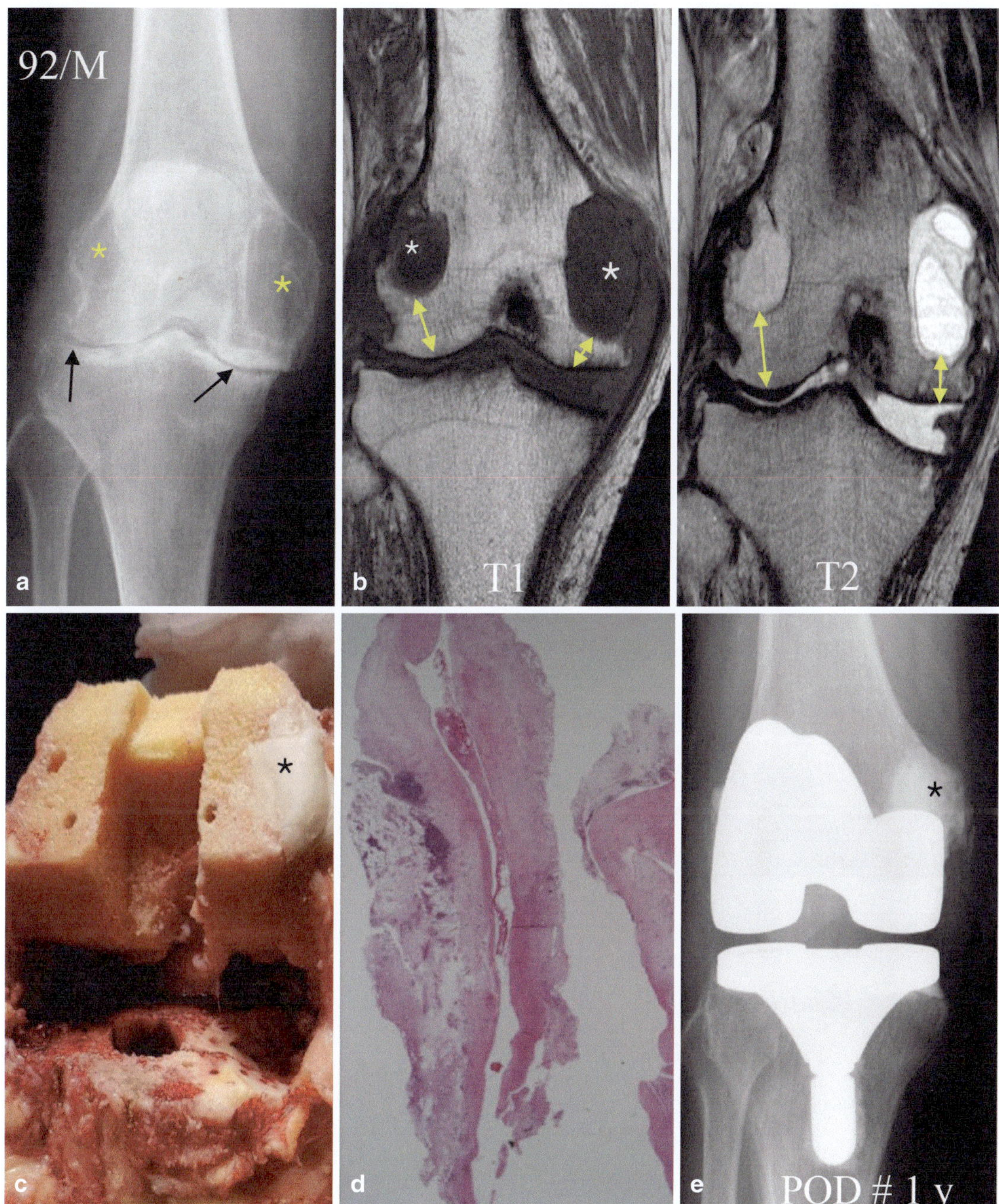
92/M
a
b
T1
T2
c
d
e
POD # 1 y

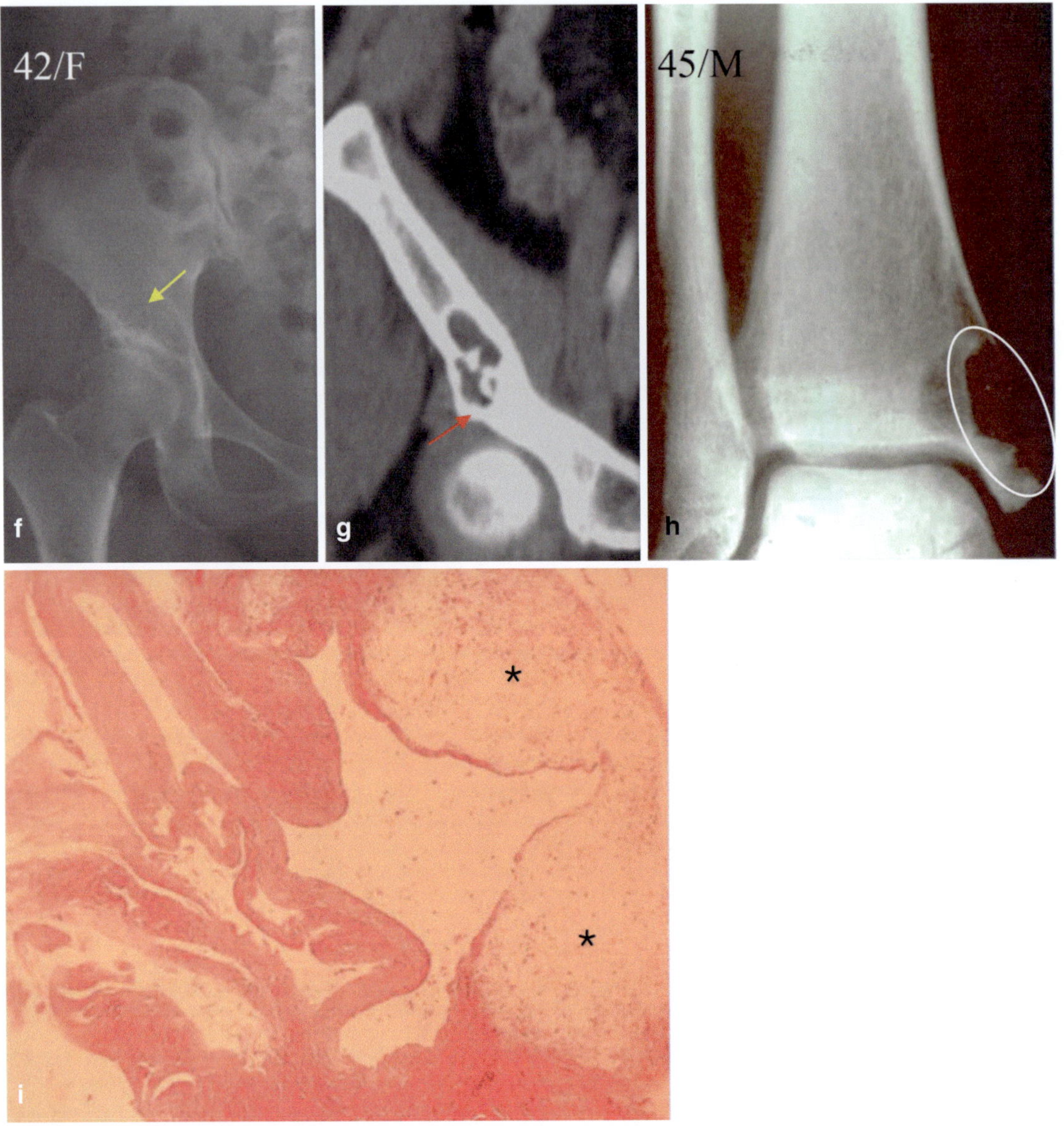

Fig. 13.2 (continued)

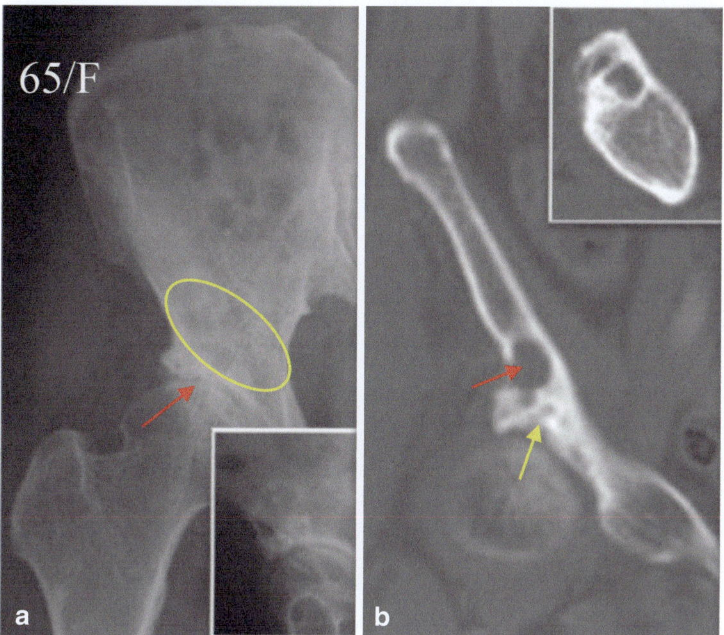

Fig. 13.3 ***Degerative subchondroal cyst*** (**a**) Radiograph taken for right inguinal pain of 3-month duration in 65-year-old woman shows a faint multi-lobulated radiolucent lesion in the acetabulum (circle) with and subchondral sclerosis, irregular joint surface, and narrowing of hip joint space (arrow) indicating degenerative arthritis. (**b**) CT scan reveals a larger cystic lesion (red arrow) with irregular articular surface, narrowing of joint space, and subchondral sclerosis as well as multiple tiny cysts connecting to the hip joint (yellow arrow). (**c**) MR images demonstrate a well-defined cystic lesion with low SI on T1-weighted image and high SI on T2-weighted image. (**d**) Follow-up radiograph at 1 year after curettage and allo-chip bone grafting for the cystic lesion notes consolidation of the lesion (circle), but the degenerative arthritis becomes severe and severely aggravates the hip pain. Total hips replacement was performed. (**e**) Follow-up radiograph at 3 years after surgery shows good maintenance of the prosthesis and consolidation of the acetabular subchondral cystic lesion (circle). ***Peri-prosthetic pseudocyst*** (**f**) Radiograph taken for right hip pain of 4-month duration in 52-year-old man shows a rarefaction with sclerosis in the femoral head and narrowing of joint space suggesting avascular necrosis of the femoral head with secondary osteoarthritis. (**g**) Follow-up radiograph at 5 years after total hip replacement using metal-on-metal bearing type reveals good maintenance but with a suspicious radiolucent area (asterisk). But the patient was free of pain at that time. (**h**) Follow-up radiograph at 9 years after surgery notes a more clearly visible radiolucent lesion (asterisk) surrounded by a thin rim of sclerosis (yellow arrow). He presented moderate degree of pain in right inguinal area and buttock. (**i**) CT scan demonstrates a clearly visible multi-lobulated cystic lesion surrounded by a thin rim of sclerosis (yellow arrows). The cystic lesion is complicated probably due to metal ion release from a femoral-acetabular articulation (red arrow). (**j**) Microscopic examination shows a cystic wall structure of variable thickness without lining cells suggesting pseudocyst. There are prominent hemosiderin-laden foamy macrophages, a few scattered multinucleated macrophages and aggregation of lymphocytes in the wall (inset). (**k**) Radiograph at 6 months after curettage and allo-chip bone graft notes some consolidation of the lesion (asterisk)

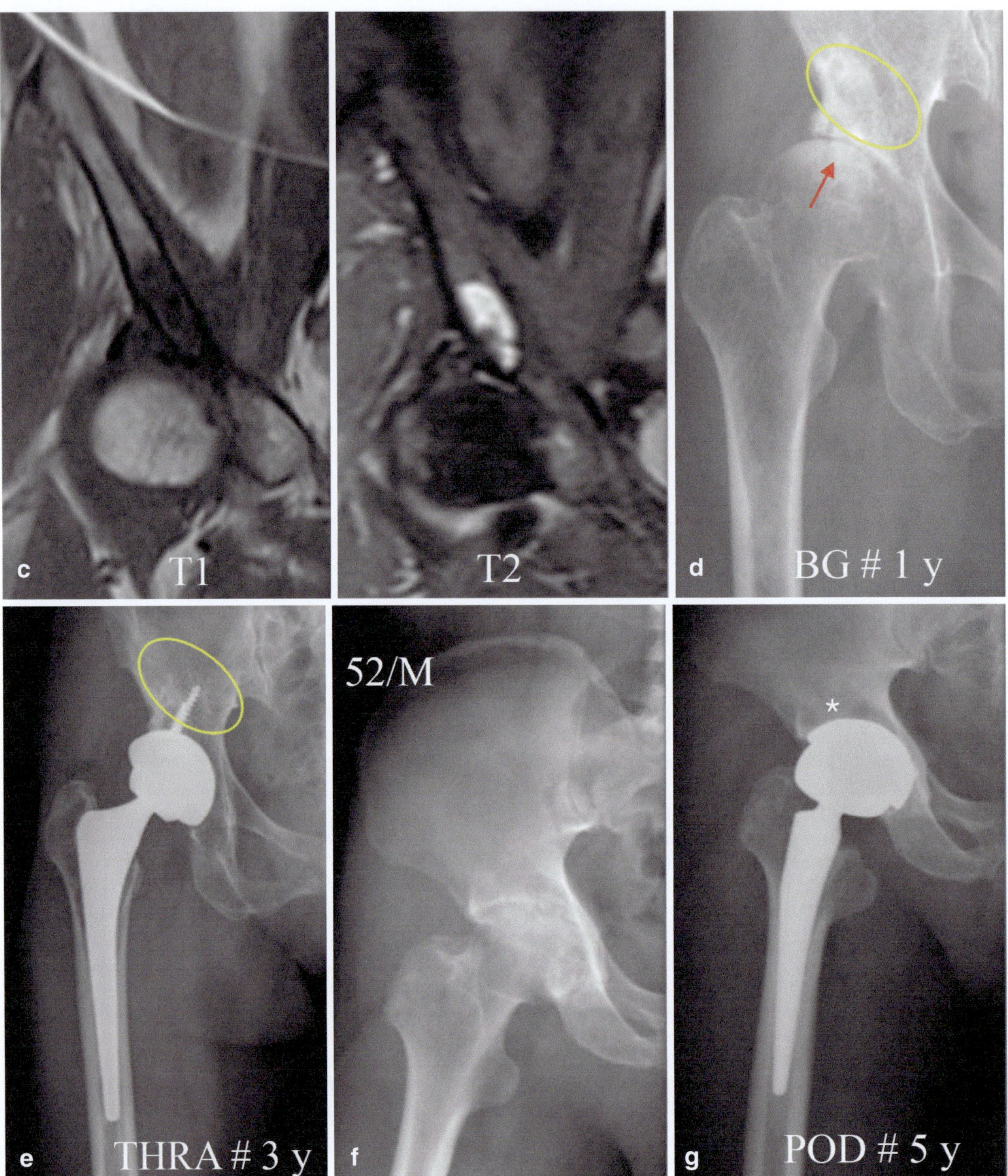

Fig. 13.1 (continued)

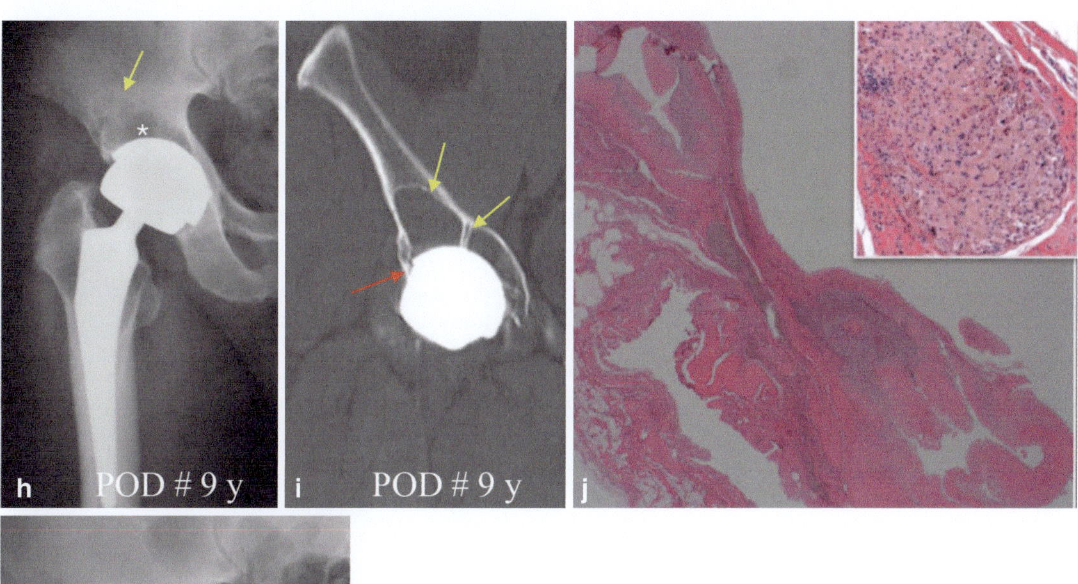

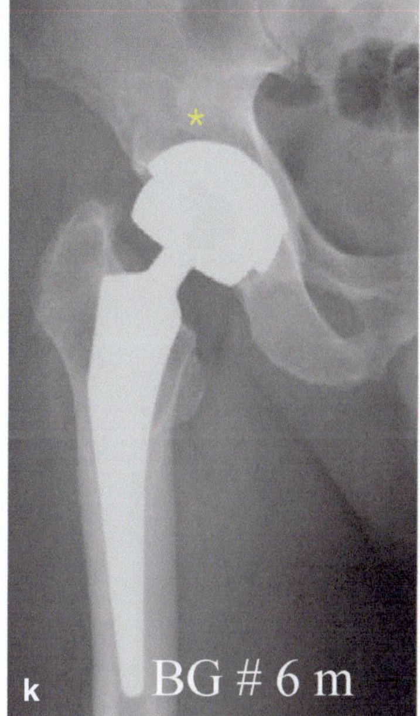

Fig. 13.1 (continued)

13.8 Management

Asymptomatic smaller lesions do not require any treatment. Simple curettage with or without bone graft depending on a size of the lesion is choice of the treatment for painful larger lesions.

13.9 Prognosis

Recurrence is barely expected even after simple curettage.

References

1. Schajowicz F, Clavel Sainz M, Slullitel JA. Juxta-articular bone cysts (intra-osseous ganglia): a clinicopathological study of eighty-eight cases. J Bone Joint Surg Br. 1979;61(1):107–16.
2. Czerniak B. Cystic lesions. In: Dorfman HD, Czerniak B, editors. Dorfman and Czerniak's bone tumors. 2nd ed. Amsterdam: Elsevier; 2016. p. 1055–99.
3. Mirra JM. Intraosseous ganglion cyst. In: Mirra JM, editor. Bone tumors: clinical, radiologic, and pathologic correlation. 2nd ed. Philadelphia, PA: Lea & Febiger; 1989. p. 1320–5.
4. Kambolis C, Bullough PG, Jaffe HL. Ganglionic cystic defects of bone. J Bone Joint Surg Am. 1973;55(3):496–505.
5. Feldman F, Johnston A. Intraosseous ganglion. Am J Roentgenol. 1973;118(2):328–43.
6. Menges V, Prager P, Cserhati MD, Becker W, Griss P, Wuster K. Das Intraossäre Ganglion. Zeitschift für Orthopädie und ihre Grenzgebiete. 1977;115:67–75.

14 Epidermal Inclusion Cyst

(***intraosseous*** "within bone" + ***epi*** "on" + ***derma*** "skin" + ***inclusio*** "enclosing" + ***kystis*** "sac")

14.1 Definition

Intraosseous epidermal inclusion cyst (IEIC) is a displacement of squamous epithelial cells into the bone and proliferation to form mass with keratin, which is histologically identical to that within a confined space in the dermis or subdermis

14.2 Synonyms

Epidermal or epidermoid cyst/keratin cyst/infundibular cyst.

14.3 Incidence

EIC is a relatively common benign tumors of the skin, but IECI primarily involving bone is exceedingly rare.

14.4 Age

The reported patients are usually young and middle-aged adults between third and sixth decades of age [1–6], although children [1, 7] and elderly patients over eighth decade [8, 9] have been reported.

14.5 Location

IECI almost always occurs in either the distal phalangeal tuft or the skull. It overwhelmingly affects the distal tuft of the terminal phalanx of finger, occupying over 95% of cases, and the rest involve toes or amputee of the residual end of fingers [10].

14.6 Clinical Presentation

Symptoms include a mildly enlarged finger or slowly growing mass with a rubbery to firm texture, pain, and tenderness. If they rupture, a local inflammatory response to the necrotic debris released can mimic infection. Pathologic fracture can be associated. Many cases are related to penetrating injury to the distal finger which has the tight subcutaneous compartment and the proximity to the distal phalanx.

14.7 Radiologic Findings

The lesion typically shows a sharply defined, mildly expanding, "punched-out" lytic defect with a sclerotic margin. The cortex can be markedly thinned often with cortical breakage or fracture line (Fig. 14.1a). **Pinhole bone scan**

W.-J. Bahk, *Diagnosis and Management of Primary Bone Tumors*,
https://doi.org/10.1007/978-981-99-5498-8_14

demonstrates a peripheral hot uptake with a central photon defect area, so-called "doughnut sign", as other cystic disease (Fig. 14.1b). **MR images** reveal a well-circumscribed round to ovoid cystic lesion with low to intermediate SI on T1-weighted image and intensely high or bright SI on T2-weighted image. The lesion usually shows a thin peripheral enhancement without internal enhancement by contrast media. When ruptured, the cyst may have septa with thick and irregular rim enhancement and can be accompanied by a focal internal enhancement as well as fuzzy surrounding adjacent bone marrow and subcutaneous tissues enhancement (Fig. 14.1c). **Histologic findings** are identical to EIC of skin, which characteristically shows cystic walls composed of keratinizing stratified squamous epithelium with abundant keratin debris. Rupture of the cyst can leak the keratin material into the adjacent soft tissue, which stimulates an inflammatory response to recruit the inflammatory cells and to produce multinucleated giant cells (Fig. 14.1d).

Fig. 14.1 (**a**) Radiograph taken for right ring finger tip pain of 1-month duration developed by lifting a heavy object in 55-year-old man shows a well-defined round to ovoid expansile lytic lesion within the terminal phalanx of the ring finger. There is an outer complete thin shell of bone with a fine cortical breakage (arrows). (**b**) Pinhole bone scan reveals a hot uptake along the periphery of the lesion with a central photon defect, so-called "doughnut sign" (asterisk). (**c**) MR images demonstrate a well-defined round to oval cystic lesion with low SI on T1-weighted image and intermediate and high SI on T2-weighted image. There are areas with internal high signal (red arrows) on both sequences, which are well enhanced by contrast media (white arrow) suggesting inflammation and foreign body reaction by rupture of the lesion. Note focal rupture of the lesion (yellow arrows) with adjacent marrow and soft tissue edema, which is well enhanced (red arrows). The lesion itself is peripherally enhanced. (**d**) Microscopic examination. (Left) The cyst wall is composed of a capsule lined by cornified epithelial cells with distinct granular layer and contains lamellate keratin without calcification. (Right) There is another area consisting of inflammatory cells and foreign body type multinucleated giant cells, suggesting foreign body reaction by ruptured lesion seen on MRI. (**e**) Follow-up radiograph at 1 year after curettage and allo-chip bone graft shows consolidation without local recurrence (arrows)

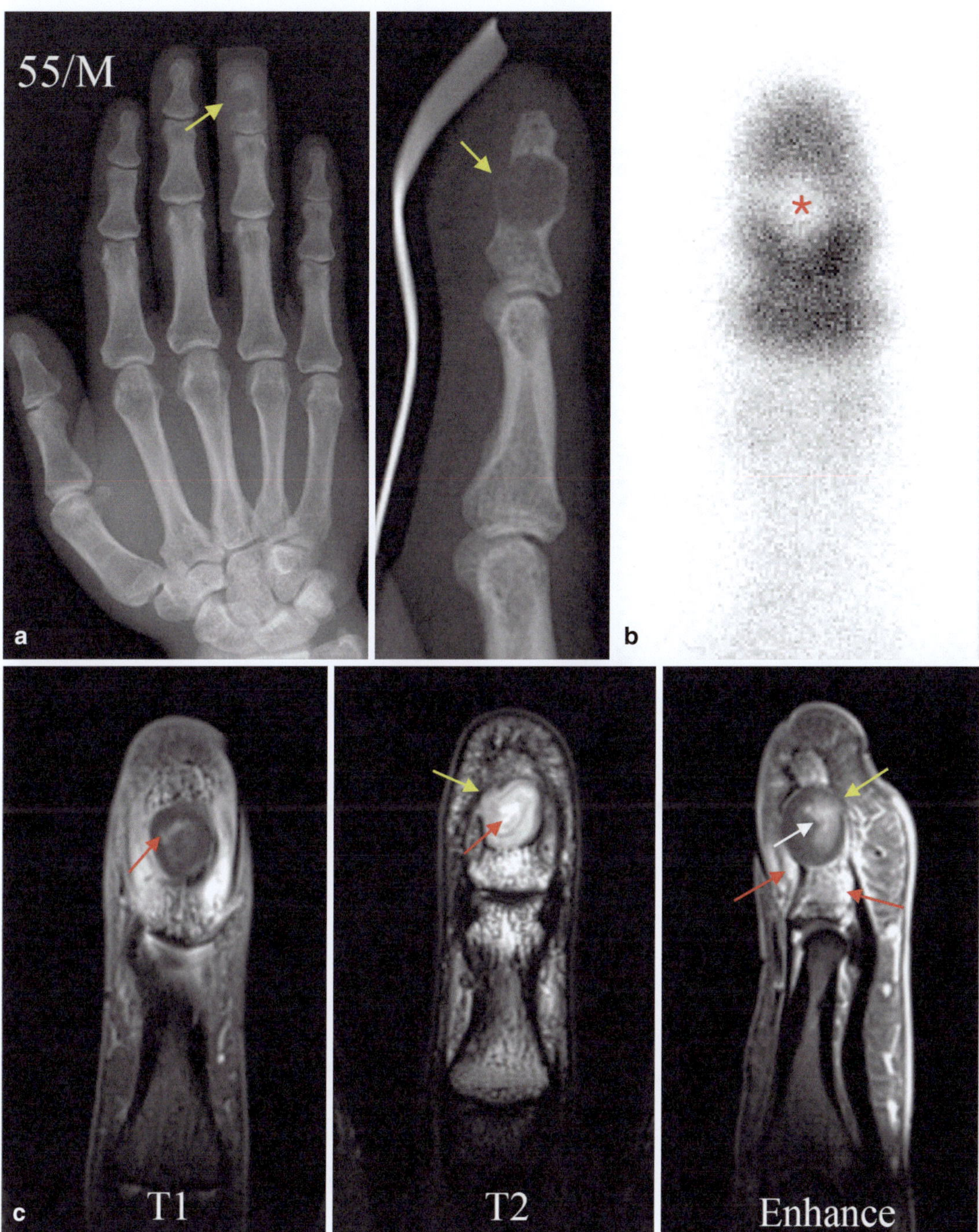
55/M
a
b
c
T1
T2
Enhance

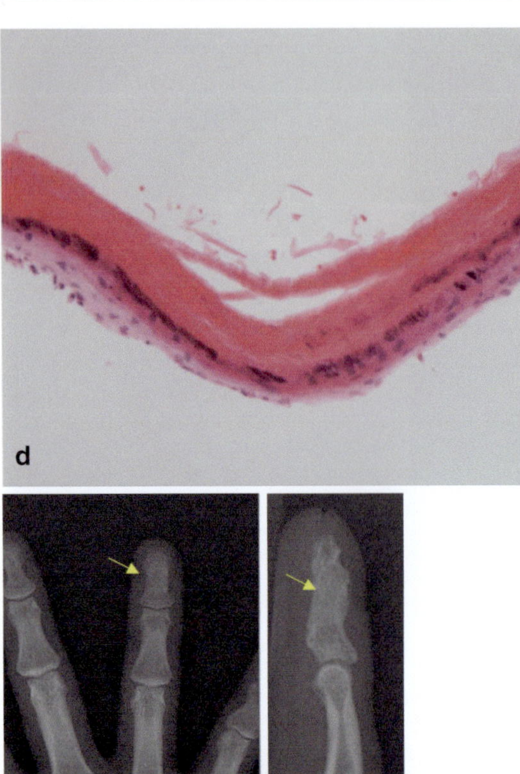

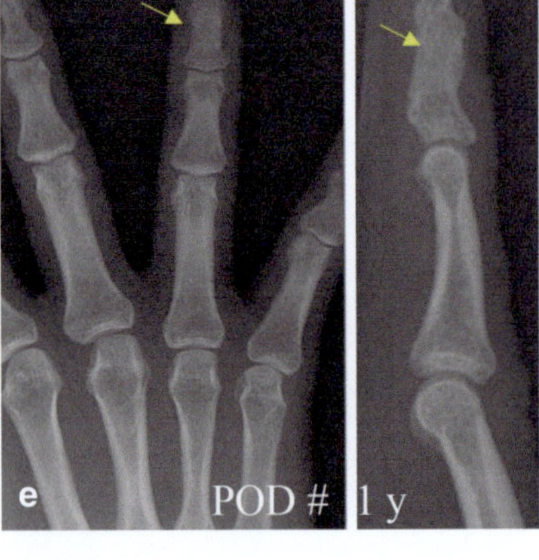

Fig. 14.1 (continued)

14.8 Management

Simple intralesional curettage with or without bone graft is choice of the treatment.

14.9 Prognosis

No recurrence is to be expected if the lesion is completely removed (Fig. 14.1e).

References

1. Kong GM, Kim JY, Kim JH, Park DH, An KH. Intraosseous epidermal cyst of the distal phalanx: a case report. J Korean Bone Joint Tumor Soc. 2014;20(1):22–6.
2. Hinrichs RA. Epidermoid cyst of the terminal phalanx of the hand: case report and brief review. J Am Med Assoc. 1965;194(11):1253–4.
3. Ruchelsman DE, Laino DK, Chhor KS, Steiner GC, Kenan S. Digital intraosseous epidermoid inclusion cyst of the distal phalanx. J Hand Microsurg. 2010;2(1):24–7.

4. Wang BY, Eisler J, Springfield D, Klein MJ. Intraosseous epidermoid inclusion cyst in a great toe: a case report and review of the literature. Arch Pathol Lab Med. 2003;127(7):e298–300.
5. Patel K, Bhuiya T, Chen S, Kenan S, Kahn L. Epidermal inclusion cyst of phalanx: a case report and review of the literature. Skelet Radiol. 2006;35(11):861–3.
6. Paparella T, Fallat L. A rare presentation of a giant epidermoid inclusion cyst mimicking malignancy. J Foot Ankle Surg. 2018;57(2):421–6.
7. Hensley CD Jr. Epidermoid cyst of the distal phalanx occurring in an eight-year-old child. A case report. J Bone Joint Surg Am. 1966;48(5):946–8. PMID: 5942810.
8. Dumitru A, Costache M, Şerban B, Japie I-M, Anghelescu D, Condrea C, et al. Posttraumatic intraosseous epidermoid inclusion cyst. A case report and short literature review. Rom J Orthop Surg Traumatol. 2020;3(1):3–8.
9. Sugimoto H, Yasue K, Hara M, Takakuma S, Yumura W, Arai T, et al. Intraosseous epidermal cyst of the great toe that was difficult to distinguish from chronic osteomyelitis: a case report and literature review. Clin Case Rep. 2021;9(4):1890–5.
10. Mirra JM. Epidermoid and dermoid cysts. In: Mirra JM, editor. Bone tumors: clinical, radiologic, and pathologic correlation. 2nd ed. Philadelphia, PA: Lea & Febiger; 1989. p. 1263–7.

Part V

Vascular Tumors

Hemangioma

15

(***intraosseous*** "within bone" + ***haima*** "blood" + ***angeion*** "vessel" + ***ōma*** "forming")

15.1 Definition

Intraosseous hemangioma (IH) is a benign vascular tumor with proliferation of capillary or cavernous type of vessels affecting the bones. The lesion can involve two or more noncontiguous bones, so-called "hemangiomatosis." Hamangioma may affect bone, subcutanous tissue, soft tissue, or skin at the same time. *Gorham-stout disease*, vanishing or phantom bone disease, is a rare bone disorder characterized by resorption (osteolysis) and replacement of bone with angiomas and/or fibrosis due to an increased number of osteoclasts along with a proliferation of distended thin-walled vascular channels.

15.2 Incidence

IH has been reported to be rare, accounting for less than 1% of all primary bone tumor [1–3]. However, Schmorl and Jurgens [4] reported an incidence of about 11% in 3892 autopsied spines in their study. The incidence should be more with increased use of MR images for spine evaluation for various reasons because most lesions are asymptomatic.

15.3 Age

The lesion can be found in any age group, ranging from the first to eighth decades of life. But over 70% of the patients diagnosed in adulthood between 30 and 60 years of age [2, 5].

15.4 Location

IH most frequently affects the craniofacial bones, mostly the calvarium (approximately half of the cases), followed by body of thoracic and lumbar spine (some 30%) [2, 5]. Metaphysis or diaphysis of the major long bones can be also affected.

15.5 Clinical Presentation

Most lesions are asymptomatic and found incidentally on imaging studies for other spinal problem. Rarely, the lesion may produce pain or neurological symptoms if a large lesion compresses neve root or spinal cord. There can be compression fracture of spines. Swelling or palpable mass can be associated in the skull, and jaw lesion may lead in loosening of the teeth.

W.-J. Bahk, *Diagnosis and Management of Primary Bone Tumors*,
https://doi.org/10.1007/978-981-99-5498-8_15

Hemangiomatosis of the bone is subdivided into two categories including multiple primary hemangiomas of bone and diffuse cystic angiomatosis or diffuse skeletal hemangiomatosis. The majority of latter also have hemangiomas of the viscera [6], where clinical features may vary depending on the involving organs. A large lesion particularly affecting weight-bearing bone or lesion with numerus holes weakening the cortex often produces pain or even pathologic fracture of long bone.

15.6 Radiologic Findings

The lesion in vertebra usually presents only nonspecific rarefaction or osteopenia but often presents vertically oriented multiple striations of bone trabeculae particularly on lateral view (Fig. 15.1a). The finding is best observed on CT scan or MR images (Figs. 15.1 and 15.2). When flat bone is affected, the bone can be significantly expanded, and the overlying cortex can be thinned. However, the cortex is not usually

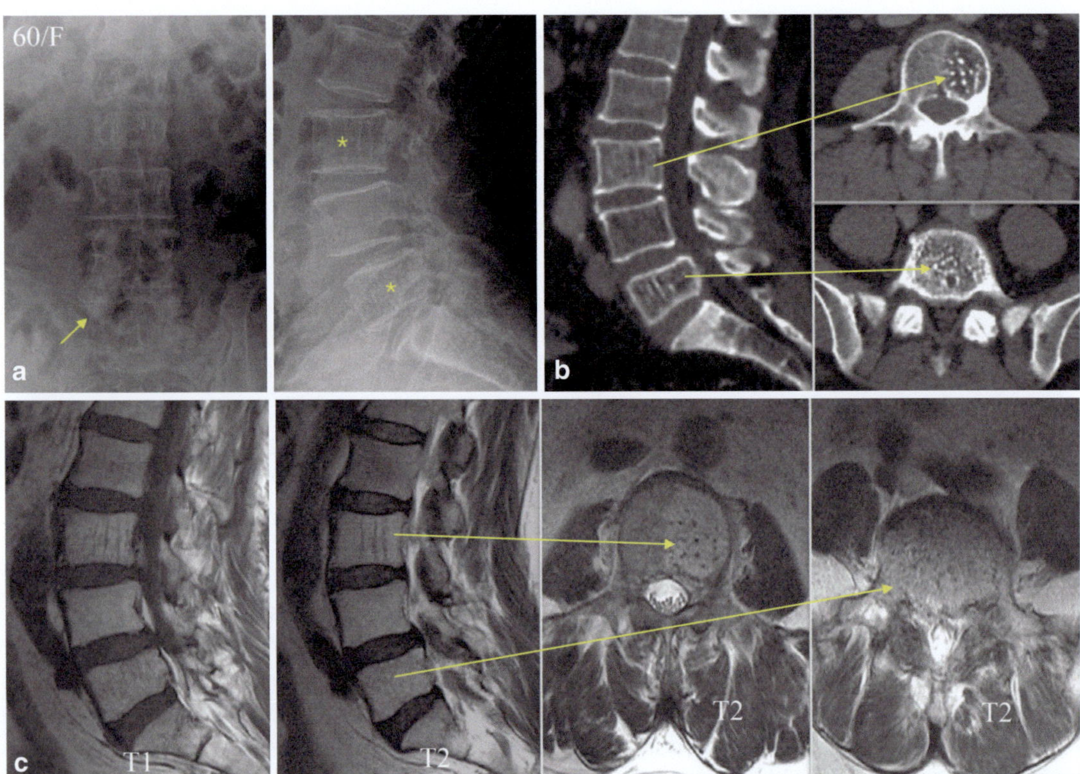

Fig. 15.1 (**a**) Radiograph taken for low back pain after traffic accident in 60-year-old woman shows no unequivocal abnormal findings except nonspecific degrative dense area in the L5 lumbar vertebrae on anteroposterior view. However, lateral view incidentally reveals vertically oriented multiple striations of bone trabeculae with radiolucent background in L3 and L5 vertebral bodies (asterisks). (**b**) CT scan more clearly demonstrates dense vertical striations in the low signal background, so-called *"corduroy"* or *"jail bar"* sign, on sagittal view. There are round multiple foci of high signal indicating thickened vertical trabeculae in the low signal background suggesting of rich fat component, so-called *"polka-dot"* sign, on axial views. Both signs are pathognomonic for vertebral hemangioma. (**c**) MR images also notes multiple vertically running striations in L3 and L5 vertebral bodies with low SI on both T1- and T2-weighted images. T2-weighted axial images show multiple tiny black dots suggesting thickened trabeculae in the intermediate to high signal background. The back pain was controlled by painkiller

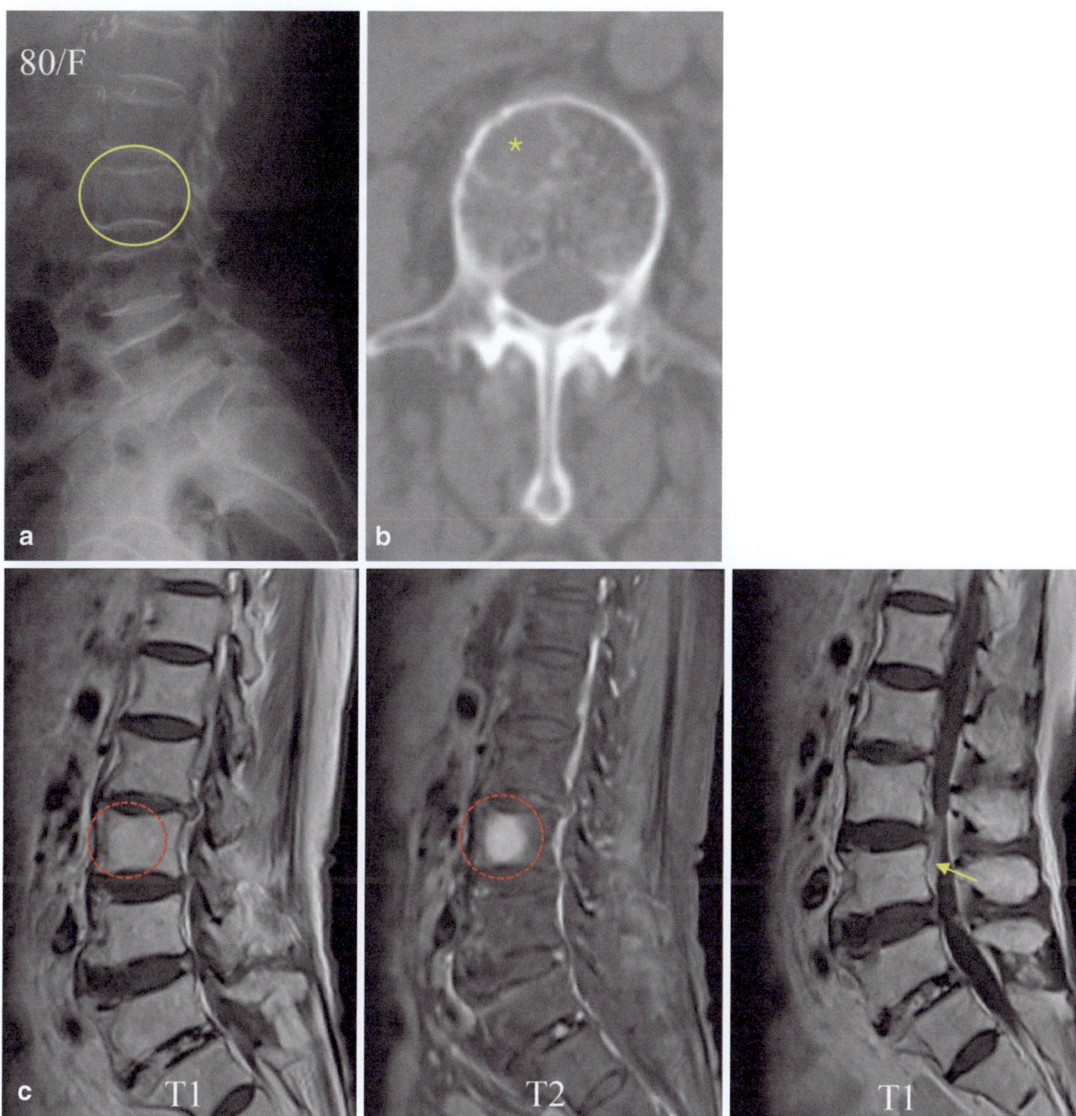

Fig. 15.2 (**a**) Radiograph taken for low back pain radiating to both legs in 80-year-old woman shows diffuse osteopenia and degenerative changes but no definite abnormal findings in the L3 vertebral body (circle). (**b**) However, CT scan reveals a well-defined oval osteolytic lesion (asterisk) surrounded by an irregular rim of sclerosis in the anterolateral aspect of L3 vertebral body. (**c**) MR images demonstrate a relatively well-defined round to oval medullary lesion (dotted circle) with intermediate SI on T1-weighted image and high SI on T2-weighted image in the L3 vertebral body. There is another lesion with intermediate to high signal of extruded disc material with significant thecal sac compression (yellow arrow) producing a severe central spinal stenosis, which is believed to be the main cause of her radiating symptom (yellow arrow). (**d**) Bone scan notes a focal moderately increased uptake at right side of L3 vertebral body indicating active bony lesion (red arrow) with milder uptake in the end plate of L4,5 vertebrae probably suggesting degenerative change (yellow arrow). (**e**) PET/CT scan shows focal FDG uptake (SUVmax 3.8) in the same location suggesting a possible malignant tumor. (**f**) Decompression laminectomy and posterolateral fusion with instrumentation in the L4,5 vertebrae for spinal stenosis were performed and transpedicular biopsy to obtain the specimen for histologic diagnosis of the L3 vertebra lesion. (**g**) Microscopic examination of the biopsy material. (Left) Lower-power magnification reveals numerous dilated thin-walled cavernous vascular spaces of varying size. The vessels permeate the bone marrow and entrap the pre-existing trabeculae (asterisk). The most lumens are filled with red blood cells, but some are containing amorphous proteinaceous material or empty. (Right) Higher-power magnification notes vascular spaces lined by a single layer of flat to mildly plum endothelial cells as well as prominently unmasked fat cells in the interstitial tissue (asterisks)

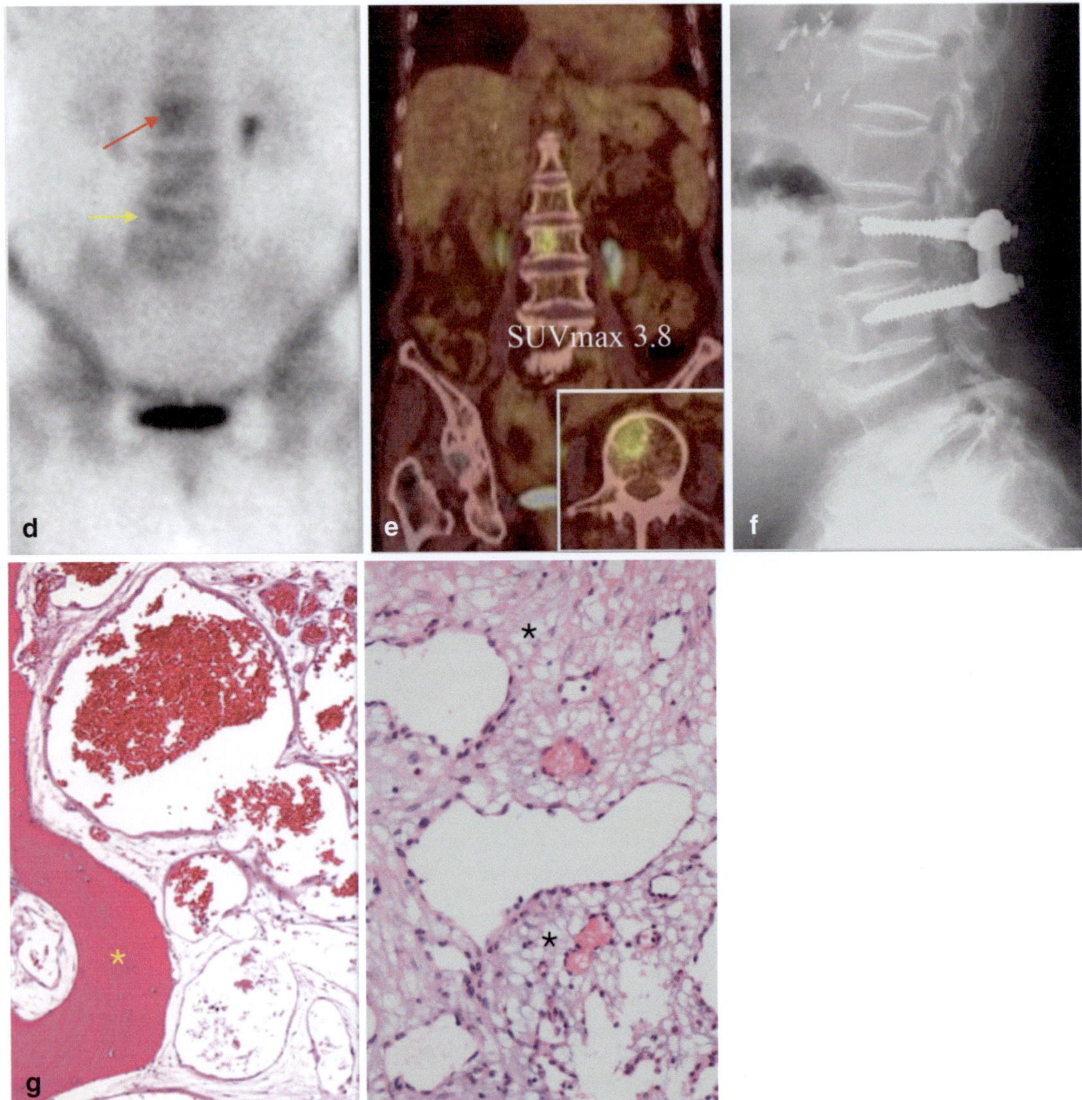

Fig. 15.1 (continued)

destructed and does not extend into soft tissue. Numerous fine spikes of periosteal new bone, which radiate perpendicularly to the skull plate, so-called *"sunburst appearance,"* can be observed. A bubbly or honeycomb appearance of trabeculated bone suggesting vascular nature of the lesion is often seen. Radiographic appearance of IHs affecting long bones is non-specific with ill-defined multiple radiolucent holes of varying size which may simulate moth-eaten to permeative destruction (Fig. 15.3a), and is often misdiagnosed radiologically as malignant tumor. **Bone Scan** Uptake is varied from none to moderate uptake depending on the amount of fat component (Figs. 15.2d) and 15.3c). Typically, the lesion appears normal, but it may show moderately increased or even decreased uptake. **CT scan** reveals typically the multiple round sclerotic dots representing thickened vertical trabeculae within the low signal background of a rich fat component in vertebral bodies, so-called *"polka-dot"* sign, on axial image. It is a characteristic finding of the vertebral hemangioma, which is the axial equivalent of the *"corduroy"*

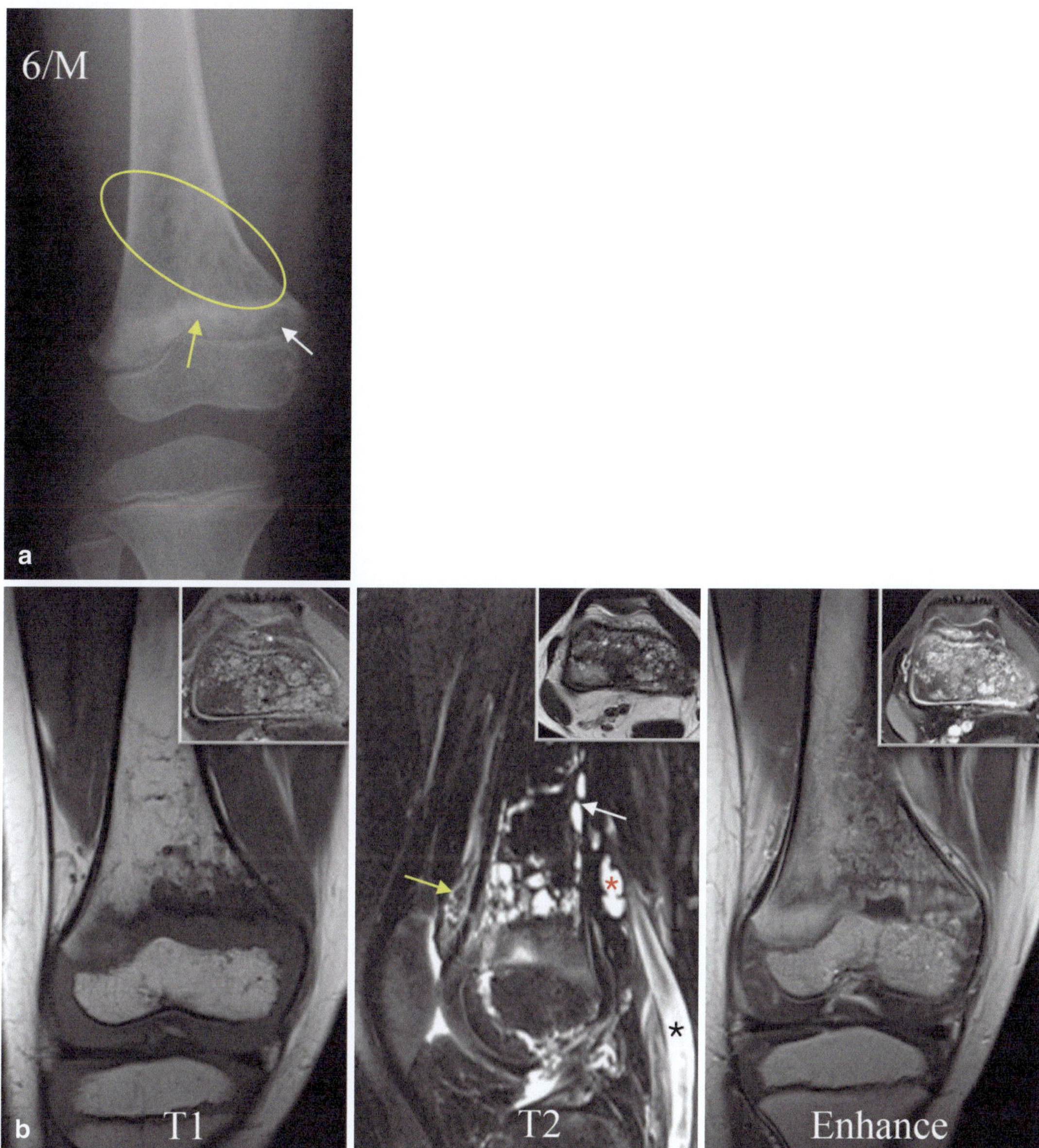

Fig. 15.3 (**a**) Radiograph taken for night pain of right knee of 1-year duration in 6-year-old boy shows ill-defined lesion with multiple radiolucent holes of varying size simulating a moth-eaten to permeative destruction (circle) in the metaphyseal area of the distal femur. Note irregular sclerosis and widening of the growth plate (yellow arrow) with radiolucent defect in the metaphyseal side (white arrow). (**b**) MR images reveal an ill-defined tubular and nodular infiltration with low and intermediate SI on T1-weighted image and low and high SI on T2-weighted image mainly in the metaphyseal area and focally in the epiphysis. The epiphyseal plate is markedly widened with separation. Note cortical erosion with intracortical involvement (white arrow) and focal extension to soft tissue posteriorly (red asterisk) as well as subperiosteal involvement through cortical breaches anteriorly (yellow arrow). There is neighboring vascular engorgement (black asterisk). The lesion is heterogeneously enhanced. (**c**) Bone scan notes no remarkable increased uptake (circle). (**d**) Radiograph at 3-year follow-up shows a progression of the lesion with increased number and size of holes in the meta-diaphysis (yellow circle) as well as more clear visible tiny holes in the epiphysis (white circle). (**e**) Follow-up MR images also reveal a progression of the lesion with markedly increased degree of infiltration into epiphyseal plate and epiphysis. (**f**) A scannogram at 4-year follow-up when he was 10 years old notes shortening of the right femur by 3 cm. Epiphysiodesis of contralateral left distal femur was performed. (**g**) Follow-up radiograph at 3 years after epiphysiodesis (yellow arrow) when he was 13 years old shows no further leg length discrepancy with marked regression of the lesion (circle). The patient is free of pain with mild limp, which is managed by right-sided shoe elevation

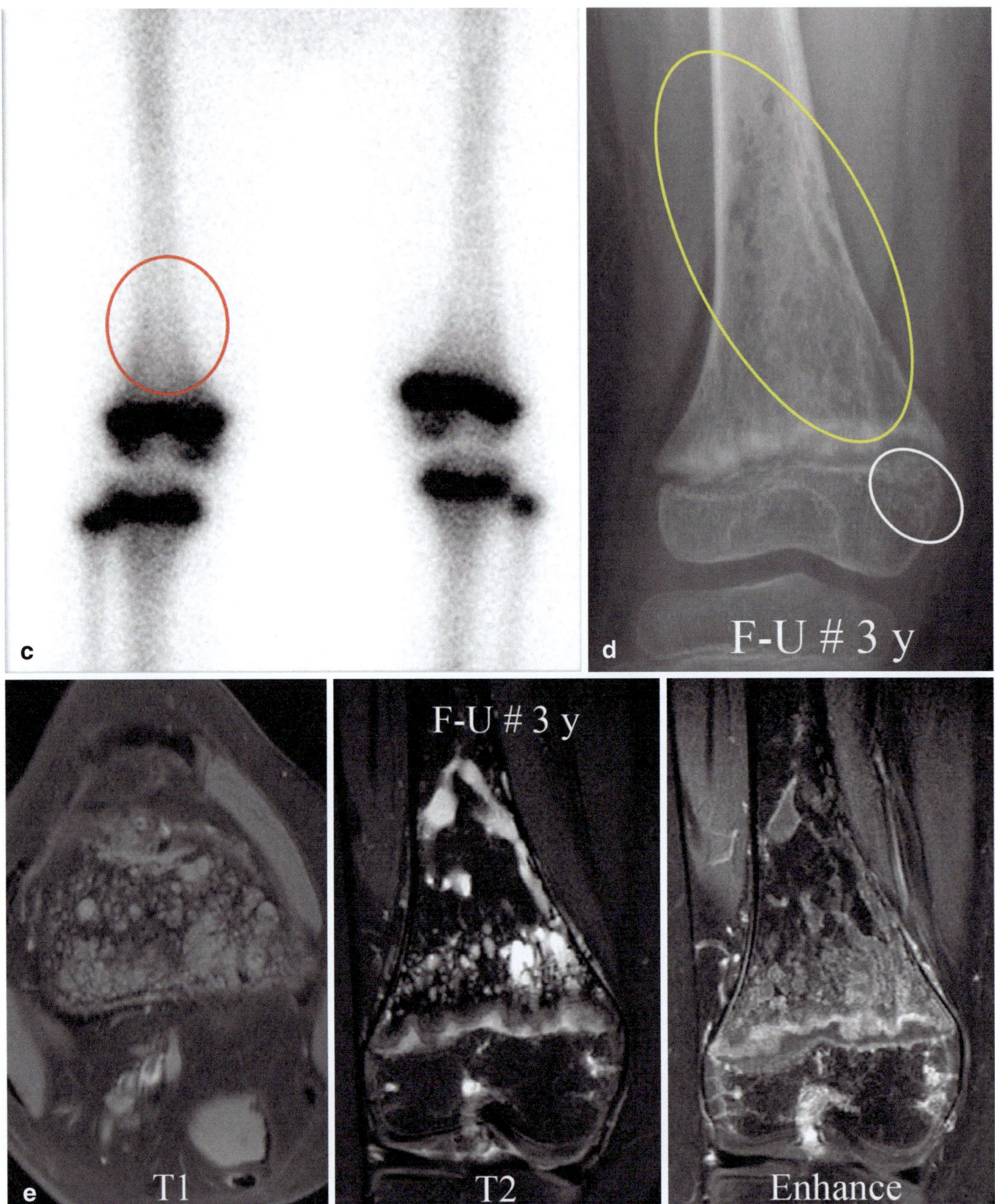

Fig. 15.3 (continued)

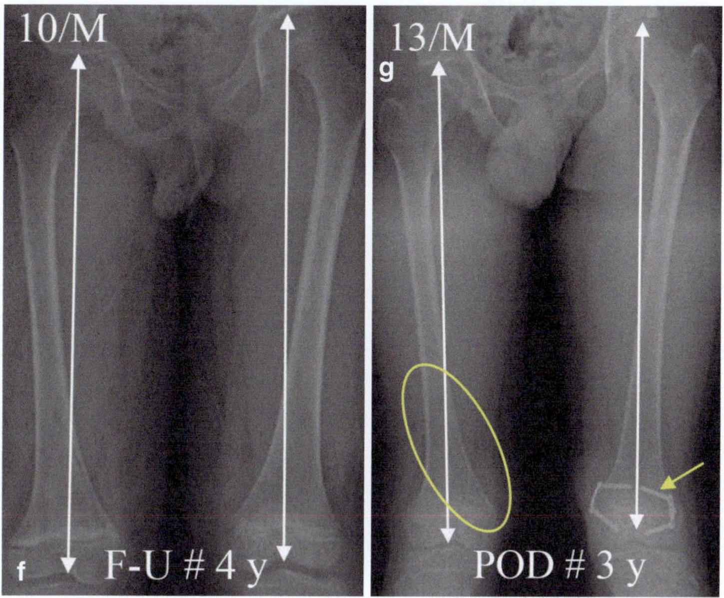

Fig. 15.3 (continued)

or *"jail bar"* sign of vertically striated appearance seen on sagittal and coronal images (Figs. 15.1b and 15.2b). **MR images** are the best modality to evaluate fatty component of the lesion and the mass-related complications such as extra-osseous extension and neural impingent as well as other spinal cause of symptoms. The signal intensity (SI) is variable depending largely on the amount fat and vascular component. The SI is low to intermediate in the fat-scanty lesion but high in the fat-rich lesion on T1-weighted image and intermediate to high on T2-weighted axial image with focal black dots of thickened trabeculae corresponding to *"polka-dot"* sign on CT scan. The high signal on T2-weighted images reflects a rich blood component of the tumor vasculature. The thickened trabeculae can be appeared as vertical striations, so-called *"corduroy"* or *"jail bar"* sign, with low SI in both T1- and T2-weighted coronal and sagittal images (Figs. 15.1c and 15.2c). If the lesion consists of abundant vasculature but scanty fatty component, the lesion is heterogeneously well enhanced by contrast media. In long bone, MR images demonstrate an ill-defined infiltrative lesion with heterogeneous low and intermediate SI on T1-weighted image and heterogeneous low and high SI on T2-weighted image, generally in the metaphysis or diaphysis (Fig. 15.3b).

15.7 Histologic Findings

Hemangioma of soft tissue usually consists of dilated thin-walled blood vessels of capillary or cavernous type. Hemangioma of bone is usually *cavernous type* containing dilated open channels and less frequently *capillary type* with tiny capillary-sized vessels. Both types can be often mixed. In general, the size of vascular spaces is relatively regular in size but may vary. The luminal spaces are lined by a single layer of flat to mildly plump endothelium-like cells and may be filled with red blood cells or empty or contain amorphous proteinaceous material. The intercellular tissue consists of loose connective tissue sometimes with myxoid change. In some field, fat cells are significantly increased with loss of hematopoietic cells by the lesion (Fig. 15.2g), which produce focal high signal area on T1-weighted image. Intraluminal shedding of individual or clusters of individual cells into the lumen is absent, which is a hallmark of angiosarcoma and lymphangiosarcoma [2]. The vessels permeate the bone marrow and entrap the pre-existing trabeculae (Fig. 15.2g), which can be almost completely resorbed and should not be automatically considered as sarcoma permeation pattern. Those characteristic features are easy to recognize in most cases. However, secondary changes including thrombosis, calcification, and papillary endothelial hyperplasia may alter the classic microscopic findings and make the diagnosis confusing.

15.8 Special Stains

Endothelial cells lining the vascular lumens are uniformly stained for endothelial cell markers such as CD31, CD34, Factor VIII-related antigen, ERG, and FLI-1.

15.9 Management

Incidentally found lesion without symptoms with characteristic features on image studies does not require either a biopsy or any treatment. Curettage with or without bone graft is necessary for symptomatic lesion or large lesion impending pathologic lesion. Surgical decompression with preoperative transarterial embolization to reduce intraoperative bleeding can be indicated for symptomatic spine lesion. Curettage or even a biopsy without preoperative embolization may result in intense and life-threatening bleeding [7]. A thorough preoperative preparation for adequate and enough blood transfusion as well as in advance use of recombinant human erythropoietin and iron products is indispensable. Radiotherapy may be indicted for inaccessible lesion and Gorham's disease. **Prognosis** is excellent with a low rate of local recurrence.

References

1. Dorfman HD, Steiner GC, Jaffe HL. Vascular tumors of bone. Hum Pathol. 1971;2(3):349–76.
2. Mirra JM. Focal hemangioma: conventional and "cellular" variants. In: Mirra JM, editor. Bone tumors: clinical, radiologic, and pathologic correlation. 2nd ed. Philadelphia, PA: Lea & Febiger; 1989. p. 1338–62.
3. Heckl S, Aschoff A, Kunze S. Cavernomas of the skull: review of the literature 1975–2000. Neurosurg Rev. 2002;25(1):56–62.
4. Schmorl G, Junghanns H. The human spine in health and disease. New York: Grune and Strattiön; 1971. (2nd American edition translated and edited by Besemann EF).
5. Czerniak B. Vascular lesions. In: Dorfman HD, Czerniak B, editors. Dorfman and Czerniak's bone tumors. 2nd ed. Amsterdam: Elsevier; 2016. p. 903–89.
6. Karlin CA, Brower AC. Multiple primary hemangiomas of bone. Am J Roentgenol. 1977;129(1):162–4.
7. Campanacci M. Hemangioma. In: Campanacci M. editor. Bone and soft tissue tumors. Wien Newyork: Springer; 1999. p. 599–618.

16 Epithelioid Hemangioma

(***intraosseous*** "within bone" + ***epi*** "on" + ***thēlē*** "nipple" + ***haima*** "blood" + ***angeion*** "vessel" + ***ōma*** "forming")

16.1 Definition

Intraosseous epithelioid hemangioma (IEH) is a benign but locally aggressive, rare variant of hemangioma with well-formed, capillary-sized vessels lined by endothelial cells with plump epithelioid morphology. **Incidence** is extremely rare, but the exact incidence is unknown.

16.2 Incidence

Incidence is extremely rare, but the exact incidence is unknown.

16.3 Age

The lesion occurs with a wide range in almost all age groups but is found most frequently between 30 and 50 years of age [1].

16.4 Location

IEH occurs most frequently in the metaphysis and diaphysis of long bones, followed by the short tubular bones of the hand and feet, flat bones, and spine [1]. Epiphyseal involvement is very rare but rather more common in children [2]. Multiple involvements have been reported in approximately 20–25% of the cases [1, 3, 4].

16.5 Clinical Presentation

Pain is the most common presentation and is often intractable particularly at night. Rarely, it can be identified incidentally without any symptoms.

16.6 Radiologic Findings

IEH reveals no distinguishing radiologic features (Fig. 16.1a) and usually manifests as a well-defined radiolucent, sometimes expansile lesion. However, it can also show a mixed lytic and sclerotic appearance with septations, partial cortical destruction, and thick periosteal reactive bone formation. Rarely, the lesion may erode and focally destruct the cortex extending into the adjacent soft tissue particularly when short tubular bone or spine is affected. **CT scan** shows a well-defined radiolucent lesion with an inner soft tissue component usually slightly lower than muscle density and no calcified or osteoid matrix. There can be internal septa, endosteal scalloping, focal cortical destruction, and bony expansion. **MR images** are also nonspecific.

W.-J. Bahk, *Diagnosis and Management of Primary Bone Tumors*,
https://doi.org/10.1007/978-981-99-5498-8_16

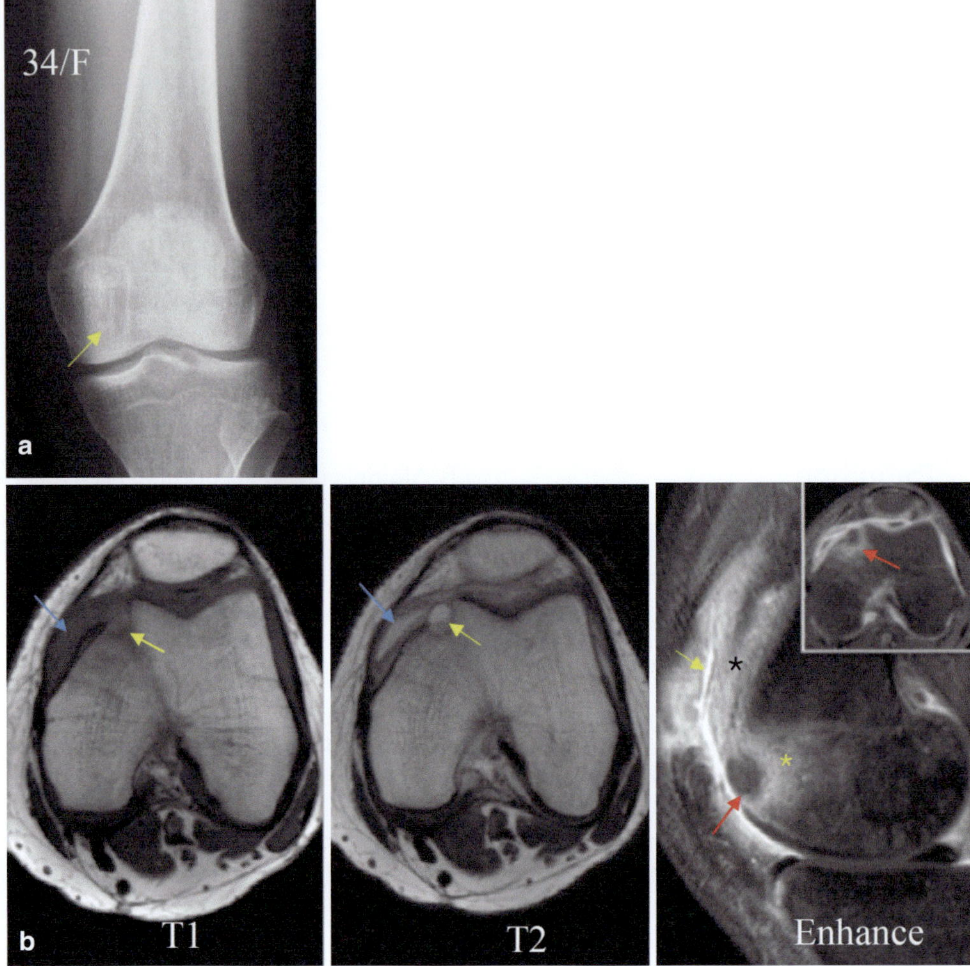

Fig. 16.1 (**a**) Radiograph taken for left knee pain of 1-year duration in a 34-year-old woman shows no definite lucent lesion to a suspicious hazy tiny lucent hole in the medial condyle of the femur (arrow). (**b**) However, MR images clearly reveal a small, 0.7 × 0.8 × 0.8 cm sized, unilocular, round to oval, subcortical cystic lesion with low to intermediate SI on T1-weighted image and intermediate and high SI with a *"fluid-fluid"* level of different densities on T2-weighted image in the antero-medical femoral condyle epiphysis (yellow arrows). There is edema of prefemoral fat pad and synovial hypertrophy with joint effusion (blue arrows). The lesion is peripherally enhanced (red arrows). Note significant edema of perilesional bone marrow (yellow asterisk) and surrounding soft issues (black asterisk) with an adjacent engorged vascular structure (yellow arrow), which is more extensive than expected when consideration of a small size of the lesion. (**c**) The excised specimen is 0.8 × 0.8 cm in size with and dark brown to black in color. (**d**) Microscopic examination. (Left) Low-power magnification notes the tumor grows in lobular pattern with well-defined borders. Several foci of hemorrhage (white asterisks) are visible in the lesion. (Right) Higher-power magnification of one lobule shows the tumor cells replace the bone marrow cavity with permeation of host bony trabeculae (yellow asterisks). The individual tumor cells are large and polyhedral epithelioid with abundant eosinophilic cytoplasm. The nuclei are vesicular, round to oval, and some kidney- or bean-shaped with cleavage. Many cells have more than one clear vacuoles within the cytoplasm, which merge together with neighboring vacuoles and create vascular lumens sometimes containing red blood cells. The stroma consists of loose fibrous tissue with focal areas of basophilic matrix and prominent inflammatory cells at periphery. Note well-formed vascular space lined by epithelioid cells, which bulge into the lumen in regular row of *"tombstone" or "hobnail-like"* fashion (red circle in inset) without cells shedding into the lumen in contrast to angiosarcoma with irregular row of individual cells shedding into the lumens (Fig. 19.3 in Chap. 19). (**e**) Immunohistochemical stain for CD 31 is strongly positive. (**f**) Follow-up radiograph at 6 months after excision of the lesion shows a hazy radiolucent defect (yellow arrow) which is not seen on initial radiograph (**a**). The patient is free of pain after surgical removal of the lesion

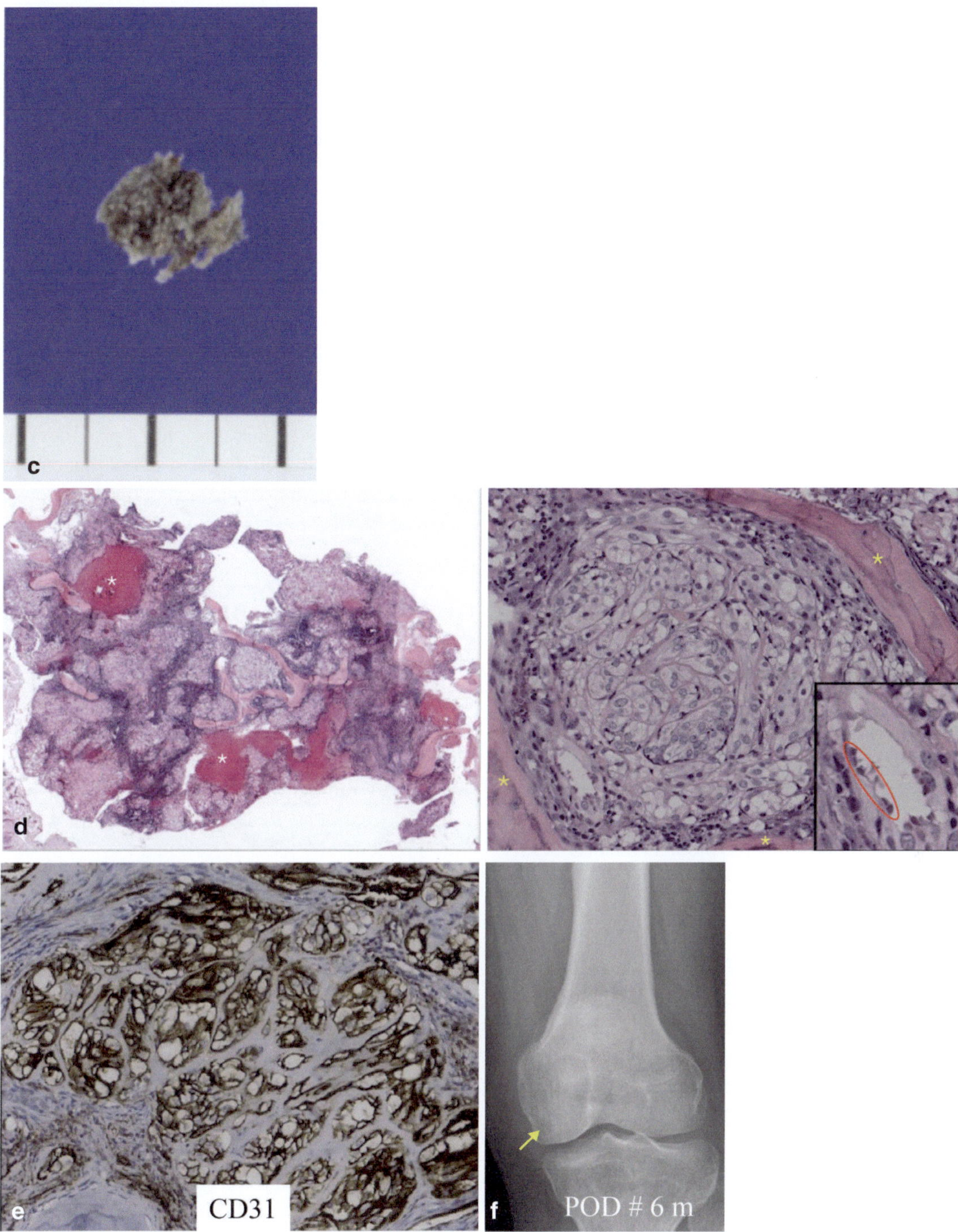

Fig. 16.1 (continued)

The lesion usually shows a lobulated lesion with low to intermediate SI on T1-weighted image and heterogeneous intermediate to high SI on T2-weighted image. It can exhibit mixed lytic and sclerotic appearance with septations and rarely partial cortical destruction with soft tissue extension as well as thick periosteal reactive bone formation. Intralesional flow void of prominent vessels and internal *"fluid-fluid"* level can be found (Fig. 16.1b). Variable degree of bone marrow and soft tissue edema can be often accompanied. The lesion is peripherally or heterogeneously enhanced.

16.7 Histologic Findings

The tumor grows in a lobulated pattern with well-demarcated or infiltrative border and replaces the bone marrow cavity and often permeate pre-existing bony trabeculae (Fig. 16.1d). Individual tumor cells are large and sometimes polygonal with abundant densely eosinophilic cytoplasm. The nuclei are vesicular, round to oval, kidney-, or bean-shaped and contain fine chromatin. Some cells have intracytoplasmic clear vacuole, which may fuse together with neighboring vacuoles to create vascular lumens sometimes containing red blood cells. Frequently, there are numerous well-formed vessels lined by epithelioid cells which may bulge into the lumen in regular row of *"tombstone"* or *"hobnail-like"* fashion in the absence of individual or clusters of individual cells shedding into the lumen being a hallmark of angiosarcoma (Fig. 16.1d). The stroma is composed of loose connective tissue with focal areas of basophilic matrix but no hyalinized or myxoid matrix. Occasionally, inflammatory cell infiltration can be prominent even simulating osteomyelitis.

16.8 Special Stains

Tumor cells are strongly stained for endothelial cell markers such as CD31 (Fig. 16.1e), CD34, factor VIII-related antigen, ERG, and FLI-1. Epithelioid endothelial cells may also exhibit intense and extensive positive staining for keratin and epithelial membrane antigen (EMA).

16.9 Molecular Gene Analysis

The classification of epithelioid vascular tumors including epithelioid hemangioma (EH) and hemangioendothelioma (EHE) remains challenging due to considerable morphological overlap between tumor subtypes with the spectrum from benign to malignant categories. The identification of WWTR1-CAMTA1 by fusion FISH or RT-PCR analysis, as the genetic hallmark of EHE regardless of anatomic location, provides an objective and powerful diagnostic tool that can be used to distinguish both entities in limited biopsy material [5, 6].

16.10 Management

Curettage with or without bone graft is choice of treatment (Fig. 16.1f). Radiotherapy can be considered for inaccessible locations or multicentric lesions. Asymptomatic patients can be carefully monitored radiographic follow-up without any surgical treatment. **Prognosis** is excellent with a low incidence of local recurrence [1, 7]. In one series including 12 patients with IEH, no patients died of disease including the four patients with multifocal involvement [4]. The authors emphasized the importance of distinguishing IEH from other malignant epithelioid vascular tumors due to different management and clinical outcome.

References

1. Nielsen GP, Srivastava A, Kattapuram S, Deshpande V, O'Connell JX, Mangham CD, et al. Epithelioid hemangioma of bone revisited: a study of 50 cases. Am J Surg Pathol. 2009;33(2):270–7.
2. Schenker K, Blumer S, Jaramillo D, Treece AL, Bhatia A. Epithelioid hemangioma of bone: radiologic and magnetic resonance imaging characteristics with histopathological correlation. Pediatr Radiol. 2017;47(12):1631–7.
3. Sung MS, Kim YS, Resnick D. Epithelioid hemangioma of bone. Skelet Radiol. 2000;29(9):530–4.

4. Errani C, Zhang L, Panicek DM, Healey JH, Antonescu CR. Epithelioid hemangioma of bone and soft tissue: a reappraisal of a controversial entity. Clin Orthop Relat Res. 2012;470(5):1498–506.
5. Errani C, Zhang L, Sung YS, Hajdu M, Singer S, Maki RG, et al. A novel WWTR1-CAMTA1 gene fusion is a consistent abnormality in epithelioid hemangioendothelioma of different anatomic sites. Genes Chromosomes Cancer. 2011;50(8):644–53.
6. Tanas MR, Sboner A, Oliveira AM, Erickson-Johnson MR, Hespelt J, Hanwright PJ, et al. Identification of a disease-defining gene fusion in epithelioid hemangioendothelioma. Sci Transl Med. 2011;3(98):98ra82.
7. O'Connell JX, Nielsen GP, Rosenberg AE. Epithelioid vascular tumors of bone: a review and proposal of a classification scheme. Adv Anat Pathol. 2001;8(2):74–82.

17 Glomus Tumor

(***intraosseous*** "within bone" + ***glomus*** "ball" + ***tumere*** "to swell")

17.1 Definition

Intraosseous glomus tumor (IGT) is a rare benign vascular tumor of bone arising in the normal "glomus body," which is histologically identical to GT of subungual areas of finger and toe. The "glomus body" is a specialized form of arteriovenous anastomosis playing a role in thermal regulation with distinct large glomus cells, which is invested with a fine network of capillaries and nerve fibers.

17.2 Incidence

True IGT arising primarily within the bone is exceedingly rare. Osseous abnormalities such as shallow erosion, scalloping, or cortical defects in the tuft of the distal phalanges adjacent to the subungual glomus tumors have been reported with a wide range of incidence [1–4]. Many, if not all, cases reported to be arising in bones may not be primary IGT but secondary erosion of bone by subcutaneous GT [5, 6].

17.3 Age

True IGT occurs most frequently in young to middle-aged adults between 20 and 50 years of age, presenting approximately 80% of reported patients in the literatures [5].

17.4 Location

Normal glomus body is distributed in the dermis layer of the skin throughout the body but most numerous in the fingers and toes. The most common sites of glomus tumor reflect the normal glomus body distribution. Early in 1959, Jaffe [7] recognized that glomus bodies occasionally exist in the medullary cavity of the terminal phalanx, accounting for IGT arising in this bone although extremely rare. Later, Enzinger and Weiss [8] described that the tumor may occur even in sites where the normal glomus body is sparse or even absent. The most frequently reported sites are short tubular bones of hands [1–4, 9–12] followed by spines [13–18]. Fibula, ulna, and calcaneus are also sporadically reported [5, 19–21].

17.5 Clinical Presentation

The classic symptom triads include acute localized pain, tenderness to pressure, and cold hypersensitivity. Characteristically, the pain is often severe out of proportion with the size of the lesion and can be triggered or aggravated by exposure to cold or pressure, even minimal touch.

W.-J. Bahk, *Diagnosis and Management of Primary Bone Tumors*,
https://doi.org/10.1007/978-981-99-5498-8_17

17.6 Radiologic Findings

GT in soft tissues often compresses the underlying distal phalanx to produce a shallow cortical erosion/thinning or well-demarcated small osseous defects probably vascular pulsation from the soft tissue mass [22], some of which may be erroneously considered as IGT particularly when the location is subungual. Exceptionally rare true IGT shows a well-circumscribed, round to ovoid, radiolucent lesion confined to the bone (Fig. 17.1a, b). The lesion can be eccentrically or centrally located with often sclerotic internal rim. It can be eccentrically located in the cortex and expand the bone with an outer complete thin shell of bone when the lesion involves bones other than phalanges (Fig. 17.1b). **MR images** reveal a well-circumscribed round to ovoid cystic lesion with low to intermediate SI on T1-weighted image and intense high SI on T2-weighted image. The lesion is avidly enhanced by contrast media due to its' high vas-

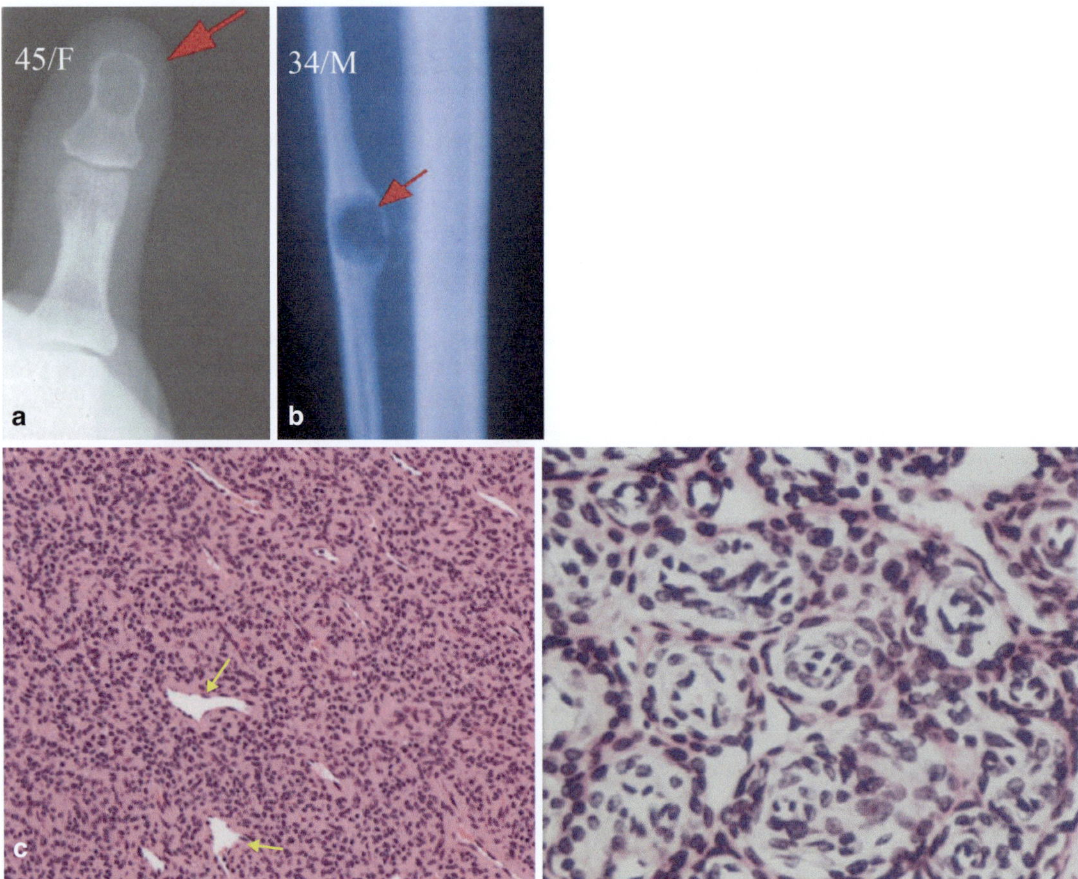

Fig. 17.1 (**a**) Radiograph taken for severe thumb pain, which is aggravated when exposed to cold weather or cold water in 45-year-old housekeeper shows a well-defined, centrally located, round to ovoid, radiolucent lesion confined to the distal phalanx (arrow). (**b**) Radiograph taken for quite severe pain in her right leg of 1-month duration in 34-year-old lady reveals a well-defined, ovoid, mildly expansive radiolucent lesion with an outer complete thin shell of bone in the mid-shaft of fibula (arrow). (**c**) Microscopic examination. (Left) Low-power magnification notes nests mostly composed of small round to ovoid cells arranged in solid sheet pattern and endothelial-lined dilated or branching vascular structure (arrows), often simulating those of hemangiopericytoma. (Right) Higher-magnification shows nests or ball-like masses of paravascular glomus cells, which have round to oval nuclei set in granular pink cytoplasm. There is no unequivocal anaplasia, and mitotic activity is low and typical. The lesion is extremely rich in reticulin, and individual cells were encased by thin reticulin fibers (not shown here). The patient was symptom free without evidence of local recurrence for 3 years after surgical excision of the tumor

cularity. **Bone scan** usually demonstrates heterogeneously hot uptake.

17.7 Histologic Findings

The key feature is nests or sheets of epithelioid glomus cells and rich vascular channels often in hemangiopericytoma-like pattern (Fig. 17.1c). It can be densely packed forming a highly cellular solid mass or separated sheet by strands of fibrous tissue. The lesion is histologically composed of varying proportions of glomus cells, vascular structures, and smooth muscle tissue forming masses, short chords, and trabeculae. The *glomus cells* are small and uniform, round to oval shaped, with distinctive cell borders, centrally located punched-out nuclei with light to deep eosinophilic cytoplasm. The *vascular structures* are usually thin-walled, capillary sized, dilated, or branching. The *smooth muscle* cells are elongated, mature looking. According to the relative proportions, soft tissue GT can be divided into three distinct subtypes including *glomus tumor proper*, *glomangioma*, and *glomangiomyoma*. A "*glomus tumor proper*" is composed of densely packed solid masses or sheets of epithelioid glomus cells separated by broad bands of loose-textured tissue. There are relatively small amount of connective tissue and a few vessels with small lumens. A "*glomangioma*" consists of a prominent vascular component with abundant cavernous spaces surrounded by small clusters or rare layers of glomus cells. A "*glomangiomyoma*" has prominent vessels and smooth muscle cells with gradual transition from glomus cells to smooth muscle cells. However, all IGTs reported to date have been of the "*glomus tumor proper*" category [6].

17.8 Management

Simple curettage or excision of the lesion with or without bone graft is choice of the treatment. More recently, percutaneous CT-guided radiofrequency ablation was introduced for spinal bone tumors [13].

17.9 Prognosis

No recurrence is to be expected if the lesion is completely removed. A small number of purportedly malignant GT have been described in deep soft tissue [23], but have not been reported in bone to date by literature search.

References

1. Lattes R, Bull DC. A case of glomus tumor with primary involvement of bone. Ann Surg. 1948;127(1):187.
2. Lehman W, Kraissl C. Glomus tumor within bone. Surgery. 1949;25(1):118–21.
3. Mackenzie D. Intraosseous glomus tumours. J Bone Joint Surg Br. 1962;44(3):648–51.
4. Bjorkengren A, Resnick D, Haghighi P, Sartoris D. Intraosseous glomus tumor: report of a case and review of the literature. Am J Roentgenol. 1986;147(4):739–41.
5. Bahk WJ, Mirra JM, Anders KH. Intraosseous glomus tumor of the fibula. Skelet Radiol. 2000;29(12):708–12.
6. Czerniak B. Vascular lesions. In: Dorfman HD, Czerniak B, editors. Dorfman and Czerniak's bone tumors. 2nd ed. Amsterdam: Elsevier; 2016. p. 903–89.
7. Jaffe HL. Tumors and tumorous conditions of the bones and joints. Acad Med. 1959;34(1):72.
8. Enzinger FM, Weiss SW. Perivascular tumors. In: Soft tissue tumors. 3rd ed. St. Louis: CV Mosby Co.; 1995. p. 701–13.
9. Chan C-W. Intraosseous glomus tumor—case report. J Hand Surg. 1981;6(4):368–9.
10. Siegel M. Intraosseous glomus tumor. A case report. Am J Orthop. 1967;9(4):68–9.
11. Sugiura I. Intra-osseous glomus tumour: a case report. J Bone Joint Surg Br. 1976;58(2):245–7.
12. Johnson DL, Kuschner SH, Lane CS. Intraosseous glomus tumor of the phalanx: a case report. J Hand Surg. 1993;18(6):1026–8.
13. Becce F, Richarme D, Letovanec I, Gilgien W, Theumann N. Percutaneous radiofrequency ablation of primary intraosseous spinal glomus tumor. Skelet Radiol. 2012;41(4):467–72.
14. Bambakidis NC, Gore P, Eschbacher J, Coons S, Albuquerque FC. Intraosseous spinal glomus tumors: case report. Neurosurgery. 2007;60(6):E1152–E3.
15. Bessho Y, Kataoka O, Sho T, Kitazawa S, Okada S. Intraosseous glomus tumor in the upper thoracic spine complicating compression myelopathy: a case report. Spine. 1991;16(8):988–9.
16. Kobayashi Y, Kawaguchi T, Imoto K, Yamamoto T. Intraosseous glomus tumor in the sacrum: a case report. Pathol Int. 1990;40(11):856–9.

17. Payer M, Grob D, Benini A, Varga S, Hodler J, Martin J-B. Intraosseous glomus tumor of the thoracic spine: case illustration. J Neurosurg Spine. 2002;96(1):137.
18. Robinson JC, Kilpatrick SE, Kelly DL. Intraosseous glomus tumor of the spine: case report and review of the literature. J Neurosurg. 1996;85(2):344–7.
19. Rozmaryn L, Sadler AH, Dorfman H. Intraosseous glomus tumor in the ulna. Clin Orthop Relat Res. 1987;220:126–9.
20. Urakawa H, Nakashima H, Yamada Y, Tsushima M, Ohta T, Nishio T. Intraosseous glomus tumor of the ulna: a case report with radiographic findings and a review of the literature. Nagoya J Med Sci. 2008;70(3–4):127–33.
21. Massari L, Caruso G, Chinni C, Ferron P, Gaban A, Traina F. Intraosseous glomus tumor of the ankle: a case report and review of the literature. Foot Ankle Int. 2006;27(12):1148–51.
22. Drapé J-L, Idy-Peretti I, Goettmann S, Guérin-Surville H, Bittoun J. Standard and high resolution magnetic resonance imaging of glomus tumors of toes and fingertips. J Am Acad Dermatol. 1996;35(4):550–5.
23. Folpe AL, Fanburg Smith JC, Miettinen M, Weiss SW. Atypical and malignant glomus tumors: analysis of 52 cases, with a proposal for the reclassification of glomus tumors. Am J Surg Pathol. 2001;25(1):1–12.

18 Epithelioid Hemangioendothelioma

(***epi*** "on" + ***thēlē*** "nipple" + ***haima*** "blood" + ***angeion*** "vessel" + ***endon*** "within" + ***thēlē*** "nipple" + ***ōma*** "forming")

18.1 Definition

Intraosseous epithelioid hemangioendothelioma (IEHE) is a very rare, well-differentiated, low to intermediate malignant vascular tumor of bone with epithelioid appearance of its endothelial cells within a distinctive myxohyaline stroma. EHE can arise in many other organs and tissues including soft tissue, lungs, liver, and bone with a biologic behavior between angiosarcoma and hemangioma.

18.2 Classification

EHE can be subclassified into two types: EHE with WWTR1-CAMTA1 gene fusion (classic type, non-vasoformative) and EHE with YAP1-TFE3 gene fusion (vasoformative).

18.3 Incidence

IEHE occurring is extremely rare, but the true incidence is not unknown. Thus, there is a paucity of documentations regarding the clinicopathological features and outcomes of these patients.

18.4 Age

It can occur in any age group between 10 and 77 years but typically occurs in patients between the ages of second and third decades of life [1, 2].

18.5 Location

Long bones in lower extremities, particularly tibia and femur, are most frequently affected location, followed by axial skeleton including pelvis, spine, and ribs. Short tubular bones of hands and feet can be also involved [1]. More than half of the cases were reported to be multicentric involvement. Synchronous or metachronous multiple involvement within multiple bones is three times more common than that in a single bone. Occasionally, the lesion in soft tissues, liver, or lung may be associated at time of diagnosis of skeletal involvement.

18.6 Clinical Presentation

Localized pain or swelling is the most common symptoms but asymptomatic in some patients. On occasion, vascular symptoms including

W.-J. Bahk, *Diagnosis and Management of Primary Bone Tumors*,
https://doi.org/10.1007/978-981-99-5498-8_18

edema or thrombophlebitis can occur when the lesion arise from a vein. Pathologic fracture is also rarely associated.

18.7 Radiologic Findings

Radiographic appearance is variable and not specific. The lesion usually reveals a predominantly lytic lesion without mineralized matrix. Often, the lytic defects are multifocal and typically tend to affect bones of one side of extremity. The lesion may be expansile with bubbly appearing trabeculations, cortical erosion, or varying degree of marginal sclerotic rim (Fig. 18.1a). Occasionally, it appears as more aggressive lesion with moth-eaten or permeative growth pattern and a wider margin of transition. Uncommonly, cortical disruption and extension into soft tissues can be present. Periosteal reaction is rare in the absence of pathologic fracture. Multiple involvement confined to one side of extremity may provide a suspicion of IEHE. **CT scan** usually shows expansile purely lytic lesions usually with no mineralized matrix or periosteal reaction. Cortical disruption with soft tissue mass is often seen (Fig. 18.1b). **MR images** demonstrate no specific pattern of intramedullary multinodular mass-like lesion with low to intermediate SI iso to muscle or hyaline cartilage on T1-weighted image and heterogeneous high on T2-weighted image (Fig. 18.1c). Numerous nodules are outline by low signal intensity with all pulse sequences. Serpentine flow void, which is characteristic finding of vascular tumor, is usually not observed in the lesion of bone probably because of small-sized vascular channel and increased cellularity [3, 4]. Perilesional bone marrow and adjacent soft tissue edema may be present. But periosteal reaction is rare. The lesion is usually homogeneously enhanced. **PET/CT and bone scan** reveal heterogeneously increased uptake in the lesion (Fig. 18.1d). They are useful to detect other bony lesions or other organ including soft tissue, lung, and liver lesions because of high incidence of multi-focal lesions.

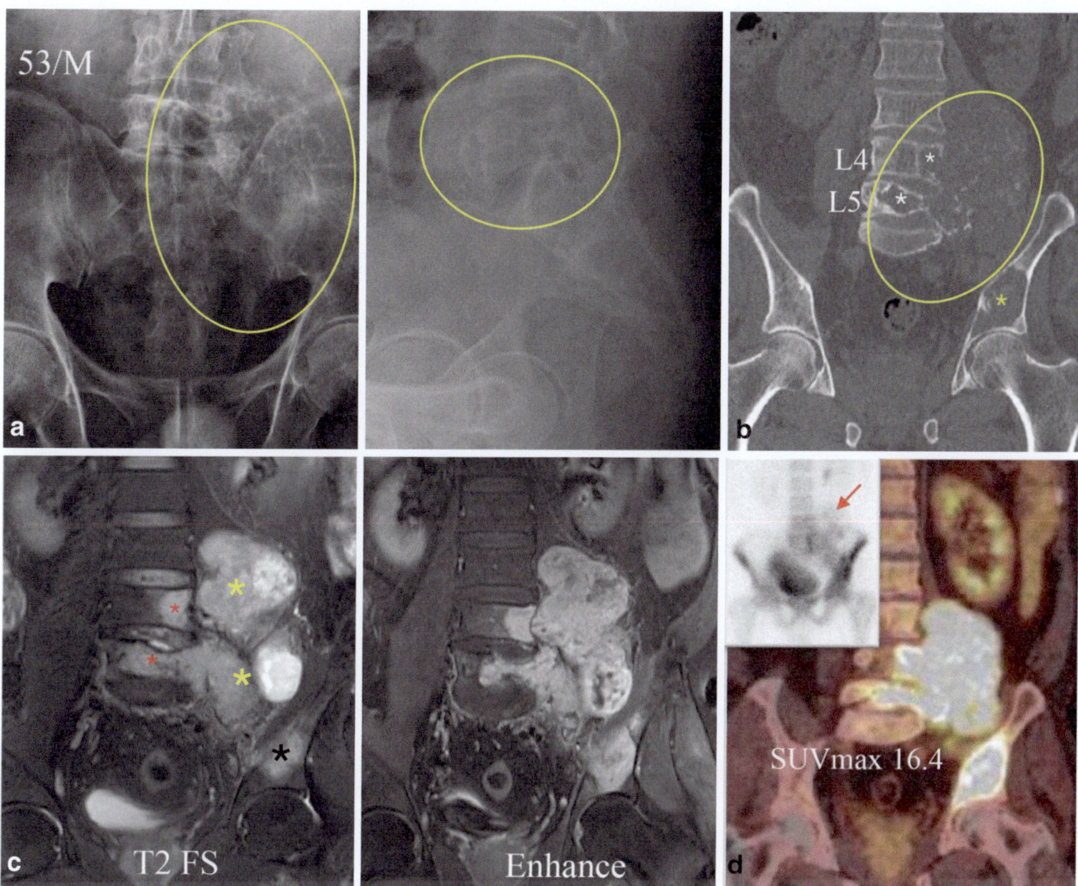

Fig. 18.1 (**a**) Radiograph taken for LBP with radiating pain to lower extremity of 3-year duration in 53-year-old man shows a huge, lytic, expanding lesion with bubbly appearing trabeculations, thin surrounding sclerosis and spotty internal calcification mainly in the body of the L5 lumbar vertebra and left iliac bone (circles). (**b**) CT scan reveals purely lytic destructive lesions (white asterisks) mainly affecting L5 and focal area of L4 vertebral bodies with significant soft tissue extension and focal internal calcifications (circle). There is another osteolytic lesion in the left iliac bone (asterisk). (**c**) MR images demonstrate intramedullary geographically destructive lesions affecting L5 and focal area of L4 vertebral bodies (red asterisks) and left ilium (black asterisk) with low SI on T1-weighted image and heterogeneous intermediate and high to bright SI on fat saturated T2-weighted image. Note prominent soft tissue mass formation (yellow asterisks) with focal internal calcifications. The bone and soft tissue lesions are homogeneously well enhanced. (**d**) PET/CT scan notes intensely hypermetabolic lesion with high FTG uptake (SUVmax16.4) in the L4,5 vertebrae and left para-spinal region as well as left iliac bone. Bone scan shows inhomogeneous hot uptake in the L4,5 vertebrae and left ilium (inset). Localized increased activity is seen in left lower para-lumbar spine region (red arrow), suggesting a soft tissue mass formation. (**e**) Microscopic examination. (Left) Low-power magnification reveals the tumor consists of mainly epithelioid and some spindle cells arranged in solid nest with a few small primitive vascular lumens. However, well-formed blood vessels are not prominent indicating non-vasoformative form. (Right) Higher-magnification notes mostly large epithelioid and some spindle-shaped endothelial cells with elongated vesicular or oval nuclei, prominent nucleoli, and abundant eosinophilic cytoplasm. The tumor cells are mild to markedly pleomorphic in size and shape, but mitotic activity is low. The stroma is fibrous and myxoid to hyalinized. Note a large vacuole displaces the nucleus peripherally to create a *"signet ring-like"* appearance (arrow). (**f**) Immunohistochemical stain for CD 31 is strongly positive. (**g**) En bloc resection of the lesion in the L4,5 vertebrae followed by posterior interbody fusion was performed and extended curettage and cementation with S-pins and iliac screw fixation was simultaneously done for the iliac bone lesion

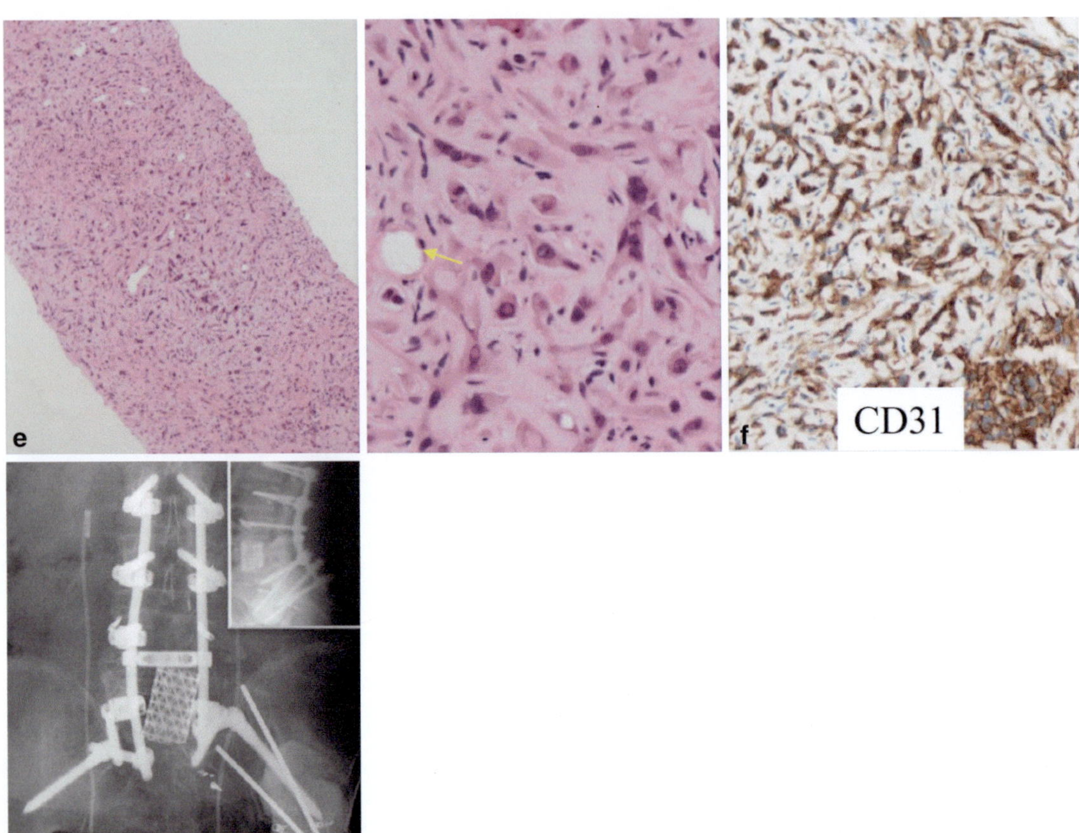

Fig. 18.1 (continued)

18.8 Histologic Findings

The tumor cells are arranged in solid nests or anastomosing cords of epithelioid cells forming irregular vascular channels without a lobular architecture unlike epithelioid hemangioma, which typically have a lobular architecture (Fig. 18.1e). The individual tumor cells are mainly large epithelioid and some spindle-shaped endothelial cells with round or oval to elongated vesicular nuclei, small prominent nucleoli, and deeply stained abundant cytoplasm. Typically, some epithelioid cells have one or more intracytoplasmic clear vacuoles, which may coalesce together with neighboring vacuoles to form primitive vascular lumens of variable size. Well-formed blood vessels are not prominent in most classical EHE (non-vasoformative form), but prominent in the lesion with YAP1-TFE3 gene fusion (vasoformative form). Sometimes, a large vacuole can displace the nucleus peripherally to create a *"signet ring-like"* appearance (Fig. 18.1e). The stroma is variable from fibrous to myxoid or hyalinized with focal areas of basophilic matrix-simulating hyaline cartilage. Cytologic atypism and mitotic activity are usually low. However, occasional pleomorphism with nuclear hyperchromasia and frequent mitoses can make it complicated to differentiate IEHE from high-grade angiosarcoma.

18.9 Special Stains

The tumor cells diffusely express endothelial markers such as CD34, CD31 (Fig. 18.1f), factor VIII-related antigen, ERG, and FLI-1. On occasion, epithelioid endothelial cells may also exhibit intense and focally positive staining for keratin and EMA in 50% and 25% of cases, respectively.

18.10 Molecular Gene Analysis

The identification of consistent WWTR1-CAMTA1 fusion and alternate *YAP1-TFE3* fusion by FISH or RT-PCR analysis gives a high diagnostic value in diagnosis of EHE with limited biopsy material, but the fusion gene is never identified in epithelioid hemangioma (EH) [5–7]. Thus, it can distinguish to EHE from EH and can provide a guide for adequate Treatment.

18.11 Management

Wide resection with adequate margin followed by reconstruction is management of choice. En bloc resection and interbody fusion using cage can be indicated for spine body lesion (Fig. 18.1g). Chemotherapy and/or radiotherapy can be considered for inaccessible lesion, multifocal disease, and incomplete resection.

18.12 Prognosis

A favorable prognosis of IEHE has been reported in the majority of data. The survival of patients with IEHE involving single bone was reported to be 89% and 97%, compared to 50% and 74% in IEHE involving multiple bones in the large series [1, 8]. About 10% of patients with uni-focal tumor progressed to multi-focal disease. The data suggested that multi-focal disease shows a much worse prognosis because many patients with multi-focal EHE also had involvement of parenchymal organs that seems to be the most important prognostic factor in IEHE. The disease-specific probability of survival is 64% at 5 years in most recent study of 50 cases from the Surveillance, Epidemiology and End Results (SEER) database, suggesting that the outcomes of IEHE are more consistent with an intermediate-grade tumor than a low-grade tumor of bone [9].

References

1. Kleer CG, Unni KK, McLeod RA. Epithelioid hemangioendothelioma of bone. Am J Surg Pathol. 1996;20(11):1301–11.
2. Weissferdt A, Moran CA. Epithelioid hemangioendothelioma of the bone: a review and update. Adv Anat Pathol. 2014;21(4):254–9.
3. Ignacio EA, Palmer KM, Mathur SC, Schwartz AM, Olan WJ. Residents' teaching files: epithelioid hemangioendothelioma of the lower extremity. Radiographics. 1999;19(2):531–7.
4. Larochelle O, Périgny M, Lagacé R, Dion N, Gigue're C. Epithelioid hemangioendothelioma of bone. Radiographics. 2006;26:265–70.
5. Errani C, Zhang L, Sung YS, Hajdu M, Singer S, Maki RG, et al. A novel WWTR1-CAMTA1 gene fusion is a consistent abnormality in epithelioid hemangioendothelioma of different anatomic sites. Genes Chromosomes Cancer. 2011;50(8):644–53.
6. Flucke U, Vogels RJ, de Saint Aubain Somerhausen N, Creytens DH, Riedl RG, van Gorp JM, et al. Epithelioid Hemangioendothelioma: clinicopathologic, immunhistochemical, and molecular genetic analysis of 39 cases. Diagn Pathol. 2014;9(1):1–12.
7. Tanas MR, Sboner A, Oliveira AM, Erickson-Johnson MR, Hespelt J, Hanwright PJ, et al. Identification of a disease-defining gene fusion in epithelioid hemangioendothelioma. Sci Transl Med. 2011;3(98):98ra82.
8. Angelini A, Mavrogenis AF, Gambarotti M, Merlino B, Picci P, Ruggieri P. Surgical treatment and results of 62 patients with epithelioid hemangioendothelioma of bone. J Surg Oncol. 2014;109(8):791–7.
9. Gusho CA, Tepper SC, Gitelis S, Blank AT. Epithelioid hemangioendothelioma of bone: a survival analysis of 50 cases from the SEER database (1992–2016). Rare Tumors. 2021;13:20363613211005593.

19 Angiosarcoma

(***angeion*** "vessel" + ***sarkos*** "flesh" + ***ōma*** "forming")

19.1 Definition

Intraosseous angiosarcoma (IAS) is a rare intermediate to high-grade malignant bone tumor arising from the endothelial cells that line the walls of blood vessels or lymphatics. Most IAS is primary tumor and rarely secondary to pre-existing condition such as chronic lymphatic stasis, bone infarction, Paget's disease, fibrous dysplasia, surgical implants near the tumor site, or exposure radiation and chemical carcinogen, and long-term use of steroids [1]. It can be solitary variant and multifocal contiguous or noncontiguous, or even disseminated variant by intravascular spreading, so-called "angiotropic" AS.

19.2 Incidence

IAS is extremely rare, accounting for less than 1.4% (36 of 2627 patients) of primary malignant bone tumors collected by SEER program during the period 1973–1987 study [1].

19.3 Age

The lesions usually occur in older patients with the highest incidence between the ages of 50 and 70 [2, 3].

19.4 Location

AS occur most frequently in the dermis and subcutis followed by breast, liver, and spleen, but extremely rarely in bone. IAS is usually solitary. The most common locations of solitary tumor are the long tubular bones including femur, tibia, and humerus, followed by the pelvis, and trunk. However, about one third of cases are multifocal with two clinical forms of contiguous and distant variants [3, 4]. Approximately two third of multifocal cases involve contiguous bone that is unique for primary malignant bone tumor, and rest of one third cases affect noncontiguous distant bones.

W.-J. Bahk, *Diagnosis and Management of Primary Bone Tumors*,
https://doi.org/10.1007/978-981-99-5498-8_19

19.5 Clinical Presentation

The most common presentation is dull, insidious pain and/or enlarging mass of relatively long duration.

19.6 Radiologic Findings

The lesion is usually an ill-defined purely osteolytic destruction of geographic pattern with or without surround rim of sclerosis. Lower-grade IAS may show well-defined areas of lysis surrounded by sclerotic rims and mild expansion of the underlying bone without cortical destruction. The lesion can be multi-lobulated or appeared bubbly. High-grade tumor usually exhibit cortical erosion or destruction with extension into the soft tissue. However, a periosteal reaction is usually absent, which is unusual for primary bone sarcoma (Figs. 19.1 and 19.2). In some cases, multiple, tiny to small, lytic holes area diffusely concentrated in the almost entire bone with or without contiguous bone (Fig. 19.3). The vascular nature of the lesion is suggested by synchronous multi-focal (non)contiguous involvement in one extremity or one anatomic region. The multifocal contiguous variant exhibits osteolytic lesions with multiple punch-out holes in neighboring bones simulating multifocal Langerhans cell histiocytosis, myeloma, or metastasis. If a destructive lesion with multiple tiny punch-out holes in metaphysis and diaphysis of neighboring or kissing bones is not accompanied by periosteal reaction in older patient, multifocal contiguous IAS should be considered (Fig. 19.3). On occasion, IAS may be radiographically occult as in myeloma. Radiographically occult lesion was reported in 16% of lesions, which were detected on CT or MR on one series [5]. **Bone scan** notes moderate to severe increased uptake along the margins of the lesion (Fig. 19.2b). Bone scan is necessary to detect the other bony lesions because about one third of cases are multifocal (Fig. 19.3c). **CT scan** shows osteolytic destruction usually without mineralized matrix and periosteal reaction. Cortical destruction and soft tissue mass formation can be seen more clearly or extensively on CT scan than appreciated on radiograph (Figs. 19.2d and 19.3e). On occasion, CT scan may reveal a periosteal reaction where no reaction is seen on radiograph. **MR images** demonstrate an ill-defined destructive lesion of geographic destruction pattern frequently with cortical destruction and soft tissue extension, which is sometimes not seen on radiograph (Figs. 19.1b, 19.2c). The SI is heterogeneous low on T1-weighted image and high on T2-weighted image. *"Fluid-fluid"* levels may be present due to hemorrhage and necrosis. Extensive ill-defined perilesional reactive change with high SI on T2-weighted image can be often seen beyond the tumor margin in the bone, periosteum and surrounding soft tissues [5], which is not usually seen in metastatic carcinoma to the bone [6]. Therefore, the extensive reactive change is useful to differentiate IAS from bone metastasis if existed (Fig. 19.3f). The bone lesion and soft tissue mass as well as reactive change are heterogeneously well enhanced by contrast media.

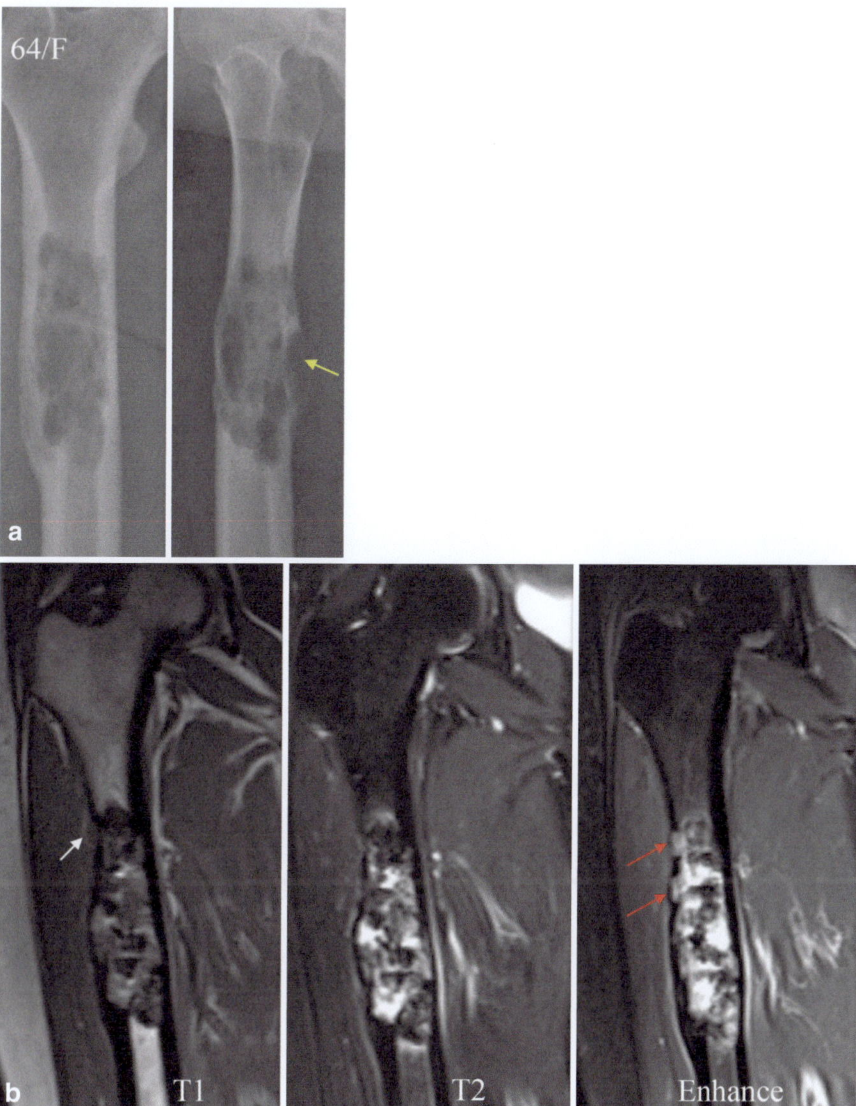

Fig. 19.1 ***Solitary variant*** (**a**) Radiographs taken for right thigh pain of 2-year duration in 64-year-old woman show a relatively well-defined, multi-lobulated or bubbly, osteolytic destruction of geographic pattern in the diaphysis of proximal femur. The lesion is mildly expansile, and the cortices are scalloped or eroded. Anterior cortex seems to be markedly thinned and almost destroyed (yellow arrow). Note the absence of periosteal reaction, which is unusual for primary malignant bone tumor when consideration of the aggressiveness of destruction. (**b**) MR images reveal a well-defined multi-lobulated intramedullary mass-like lesion with low to intermediate and focal high SI on T1-weighted image and heterogeneous intermediate and high SI on T2-weighted image. There are internal foci of dark signals on both sequences suggesting calcification. The underlying femur is slightly expanded, and the cortices are significantly eroded with focally breached and tiny soft tissue mass formation (white arrow) but no distinct periosteal reaction. The lesion is heterogeneously well enhanced by contrast media. Note cortical invasion of the tumor tissues, which are more clearly seen by contrast enhancement (red arrows). (**c**) Wide resection including surrounding soft tissue and muscle was performed under a diagnosis of IAS by incisional biopsy. Bone scan and PET/CT scan presents no other lesions than femur leison. (**d**) Microscopic examination. (Left) Low-power magnification shows irregular anastomosing channels of varying size in the high cellular stroma. (Middle) The tumor cells replace marrow space and entraps the host lamellar bone (L). (Right) Higher-power magnification demonstrates highly pleomorphic and atypical cells, which are mostly epithelioid and less frequently spindled in shape. The cytoplasm is deeply eosinophilic, and some cells show one or more vacuoles. Note a large vacuole displaces the nucleus peripherally to create a *"signet-ring"*-like appearance (black arrow in inset). Mitotic activity is brisk including a few abnormal mitoses. (**e**) Stain with epithelial marker, CD31, is strongly positive. (**f**) Follow-up radiograph at 4 years after surgery reveals no evidence of local recurrence

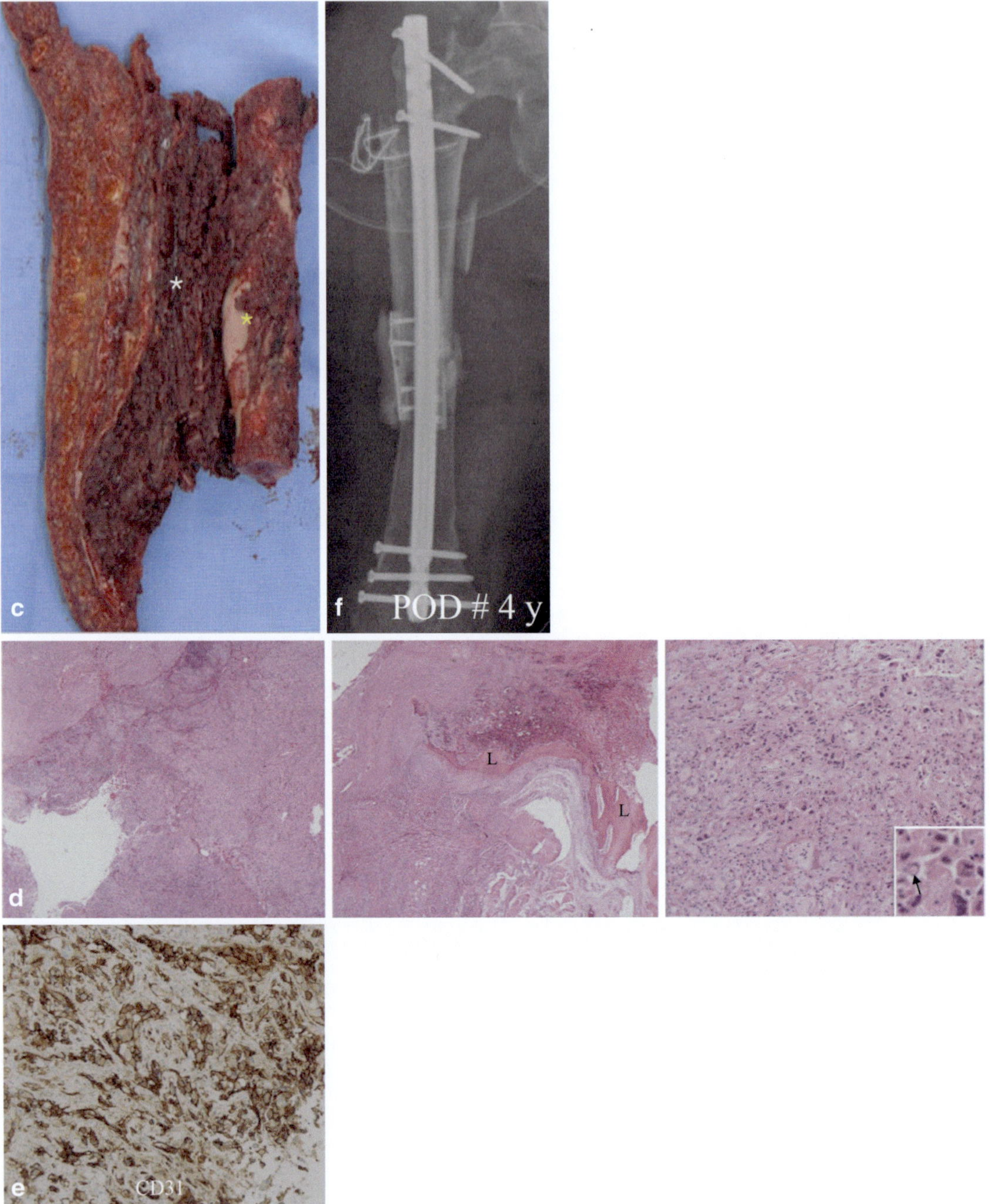

Fig. 19.1 (continued)

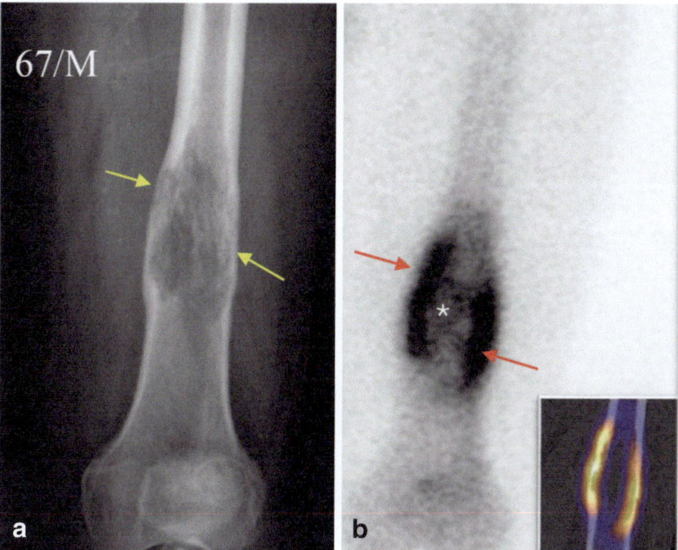

Fig. 19.2 ***Solitary variant with lung metastasis*** (**a**) Radiograph taken for left thigh pain of 3-month duration in 67-year-old man shows a relatively ill-defined, osteolytic destruction of geographic and focally moth-eaten pattern with honeycomb appearance in the diaphysis of distal femur. The lesion notes mild to moderate expansion with cortical erosion and significant thinning but no distinct cortical destruction (yellow arrows). There is also no visible periosteal reaction, which is unusual for primary malignant bone tumor in consideration of the degree of destruction. (**b**) Bone scan reveals strong uptake at cortical lesion (red arrows) with moderate uptake at central medullary lesion (asterisk). Bone SPECT/CT notes an increased uptake at cortical and periosteal regions (inset). There is no increased uptake in other bones. (**c**) MR images demonstrate a well-defined multi-lobulated lesion with heterogeneous low and intermediate SI with focal high signal on T1-weighted image and intermediate with high SI on T2-weighted image. The cortex is markedly thinned and focally perforated with soft tissue extension (white arrows) and marked periosteal edema (yellow arrows). The bony lesion is heterogeneously strongly enhanced, and soft tissue edema is also strongly enhanced by contrast media. (**d**) CT scan images after incision biopsy note a medullary lesion with cortical thinning and endosteal scalloping. The cortex is focally perforated medially with soft tissue mass formation (red arrows). Focal bone defect (white arrow) with low density in the soft tissue suggesting air shadow in the biopsy site (yellow arrow). (**e**) PET/CT scan shows a heterogeneously increased FDG uptake (SUVmax 14.8) in the distal femur as well as another homogeneous intense uptake in the lung, suggesting pulmonary metastasis (inset). (**f**) Wide resection and reconstruction with allogenic bone graft (between yellow arrows) were performed. VATS wide wedge resection was done for lung mass, which was histologically proved as metastatic AS. (**g**) Follow-up radiograph at 3 years after surgery reveals no evidenced of local recurrence with complete union of the graft-host junction (yellow arrows). He is also free of disease in the lung

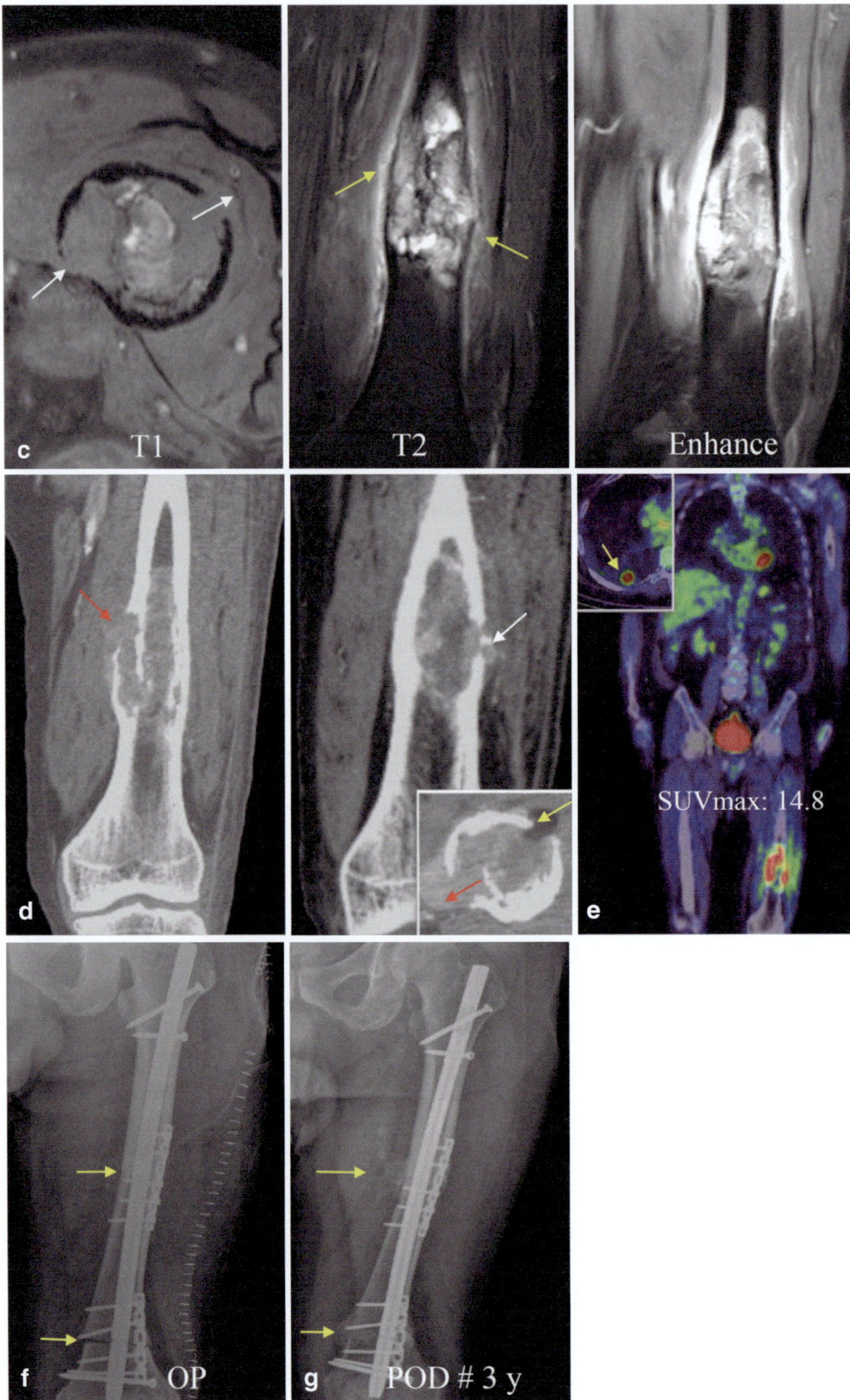

Fig. 19.2 (continued)

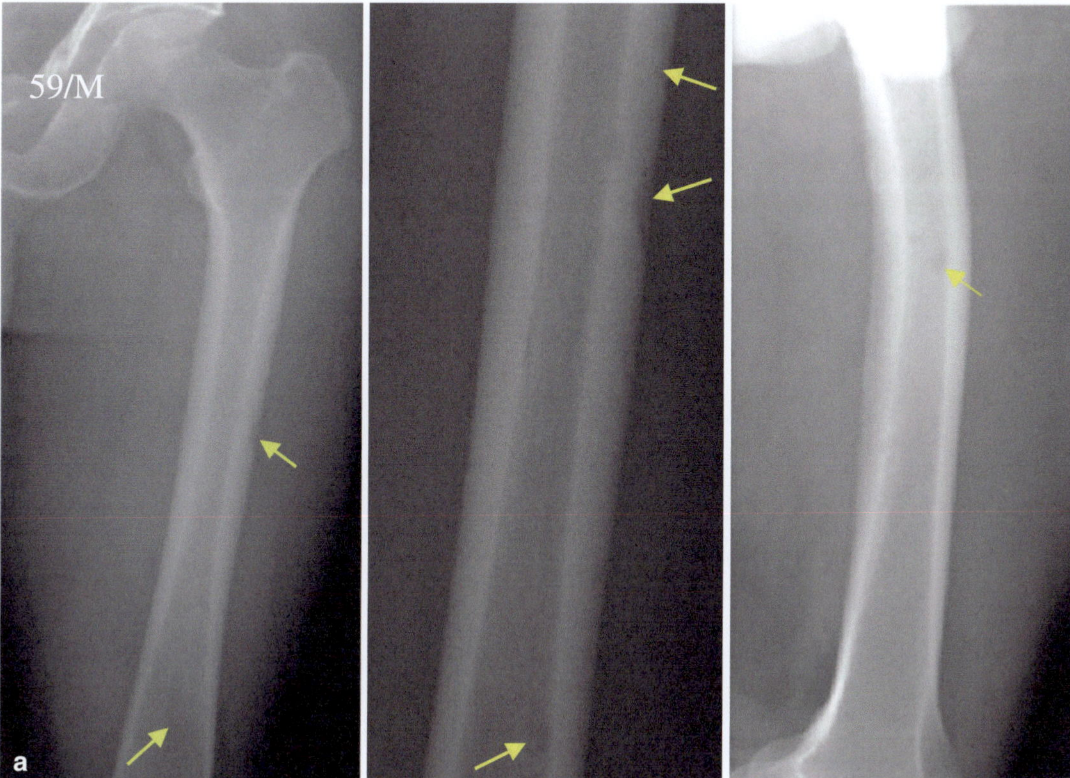

Fig. 19.3 ***Multi-focal (non)contiguous or disseminated variant*** (**a**) Radiograph taken for left thigh pain of 2-week duration in 59-year-old man shows hazy numerous tiny punch-out holes throughout the left femur (yellow arrows). (**b**) MR images reveal multiple variable-sized round to oval lesions in the trochanteric area (blue arrows) and multiple tiny punch-out holes in the shaft (yellow arrows) as well as in the kissing acetabulum (red arrows). The lesions are well enhanced. (**c**) Bone scan reveals subtle to mild uptake in both proximal femurs and shaft (yellow arrows) and moderately increased uptake in the kissing acetabulum and iliac bone (red arrows). (**d**) PET/CT scan demonstrates multiple hypermetabolic lesions in L4 vertebra, sacrum, left iliac, bilateral ischial, and pubic bones, both proximal femurs (white circle) as well as in abdominal aorta (white arrow in inset) anterior to L4 body just above bifurcation level (SUVmax 5.5). In addition, multiple hypermetabolic nodular or irregular shaped lesions are observed in left thigh and calf muscles (white arrows, Right), suggesting multi-focal or disseminated variant. (**e**) CT scan shows a small round osteolytic lesion in the L4 vertebral body (red arrow) as well as a large geographic destruction with cortical destruction and satellite smaller lytic lesions in the iliac bone (yellow circle). (**f**) MR images reveal a large geographic destruction with low SI on T1-weighted image and heterogeneous intermediate and high SI on T2-weighted affecting left iliac wing. There are cortical destruction and soft tissue mass formation as well as extensive ill-defined perilesional reactive change (white circles). There are neighboring several small lesions (yellow arrows). The larger main lesion and satellite small lesions are heterogeneously enhanced by contrast media. (**g**) Two strands of biopsy specimen are obtained by trocar biopsy from the iliac wing. (**h**) Microscopic examination. (Left) Lower-power magnification shows the pleomorphic tumor cells are mostly epithelioid and less frequently spindled, which are growing with solid nest pattern in association with irregular and haphazard anastomosing vascular channels. (Middle) Medium-power magnification reveals the individual tumor cells have enlarged pleomorphic nuclei, prominent nucleoli, and brisk mitotic activity including abnormal mitoses. (Right) Higher-power magnification notes plump cells intruding into the slit-like anastomosing channels in irregular *"hobnail-like"* pattern (yellow arrows). Some individual cells begin to shed into the lumens (red arrow), and they merge together to form intraluminal masses (white circle), which are virtually pathognomonic of IAS but are not ordinary in hemangioma (Fig. 16.1d in epithelioid hemangioma). (**i**) Immunochemical stains for CD31 and ERG are strongly positive

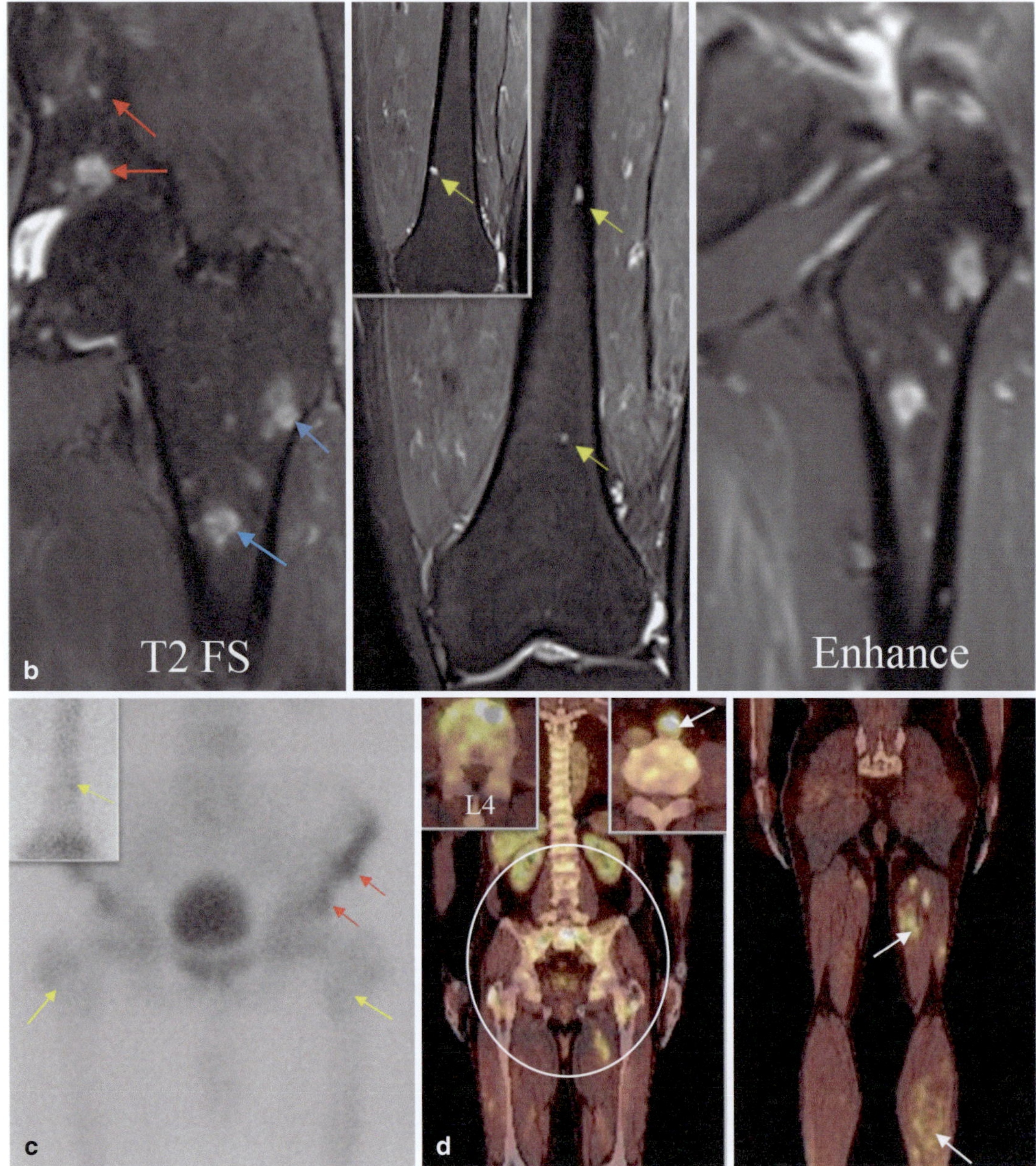

Fig. 19.3 (continued)

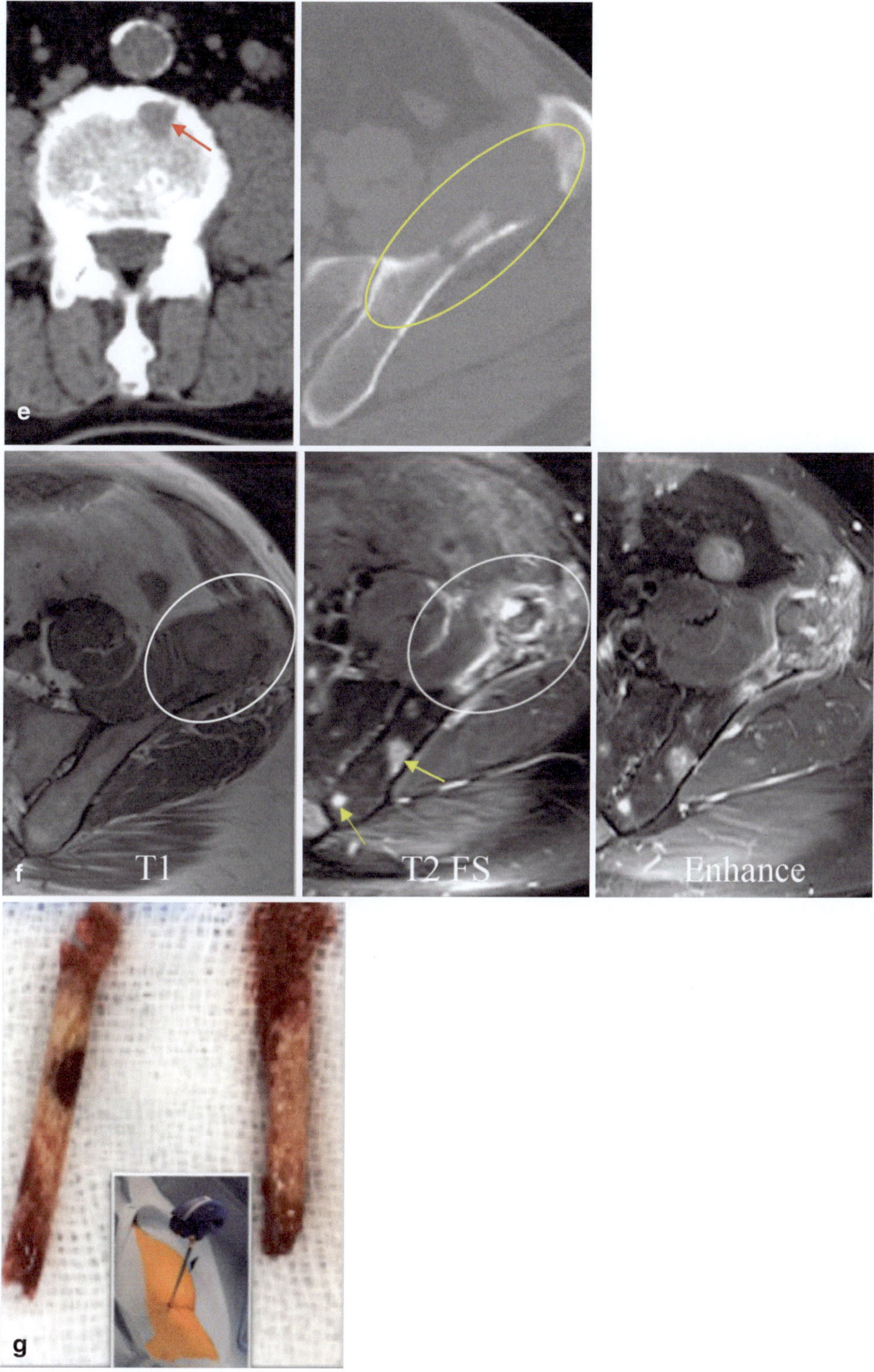

Fig. 19.3 (continued)

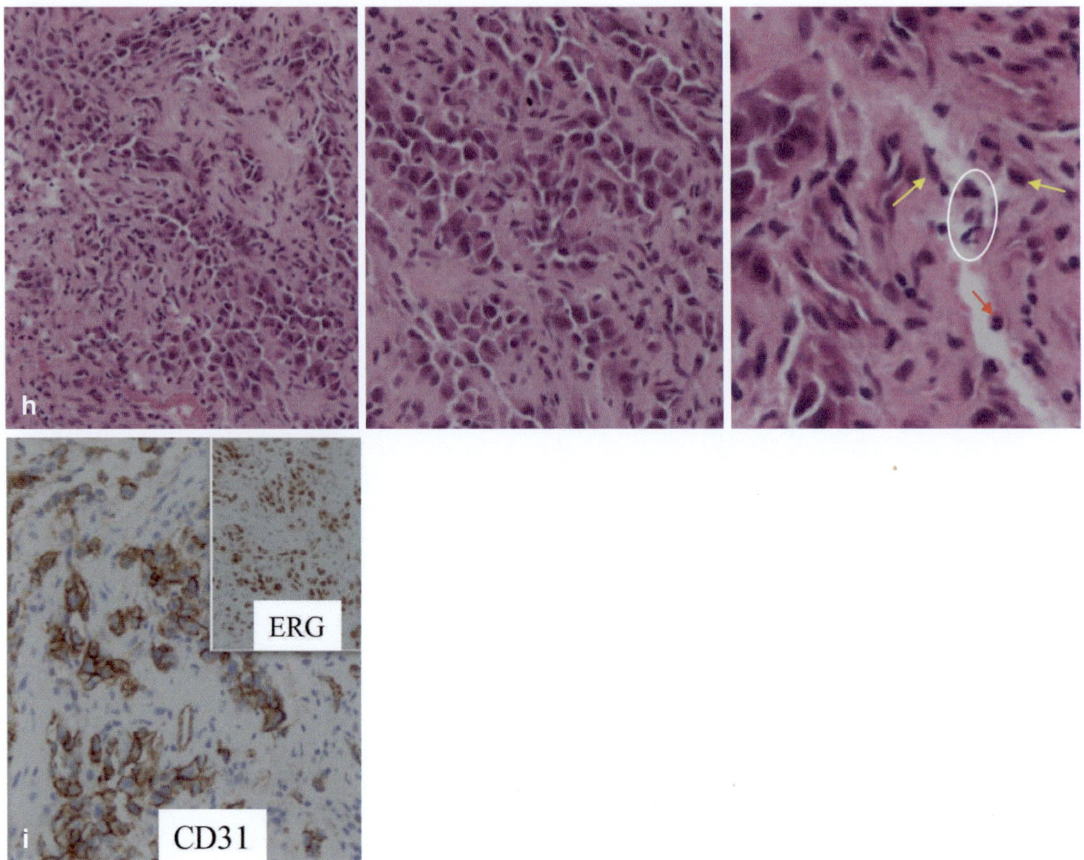

Fig. 19.3 (continued)

19.7 Histologic Findings

IAS characteristically consists of irregularly haphazard blood-filled anastomosing vascular channels and other areas of solid sarcoma. Most lesions show more significant variations in size, shape, and organization of the vascular channels than hemangioma. The vascular channels are lined by atypical malignant endothelial cells. The characteristic abnormal endothelial patterns are plump cells intruding into the anastomosing channels in irregular row of *"tombstone" or "hobnail-like"* fashion. In addition, varying numbers of intruding epithelial cells are shedding into the lumens, and they merge together to produce syncytial cell tuft or masses of several cells in the lumen, which is virtually pathognomonic of IAS (Fig. 19.3h). The similar finding can be also observed in epithelioid hemangioma, but it shows the regular row of *"tombstones"* pattern, small syncytial mass of two to three cells in the absence of individual cells or clusters of individual cells shedding into the lumen (Fig. 16.1d in epitheliod hemangioma Chapter). High-grade IAS reveals variable-sized areas of solid sarcoma consisting of large, round to polygonal highly atypical nuclei. The malignant cells are mostly epithelioid and less frequently spindled in shape with enlarged nuclei, prominent nucleoli, and brisk mitotic activity including abnormal mitoses. The cytoplasm is deeply eosinophilic, and some cells may have one or more vacuoles, which are usually clear but may contain red blood cells. Numerous extravasated erythrocytes can be exhibited in association with hemosiderin deposition. Inflammatory cells including neutrophils, lymphocytes, and eosinophils may be infiltrated.

19.8 Special Stains

The tumor cells with vasoformative feature are usually stained for endothelial markers including CD31, ERG, and FLI-1 (Fig. 19.3i) but less frequently for CD34 and factor VIII-related antigen. Additionally, the epithelioid tumor cells can be often stained epithelioid markers such as keratin and EMA when the tumor cells have epithelioid morphology.

19.9 Management

Wide resection with adequate margin followed by reconstruction is the management of choice. Immediate amputation would be necessary for multifocal variant to prevent rapid intravascular spread from bone to bone. Radiation therapy can be considered for the patients with multifocal and/or surgically inaccessible tumors, or those with adequate margin. Although its role has not been proved, adjuvant chemotherapy can be also considered for the patients with inadequate margin or metastatic disease.

19.10 Prognosis

In higher-grade IAS, survival is poor due to extremely aggressive behavior and early distant metastasis. A multicenter study including 80 patients in nine centers showed that a 5-year overall survival was 41% for localized disease and only 8% in metastatic disease [7]. Another analysis of 60 patients from two major institutes reported 46% of 5-year overall survival in patients achieving surgical complete remission, whereas all patients who did not had surgical remission died at 5 years. The authors conducted complete surgical resection with adjuvant chemotherapy based on cisplatin, doxorubicin, and ifosfamide, which are essential for an improved survival outcome [8].

References

1. Dorfman HD, Czerniak B. Bone cancers. Cancer. 1995;75(S1):203–10.
2. Bovée JV, Rosenberg AE. Angiosarcoma. In: Fletcher CDM, Bridge JA, editors. Pathology and genetics of tumours of soft tissue and bone. World Health Organization classification of Tumours. 4th ed. Lyon: International Agency for Research on Cancer (IARC) Press; 2013. p. 337–8.
3. Verbeke SL, Bertoni F, Bacchini P, Sciot R, Fletcher CD, Kroon HM, et al. Distinct histological features characterize primary angiosarcoma of bone. Histopathology. 2011;58(2):254–64.
4. Deshpande V, Rosenberg AE, O'Connell JX, Nielsen GP. Epithelioid angiosarcoma of the bone: a series of 10 cases. Am J Surg Pathol. 2003;27(6):709–16.
5. Vermaat M, Vanel D, Kroon HM, Verbeke SL, Alberghini M, Bovee JV, et al. Vascular tumors of bone: imaging findings. Eu J Radiol. 2011;77(1):13–8.
6. Mulder J, Schütte H, Kroon H, Taconis W. Radiologic atlas of bone tumors. Cancer Genet Cytogenet. 1993;71:132–8.
7. Palmerini E, Leithner A, Windhager R, Gosheger G, Boye K, Laitinen M, et al. Angiosarcoma of bone: a retrospective study of the European musculoskeletal oncology society (EMSOS). Sci Rep. 2020;10(1):1–8.
8. Palmerini E, Maki RG, Staals EL, Alberghini M, Antonescu CR, Ferrari C, et al. Primary angiosarcoma of bone: a retrospective analysis of 60 patients from two institutions. Am J Clin Oncol. 2014;37(6):528.

Part VI

Neurogenic Tumors

20 Neurilemmoma

(***neuron*** "nerve" + ***lemma*** "rind" + ***ōma*** "forming")

20.1 Definition

Intraosseous neurilemmoma (IN) is a rare benign tumor arising from the Schwann cells of peripheral nerve sheath within the medullary cavity of the bone.

20.2 Synonym

Schwannoma.

20.3 Incidence

It is extremely rare, only accounting less than 0.2% of primary bone tumor [1–3].

20.4 Age

The lesion can be found in any age group with a high incidence in adulthood between 30 and 50 years of age.

20.5 Location

Most commonly affected locations are mandible and sacrum, where the major myelinated nerve trunk is in close proximity or passes through the foramina [4, 5]. On the contrary, the lesion is exceedingly rare in the bones of the extremities because most intraosseous nerves are nonmyelinated and participate in vasomotor functions [6]. Other involved bones that have been sporadically reported include vertebral bodies and long bones including femur, tibia, fibula, and ulna [2, 7–10].

20.6 Clinical Presentation

Due to slow-growing nature, the lesion can be often discovered incidentally on radiologic examination for other reasons. Local pain of insidious and long period is the most common symptom. Rarely, localized swelling over the affected region can be accompanied. Radiculopathy or neurogenic symptoms such as sciatica are often associated particularly in the sacrum lesion due to close proximity or passing through the foramen of the major myelinated nerve trunk (Fig. 20.1a). Rare patents may present with a pathological fracture.

W.-J. Bahk, *Diagnosis and Management of Primary Bone Tumors*,
https://doi.org/10.1007/978-981-99-5498-8_20

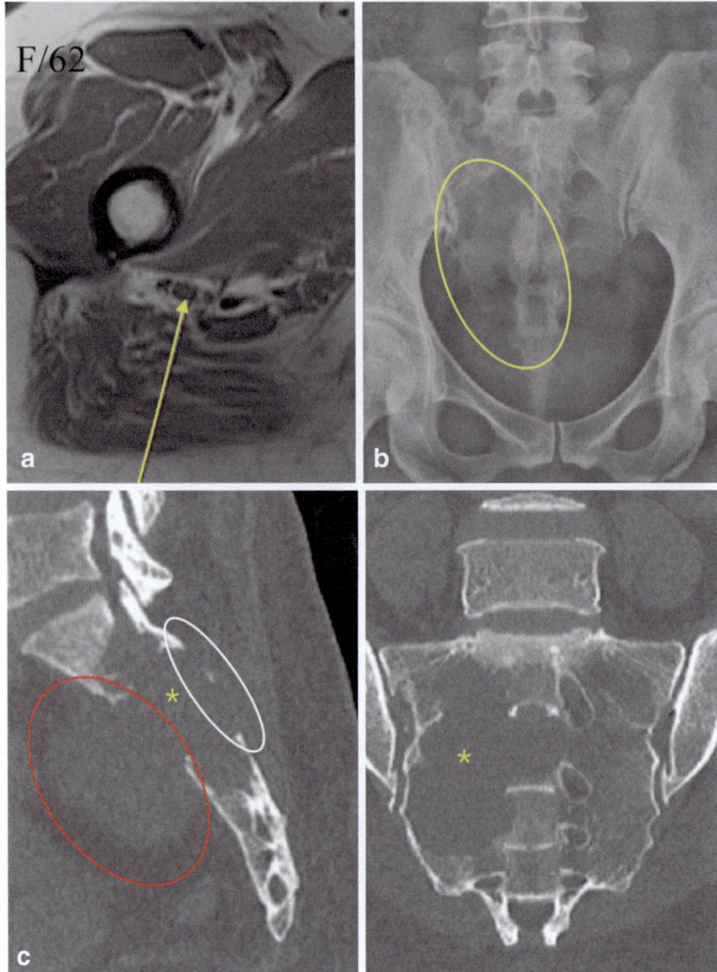

Fig. 20.1 (**a**) T1-weighted MR image of the thigh taken for right posterior thigh tingling and discomfort of 2-month duration in 59-year-old man shows no bony abnormality but mild thickening of sciatic nerve at proximal femur level with internal signal change, suggesting sciatic neuropathy (arrow). EMG reveals findings indicative of right sciatic neuropathy. (**b**) However, pelvis radiograph presents a relatively well-defined osteolytic destruction in right sacrum (circle). (**c**) CT scan demonstrates a huge geographic destruction (asterisks) with anterior cortical destruction and ventral naked soft tissue mass (red circle) as well as posterior cortical destruction but no distinct soft tissue mass (white circle). (**d**) Bone scan reveals a moderately increased uptake along the periphery of the lesion (arrow) with a large photon defect (asterisk) in the right side of sacrum. (**e**) Pelvic bone MR images show a huge intramedullary mass-like lesion with marked soft tissue extension in the body of right side of sacrum (asterisks). The signal is low on T1-weighted image and intermediate and high on fat saturated T2-weighted image. The lesion is heterogeneously enhanced (inset). The lesion involves neural foramen of right S1–3 and displaces the emanating nerve roots, which may contribute for his right thigh pain. (**f**) Microscopic examination. (Left) Lower-power magnification reveals a characteristic feature of spindle cells with elongated nuclei. There is a typical alternation of Antoni A (hypercellular) and Antoni B (hypocellular) areas. (Right) Higher-power magnification of hypercellular area notes compactly arranged spindle cells with focally palisading or paralleling rows of nuclei (circle). Note another typical finding with nuclear palisading that radiate in parallel toward the center, so-called *"Verocay bodies"* (inset). (**g**) Follow-up CT scan at 8 months after curettage and decompression laminectomy notes an ill-defined soft tissue density in right ala of S1–2-3, extending to erector spinae muscle and presacral space, suggesting remnant tumor or a possible local recurrence (asterisks). However, the patient is free of symptom, and thus, he wants periodic observation without further surgical management

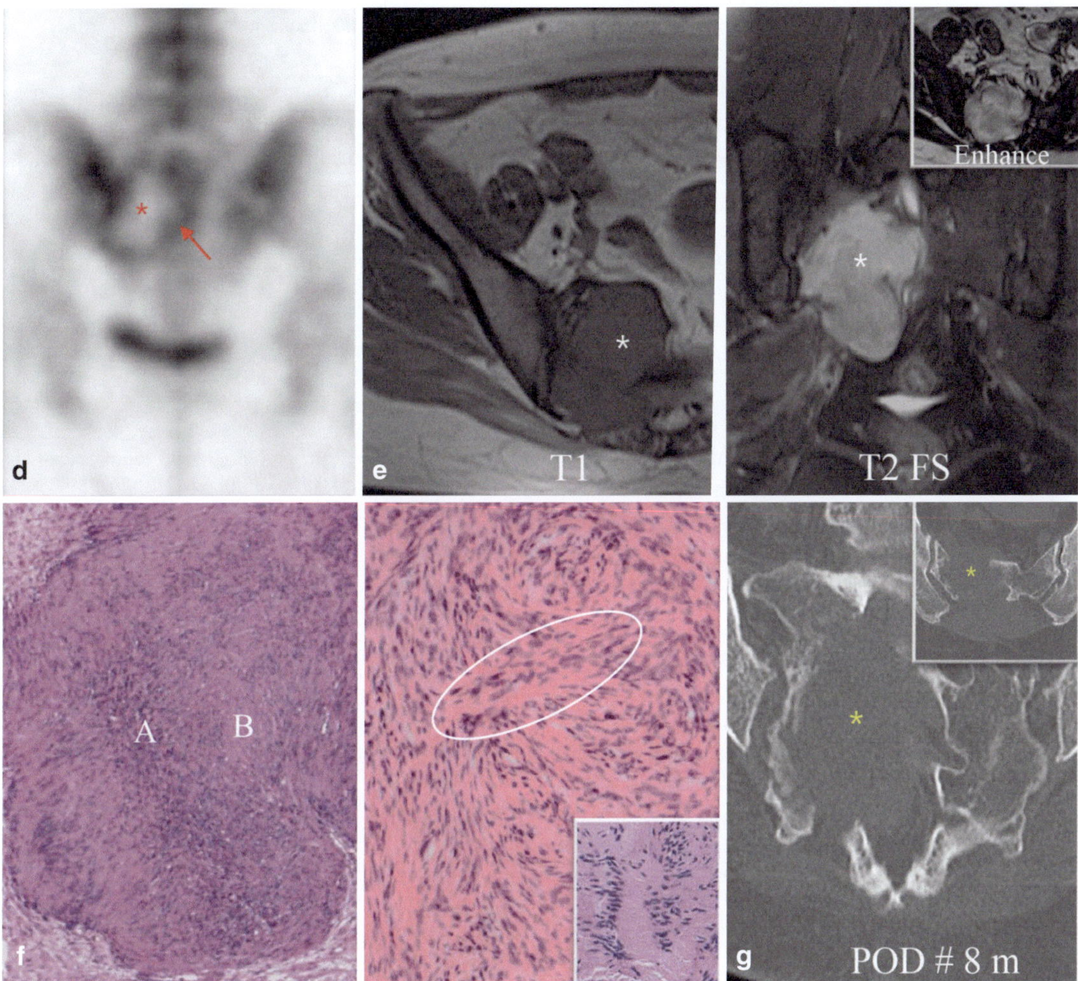

Fig. 20.1 (continued)

20.7 Radiologic Findings

Radiologically, the lesion is not specific. IN usually manifests a well-defined lytic bony lesion sometimes with a sclerotic margin but no internal calcification or bone formation within the lesion. The lesion can be lobulated or trabeculated in contour, and the underlying bone can be expanded with cortical thinning but no periosteal reaction. On occasion, cortical destruction with soft tissue mass formation simulating locally aggressive or even malignant tumor can be seen (Fig. 20.1b). **CT scan** facilitates detection and delineation of the lesion, which is a well-defined expansile osteolytic with cortical thinning or even destruction, but no calcification or bone formation within the lesion (Fig. 20.1c). On occasion, the cortical destruction with extension of the tumor into soft tissue simulating malignant tumor, which is not detected on plain radiograph, can be observed. The density of the tumor is homogeneously hypodense being similar to muscle. **Bone scan** may show varying degree of increased uptake with internal photon defect (Fig. 20.1d). **MR images** usually demonstrate a well-defined expansile intramedullary mass-like lesion with isointense to adjacent muscle on T1-weighted image and intermediate to high SI on T2-weighted images. The lesion can invade into the cortex and occasionally destruct the cortex and extend into soft tissue (Fig. 20.1e). Cystic component with *"fluid-fluid"* level can be seen in rare cases of old or ancient lesion with different stage of hemorrhage. The lesion is heterogeneously enhanced by contrast medium.

20.8 Histologic Findings

IN is histologically identical to its' soft tissue counterpart (Fig. 20.1f). It is characteristically composed of spindle cells with an alternation of hypercellular areas (Antoni A) and hypocellular areas (Antoni B). In hypercellular area, spindle cells are compactly arranged in a focal fascicular pattern with nuclear palisading that radiate in parallel toward the center, so-called *"Verocay bodies."* In hypocellular area, the tumor cells are disorderly arranged in loosely textured to myxoid matrix. Varying degree of ancient or degenerative change including cystic change, calcification, hemorrhage, stromal hyalinization, or xanthoma-like cells may be observed. Occasional degenerated cells can exhibit nuclear pleomorphism with enlarged and hyperchromatic nuclei but no abnormal mitosis.

20.9 Management

Complete curettage of the lesion with or without bone grafting is a choice of the treatment (Fig. 20.1g). Incidentally found asymptomatic quiescent lesion affecting the sacrum can be monitored by periodic follow-up without surgery with a histologic confirmation with an exclusion of locally more aggressive or malignant tumors including giant cell tumor, chordoma or other sarcomas.

20.10 Prognosis

Local recurrence is uncommon if the lesion is completely removed. However, a high recurrence rate (16%) was reported in cases with incomplete tumor excision [11].

References

1. Fawcett KJ, Dahlin DC. Neurilemmoma of bone. Am J Clin Pathol. 1967;47(6):759–66.
2. Ida CM, Scheithauer BW, Yapicier Ö, Carney JA, Wenger DE, Inwards CY, et al. Primary schwannoma of the bone: a clinicopathologic and radiologic study of 17 cases. Am J Surg Pathol. 2011;35(7):989–97.
3. Unni KK, Inwards CY, Bridge JA, et al. Miscellaneous tumors. In: Silverberg SG, Sobin LH, editors. Tumors of the bones and joints. Washington, DC: American Registry of Pathology and Armed Forces Institute of Pathology; 2005. p. 309–19.
4. Jaffe HL. Tumors and tumorous conditions of the bones and joints. Acad Med. 1959;34(1):72.
5. De la Monte SM, Dorfman HD, Chandra R, Malawer M. Intraosseous schwannoma: histologic features, ultrastructure, and review of the literature. Human Pathol. 1984;15(6):551–8.
6. Gordon EJ. Solitary intraosseous neurilemmoma of the tibia: review of intraosseous neurilemmoma and neurofibroma. Clin Orthop Relat Res. 1976;117:271–82.
7. Cohen D, Dahlin DC, MacCarty CS. Apparently solitary tumors of the vertebral column. Mayo Clin Proc. 1964;39:509.
8. Wang XJ, Hartley K, Holt GE, Fadare O, Cates JM. Intracortical schwannoma of the femur. Skelet Radiol. 2014;43(5):687–91.
9. Verma R, Khan M, Davies A, Mangham D, Grimer R. Subperiosteal schwannomas of the femur. Skelet Radiol. 2002;31(7):422–5.
10. Sanado L, Ruiz J, Laidler L, et al. Femoral intraosseous neurilemoma. Arch Orthop Trauma Surg. 1991;110(4):212–3.
11. Wirth W, Bray C Jr. Intra-osseous neurilemoma. Case report and review of thirty-one cases from the literature. J Bone Joint Surg. 1977;59(2):252–5.

Neurofibroma

21

(***neuron*** "nerve" + ***fibra*** "fiber" + ***ōma*** "forming")

21.1 Definition

Intraosseous neurofibroma (INF) is a rare benign tumor arising from nerve fascicles supplying the periosteum or nerves entering foramina in the bone.

21.2 Incidence

A solitary INF purely affecting a single bone in patients with no neurofibromatosis or von Recklinghausen's disease is extraordinarily rare, although secondary involvement of the bone surface by soft tissue NF is not uncommon. The incidence was reported to be 0.06% of biopsy-proven primary bone tumors in a large personal series [1].

21.3 Age

Most reported patients are adults between 20 and 40 years of age [1].

21.4 Location

The most frequently involved sites are mandible, maxilla, and sacrum probably because of close proximity of the nerve with ramification to the teeth or passage through the foramina as in intraosseous neurilemmoma [2]. Solitary NF involving a long bone is extremely rare because nerve sheath or myelinated nerve is not existing in the bone marrow space. Pure INFs outside of the mandibular location were exceptionally reported in the tibia [3, 4], femur [5], humerus [6] (Fig. 21.1), and clavicle [7].

W.-J. Bahk, *Diagnosis and Management of Primary Bone Tumors*,
https://doi.org/10.1007/978-981-99-5498-8_21

Fig. 21.1 ***Solitary INF in the setting of NF 1*** (**a**) Radiograph taken for left elbow pain of 3-month duration in 62-year-old woman shows a well-defined, eccentric, multi-lobulated, radiolucent lesion surrounded by a thin rim of sclerosis mainly in the meta-diaphysis of distal humerus. Note cortical thinning and focal breakage with mild expansion (arrow). She had a history of type 1 neurofibromatosis (NF 1) with Café-au spots, whole body multiple nodules, and back mass since her young age. (**b**) MR images reveal a well-defined, eccentric, multi-lobulated intramedullary lesion with intermediate SI (iso to muscle) on T1-weighted image and high SI with focal dark signals on T2-weighted image in the meta-diaphysis of distal humerus. There is cortical thinning and breakage with soft tissue extension (red arrows). Note multiple small nodules with similar signals to the bony lesion in the subcutaneous layer (yellow arrows) suggesting pre-existing neurofibromatosis. The bony lesion and soft tissue mass (red asterisks) as well as subcutaneous nodules (red arrow) are homogeneously well enhanced. (**c**) PET/CT scan demonstrates intense a localized FDG uptake (SUVmax 7.6) in left distal humerus, suggesting a possible malignancy. (**d**) Microscopic examination of incision biopsy material from the humerus lesion notes a hypocellular proliferation of spindle cells with rich networks of collagen fibers. There are interlacing bundles of wavy, elongated cells with hyperchromatic nuclei with mild to moderate atypism within range of INF. Higher-power magnification additionally presents no true anaplasia features such as nuclear plumpness, prominent nucleoli, and atypical mitosis (inset). Curettage and cementation was performed. ***Malignant transformation of pre-existing neurofibromatosis.*** (**e**) The patient also presents a recurrent back mass, which was locally recurred twice at 1 and 4 years after surgical excision. The pathologic diagnoses were benign NF each time. (**f**) MR image of recurrent mass notes an ill-defined, infiltrative, multi-lobulated, subcutaneous mass with similar signal to the bony lesion as well as homogeneous intense enhancement. Other multiple small nodules with similar enhancement are scattered in the skin (yellow arrows) indicating pre-existing NFs. (**g**) PET/CT scan shows a more intense localized FDG uptake (SUVmax 11.5) in the recurred mass indicating a malignant transformation of NF. (**h**) Microscopic examination. (Left) Lower-power view notes overall cellular shape and architectural arrangement similar to those of fibrosarcoma. There are high number of tumor cells arranged in alternating cellular and less cellular fascicles with whirling or palisading structure with focal "*herringbone*" pattern. Scattered thin-walled, anastomosing vessels are richly present. (Right) Higher-power magnification shows predominant spindle cells and occasional polygonal cells with prominent nuclear atypism. The individual cells appear as round to oval on perpendicular sections while blunt-ended or comma-shaped on longitudinal sections. Mitotic activity is brisk including abnormal mitoses indicating malignant peripheral nerve sheath tumor (MPNST). Wide resection and coverage with local skin flap was performed followed by external radiation therapy. (**i**) Follow-up radiograph at 4 years after curettage and cementation for INF of distal humerus reveals no evidence of local recurrence. However, she died of multiple metastases of MPNST to lung, liver, pancreas, and adrenal gland at 4 years after wide excision and fap coverage

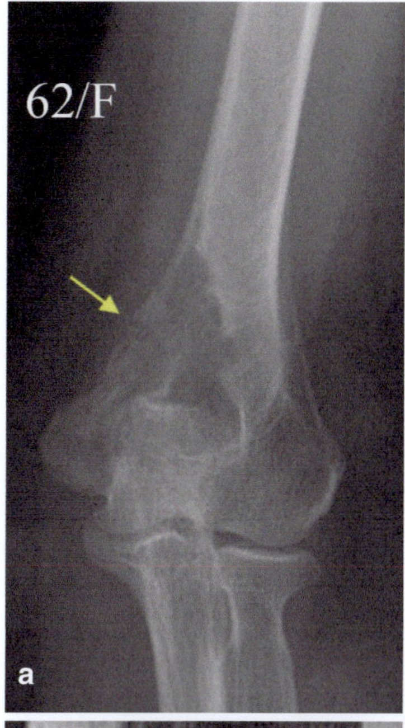
62/F
a

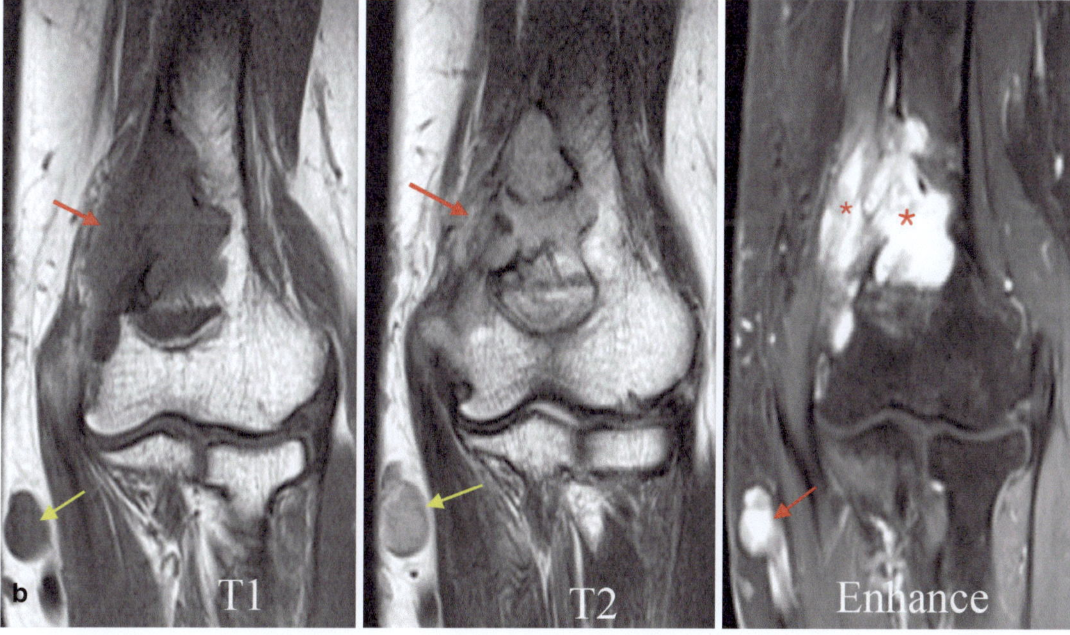
b
T1
T2
Enhance

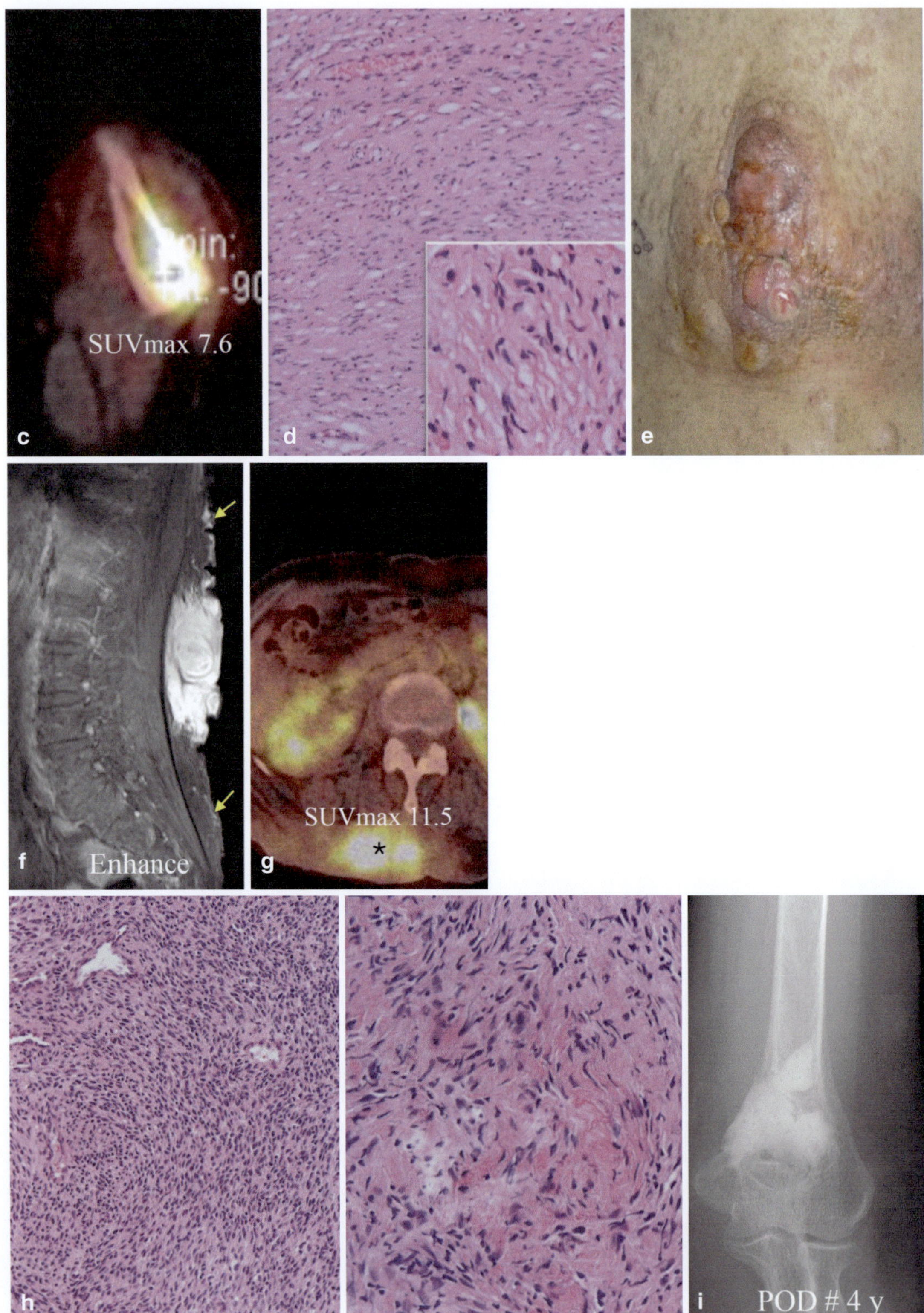

Fig. 21.1 (continued)

21.5 Clinical Presentation

Solitary INF often occurs in the setting of neurofibromatosis (Fig. 21.1). Clinical symptoms depend on the location, size, and extension. Due to slow-growing nature, the lesion can be an incidental finding on radiologic examination for other problems, and a chronic mild pain of long duration is the most common symptom. Localized swelling can be associated in larger lesion. Radiculopathy or neurogenic symptoms are often accompanied in the sacrum lesion.

21.6 Radiologic Findings

Radiologically, the lesion is not specific, but it usually manifests a well-defined, eccentric, multilobulated, lytic bony lesion sometimes with a variable thickness of sclerotic margin (Fig. 21.1a). There is no internal calcification or bone formation within the lesion. The cortex is thinned with focal erosion with no evident periosteal reaction. **MR images** usually demonstrate a well-defined expansile intramedullary lesion with isointense to muscle on T1-weighted image and heterogeneous intermediate and high on T2-weighted images. The lesion can invade into the cortex and rarely destruct the cortex and extend into the soft tissue. The lesion is heterogeneously enhanced by contrast medium (Fig. 21.1b).

21.7 Histologic Findings

INF is histologically identical to its soft tissue counterpart (Fig. 21.1d). The lesion consists of interlacing fascicles or bundles of usually wavy, elongated cells often containing a rich network of collagen fibers. The stroma is typically myxoid with varying amount from meager to copious, which is one hallmark of the INF. The individual cells may have hyperchromatic nuclei with mild to moderate cytologic atypism. However, there are absent of frank anaplastic features such as nuclear plumpness, prominent nucleoli, and atypical mitosis. The nuclei are ovoid, short to long, and thin. Nuclei in myxoid areas tend to be smaller, more ovoid, and shorter as compared to longer and as wavy as adjacent collagen bundles in collagenized areas. Mitosis is absent to rare and typical.

21.8 Management

Complete curettage of the lesion followed by bone grafting is a choice of the treatment (Fig. 21.1i).

21.9 Prognosis

Local recurrence is uncommon if the lesion is completely removed.

References

1. Mirra JM, Eckardt JJ. Solitary neurofibroma: conventional and "cellular" variants. In: Mirra JM, editor. Bone tumors: clinical, radiologic, and pathologic correlation. 2nd ed. Philadelphia, PA: Lea & Febiger; 1989. p. 803–11.
2. Prescott G. Solitary, central neurofibroma of the mandible. J Oral Surg. 1970;28:305–9.
3. Suvarna S, Smith J, Barrington N. Case report: periosteal neurofibroma mimicking osteochondroma. Clin Radiol. 1995;50(11):800–2.
4. Huang GS, Lee CH, Lee HS, Chang WC, Juan CJ, Chen CY. Solitary intraosseous neurofibroma of the tibia. Skeletal Radiol. 2005;34(5):303–6.
5. Chin D, Gubbay S, Foster J. Femoral pain of solitary neurofibromatous origin: a report of three cases. J Neurol Neurosurg Psychiatry. 1983;46(3):277–9.
6. Paksoy Y, Sahin M, Avunduk M, Aksoy F, Ödev K. Solitary juxtacortical neurofibroma of the humerus. Skeletal Radiol. 2002;31(2):112–5.
7. Soodan V. Intraosseous neurofibroma of the clavicle. Acta Orthop Scand. 1976;47(4):370–2.

22 Neurofibromatosis Affecting Bone

22.1 Definition

Neurofibromatosis (NF) is a hereditary or familial disease caused by the mutation of neurofibromin, a gene on chromosome 17 presenting with neurogenic masses and other associated abnormalities of the skin, nervous system, bones, and soft tissues. Clinically and genetically, NF is classified in three distinct forms: peripheral type 1 (NF1), central type 2 (NF2), and Schwannomatosis which is a neurocutaneous syndrome that is clinically and genetically distinct from NF1 and NF2. It is characterized by multiple schwannomas in the absence of the tumor on both vestibular nerves [1].

22.2 Synonym

von Recklinghausen's disease.

22.3 Incidence

Musculoskeletal manifestations of NF are relatively common.

22.4 Age

NF may begin at any age but usually occurs in early childhood or adolescence subsequent to detection of café au lait spots, which are identified usually within the first several years of life [2–6]. Schwannomatosis is recognized most often in people over the age of 30.

22.5 Skeletal Distribution

Spine, skull, long bone, and rib are commonly affected.

22.6 Clinical Presentations

In general, the younger the patient with clinical manifestations, the severer the disease in adult life. NF1 is the most common type and presents a classic symptom triad of (1) multiple soft small cutaneous elevated masses (fibroma molluscum); (2) neurofibroma masses of peripheral nerves, which are frequently palpable in the subcutaneous tissue; and (3) multiple cutaneous pigmentations, so-called *"café-au-lait"* spots, which occur most often over the trunk and axillary area (Fig. 22.1a). The spots of skin pigmentation show the regular smooth borders resembling "the coast of California" in contrast to the irregular serrated borders of "the coast of Maine" in polyostotic fibrous disease or McCune-Albright syndrome. They do not usually confluent to the extent that of latter conditions. Localized or rarely diffuse mass lesions may involve deep soft tissue, viscera, brain and spinal cord, and vascular and endocrine

W.-J. Bahk, *Diagnosis and Management of Primary Bone Tumors*,
https://doi.org/10.1007/978-981-99-5498-8_22

organ. Thus, clinical symptoms depend on locations of the lesion including skin lumps, urinating difficulty or bowel dysfunction, facial weakness, headaches, numbness, vision changes, mental deficiency, weakness, and even hypertension. It can also cause erosion, atrophy, or deformation of the long bones and scoliosis of the spine. In addition, variable-sized bump can be formed over the nerve surface, which may result in enormous hypertrophy of the limb or buttock with redundant skin fold, so-called *"elephantiasis neuromatosa"* (Fig. 22.1a). Deformities on the underlying bones can be associated with mass effect and pressure-induced changes by the skin and soft tissue enlargement in severe plexiform neurofibromatosis. Occasionally, the lesions affect the brain, cranial nerves, or spinal cord, and the patients have learning disabilities or mental retardation. NF2 is much less common than NF1 and presents hearing loss by pressure of tumors on the bilateral acoustic nerves. NF2 can exhibit the same type of skin symptoms as type 1, but not necessarily in every case. Schwannomatosis is considered as a distinct clinical entity with a localized intense pain induced by more pressure due to nearby tumors.

Fig. 22.1 (**a**) Note numerous cutaneous elevated small masses (fibroma molluscum) on whole body, *"cafe-au-lait"* skin pigmentation with regular borders resembling "the coast of California" (arrow), and enormous hypertrophy of left buttock with redundant skin fold, so-called *"elephantiasis neuromatosa"* (asterisk). (**b**) Radiograph taken for rapidly growing mass of left buttock after blunt trauma in 29-year-old man shows a hyperplastic enlarged proximal femur with thickening of the lateral cortex (yellow arrow), elongation of the femoral neck and indentation from outside (red arrow) as well as surrounding huge soft tissue densities (asterisks). However, the contralateral femur is markedly hypoplastic or atrophied (white arrow). There are cortical indentation and erosion by the soft tissue mass in the proximal tibia (red arrow) and distal femur (yellow arrow) as well as cortical thickening (asterisks). (**c**) MR images demonstrate an ill-defined huge extensive subcutaneous mass (asterisks) with low SI on T1-weighted image and heterogeneous intermediate and high SI on T2-weighted image. Note indentation and deformation of the femoral neck due to compression by adjacent soft tissue mass with similar SI as the buttock and thigh mass (red arrows). All lesions are heterogeneously well enhanced by contrast media (yellow arrows). (**d**) Microscopic examination. (Left) Medium-power magnification reveals varying size of multiple nodules of thickened tortuous nerve branches consisting of haphazardly arranged spindle cells with increased amount of myxoid matrix (black asterisks). They are growing in between skeletal muscle bundles (yellow asterisk). (Right) High-power magnification shows increased cellularity within myxoid stroma. (inset) There are distinctive delicate wavy collagen bundles embedded in the myxoid stroma with scanty cells having thin ovoid nuclei, indicating subcutaneous NF

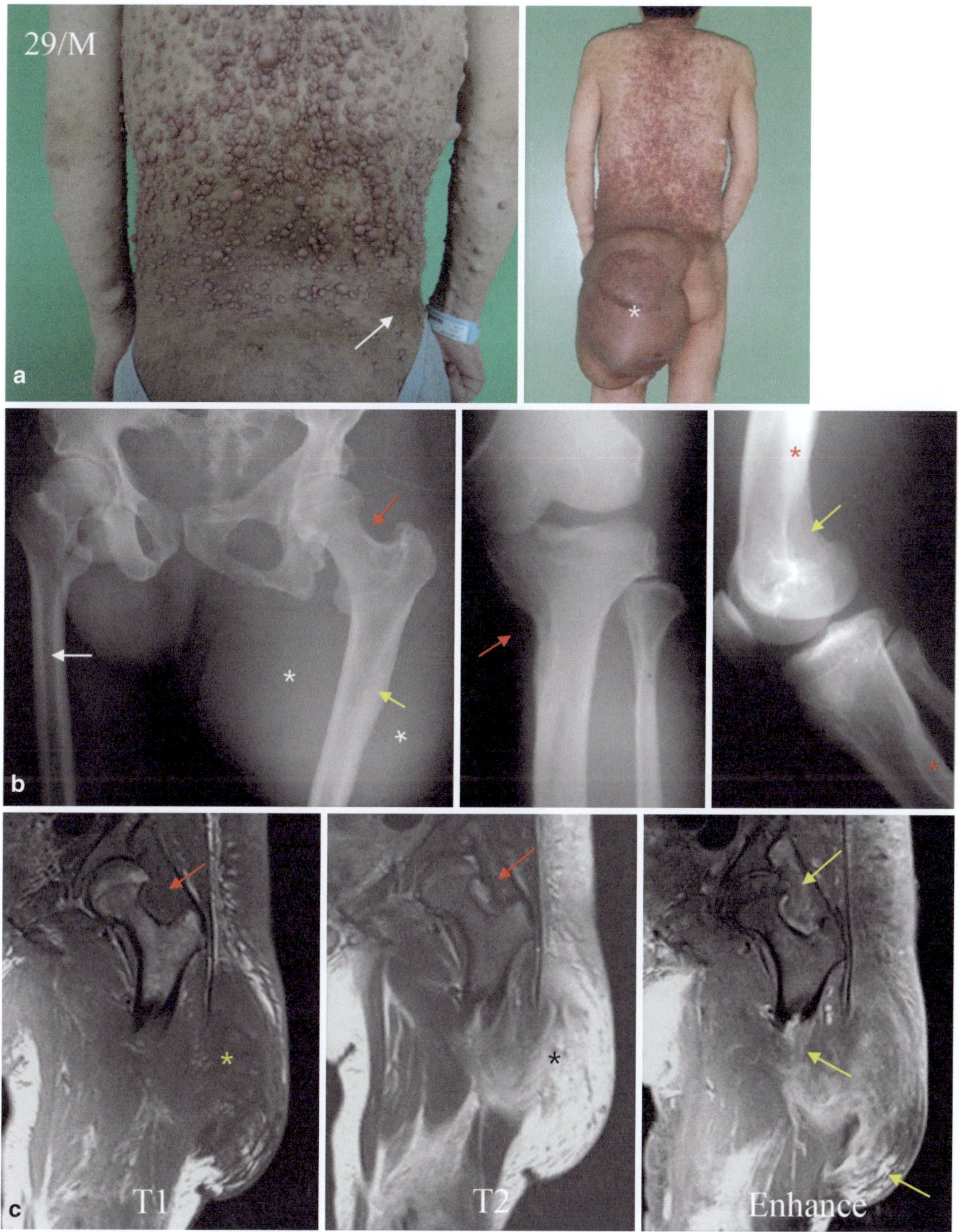
29/M
a
b
c
T1
T2
Enhance

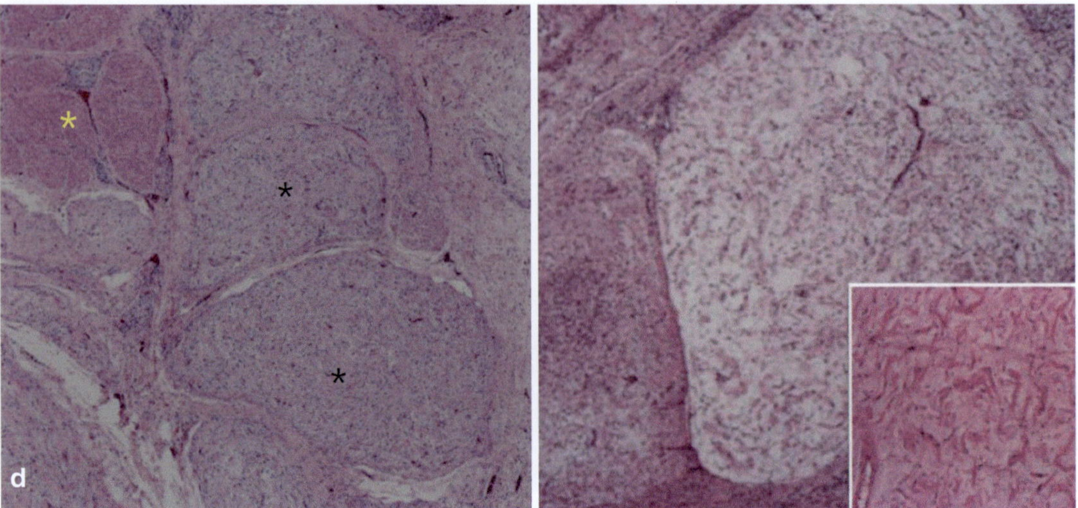

Fig. 22.1 (continued)

22.7 Radiologic Findings

NF affects multiple organ systems with protean skeletal abnormalities seen in over half of patients. Spinal deformities occur in up to 50% of patients with NF1 [3]. Scoliosis is the most common osseous complication of NF1, affecting some 20% of patients [7]. Kyphosis often predominates over scoliosis with sharply angulated segments in association with vertebral scalloping, neuroforaminal widening, transverse process spindling, and rib penciling [7]. The effects of mesodermal dysplasia and extrinsic pressure may result in deficient bone formation of the pectoral and pelvic girdles as well as of the bones of the extremities [3]. The changes are varying widely from mild erosive defects to severe disfiguring anomalies including scalloping/erosive defect, subperiosteal hemorrhage, bowing/pseudoarthrosis, and hyperplasia/hypoplasia/atrophy of bones (Fig. 22.1b). Bowing and pseudarthrosis can occur in a variety of bones but most commonly affect the tibia [8]. Typically, bowing of tibia is discovered during the first years of life before other signs of NF1 are evident, and fracture usually occurs before the age of 3 years [7]. Multiple non-ossifying fibromas (NOF) are often associated with NF, predominantly affecting the metaphases of the long bones [9]. The presence of bilateral multiple symmetric NOFs of lower extremity may raise the possibility of underlying NF1 [10]. **MR Findings** Superficial NFs are usually unilateral or asymmetric and extend to the skin surface. The lesions are diffuse rather than fascicular or nodular in morphology, whereas deep NFs are more likely nodular or fascicular [11]. The SI is low to intermediate (iso to muscle) on T1-weighted image and intermediate to high on T2-weighted image. A dense central area of low signal representing bundles of residual nerve fibers and peripheral bright area of myxoid stroma, so-called *"target sign"* or *"Bull's eye sign,"* may be seen more likely in deep NFs on T2-weighted image [11]. The lesions are heterogeneously enhanced. Bones may show varying degree of indentation and deformation due to long-standing compression by adjacent NF mass (Fig. 22.1c).

22.8 Histologic Findings

The multiple neurofibromas can present in the form of localized, plexiform, or diffused NF [9]. *Localized NF* is histologically equivalent to that of solitary neurofibroma unassociated with NFs.

Multiple localized NF forming discrete nodules in the soft tissue are the most common form in well-developed cases of NF 1. The overall architecture is patternless in contrast to fascicular pattern of spindle cells with nuclear palisading in Schwannoma. *Plexiform NF* consists of a "worm-like" tortuous nerve branches irregularly expanded with multiple nodular appearance, so-called *"a bag of worms"* (Fig. 22.1d). The individual nodule consists of haphazardly arranged spindle cells with delicate wavy collagen and variable amount of myxoid matrix. The cellular composition is similar to that of localized form in association with increased myxoid stroma having delicate collagen bundles. However, increased cellularity with nuclear pleomorphism and hyperchromatism is often seen particularly in larger and older lesions, which can be at a greater risk of malignant change. *Diffuse NF* is the rarest form and characterized by a randomly infiltrative growth pattern of spindle cells with short oval nuclei embedded in non-wavy to way collagen. The nuclei can be moderately pleomorphic in size and hyperchromatic, but mitosis is extremely rare and always typical.

22.9 Management

There is no standard option of treatment, but it can include regular monitoring, physiotherapy, psychological support, and pain management. Children with NFs1 at an early age need to have an examination each year for physical and sexual development, scoliosis, signs of learning disability, and/or behavioral problems. Adult patients generally need standard physical evaluations including blood pressure, screening for hearing, and visual loss as well as any potential growth or change of the masses. Superficial NFs can be excised with marginal margin. However, it is often difficult to separate the deeply located mass from the parent nerve, which may require sacrificing of the parent nerve to ensure complete excision. Thus, benefits of excision should always be weighed against its complications. Likewise, the risks and benefits must be carefully considered if radiation therapy is chosen for an option to reduce the size.

22.10 Clinical Course

Symptoms of NF1 are usually mild, and individuals can live normal and productive lives. However, some patients are severely debilitating and may suffer cosmetic and psychological issues. Plexiform NFs are often difficult to excise completely leading to frequent recurrence. Some patients with NF1 have an increased risk of malignant transformation to a malignant peripheral nerve sheath tumor (MPNST).

References

1. MacCollin M, Woodfin W, Kronn D, Short M. Schwannomatosis: a clinical and pathologic study. Neurology. 1996;46(4):1072–9.
2. Enzinger FM, Weiss SW. Benign tumors of peripheral nerves. In: Enzinger FM, Weiss SW, editors. Soft tissue tumors. 3rd ed. St. Louis: CV Mosby; 1995. p. 821–88.
3. Patel NB, Stacy GS. Musculoskeletal manifestations of neurofibromatosis type 1. Am J Roentgenol. 2012;199(1):W99–W106.
4. Feldman F, Johnston A. Intraosseous ganglion. Am J Roentgenol. 1973;118(2):328–43.
5. Holt JF. 1977 Edward BD. Neuhauser lecture. Neurofibromatosis in children. Am J Roentgenol. 1977;130(4):615–39.
6. Riccardi VM. von Recklinghausen neurofibromatosis. N Engl J Med. 1981;305(27):1617–27.
7. Crawford AH, Schorry EK. Neurofibromatosis update. J Pediatr Orthop. 2006;26(3):413–23.
8. Friedman J, Birch PH. Type 1 neurofibromatosis: a descriptive analysis of the disorder in 1,728 patients. Am J Med Genet. 1997;70(2):138–43.
9. Czerniak B. Neurogenous tumors and neurofibromatosis affecting bone. In: Dorfman HD, Czerniak B, editors. Dorfman and Czerniak's bone tumors. 2nd ed. Amsterdam: Elsevier; 2016. p. 990–1054.
10. Howlett D, Farrugia M, Ferner R, Rankin S. Multiple lower limb non-ossifying fibromas in siblings with neurofibromatosis. Eur J Radiol. 1998;26(3):280–3.
11. Lim R, Jaramillo D, Poussaint TY, Chang Y, Korf B. Superficial neurofibroma: a lesion with unique MRI characteristics in patients with neurofibromatosis type 1. Am J Roentgenol. 2005;184(3):962–8.

23 Malignant Peripheral Nerve Sheath Tumor

23.1 Definition

Intraosseous malignant peripheral nerve sheath tumor (IMPNST) is a malignant tumor of bone arising from peripheral nerve sheath cells. It usually develops secondarily by malignant transformation in pre-existing neurofibromas, schwannomas, or following radiation therapy. However, IMPNST can extraordinarily occur primarily from the nerves within the bone.

23.2 Synonyms

Nerufibrosarcoma/malignant schwannoma/neurogenic sarcoma.

23.3 Incidence

Secondary spinal infiltration by a paraspinal MPNST is a well-known entity. However, a primary IMPNST, de novo from peripheral nerve, is extremely rare and one of the rarest bone sarcomas due to low density of sensory nerve fibers in the bone. Even secondary MPNST associated with neurofibromatosis (NF) is also very uncommon. Only less than 5% of patients with NF type 1 eventually develops MPNST [1].

23.4 Age

MPNSTs occurs mainly in adults between the ages of 20 and 50 years.

23.5 Location

They most commonly occur in the trunk (50%) followed by the extremities (30%) and the head and neck region (20%) [2]. Primary IMPNST most commonly affects mandible, maxilla, or sacrum where the major myelinated nerve trunk is in close proximity or pass through the foramina as intraosseous neurilemmoma and neurofibroma (Figs. 23.1 and 23.2). Scanty sporadic cases have been reported in long bones including the ulna [3–5] and femur [6, 7].

W.-J. Bahk, *Diagnosis and Management of Primary Bone Tumors*,
https://doi.org/10.1007/978-981-99-5498-8_23

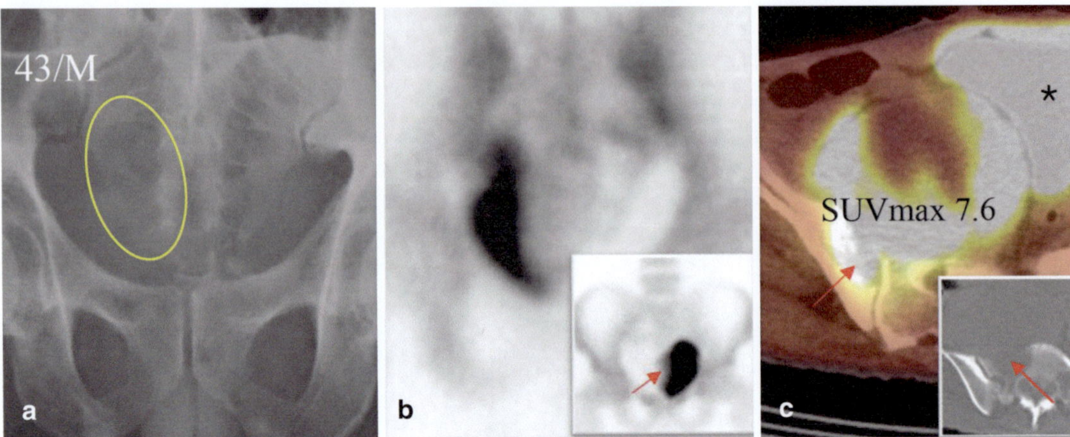

Fig. 23.1 ***Intraosseous high-grade MPNST in the setting of NF*** (**a**) Radiograph taken for right buttock pain with weakness of right lower extremity of 2-week duration in 43-year-old man shows a relatively well-defined geographic destruction affecting right upper and middle sacrum (circle). He had a history of NF1 with café-au spots and numerous nodules in the whole body since his young age, and slowly growing neck mass of 10-year duration. (**b**) Pinhole bone scan reveals a homogeneous strong uptake in the lesion. The urinary bladder with strong uptake is markedly displaced (arrow in inset) due to a huge soft tissue mass delineated in the MR images. (**c**) PET/CT scan reveals a destructive medullary lesion affecting right upper sacrum and sacroiliac joint (arrows) with a huge presacral mass. The FDG uptake is intense in the solid part of the tumor (SUVmax 7.6) with internal photon defect of cystic or necrotic change. The bladder is markedly compressed and displaced (asterisk) by the huge soft tissue mass. There is another milder uptake in the right neck (SUVmax 3.2 in **f**). Milder tiny focal uptakes (FDG 1.3) are also observed throughout the in skin of the whole body, suggesting known multiple neurofibromas. (**d**) MR images demonstrate a well-defined bone destruction of right ilium (white arrow) and upper sacrum (red arrow) producing a huge multi-lobulated presacral mass with low to intermediate SI on T1-weighted image and heterogeneous intermediate and high SI on T2-weighted image. The soft tissue mass exhibits multiple cystic changes with *"fluid levels"* of hemorrhage. The bladder is severely compressed and displaced by the huge soft tissue mass (yellow arrow) on T2-weighted image, which is also reflected in bone scan (inset in **b**). The lesion shows a markedly irregular, thick peripheral enhancement by contrast medium (yellow arrows). (**e**) En bloc resection of the mass and partial sacrectomy as well as laminectomy and SI joint resection (circle) was performed under a histo logic diagnosis of MPNST. ***Secondary MPNST developed in pre-existing NF in the same patient*** (**f**) PET/CT scan shows a milder heterogeneous FDG uptake (SUVmax 3.2) in the right lateral aspect of the neck in the same patient. He has the neck mass for 10 years. (**g**) MR images notes a relatively well-defined dumbbell-shaped mass at the right lateral neck region displacing right sternocleidomastoid muscle and right carotid artery. The signal and enhancement pattern is similar to that of sacrum and presacral mass. (**h**) Marginal resection was done. (**i**) The patient presents multiple soft small cutaneous elevated masses (fibroma molluscum) and multiple cutaneous pigmentations, so-called "café-au-lait" pigmentation with a regular border resembling "the coast of California." (**j**) Microscopic examination of pelvis lesion. (Left) Low-power magnification reveals proliferation of predominantly spindle cells arranged in whirling with a focal herringbone pattern. (Middle) Medium-power magnification notes alternating cellular and less cellular fascicles with nodular foci of spindle cells (circle). There are varying sizes of vascular channels, some of which show markedly dilated lumen with a single layer of flattened endothelium and perivascular hyalinization (red arrow). (Right) Higher-power magnification shows round to oval or blunt-ended or comma-shaped individual cells with prominent nuclear atypism and brisk mitotic activity including abnormal mitoses (white arrows), suggesting high-grade MPNST. (**k**) Microscopic examination of neck mass reveals low to moderate cellularity with blunt-ended or comma-shaped nuclei and moderate nuclear atypia as well as myxoid and degenerative change (inset), indicating low-grade MPNST. He died of lung metastasis with general weakness and aspiration pneumonia at 3 months after initial visit

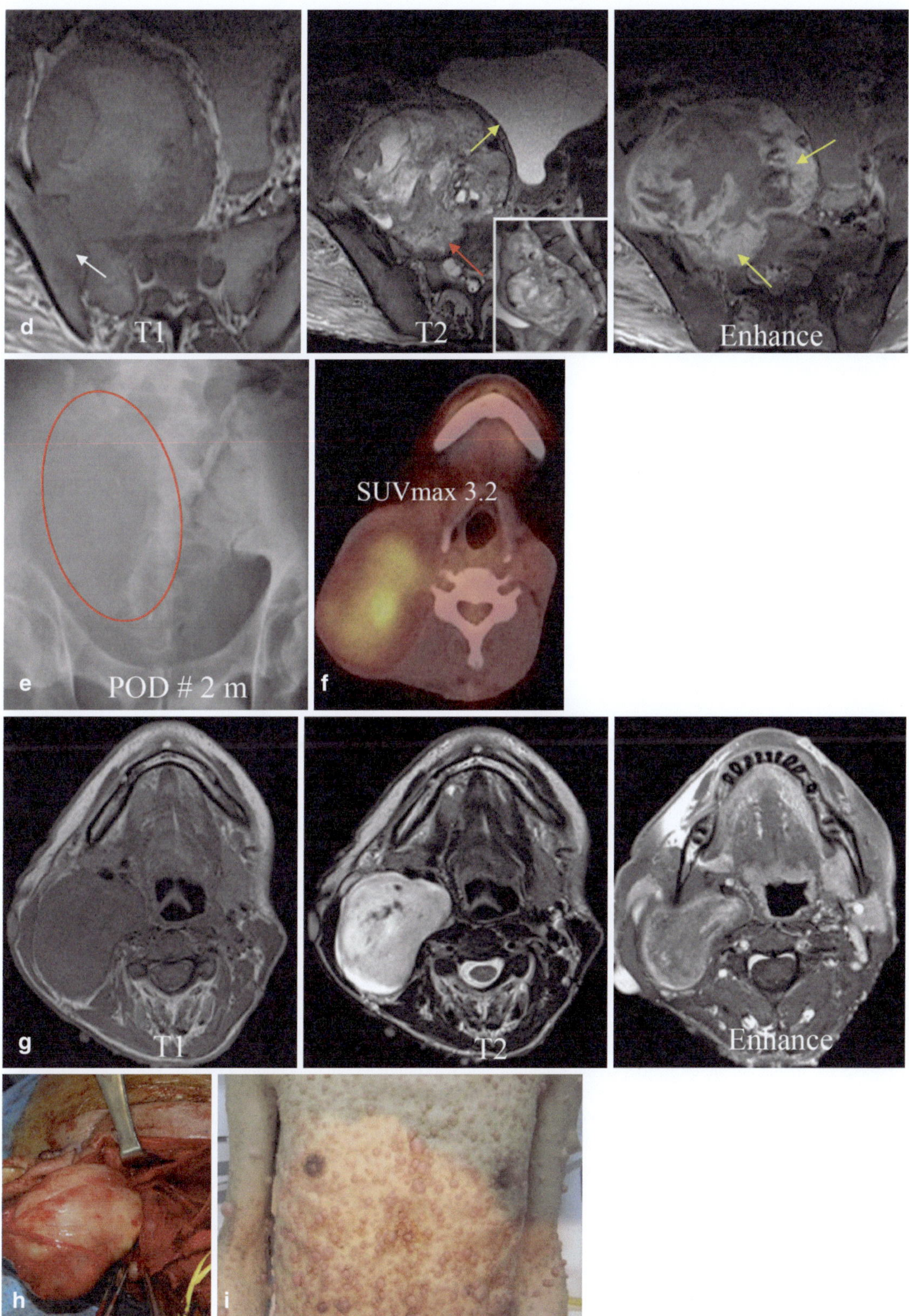

Fig. 23.1 (continued)

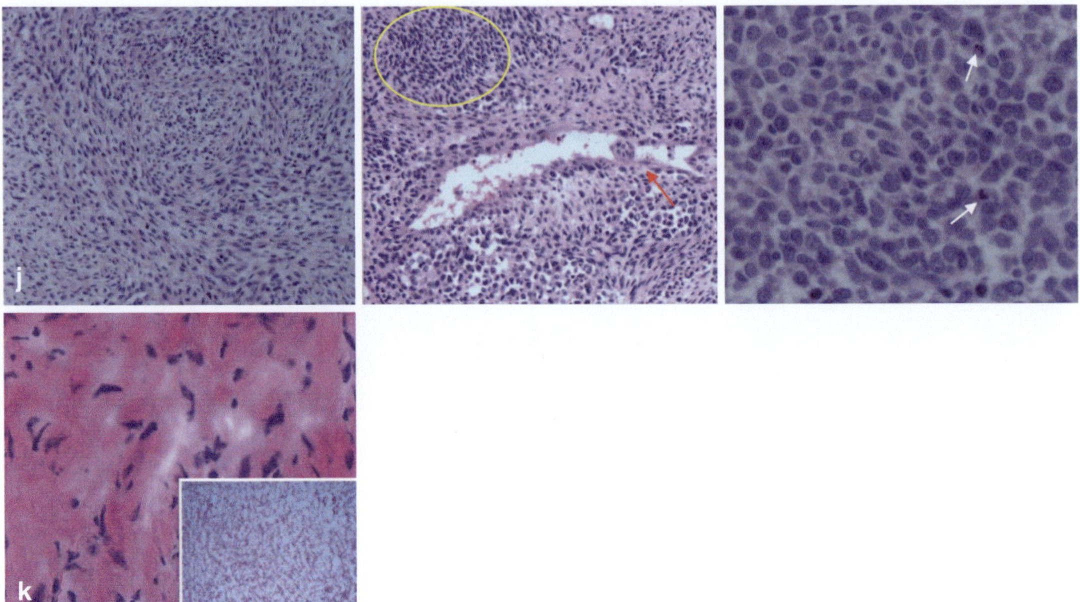

Fig. 23.1 (continued)

Fig. 23.2 ***Primary, de novo, low-grade MPNST*** (**a**) CT scan taken for urinary difficulty of 1-year duration with recent aggravation in 30-year-old woman shows a medullar occupying mass-like lesion of lower sacrum with cortical destruction (arrow) producing a huge soft tissue mass (yellow asterisk), which markedly displaces the bladder, rectum, and prostate. (**b**) Radiograph reveals a relatively well-defined multi-lobulated geographic destruction in left lower sacrum (circle). (**c**) MR images demonstrate a well-defined intramedullary mass lesion with anterior cortical destruction (yellow arrow) forming a huge presacral soft tissue mass, which compresses and displaces the bladder, rectum, and prostate anteriorly. There is posterior cortical destruction with a small mass formation as well (red arrow). The SI is low SI on T1-weighted image and heterogeneously intermediate and focal high SI on T2-weighted image. The lesion presents a homogeneous enhancement by contrast medium with internal non-enhancing foci. The lesion is believed to be primary malignant bone tumor including chordoma or neurogenic tumor such as MPNST. (**d**) Microscopic examination. (Left) Lower-power magnification shows predominantly spindle-cells arranged in whorled fascicles with a herringbone pattern. There are numerous small thin-walled anastomosing vessels with surrounding haphazard arrangement of short spindle shaped cells. (Right) Higher-power magnification reveals mild to moderately increased cellularity with bizarre nuclear atypism (yellow arrow), dark smudged, or dispersed coarse chromatin. The stroma contains abundant interlacing bundles of collagen and a moderate amount of extracellular myxoid material. Individual cells are long and spindle shaped with pale eosinophilic cytoplasm and ill-defined cytoplasmic border. The nuclei are mostly elongated, wavy, tapered, and "buckled," but some are comma-shaped (white arrows). (**e**) Immunohistochemical stain for S100 is positive. A final diagnosis of primary, de novo MPNST involving sacrum has been rendered because he had no clinical evidence of NF such as soft small cutaneous elevated masses and multiple cutaneous pigmentations as well as no other large soft tissue mass on MR images

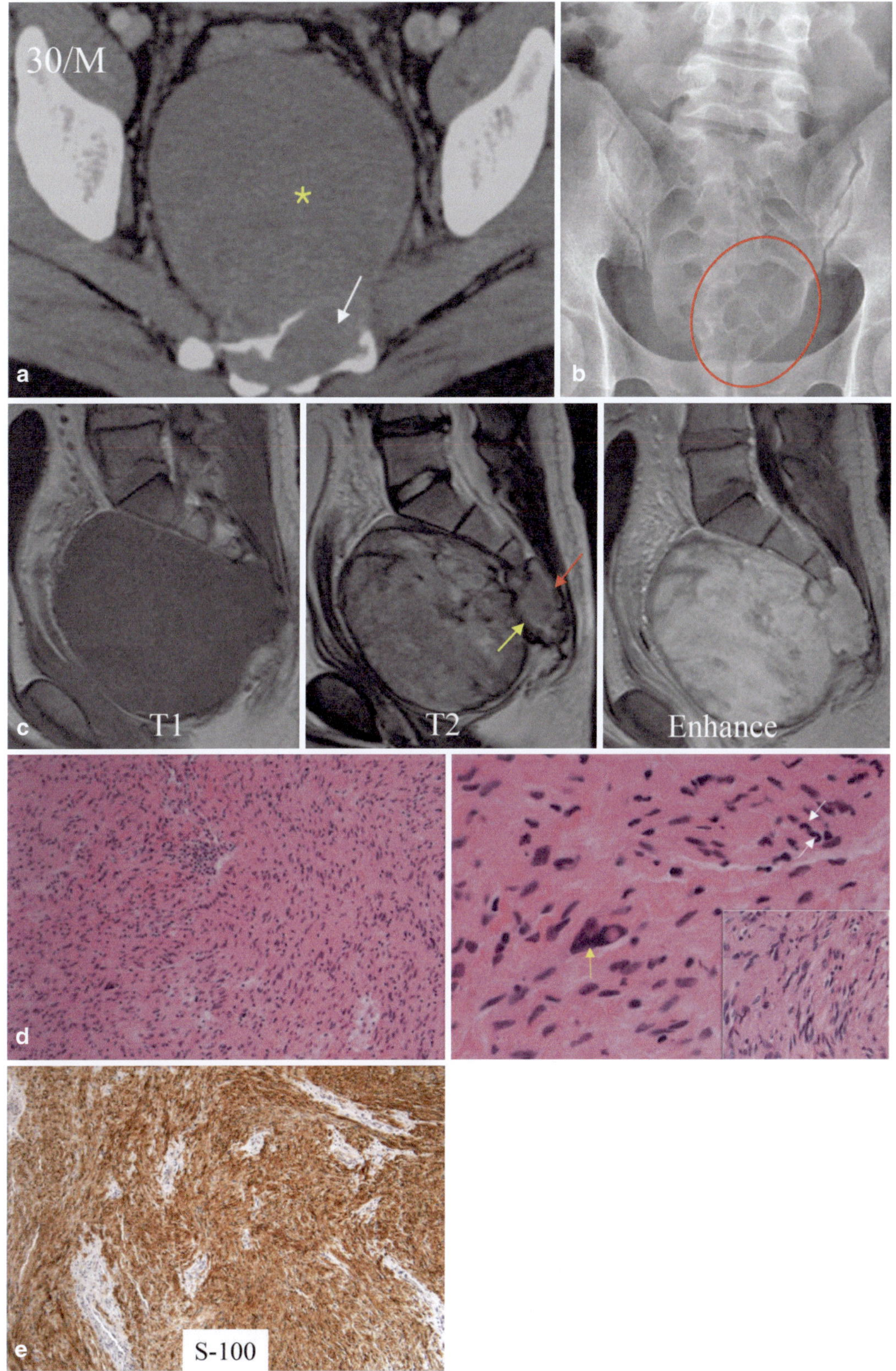
30/M
a
b
c
T1
T2
Enhance
d
e
S-100

23.6 Clinical Presentations

About half of MPNST are associated with NF1 [1]. A slowly growing mass or swelling is the most common presentation. It most frequently arises in association with major nerves such as brachial, sciatic, or sacral nerve. Bony involvement usually originates from secondary invasion into the adjacent bone, which can produce localized bone pain. Often, MPNST produce neurologic deficits in the distribution of the involved nerves by impingement or mass effect (Fig. 23.1). It can also result in urinary or defecation difficulty (Fig. 23.2).

23.7 Radiologic Findings

The IMPNST is usually a well-delineated osteolytic lesion with sharp sclerotic or partially sclerotic margins. The lesion is usually multilobulated without internal calcification or ossification (Figs. 23.1a and 23.2b). The cortex is usually destructed, and the tumor extends to the soft tissue, which may not clearly visible on routine radiograph. **CT scan** IMPNSTs clearly present as a geographic destruction with heterogeneous hypodense masse due to varying degree of degeneration and cellular density of the lesion (Figs. 23.1c and 23.2a). **MR images** reveal a well-defined intramedullary mass-like lesion with cortical destruction and large soft tissue mass formation. The SI is low to intermediate on T1-weighted image and heterogeneous intermediate and high on T2-weighted image. The signal can be low on T2-weighted image when collagen content is rich. The lesion is heterogeneously enhanced by contrast medium (Figs. 23.1 and 23.2). **Bone scan and PET/CT scan** usually show a heterogeneously avid uptake (Fig. 23.1b).

23.8 Histologic Findings

The lesion consists predominantly of spindle cells or polygonal cells with prominent nuclear atypism and variable cellularity. Those are arranged in alternating bands of longitudinal and perpendicular cut. Overall cellular shape and architectural arrangement in alternating cellular and less cellular fascicles occasionally with focal whirling or *"herringbone"* pattern are similar to those of fibrosarcoma (Figs. 23.1j and 23.2d). Most MPNSTs are higher-grade malignant tumor with prominently pleomorphic cells, but less than 20% of soft tissue MPNST were reported as low-grade in a large series [2]. The individual cells appear as round to oval on perpendicular sections while *"blunt-ended"* or *"comma-shaped"* on longitudinal sections (Figs. 23.1k and 23.2d). Mitotic activity is brisk including abnormal mitoses. On occasion, thin-walled hemangiopericytoma-like vascular channels of variable number and size with a single layer of flattened endothelium and perivascular hyalinization can be observed (Fig. 23.1j).

23.9 Special Stains

The tumor cells are patchy or focally positive for neural markers such as S-100, neurofilaments, and neuron-specific enolase (Fig. 23.1e).

23.10 Management

Wide excision with adequate margins is the mainstay of management for localized disease. The use of chemotherapy and radiotherapy for MPNST has been still debated. Doxorubicin-based cytotoxic chemotherapy remains the standard of care in the front line of treatment for unresectable, advanced, or metastatic disease [8].

23.11 Prognosis

MPNST is a highly malignant and possesses a high propensity to local recur and metastasize to distant sites, frequently lung and liver. The exact prognosis of IMPNST is not known because most cases are sporadically documented as a case report. However, the overall prognosis remains dismal particularly in patients with MPNST associated with NF. The 5-year survival was reported to be approximately double in solitary MPNSTs not associated with NF (40–50%) when compared to those associated with NF (20–30%) [2, 9–11].

References

1. Czerniak B. Neurogenous tumors and Neurofibromatosis affecting bone. In: Dorfman HD, Czerniak B, editors. Dorfman and Czerniak's bone tumors. 2nd ed. Amsterdam: Elsevier; 2016. p. 990–1054.
2. Ducatman BS, Scheithauer BW, Piepgras DG, Reiman HM, Ilstrup DM. Malignant peripheral nerve sheath tumors. A clinicopathologic study of 120 cases. Cancer. 1986;57(10):2006–21.
3. Peers JH. Primary intramedullary neurogenic sarcoma of the ulna: report of a case. Am J Pathol. 1934;10(6):811.
4. Bose K, Thakur S, Chakrabarty S, Banerjee S. Intraosseous malignant schwannoma. J Indian Med Assoc. 1970;55:383.
5. Kendi TK, Erakar A, Yildiz HY, Saglik Y, Erekul S. Intraosseous malignant peripheral nerve sheath tumor with local recurrence, lung metastases and death. Skeletal Radiol. 2004;33(4):223–5.
6. Bullock MJ, Bedard YC, Bell RS, Kandel R. Intraosseous malignant peripheral nerve sheath tumor. Report of a case and review of the literature. Arch Pathol Lab Med. 1995;119(4):367–70.
7. Terry DG, Sauser DD, Gordon MD. Intraosseous malignant peripheral nerve sheath tumor in a patient with neurofibromatosis. Skeletal Radiol. 1998;27(6):346–9.
8. Sobczuk P, Teterycz P, Czarnecka AM, Świtaj T, Koseła-Paterczyk H, Kozak K, et al. Systemic treatment for advanced and metastatic malignant peripheral nerve sheath tumors—a sarcoma reference center experience. J Clin Med. 2020;9(10):3157.
9. D'Agostino AN, Soule EH, Miller RH. Primary malignant neoplasms of nerves (malignant neurilemomas) in patients without manifestations of multiple neurofibromatosis (von Recklinghausen's disease). Cancer. 1963;16(8):1003–14.
10. D'Agostino AN, Soule EH, Miller RH. Sarcomas of the peripheral nerves and somatic soft tissues associated with multiple neurofibromatosis (von Recklinghausen's disease). Cancer. 1963;16(8):1015–27.
11. Sordillo PP, Helson L, Hajdu SI, Magill GB, Kosloff C, Golbey RB, et al. Malignant schwannoma—clinical characteristics, survival, and response to therapy. Cancer. 1981;47(10):2503–9.

Part VII

Other Mesenchymal Cell Tumors

24 Lipoma

(***lipos*** "fat" + ***ōma*** "forming")

24.1 Definition

Intraosseous lipoma (IL) is a rare benign tumor consisting of mature adipocytes arising within the medullary cavity. IL is divided into three types, namely, intramedullary, intracortical/subperiosteal, and parosteal type.

24.2 Incidence

Although lipoma is one of the most common soft tissue tumors, IL is one of the rarest primary bone tumors. Some authors have reported accounting for less than 0.1% of primary bone tumors [1–3]. However, others have reported the higher incidence up to 2.5% [4–7]. The real incidence should be higher because many patients with IP have asymptomatic to only minor pain or discomfort, and the lesions are incidentally found on radiographs for other reasons. Parosteal lipoma (PL) is extremely rare, constituting about 0.3% of all lipomas [8].

24.3 Age

It presents with extremely wide range of age between first and ninth decades of life but usually found in the fourth and fifth decades [9–11].

24.4 Location

Although it can occur essentially any bone with fat tissue, the lesion is most commonly found in calcaneus and metaphyseal regions of long bone of lower extremity including femur, tibia, and fibula (Figs. 24.1, 24.2, 24.3, 24.4, 24.5, 24.6 and 24.7). Intertrochanteric region of the femur and calcaneus is the most prevalent locations. Rarely, it is found in upper extremity, pelvis, spine, rib, skull, and mandible. Extremely rarely, it has been reported to occur in parosteal region of long bone [12–17] (Fig. 24.8).

W.-J. Bahk, *Diagnosis and Management of Primary Bone Tumors*,
https://doi.org/10.1007/978-981-99-5498-8_24

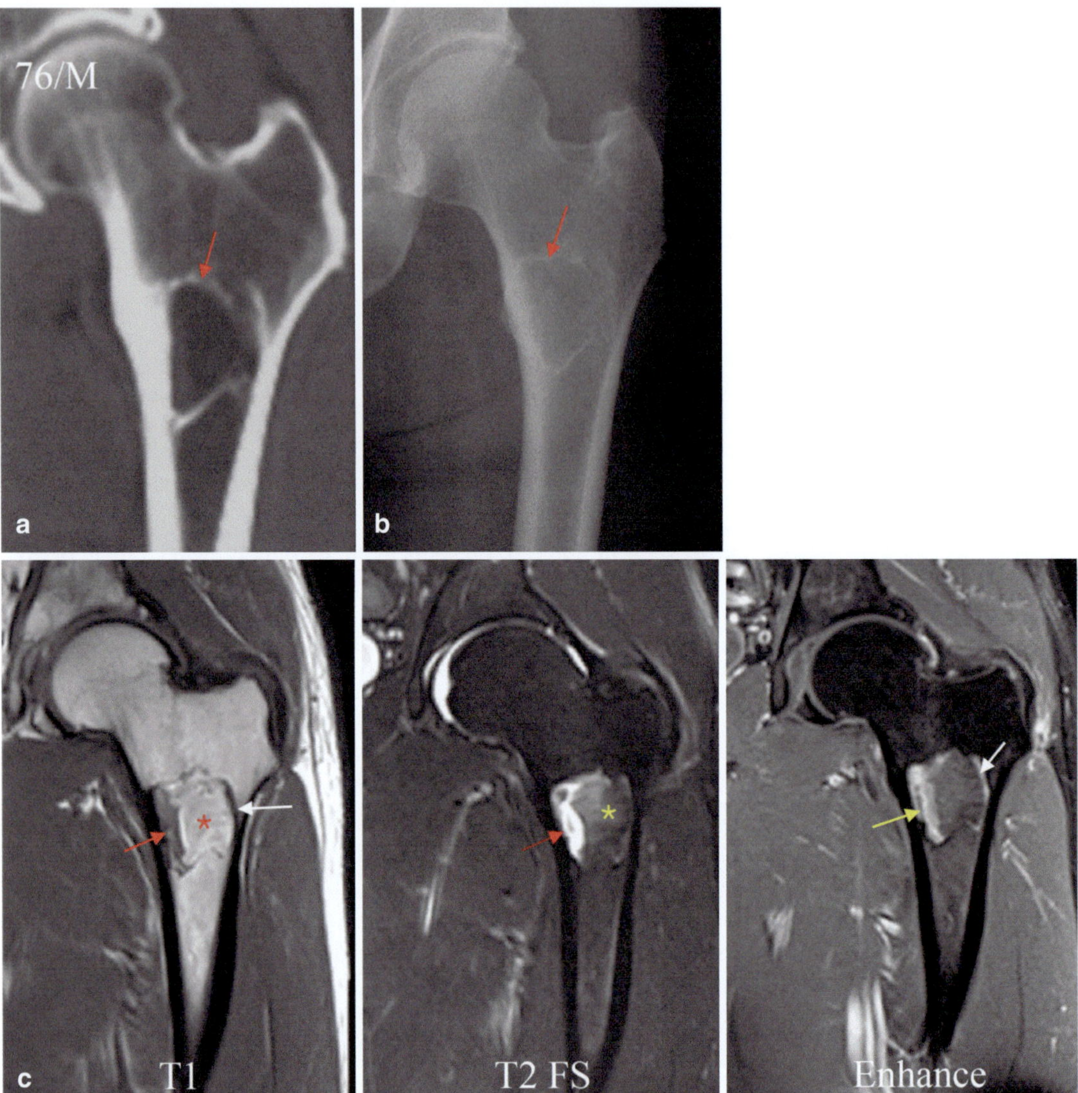

Fig. 24.1 (**a**) Abdomen and pelvis CT scan taken for an evaluation of nephropathy in 76-year-old man incidentally shows a well-defined radiolucent lesion surrounded by a complete rim of sclerosis (arrow) involving proximal femur. (**b**) Radiograph reveals the same findings as CT scan (arrow). (**c**) MR images demonstrate a well-defined intramedullary lesion with mostly high SI (red asterisk) with a focal area of low to intermediate SI (red arrow) on T1-weighted image, and the high signal portion is mostly suppressed (yellow asterisk) indicating fatty tissue component with a focal area of high signal (red arrow) suggesting myxoid or cystic change on fat saturated T2-weighted image. This focal lesion is diffusely enhanced (yellow arrow) suggesting myxoid change rather than cystic change. The lesion itself shows only peripheral thin enhancement (white arrow). (**d**) Pinhole bone scan shows normal to very subtle increased uptake at medial aspect of the lesion (red arrow). (**e**) Microscopic examination notes that most areas consist abundant fat cells, some areas of foamy macrophages, and ghost outlines of necrotic fat cells with dystrophic calcification in some areas indicating IL *(stage 2 lesion)*. No surgical management was performed

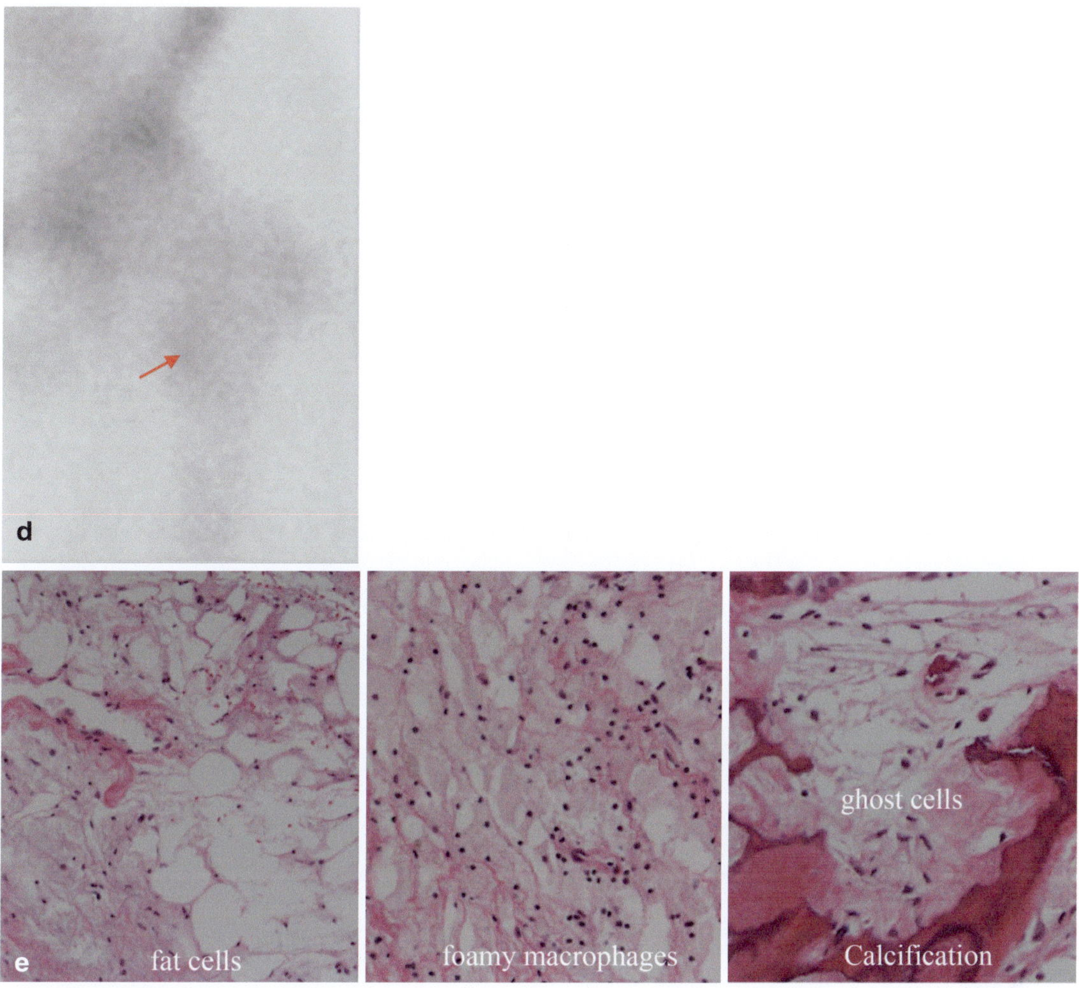

Fig. 24.1 (continued)

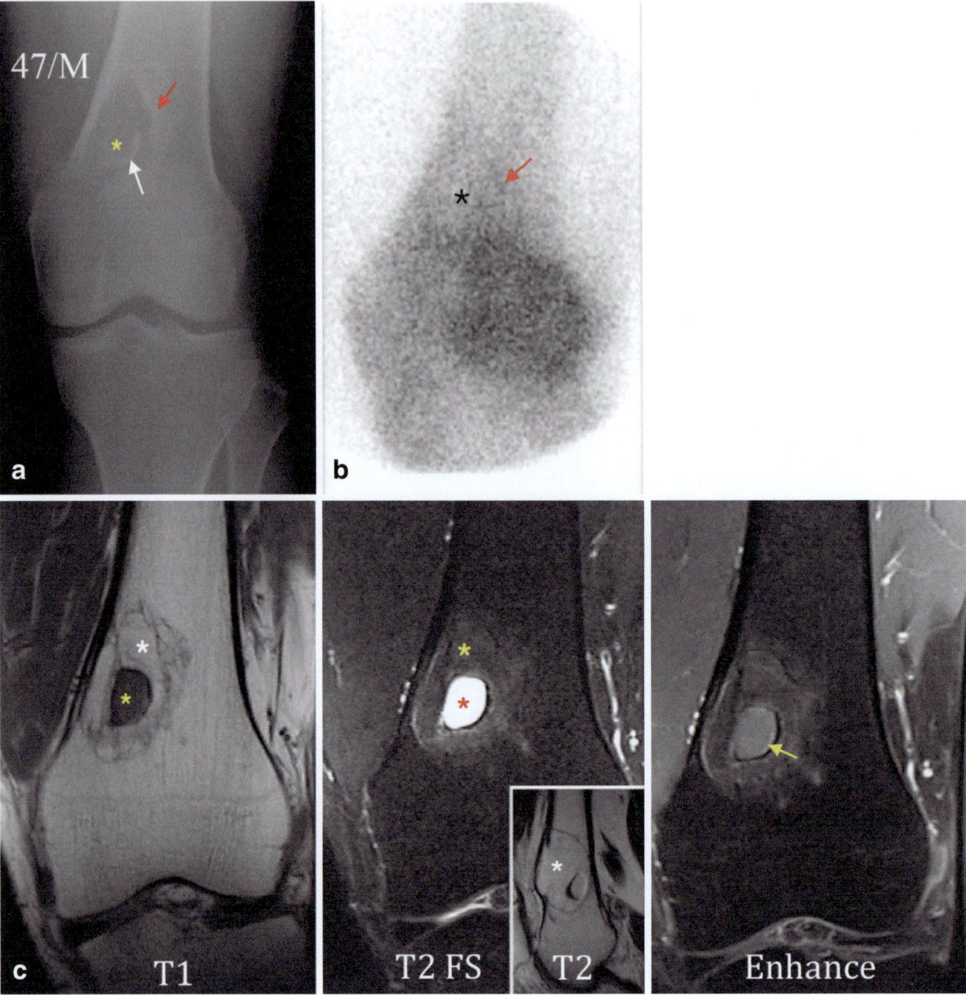

Fig. 24.2 (**a**) Radiograph taken for left distal thigh pain 47-year-old man shows a well-defined radiolucent lesion with a surround rim of sclerosis (red arrow) and central smaller, round to oval, mixed lytic and sclerotic lesion (yellow asterisk) surrounded by a thin sclerotic rim (white arrow), so-called *"bull's eye* or *"target*" appearance, in the metaphyseal area of right distal femur. (**b**) Pinhole bone scan reveals mildly increased uptake along the reactive sclerotic shell (red arrow) with internal photon defect (asterisk). (**c**) MR images demonstrate a medullary mass-like lesion with high SI (white asterisks) on both T1- and T2-weighted images (inset), which is suppressed to become low signal (yellow asterisk) on fat saturated T2-weighted image, indicating fatty component. There is a central round to oval area with low signal (yellow asterisk) on T1-weighted image and bright signal (red asterisk) on fat saturated T2-weighted image, suggesting cystic change surrounded by a thin rim of dark signal of reactive rim. The lesion is only partially enhanced along the periphery (yellow arrow). (**d**) Follow-up radiograph at 1 year after curettage and allo-chip bone graft notes under a histologic confirmation of *stage 2 IL* notes consolidation of the lesion (asterisk). (**e**) Radiograph taken for left knee pain in 64-year-old woman shows a relatively well-defined eccentric radiolucent lesion with internal irregular calcification surrounded by a thin rim of sclerosis (yellow arrows) involving the epi-metaphyseal area of medial femoral condyle. Note mild budging or expansion (white arrow) that is useful finding to distinct IL from bone infarct together with eccentric location. The more prominent heterogeneity and mild bone expansion indicate significant involution. (**f**) Bone scan reveals an internal focal hot uptake with lesser increase uptake in the periphery of the lesion (red arrows). (**g**) MR images reveal a well-defined intramedullary mass lesion with heterogeneous low and high SI on T1-weighted image. The high signal becomes low signal (white arrow) by fat suppression indicating fat component, and the bright signal without suppression (yellow arrow) suggests cystic or myxoid change on fat-saturated T2-weighted image. Focal areas of dark signal of heavy dystrophic calcification are focally noted. The lesion is heterogeneously enhanced by contrast medium (yellow arrow), which may suggest a possible malignant change. However, microscopic examination of incision biopsy notes marked involution changes such as reactive bone formation, calcification, fibrosis, myxoid degeneration change, foamy macrophages, and old hemosiderin pigments but no evidence for malignancy, indicating *stage 3 IL*

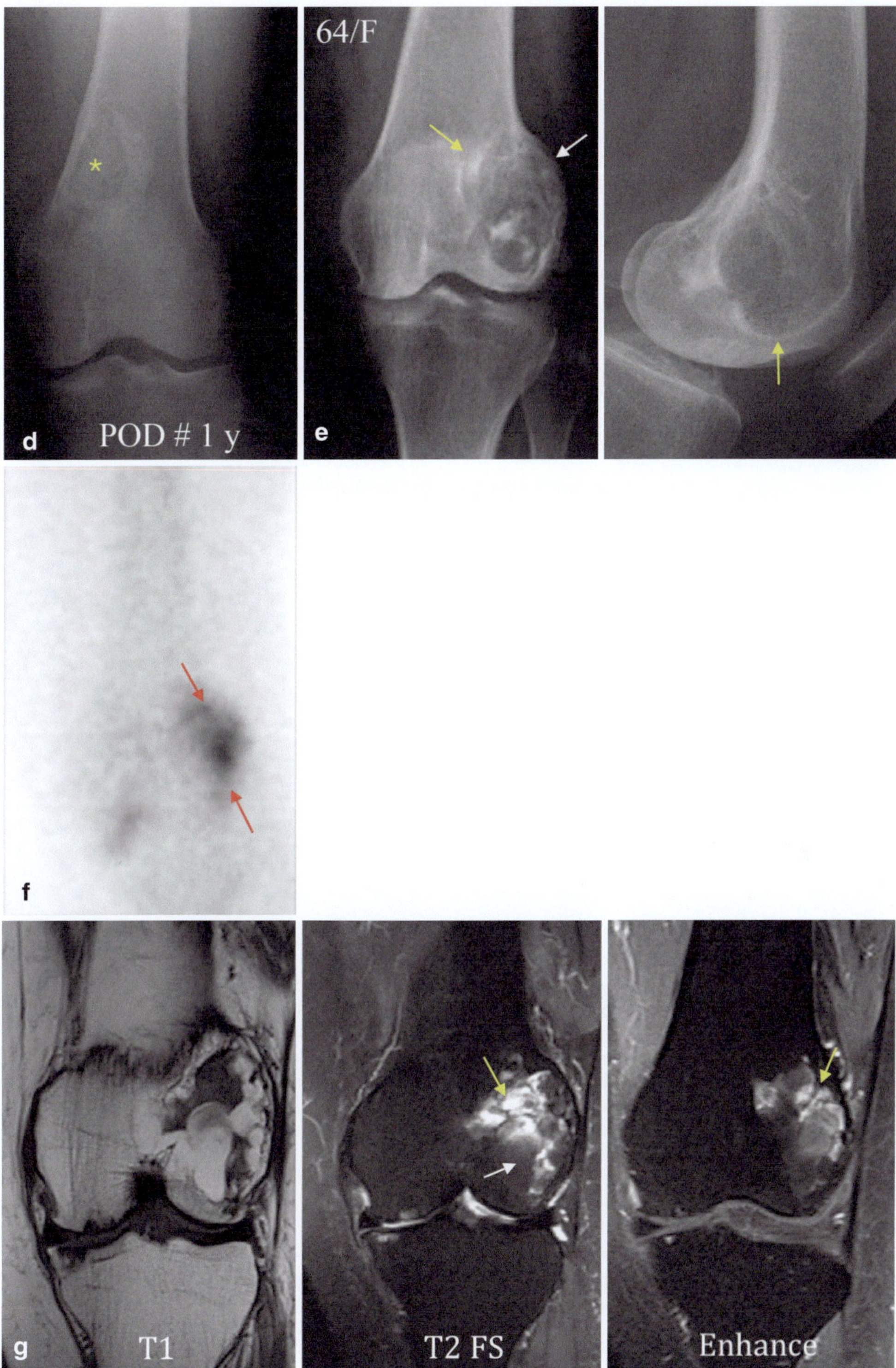

Fig. 24.2 (continued)

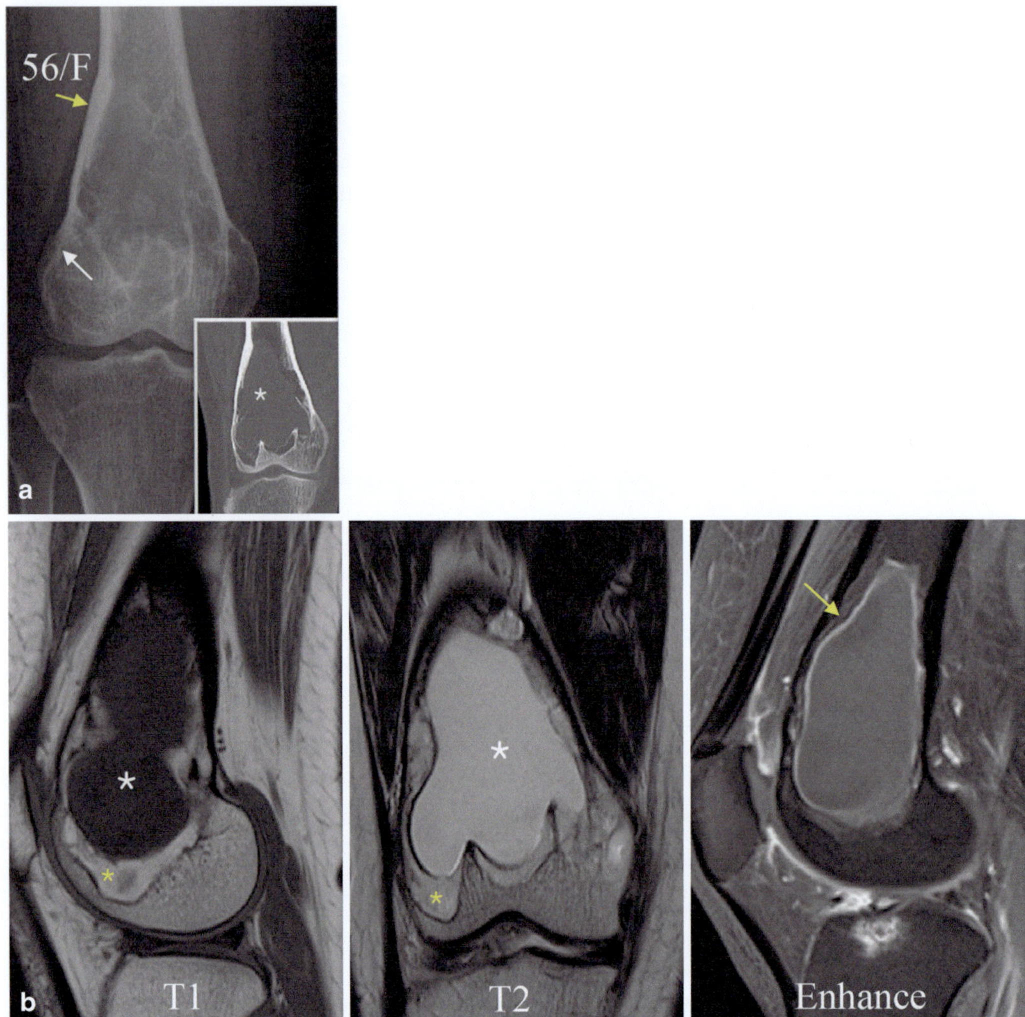

Fig. 24.3 (**a**) Radiographs taken for right knee pain of 6-month duration in 56-year-old woman shows a large multi-septated radiolucent lesion with multiple thin peripheral trabecular ridges and thin rim of sclerosis affecting the epi-metaphysis of the distal femur. Note mild expansion and cortical thickening (yellow arrow) as well as thinning with endosteal scalloping (white arrow). CT scan reveals a well-defined low density of fat tissue or cystic component surrounded by a thin rim of sclerosis (inset). (**b**) MR images demonstrate a huge medullar occupying lesion with mostly low SI on T1-weighted image and high SI on T2-weighted image (white asterisks), suggesting cystic component. There is a peripheral small area of high signal (yellow asterisks) on both T1- and T2-weighted images, indicating fatty component. The cystic lesion is peripherally enhanced (yellow arrow). (**c**) Microscopic examination notes involution changes of the entire lesion including necrotic fat with varying degree of calcification, cyst formation, and reactive new bone formation indicating *stage 3 IL.* (**d**) Follow-up radiograph at 8 months after curettage and chip-bone graft notes consolidation of the lesion. (**e**) Radiographs taken for left knee pain of 3-year duration in 55-year-old man shows an ill-defined radiolucent lesion (yellow arrow) with multiple internal calcifications. (**f**) MR images reveals a well-defined medullar occupying lesion with high SI surrounded by a thin sclerotic rim of dark signal both on T1- and T2-weighted images (red circles). The high signal is suppressed to be dark fat signal drop (yellow circle) on fat saturated T2-weighted image. In addition, there is central low signal on T1-weighted image and heterogeneous high with focal low signal on T2-weighted image that is not suppressed on fat saturated T2-weighted image, indicating involution change such as necrosis, calcification, and cystic change. The central small lesion of involution change is heterogeneously enhanced (yellow arrow). Microscopic examination notes areas of viable fat cells with focal areas of spontaneous infarction due to expansion of fat cells confined to certain part of the lesion. Some portions of fat necrosis are calcified, and primitive woven bone is deposited indicating *stage 2 IL.* (**g**) Follow-up radiograph at 6 months after curettage and chip-bone graft shows partial consolidation of the lesion

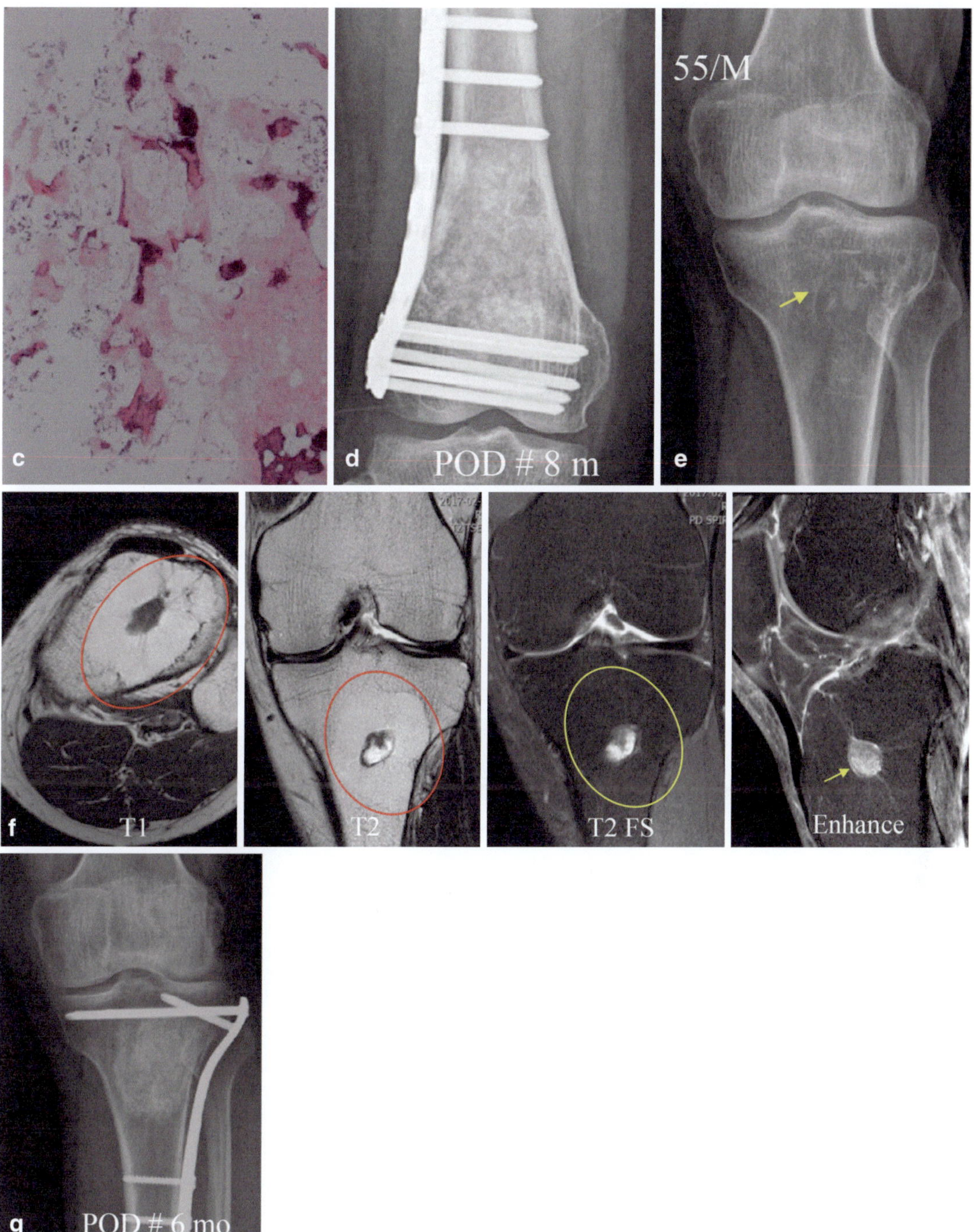

Fig. 24.3 (continued)

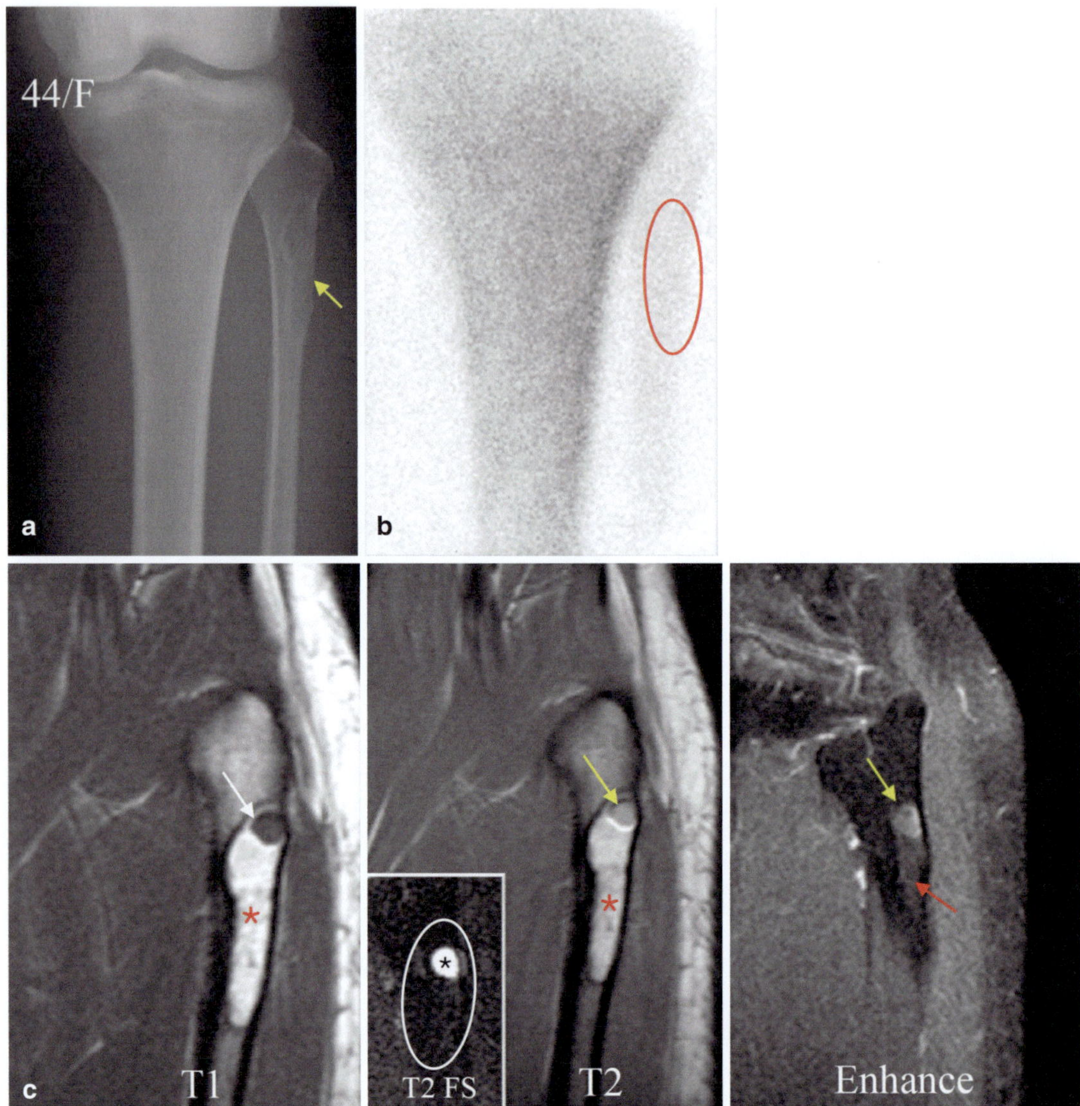

Fig. 24.4 (**a**) Radiograph taken for left proximal leg pain of 1-month duration in 44-year-old man shows a well-defined eccentric osteolytic lesion surrounded by a thin rim of sclerosis with mild expansion and cortical thinning (yellow arrow) affecting the proximal fibula. (**b**) Pinhole bone scan reveals no definite increased uptake (red circle) in the lesion. (**c**) MR images demonstrate a well-defined, elongated, eccentric lesion with intermediate and high SI both on T1- and T2-weighted images (red asterisks) indicating fat component in the meta-diaphysis of left proximal fibula. There is a focal area with low SI on T1-weighted image (white arrow) and intermediate to high SI on T2-weighted image (yellow arrow). Low signal sclerotic rim is also present on both sequences. Diffuse fat suppression (white circle) except cystic area (black asterisk) is observed on fat-saturated T2-weighted image (inset). Post-contrast image shows mild to no enhancement of most solid portion (red arrow) but a diffuse enhancement of focal cystic or myxoid area in the upper portion of the lesion (yellow arrow). (**d**) Follow-up radiograph at 12 years after curettage and allo-chip bone graft notes consolidation of the lesion (yellow arrow). (**e**) Radiograph taken for right hip discomfort of 2-week duration in 37-year-old lady shows a well-defined radiolucent lesion surrounded by a thin rim of sclerosis with internal calcification involving acetabulum (red arrow). (**f**) Pinhole bone scan reveals no definite abnormal uptake in the lesion (circle). (**g**) MR images demonstrate a well-defined mass-like lesion mainly with intermediate to high SI, which is identical to adjacent bone marrow or subcutaneous fat with a dark signal of thin sclerotic rim on both sequences involving right acetabulum. Fat-saturated T2-weighted image reveals a dark fat drop signal (yellow asterisks) in most of the lesion with focal tiny dot areas of non-suppression indicating calcification and cystic change. The lesion is focally enhanced (white arrow). (**h**) Surgical procedure including incisional biopsy was not performed, and radiograph at 1-year follow-up notes no interval change

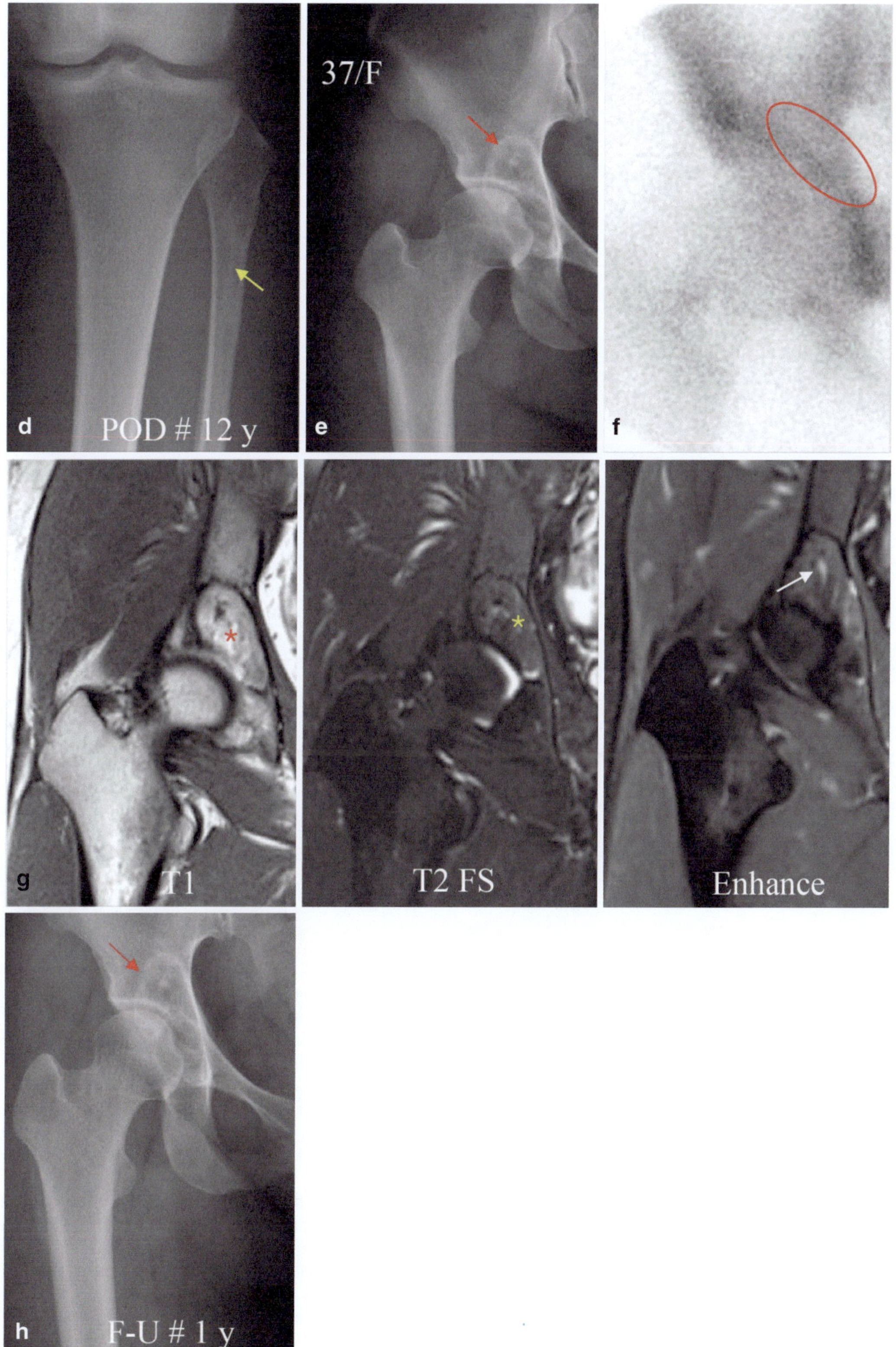

Fig. 24.4 (continued)

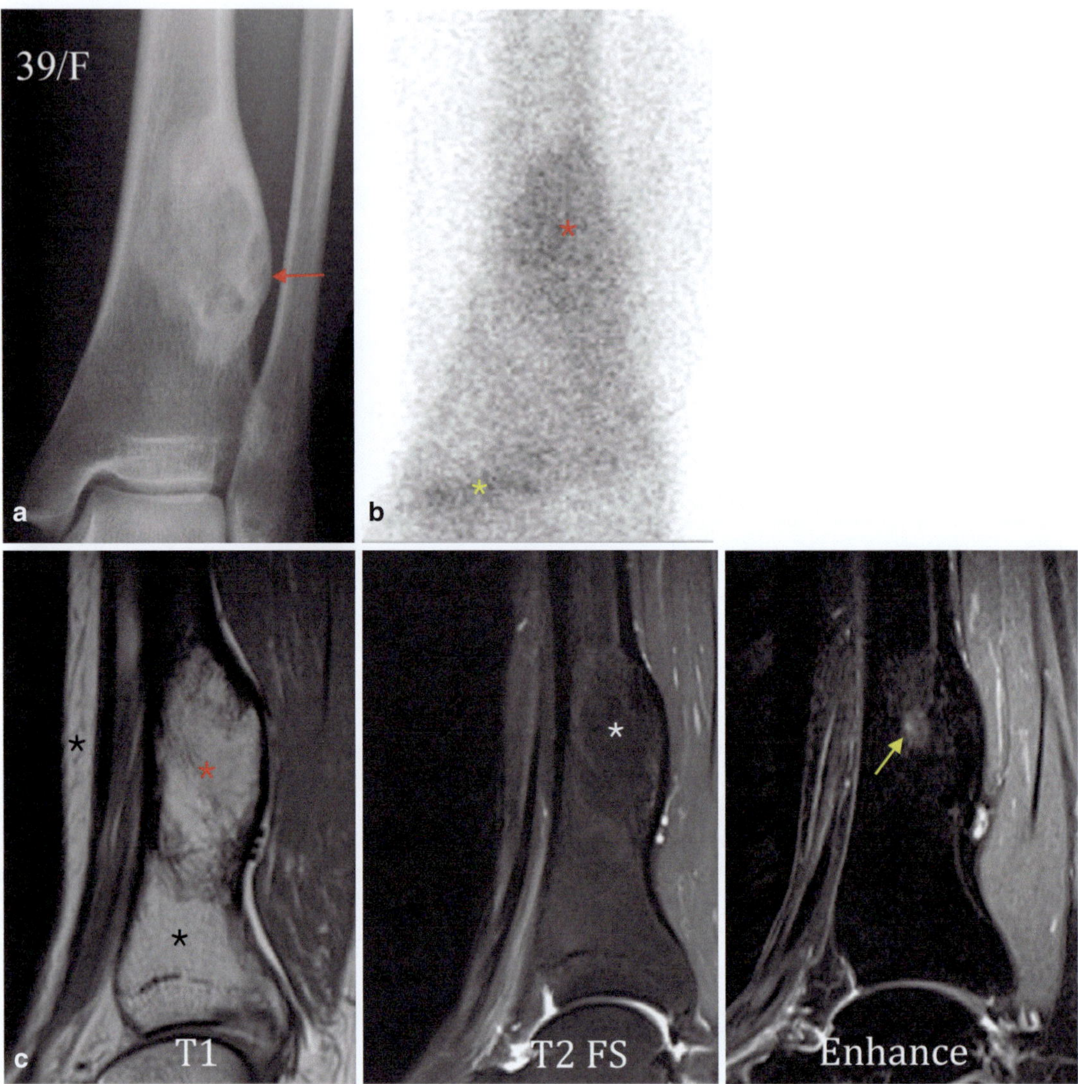

Fig. 24.5 (**a**) Radiographs taken for left ankle pain of 4-month duration in 39-year-old lady show a multilobulated, eccentric, radiolucent lesion with some internal dense areas involving the distal tibia. There is a moderate bulging with cortical thinning but no unequivocal destruction (red arrow). (**b**) Pinhole bone scan reveals a mild uptake in the lesion (red asterisk) and another linear uptake in the distal tibia (yellow asterisk) suggesting reactive change that is not reflected on MR images. (**c**) MR images demonstrate an eccentrically bulging mass-like lesion without cortical destruction in the distal tibia. The signal intensity is mainly high (red asterisk) being equivalent to adjacent bone marrow or subcutaneous fat (black asterisks) with focal low signals of involution on both T1- T2-weighted images (not shown here). The fat signal is diffusely suppressed to become low signal on fat saturated T2-weighted image (white asterisk). The lesion is focally enhanced (yellow arrow). Curettage and bone graft were performed, and histologic diagnosis of *stage 2 IL* was made. (**d**) Radiograph at 4 years after surgery notes consolidation of the lesion. (**e**) Radiographs taken for right ankle discomfort of 1-month duration in 65-year-old man show a hazy radiolucent lesion with a thin rim of sclerosis (red arrow) and internal dense oval lesion (yellow asterisk) in the meta-diaphysis of the distal tibia. (**f**) Pinhole bone scan reveals no remarkable increase of uptake in the lesion (asterisk). (**g**) MR images demonstrate a large well-defined lesion with high SI on both T1- and T2- weighted images (red asterisks), which are similar to subcutaneous fat and bone marrow (white asterisks), surrounded by a dark thin rim of sclerosis. In addition, the lesion contains mostly low signal on T1-weighted image and high signal on T2-weighted image (yellow asterisks) with tiny area of dark signal in the center of the lesion, suggesting cystic change with calcification. The lesion is partially enhanced only in the inferior part (red arrow). (**h**) Surgical procedure including incisional biopsy was not performed, and radiograph at 2-year follow-up notes no interval change

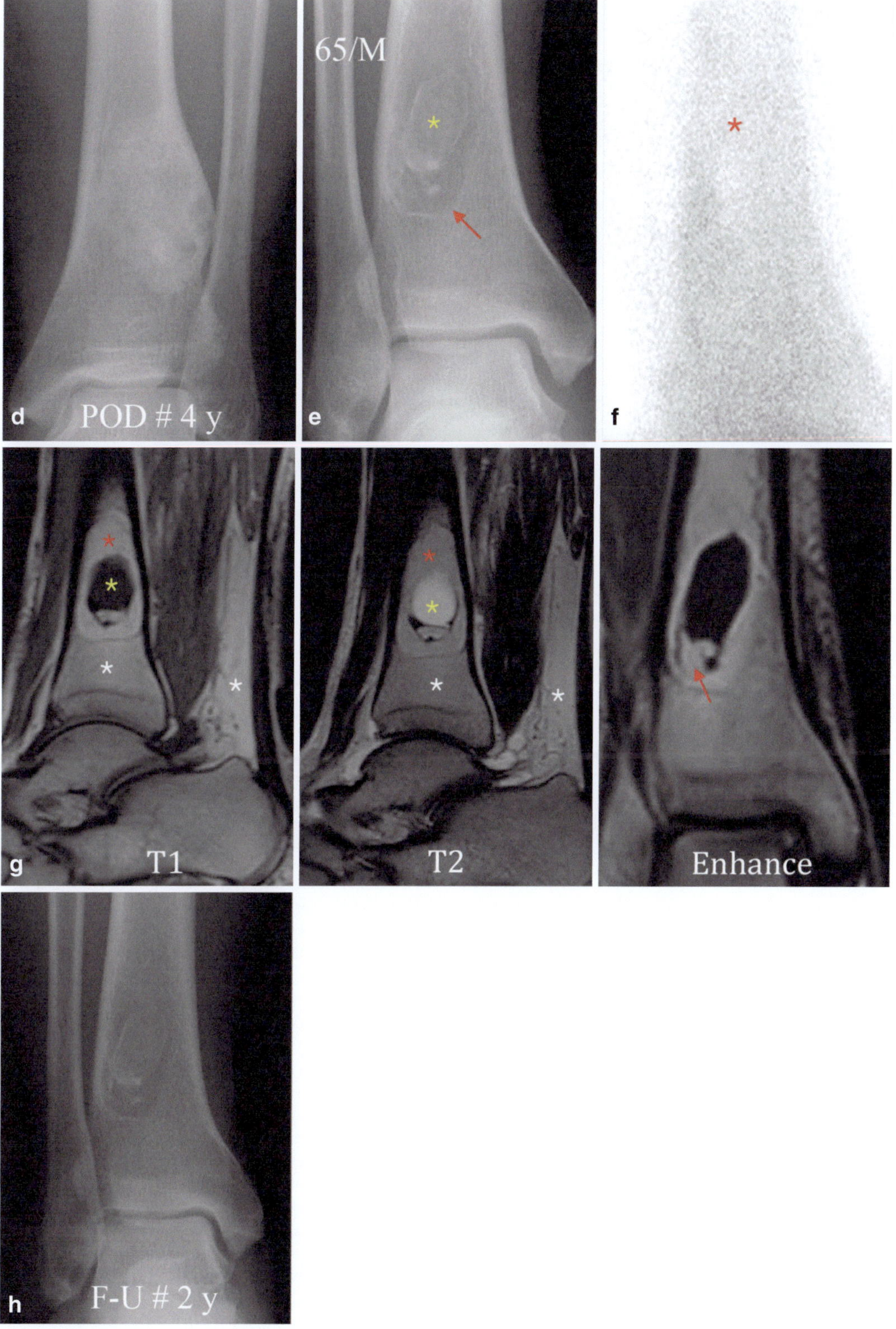

Fig. 24.5 (continued)

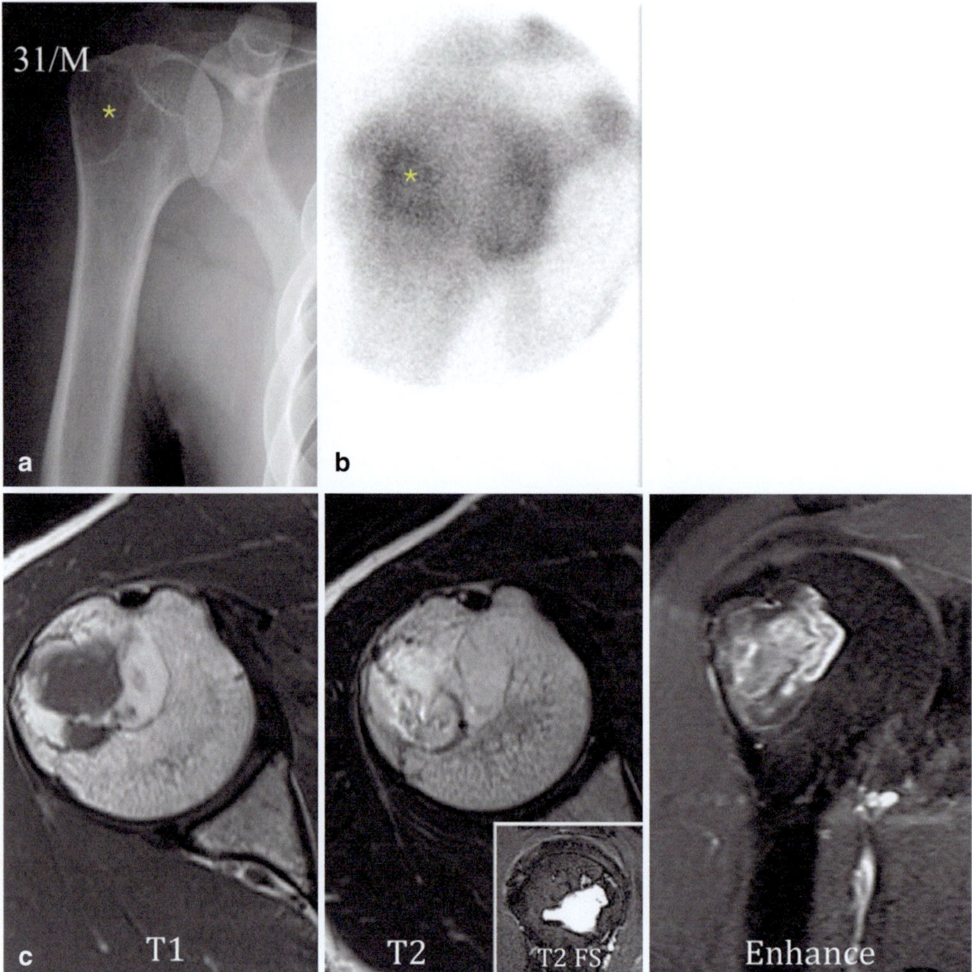

Fig. 24.6 (**a**) Radiograph taken for right shoulder pain of 1-year duration in 31-year-old man shows a multi-lobulated radiolucent lesion (asterisk) with a thin rim of sclerosis in greater tuberosity area of the humerus. (**b**) Pinhole bone scan reveals a heterogeneous moderate uptake at greater tuberosity (asterisk). (**c**) MR images demonstrate a well-defined multi-lobulated mass lesion with heterogeneous low and intermediate to high SI on both T1- and T2-weighted images. There are central areas of low signal on T1-weighted image and high to bright signal on T2-weighted image suggesting cystic change. Peripheral signal drop is noted with internal bight signal of cystic change on fat-saturated T2-weighted image (inset). The lesion is heterogeneously enhanced along the periphery with focal internal enhancement suggesting involutional changes. (**d**) Follow-up radiograph at 6 months after curettage and bone graft notes consolidation of the lesion. (**e**) Radiograph taken for right shoulder pain with acro-clavicular (AC) joint tenderness of 2-month duration in 29-year-old man shows a multi-septated osteolytic lesion with internal sclerotic areas (asterisk) in the humeral head and neck area. Note additional irregular erosion and resorption of the subchondral bone of distal end of right clavicle with widening of the acro-clavicular (AC) joint space (yellow arrow in inset), suggesting *"distal clavicle osteolysis"* that was initially neglected on this radiograph. He was a worker who undergoes repeated micro-injury of his right shoulder during setup air-conditioners on the wall. (**f**) Pinhole bone scan reveals a heterogeneous moderate to hot uptake with inner focal lesser activity (asterisk) in the lesion as well as in articular bones of right AC joint (circle). (**g**) MR images demonstrate a medullar occupying lesion with consecutive peripheral high fat signal and internal low cystic signal mainly in the metaphysis of proximal humerus on T1-weighted images. A fat signal drop is observed with high signal of cystic change on fat saturated T2-weighted image. The lesion is peripherally enhanced with internal focal enhancement. (inset) There is additional findings of irregular articular erosion of distal clavicle with widening of AC joint capsule, bone marrow, and soft tissue edema. The signal intensity is low on T1-weighted image and heterogeneously high SI on fat saturation T2-weighted image, which are diffusely well enhanced. The AC joint lesion is consistent with *"distal clavicle osteolysis"* producing AC joint tenderness. (**h**) Follow-up radiograph at 9 years after curettage and bone graft for IL notes consolidation of the lipoma lesion as well as healing of the *"distal clavicle osteolysis"* without surgical management (yellow arrow in inset). He is free of pain at last follow-up

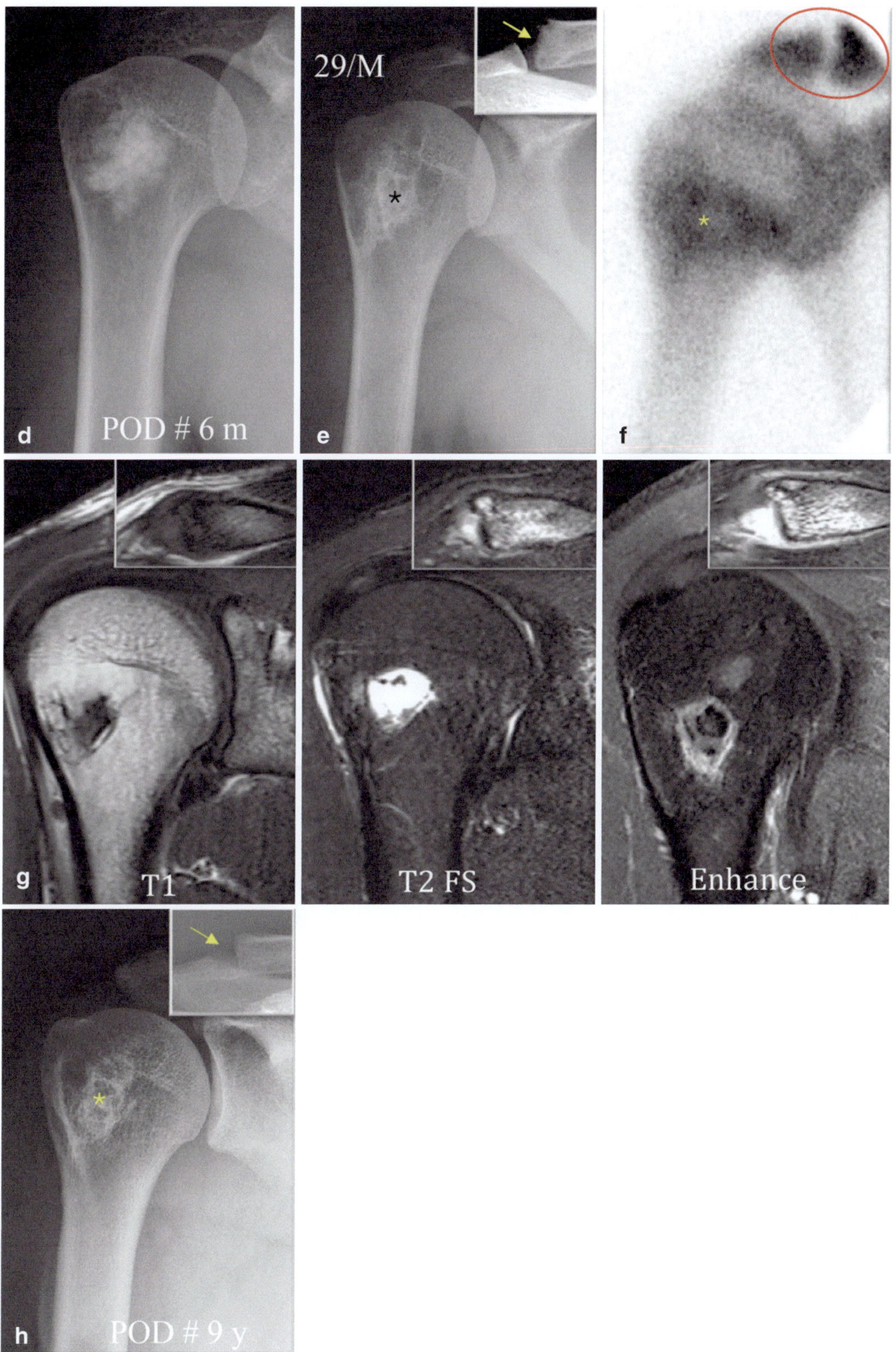

Fig. 24.6 (continued)

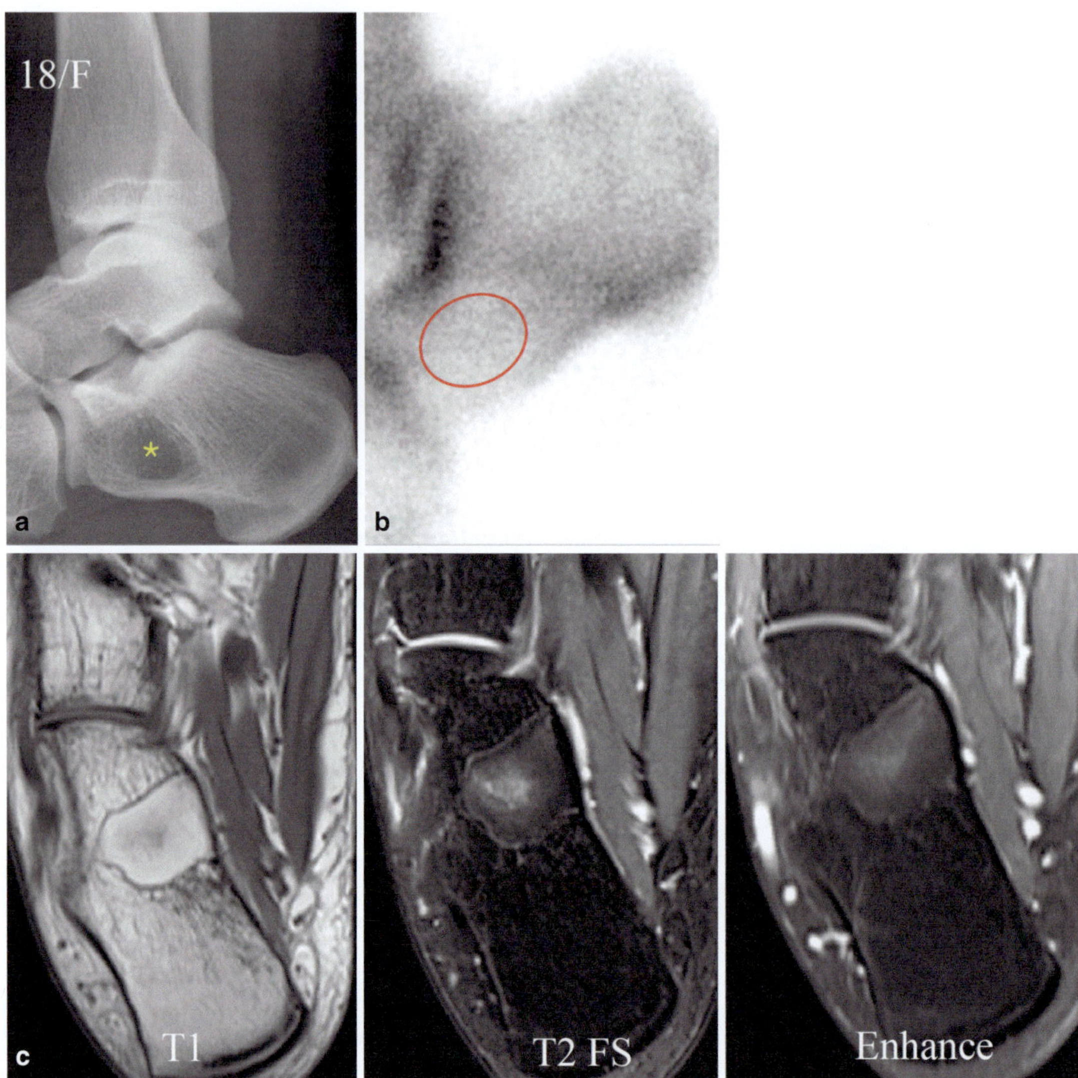

Fig. 24.7 (**a**) Radiographs taken for left ankle pain of 3-month duration in 18-year-old girl shows a well-defined round to oval radiolucent lesion affecting the calcaneus (asterisk). (**b**) Pinhole bone scan reveals no increased uptake (circle). (**c**) MR images demonstrate a well-defined mass lesion surrounded by a thin rim of sclerosis with mainly fat signal with internal focal cystic change. Fat-saturated T2-weighted image notes fat signal drop with an internal high signal of cystic change. The lesion is partially and peripherally enhanced. (**d**) Follow-up radiograph at 9 months after curettage and bone graft notes consolidation of the lipoma (asterisk). (**e**) Radiographs show various radiolucent lesions affecting calcaneus including lipoma, simple bone cyst, and secondary aneurysmal bone cyst with giant cell tumor. Lipoma arising in calcaneus shows oval to quadrangular lytic lesion with peripheral rim of sclerosis is equivalent to calcaneal cyst, but central calcification is often associated in the lipoma lesion creating a *"cockade sign"* (yellow arrows), which is typical for lipoma

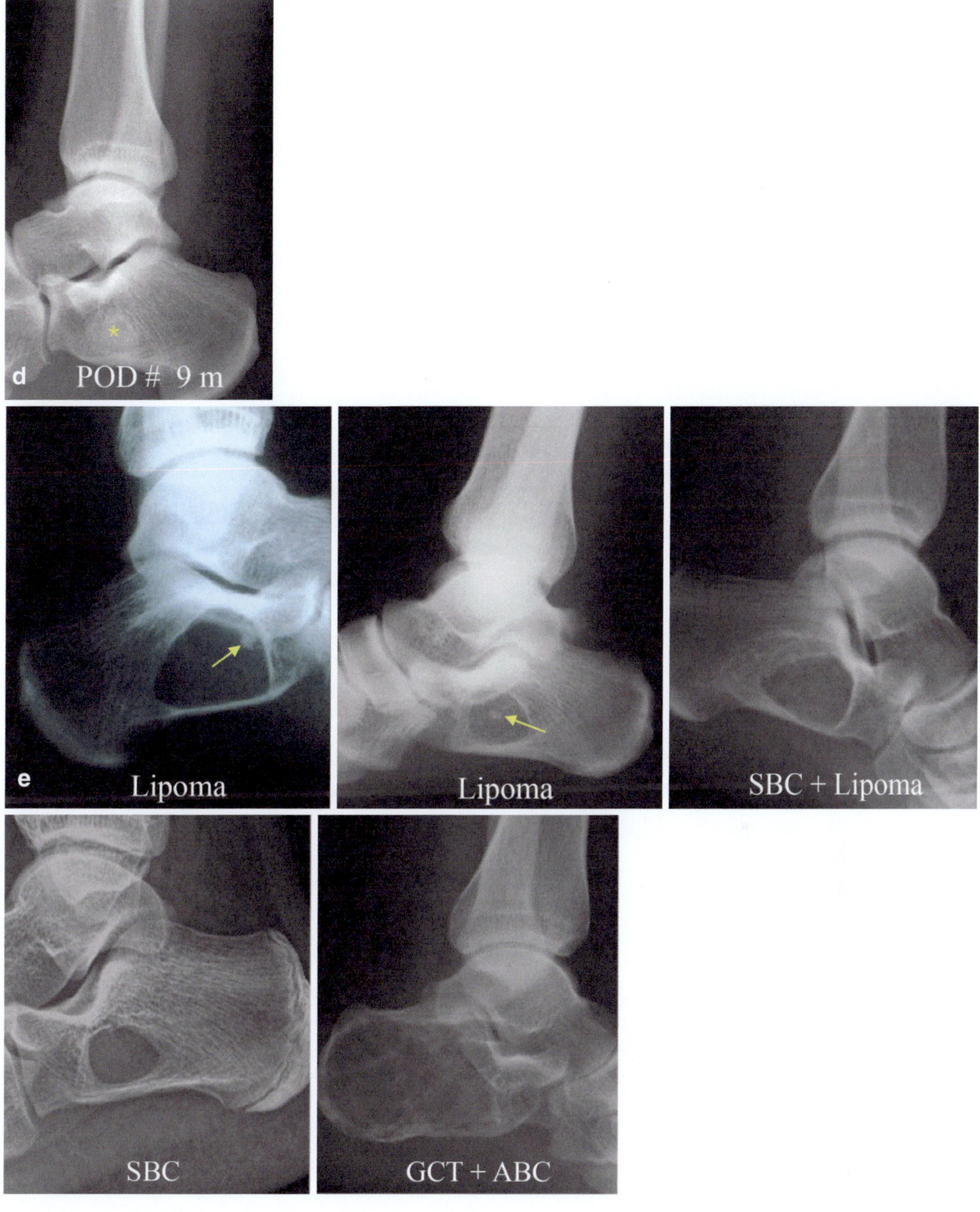

Fig. 24.7 (continued)

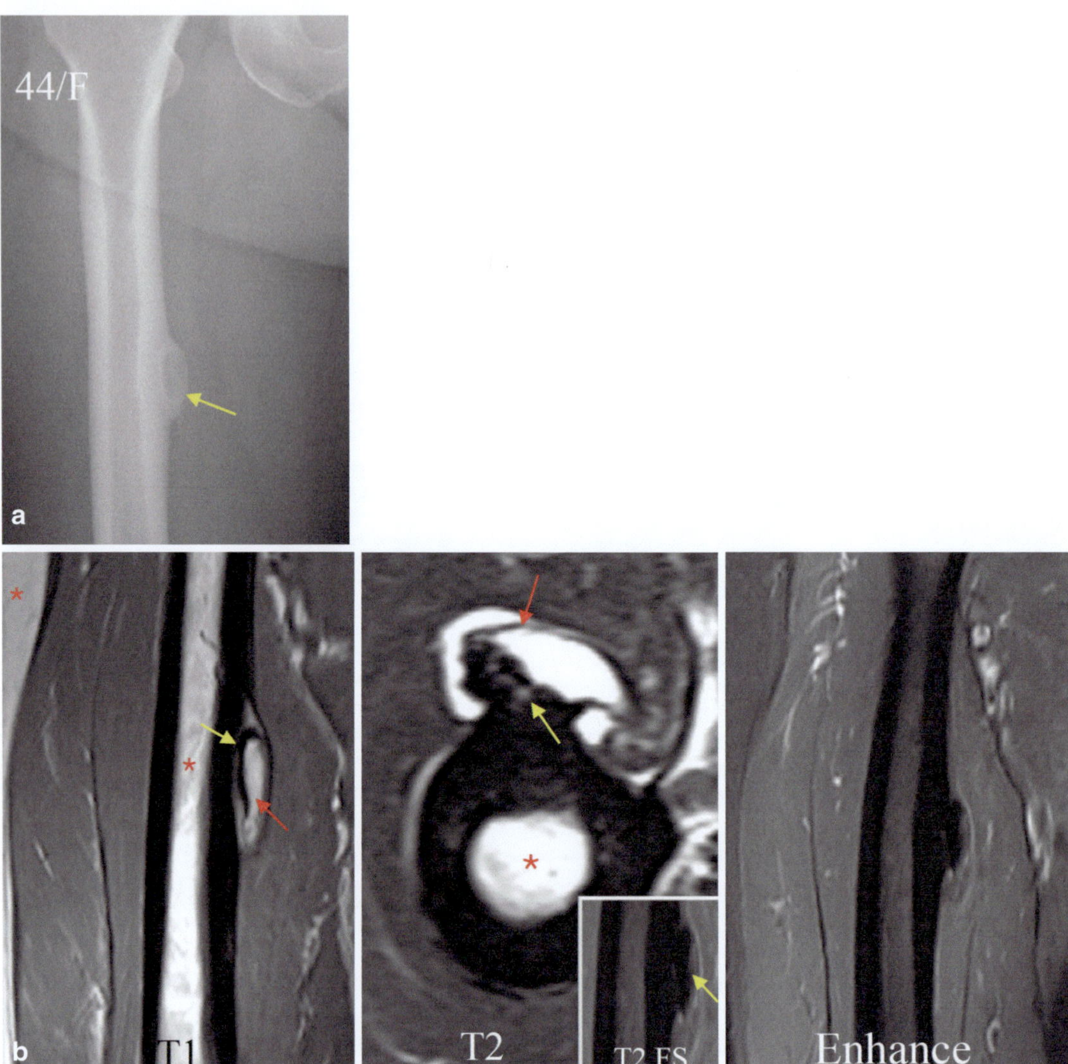

Fig. 24.8 ***Parosteal lipoma*** (**a**) Radiograph taken for right thigh mass of 6-month duration in 44-year-old woman shows a juxta-cortical lucent mass surrounded by thick sclerotic rim (arrow). (**b**) MR images reveal a periosteal protruding mass with mostly high SI of fat component (red arrows) on both T1- and T2-weighted images, being equivalent to bone marrow and subcutaneous fat (red asterisks). There is also focal areas of dark signal suggesting calcification (yellow arrows). Fat-saturated T2-weighted image shows fat signal drop (yellow arrow in inset). The mass is not communicated with marrow and not enhanced by contrast medium. (**c**) A yellowish hard mass is firmly attached to the cortex (asterisk). (**d**) Excised mass seems to be similar to soft tissue lipoma but contains several firm to hard small nodules over the mass suggesting calcification (asterisk). (**e**) Microscopic examination notes lobules of mature-appearing adipocytes (black asterisk) encasing pre-existing host bone trabeculae (white asterisk). Fibroblastic formation of collagen bundles and reactive ossification resembling primitive woven bone are deposited around the infarcted area (inset). (**f**) Follow-up radiograph at 6 months after excision shows no evidence of local recurrence (arrow)

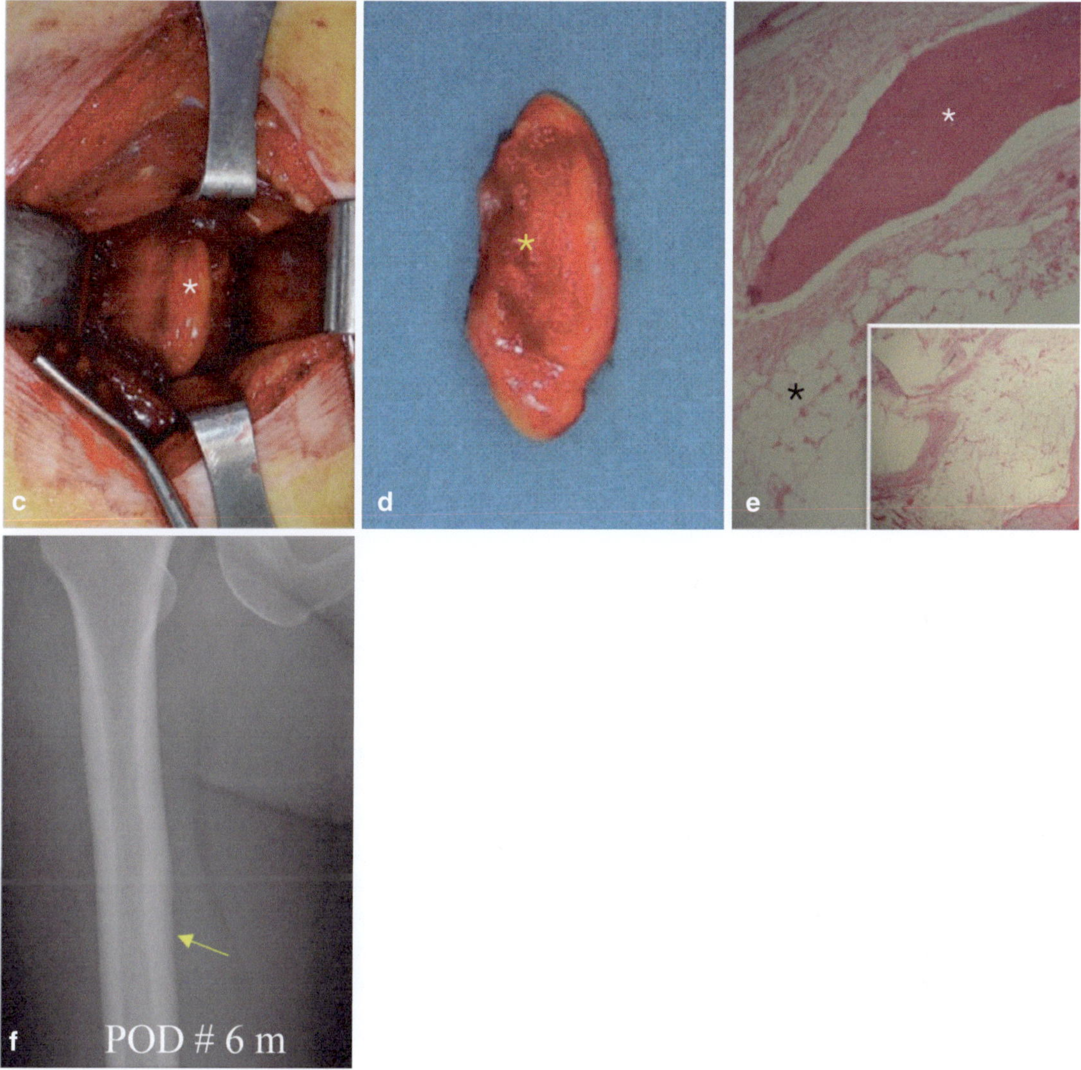

Fig. 24.8 (continued)

24.5 Clinical Presentations

Mild pain or discomfort is the most common presenting symptom in about 70% of patients [10, 18], but it can be occasionally asymptomatic and found incidentally (Fig. 24.1a). PL may present as a slowly growing mass often with local irritation and peripheral neuropathy particularly when occurring in the proximal radius [12, 14–16]. ILs are divided into three stages depending on the degree of histologic involution by Milgram [19]: Stage 1, tumors of viable fat cells; Stage 2, transitional cases composed partly of viable fat cells and fat necrosis and calcification; and Stage 3, lesions demonstrating necrotic fat, calcification of necrotic fat, variable degrees of cyst formation, and reactive woven bone formation.

24.6 Radiologic Findings

The findings on radiographs, CT scan, and MR images can vary with the stage depending on various histologic composition of fat and fibrous tissue, ossification or mineralization of bone, and cystic degeneration [8] (Figs. 24.1, 24.2, 24.3, 24.4, 24.5, 24.6 and 24.7). It is a well-defined osteolytic lesion surrounded by thin rim of sclerosis and mild focal expansion if the lesion consists of only fat component *(Stage 1 lesion)*. The finding is nonspecific and simulates other benign bone tumor such as simple bone cyst or fibrous dysplasia particularly when affecting the calcaneus or trochanter of the femur, respectively. Occasionally, it presents a smooth, fusiform, eccentric expansion that is more prominent with cortical thinning in small caliber bones including fibula, ulna, or rib. A presence of the eccentricity and expansion is useful to differentiate IL from bone infarct that does not exhibit these findings. Thin peripheral trabecular ridges can produce a multi-septated appearance. Varying degree of ossification or dystrophic calcification may be associated within area of fat necrosis in more involution cases *(Stage 2, 3 lesion)*. A central nidus-like calcification or sclerosis in the radiolucent fatty lesion can be observed as a *"bull's eye"* or *"target"* appearance (Fig. 24.2a). If arising in calcaneus, the finding of oval to quadrangular, lytic lesion with a peripheral rim of sclerosis is equivalent to calcaneal cyst, but central calcification in the lesion can make the *"cockade sign,"* which is typical for IL (Fig. 24.7e). **Bone scan** Uptake is varied from none to moderate uptake depending on the stage of lesion (Figs. 24.1, 24.2, 24.4, 24.5, 24.6 and 24.7). The lesion typically appears normal, but it may show moderately increased uptake if the lesion contains calcification of necrotic fat. However, significantly increased uptake is distinctly unusual. **CT scan** demonstrates a low density of fatty component similar to fat tissue as well as varying degrees of central necrosis, cystic change, calcifications, or ossification depending on the stages. **MR Findings** Fat signal in the lesion is similar to that of subcutaneous fat. The fatty components of IL may display varying degrees of involution and necrosis (Figs. 24.1, 24.2, 24.3, 24.4, 24.5 and 24.6). *Stage 1 Lesion*: The signal is homogeneous high SI on both T1- and T2-weighted images that can be totally suppressed on STIR or fat-saturated images. The trabecular cancellous bone pattern is typically lost within the lesion. *Stage 2 Lesion*: The signal is low on T1-weighted image and heterogeneous high due to granulation tissue or necrosis and low due to calcifications or ossification on fat-suppressed T2-weighted image. *Stage 3 Lesion:* The signal is more heterogeneous than that of *stage 2 lesion*, which may contain cystic cavity, signal-void bony septa, and rims of reactive sclerotic bone depending on the amount of various components. Over time, the lesion can be eccentrically expansile and outgrow the cortical border without destruction.

24.7 Histologic Findings

IL consists of lobules of mature adipocytes identical to its soft tissue counterpart, which replace marrow space and encase pre-existing host bone trabeculae by the tumor cells (Fig. 24.8e). Lipoma is typically composed of lobules of mature fat cells bigger than normal white adipose tissue devoid of admixed hematopoietic tissues or bony trabeculae. Each adipocyte has a single large, clear, cytoplasmic vacuole that typically displaces the nucleus to periphery making crescent-shape (Fig. 24.9a). A lobule with mature fat cells and some infarcted cells is surrounded by reactive collagen bundle and cartilage undergoing endochondral ossification (Fig. 24.9b). With time, the lesion undergoes spontaneous involution changes including granulation tissue, fat necrosis, dystrophic calcification, cystic change, ossification, or reactive bone formation. Some necrotic adipocytes have ghostlike outlines in association with extensive dystrophic calcification (Fig. 24.9c). The presence of fat necrosis with dystrophic calcification corresponds to central, nidus-like opacity on radiograph, so-called *"bull's eye"* appearance

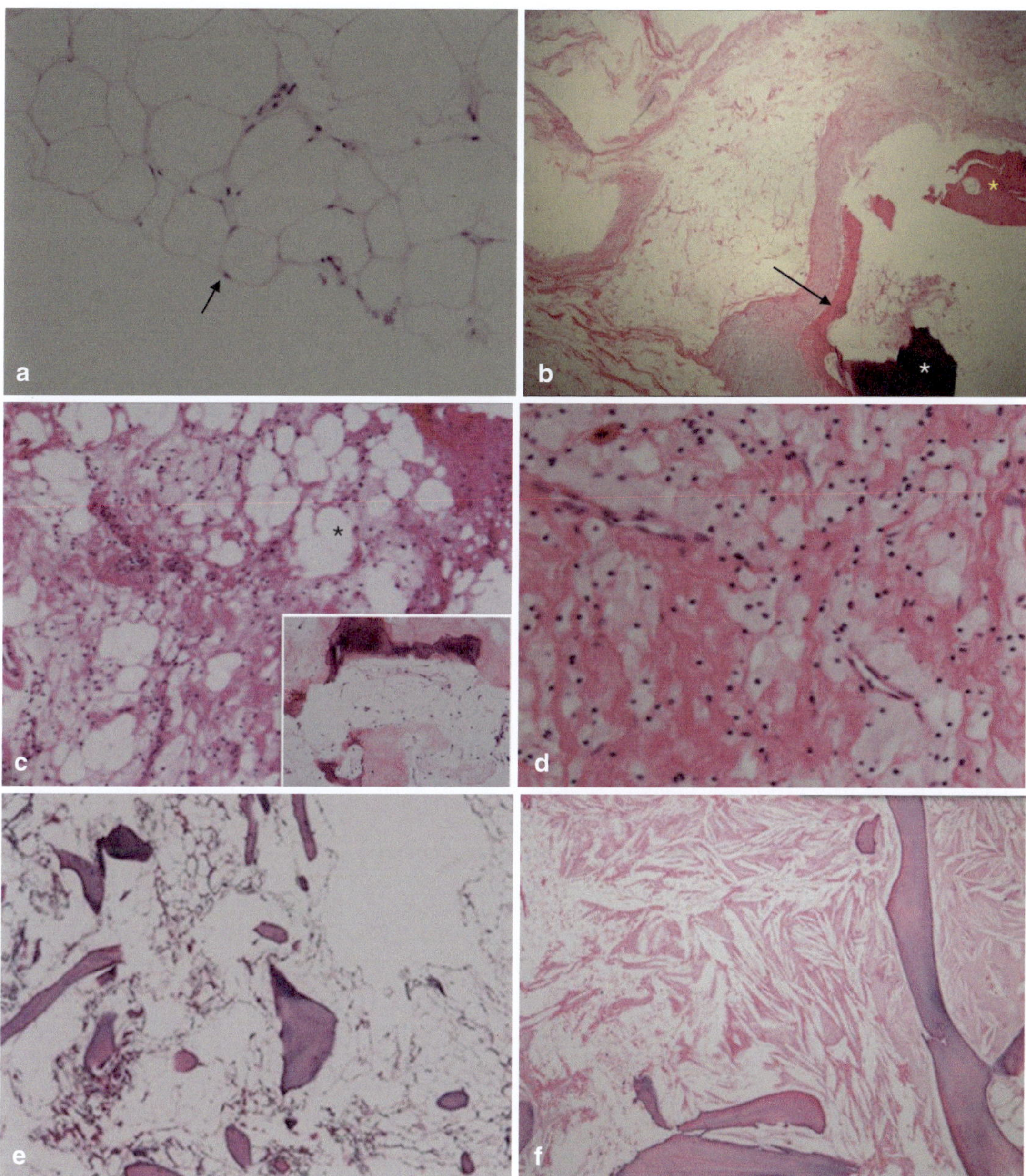

Fig. 24.9 *Microscopic features* (**a**) Lipoma is typically composed of lobules of mature fat cells bigger than normal white adipose tissue devoid of admixed hematopoietic tissues or bony trabeculae that is identical to ordinary lipoma of soft tissue. Each adipocyte shows a single large, clear, cytoplasmic vacuole that displaces the nucleus to periphery making crescent-shape (arrow). (**b**) A lobule with mature fat cells and some infarcted cells is surrounded by reactive collagen bundle and cartilage undergoing endochondral ossification (arrow). There are fragmented lamellar bone spicule (yellow asterisk) and calcium deposition with under-decalcification (white asterisk). (**c**) Mature adipose tissue is associated with dense collagenous bands of fibrosis. Note the ghost outlines of necrotic adipocytes (asterisk). There is dystrophic calcification around infarction area (inset). (**d**) Some areas of fat necrosis present reactive foamy histiocytes with abundant collagen bundle deposition. (**e**) At periphery of the lesion, an interdigitating zone with the fat lobules of the tumor among significantly thinned trabeculae of lamellar bone simulating osteoporosis is observed with focal normal-appearing bone marrow elements. (**f**) Area of cholesterol clefts formation is presented with scattered thinned host lamellar bone trabeculae

or *"cockade"* sign. Some areas of fat necrosis present reactive foamy histiocytes in association of abundant collagen bundle deposition (Fig. 24.9d). Focal fields with thinned bone trabeculae by mass effect (Fig. 24.9e) may be seen being equivalent to osteoporosis that is, however, generalized disease, and the finding should present throughout the entire fields. Areas of cholesterol cleft formation can be presented probably due to long-standing hemorrhage (Fig. 24.9f). *Stage 1 lesion* consist of sheets of fully viable fat cells without distinct cryptologic abnormalities with completely resorbed or scattered thin trabeculae of minimally remained normal bone. There is no reactive fibroblastic formation of collagen. *Stage 2 lesion* reveals solid fields of viable fat cells with focal areas of spontaneous necrosis due to expansion of fat cells within rigid osseous trabeculae confined to certain part of the lesion. Some portions of fat necrosis are calcified, and reactive ossified bone resembling primitive woven bone is deposited around the necrotic areas. *Stage 3 lesion:* Overtime, focal necrosis gradually extends to the entire lesion with involution changes such as more degree of calcification, cyst formation, and reactive peripheral or central new bone formation.

24.8 Management

The lesion is usually asymptomatic to mildly painful and does not affect bone stability. Thus, surgical management is rarely indicated. Curettage with bone graft is indicated for symptomatic patients or impending fracture.

24.9 Clinical Course

The lesion recurs very rarely after surgical management [9]. Often, the lesion spontaneously undergoes involution, but malignant transformation is extremely rare. Malignant change should be suspected when rapid bone destruction is associated. Since involuted IL may contain the similar cellular constituents as bone infarcts, it is not surprising that ILs can rarely undergo malignant change. The mechanism of malignant change is not clear, but it occurs in the reactive border of ischemic bone marrow of the lesion with secondary involution change such as fat necrosis, ischemic woven bone with calcification, and reactive ossification as malignant change in bone infarct [20]. Liposclerosing myxofirous tumor and involutional IL contain the overlapped cellular constituents including fat cell necrosis, focal calcification, and reactive ischemic bone formation ("pseudopagetoid" or "mosaic" bone). I and my colleagues previously observed that atypical cells were gradually increased in number and grade of cellular atypism as the sarcoma region was approached, and the atypical cells imperceptibly merged into the high-grade spindle cell sarcoma in infarct-associated sarcoma (IAS) [21]. I support the assumption that malignant change in IL may occur in the reactive border of ischemic areas with secondary involution change, based on our observation of IAS arising from the reparative tissues at the periphery of ancient infarcts.

References

1. Rosenberg AE, Bridge JA. Lipoma of bone. In: Fletcher CM, Uni KK, Mertens F, editors. WHO classification of tumors: pathology and genetics of tumors of soft tissue and bone. Lyon: IARC Press; 2002. p. 328–9.
2. Unni KK, Inwards CY. Lipoma and liposarcoma. In: Unni KK, Inwards CY, editors. Dahlin's bone tumors: general aspects and data on 10,165 cases. 6th ed. Philadelphia, PA: Lippincott William & Wilkins; 2010. p. 298–302.
3. Leeson MC, Kay D, Smith BS. Intraosseous lipoma. Clin Orthop Relat Res. 1983;181:186–90.
4. Chow LT, Lee KC, Intraosseous lipoma. A clinicopathologic study of nine cases. Am J Surg Pathol. 1992;16(4):401–10.
5. Hirata M, Kusuzaki K, Hirasawa Y. Eleven cases of intraosseous lipoma of the calcaneus. Anticancer Res. 2001;21(6A):4099–103.
6. Goto T, Kojima T, Iijima T, Yokokura S, Motoi T, Kawano H, et al. Intraosseous lipoma: a clinical study of 12 patients. J Orthop Sci. 2002;7(2):274–80.
7. Campbell R, Grainger A, Mangham D, Beggs I, Teh J, Davies A. Intraosseous lipoma: report of 35 new cases and a review of the literature. Skeletal Radiol. 2003;32(4):209–22.

8. Murphey MD, Carroll JF, Flemming DJ, Pope TL, Gannon FH, Kransdorf MJ. From the archives of the AFIP: benign musculoskeletal lipomatous lesions. Radiographics. 2004;24(5):1433–66.
9. Milgram JW. Intraosseous lipomas. A clinicopathologic study of 66 cases. Clin Orthop Relat Res. 1988;231:277–302.
10. Resnick D. Tumor and tumor-like diseases. In: Resnick D, editor. Diagnosis of bone and joint disorders. 4th ed. Philadelphia, PA: Saunders; 1995. p. 3745–4128.
11. Smith WE, Fienberg R. Intraosseous lipoma of bone. Cancer. 1957;10(6):1151–2.
12. Başarir K, Şahin E, Kalem M, Karaca MO, Yildiz Y, Saglik Y. Parosteal lipoma as a rare cause of peripheral neuropathy and local irritation: a report of 12 cases. Acta Orthop Traumatol Turc. 2017;51(6):474–7.
13. Ramos A, Castello J, Sartoris D, Greenway G, Resnick D, Haghighi P. Osseous lipoma: CT appearance. Radiology. 1985;157(3):615–9.
14. Moon N, Marmor L. Parosteal lipoma of the proximal part of the radius: a clinical entity with frequent radial-nerve injury. J Bone Joint Surg. 1964;46(3):608–14.
15. Berry J, Moiel R. Parosteal lipoma producing paralysis of the deep radial nerve. South Med J. 1973;66(11):1298–300.
16. Nishida J, Shimamura T, Ehara S, Shiraishi H, Sato T, Abe M. Posterior interosseous nerve palsy caused by parosteal lipoma of proximal radius. Skeletal Radiol. 1998;27(7):375–9.
17. Jacobs P. Parosteal lipoma with hyperostosis. Clin Radiol. 1972;23(2):196–8.
18. Mirra JM, Picci P. Intraossoeus lipoma. In: Mirra JM, editor. Bone tumors: clinical, radiologic, and pathologic correlation. 2nd ed. Philadelphia, PA: Lea & Febiger; 1989. p. 1480–90.
19. Milgram JW. Intraosseous lipomas: radiologic and pathologic manifestations. Radiology. 1988;167(1):155–60.
20. Milgram JW. Malignant transformation in bone lipomas. Skeletal Radiol. 1990;19(5):347–52.
21. Bahk WJ, Lee AH, Kang YK, Park JM, Chung YG, Shin DS, et al. Infarct associated sarcoma: a possible pathogenesis based on histological observation of repair tissue origin in two cases. Acta Oncol. 2010;49(6):868–72.

25 Ewing's Sarcoma

25.1 Definition

Ewing's sarcoma (ES) is a distinct highly malignant primary tumor in bone or soft tissue around the bone, typified by sheets of undifferentiated small round mesenchymal cells rich in glycogen and genetic alteration with expression of a chimeric EWSR1-FLI1 protein. Ewing sarcoma family of tumors (ESFT) is a group of high-grade small round cell tumors coming from the same type of stem cell, including bone ES, extraosseous ES, peripheral primitive neuroectodermal tumors (PNET), and Askin tumors (PNET of the chest wall). The microscopic features are similar, and a common chromosomal abnormality is consistently presented in both classical ES and PNET in parenchymal and reproductive organs. Thus, they are collectively referred to as the Ewing's sarcoma/PNET family of tumors [1]. ES of bone will be presented in this textbook.

25.2 Pathogenesis

The translocation t(11;22)(q24;q12) is the most common chromosomal translocations leading expression of a new chimeric EWSR1-FLI1 fusion protein, which contributes to ESFT pathogenesis by modulating the expression of target genes. In general, the expanded family of ES can be separated into two major groups including chimeric genes with E-26 transformation specific (ETS) and non-ETS fusion partners [1].

25.3 Incidence

ES is the second most common primary malignant bone tumor after osteosarcoma in children and adolescents and the third most frequent after osteosarcoma and chondrosarcoma in adults. It is estimated to occupy approximately 6–9% of all primary malignant bone tumors [1, 2] and about 5% of all bone tumors [3].

25.4 Age

ES typically occurs in children and adolescents between 10 and 20 years of age. Approximately 75–80% of all patients are in their first two decades of life, and about half of the patients are affected in the second decade [1, 2]. It is rare in infant and toddler younger than 3 years and in adult older than 40 years [3].

25.5 Location

Although it can occur essentially any bone, the lesion is most commonly found in major long bones including femur, tibia, humerus, fibula,

W.-J. Bahk, *Diagnosis and Management of Primary Bone Tumors*,
https://doi.org/10.1007/978-981-99-5498-8_25

and forearm in following order. The lesion characteristically affects diaphysis or meta-diaphysis of long bone but rarely involves epiphysis. In the trunk, the ilium is the most commonly involved location, followed by the spine, sacrum, scapula, rib, and clavicle.

25.6 Clinical Presentations

The initial symptom is usually localized pain, which becomes more severe and persistent. Swelling or soft tissue mass is next frequent presentation. Nonspecific constitutional symptoms such as mild fever and malaise can be associated with abnormal laboratory findings including elevated erythrocyte sedimentation rate (ESR), leukocytosis, or anemia, which can be easily confused with those in osteomyelitis [3].

25.7 Radiologic Findings

Although the radiologic appearance is protean and nonspecific, a diagnosis of ES can be reasonably suspected in correlation with clinical presentation of abovementioned age and location as well as radiographic features of intramedullary lesion affecting large segment and large soft tissue mass despite the relatively minimal cortical change, which is more extensive than expected (Figs. 25.1, 25.2 and 25.3). Bone destruction varies from geographic or nearly pure lytic pattern to ill-defined, permeative, or focally moth-eaten pattern. The latter pattern with imperceptible broad margin is the major feature mimicking other most malignant bone tumors, acute osteomyelitis, or Langerhans cell histiocytoma. Other nonspecific patterns of destruction include fine to reticulated, honeycombed, punched-out, or circumscribed patterns. Occasionally, reactive sclerotic bone is laid down faster than it is being destroyed and resorbed. The cortex may seem to be intact or subtlely changed or even thickened on plain radiograph, but the majority lesions (up to 90%) multiply breaches the cortex to make a large naked soft tissue mass best seen on CT scan or MR image (Figs. 25.1, 25.2 and 25.3). Thus, an ill-defined large soft tissue density with permeative to moth-eaten bony lesion is important clue for a diagnosis of ES as in lymphoma of bone. In general, the soft tissue mass is significantly prominent when compared to comparably smaller radiolucent bony lesion. Sometimes a *"periosteal ES"* without medullary involvement, or more commonly a subperiosteal and/or soft tissue mass may erode the outer cortex and produce a concave defect, so-called *"saucerization"* (Fig. 25.5a). The *"periosteal ES"* can extend into the adjacent soft tissue through the destructed cortex producing a large soft tissue mass (Fig. 25.5b). Periosteal reaction is another common finding particular when the diaphysis is affected in younger patient. *"Onion skinning"* is the most characteristic although not pathognomonic, which can become solid and extensively produce a fusiform enlargement of the shaft (Fig. 25.4a). A thick *"onion-skinning"* that is more extensive than would be expected from severity of bone destruction can be also observed in Langerhans cell histiocytosis (see Fig. 4.1a in that chapter). The "*Codman's triangle*" or *"sunburst"* appearance of periosteal new bone deposition is less frequently observed (Fig. 25.3a). **Bone scan** Uptake is typically avid on all three phases (Figs. 25.1, 25.3, 25.4 and 25.5). The role of the bone scan in detecting presence of metastases at presentation and during follow-up seems to be clear [4, 5]. **PET/CT scan** demonstrates a heterogeneously intense FDG uptake in the lesion (Fig. 25.3d and 25.5d). It is a valuable imaging method in the initial staging of the disease, restaging during therapy, and evaluation of therapeutic response as in other malignant bone tumors. **CT scan** can more clearly demonstrate cortical alterations particularly in anatomically complex regions such as the vertebral column and the pelvic bones due to the lack of superimposition as well as an extra-osseous extension of the tumor producing a naked soft tissue mass. The density is predominantly radiolucent with an attention coefficient similar to muscle. **MR images** most clearly identify the extent of intramedullary and extra-osseous lesion as well as skip lesion to provide more accurate preoperative plan. Typical findings include bone marrow

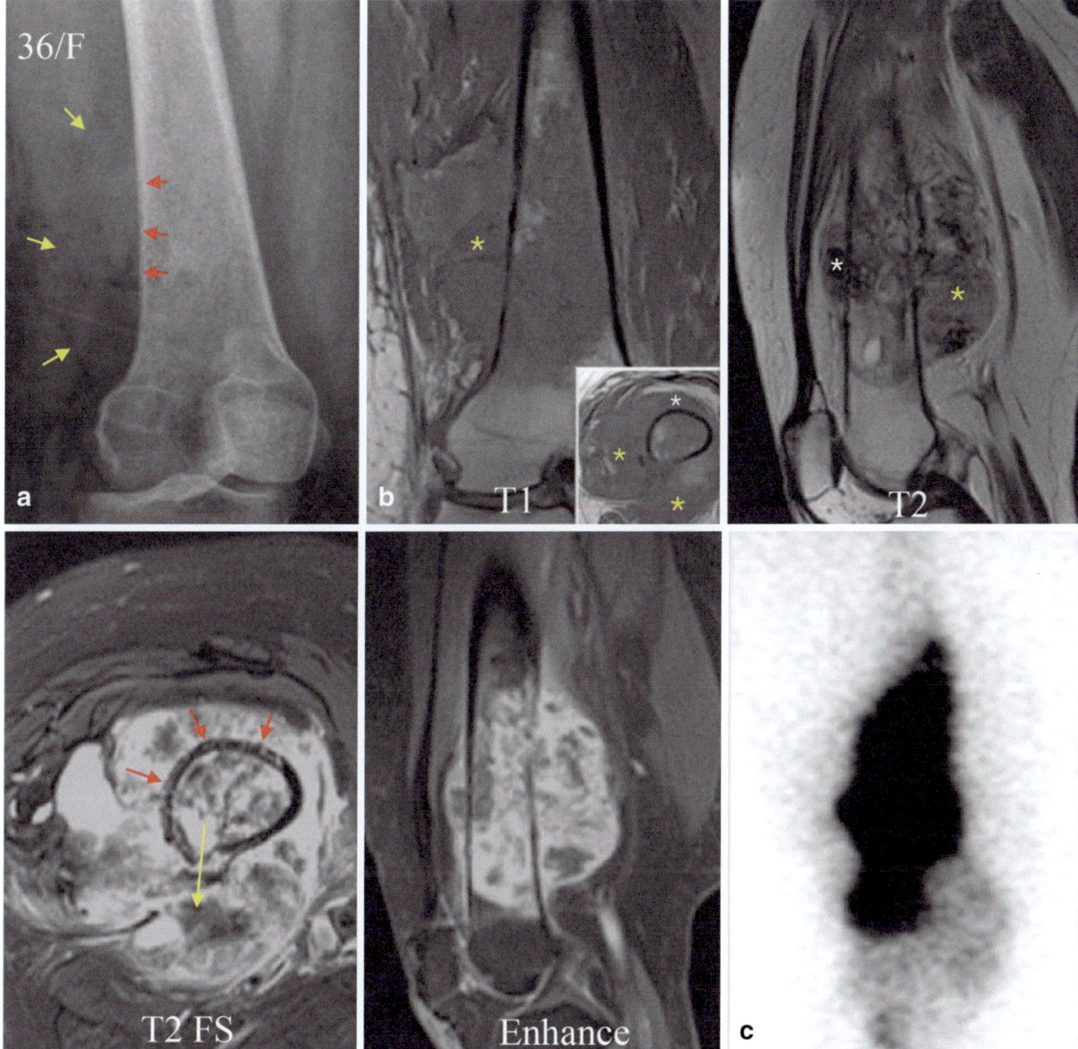

Fig. 25.1 (**a**) Radiograph taken for right distal thigh pain of 6-month duration in 36-year-old woman shows an ill-defined moth-eaten to permeative medullary lesion mainly in the diaphysis of the distal femur. Note tiny multiple medial cortical breaches (red arrows) with a hazy huge soft tissue mass (yellow arrows). (**b**) MR images demonstrate a bone marrow replacement with low SI on T1-weighted image and heterogeneous intermediate and high SI on T2-weighted image. The signal is much bright on fat saturated T2-weighted image. There are numerous breaches in the medial, anterior, and posterior cortices with a huge soft tissue mass. Medial and posterior soft tissue masses are much larger (yellow asterisks) than anterior one (white asterisks). Note numerous linear *"penetrating channels"* of high signal within the anterior and medial cortices (red arrows) as well as more prominent destruction in the posterior cortex (yellow arrow) through which larger and smaller masses are produced on fat saturated T2-weighted axial image. They merge gradually and eventually wrap around the whole femur, so-called *"wrap-around"* sign. The bony and soft tissue lesion heterogeneously well enhanced by contrast medium. The *"penetrating channels"* are linearly enhanced. (**c**) Bone scan reveals a homogeneously strong uptake in the distal femur and adjacent soft tissue mass beyond the cortex. (**d**) Wide resection including previous biopsy tract and reconstruction with tumor prosthesis as well as chemotherapy was performed. (**e**) Resected specimen shows soft and glistening viable tumor tissue with extensive necrotic and hemorrhagic patches in the medullary space (yellow asterisk)) and large soft tissue mass (white asterisk). (**f**) Radiograph taken for right thigh pain with pseudomotion after slip on 27 months after initial surgery reveals a periprosthetic fracture. (**g**) Open reduction and internal fixation with plate was done. (**h**) Follow-up bone scan at 7 years after initial surgery with chemotherapy notes periprosthetic mild uptake only in the prosthesis-host bone contact area (red arrow) and proximal end of the prosthesis (blue arrow). There is a large photon defect in the area of prosthesis body where is previous tumor site (asterisk) with a diffuse faint peri-prosthetic uptake (black arrow), indicating no local recurrence

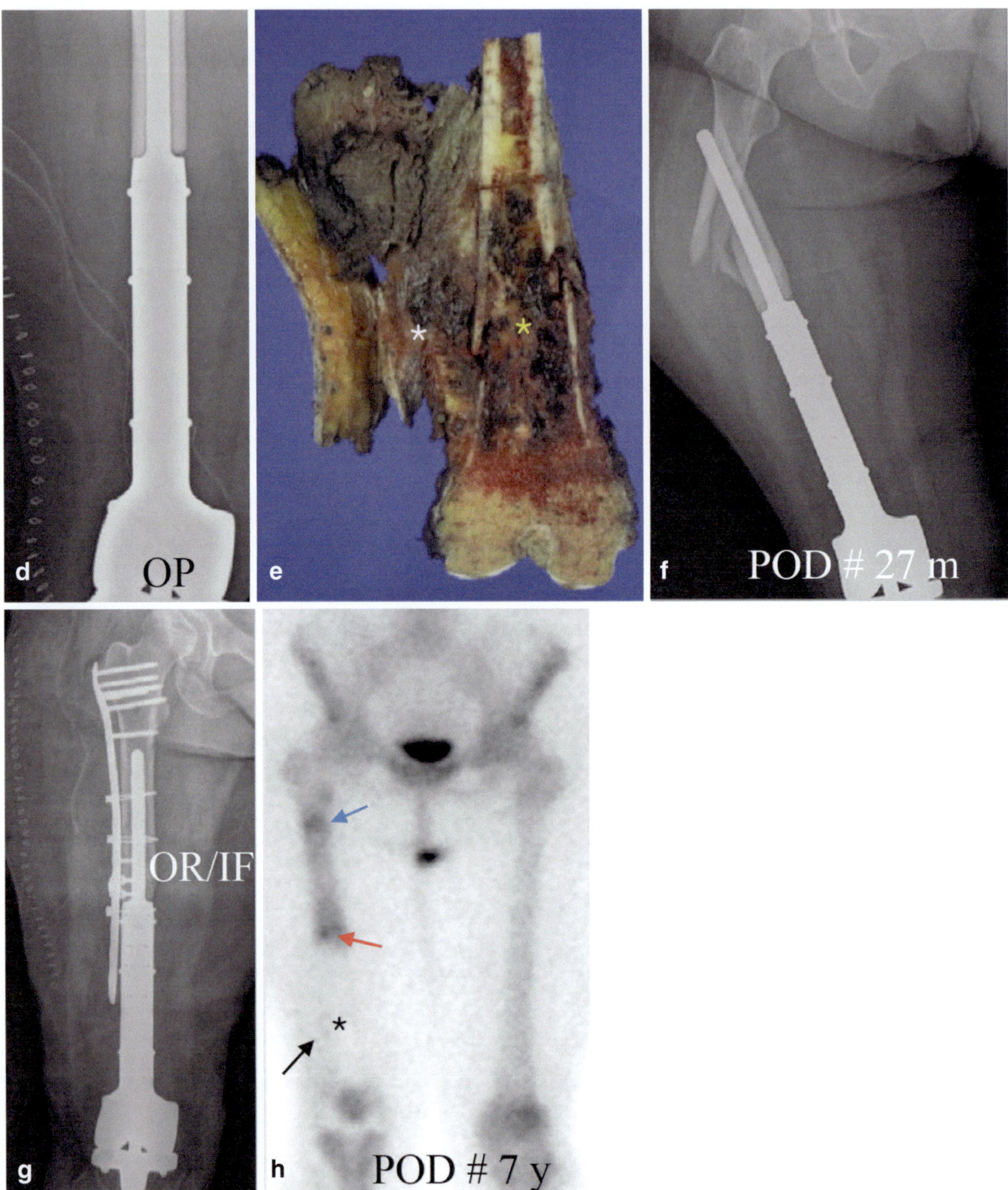

Fig. 25.1 (continued)

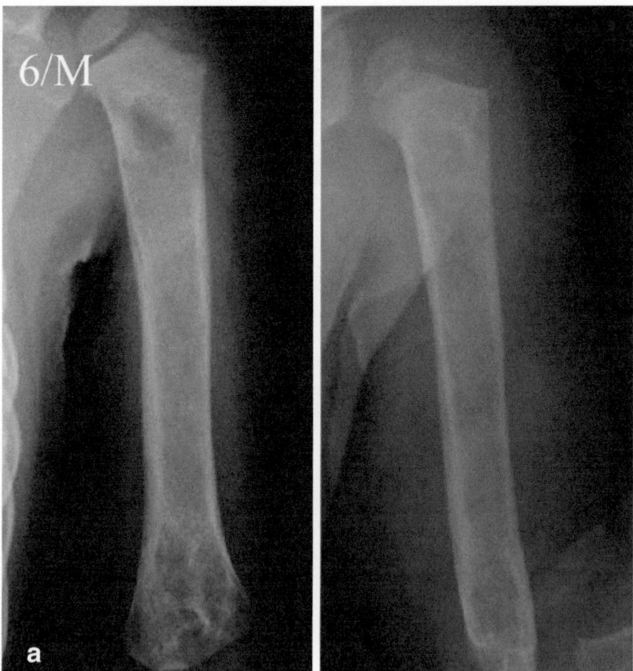

Fig. 25.2 (**a**) Radiograph taken for left upper arm painful swelling of 6- to 7-month duration in 6-year-old boy shows moth-eaten to permeative lesion with small geographic destruction and focal sclerotic areas in the almost entire humerus. The bone is mildly expanded with subtle cortical change, but periosteal reaction is not clear. (**b**) MR images reveal a bone marrow replacement with heterogeneous intermediate and high SI on fat saturated T2-weighted image. The cortex is irregularly undulated and indistinctly breached in association with subperiosteal (red asterisk) and larger soft tissue mass formation beyond the cortex (black asterisk). T2-weighted axial view clearly demonstrates the tumor extends to the subperiosteal space from the medullary cavity through the numerous tiny *"penetrating channels"* within the cortex (red circles) as well as subtle cortical breaches. The tumor cells are subperiosteally accumulated and elevate the periosteum. Then, the sub-periosteal mass extends to the surrounding soft tissue though the periosteal breakage (white arrow) and makes a large mass, which wraps around the entire circumference of the humerus (white asterisks) on T2-weighted axial image. A small focal cortical breakage is clearly observed in medial aspect of the distal humerus (yellow arrow in inset), and periosteal elevation with tiny linear dark signals (white circle in inset) may suggest early *"sunburst"* appearance of periosteal new bone deposition, which is not visible on radiograph. The bony lesion is enhanced by contrast medium in peripheral nodular pattern, and the soft tissue lesion is diffusely enhanced. The *"penetrating channels"* are linearly enhnaced. (**c**) After neo-adjuvant chemotherapy, limb-salvage surgery was performed. En bloc resection using giggly saw (white arrows) with wide margin followed by reconstruction using pasteurized auto-humerus fixed with wiring (yellow arrows) was performed. (**d**) Immediate postoperative radiograph notes well-positioned and fixed graft bone. However, allograft insertion with plate fixation was done again at 8 months after initial surgery due to proximal graft resorption and metallic failure. (**e**) Follow-up radiograph at 20 months after re-operation shows nonunion with resorption of proximal part of the graft (yellow arrow) and metallic failure. (**f**) Removal of plate and re-plate fixation with bone graft (red arrow) was performed for non-union at 3 years after initial surgery. Then, infection was complicated. (**g**) After infection control, Augmented vascularized fibular graft (VFG) was performed at 5 years after initial surgery. (**h**) Open reduction and plate fixation was performed due to fracture of grafted fibula with metallic failure at 1 year after VFG. (**i**) Corticotomy (yellow arrow) and external fixator application (asterisk) for limb lengthening were performed because of significant shortening of left upper arm at 4 years after VFG. (**j**) Follow-up radiograph at 1 year after auto-bone graft for delayed union of lengthened humerus notes a complete union. The patient is doing well with no evidence of disease at 10 years after initial surgery

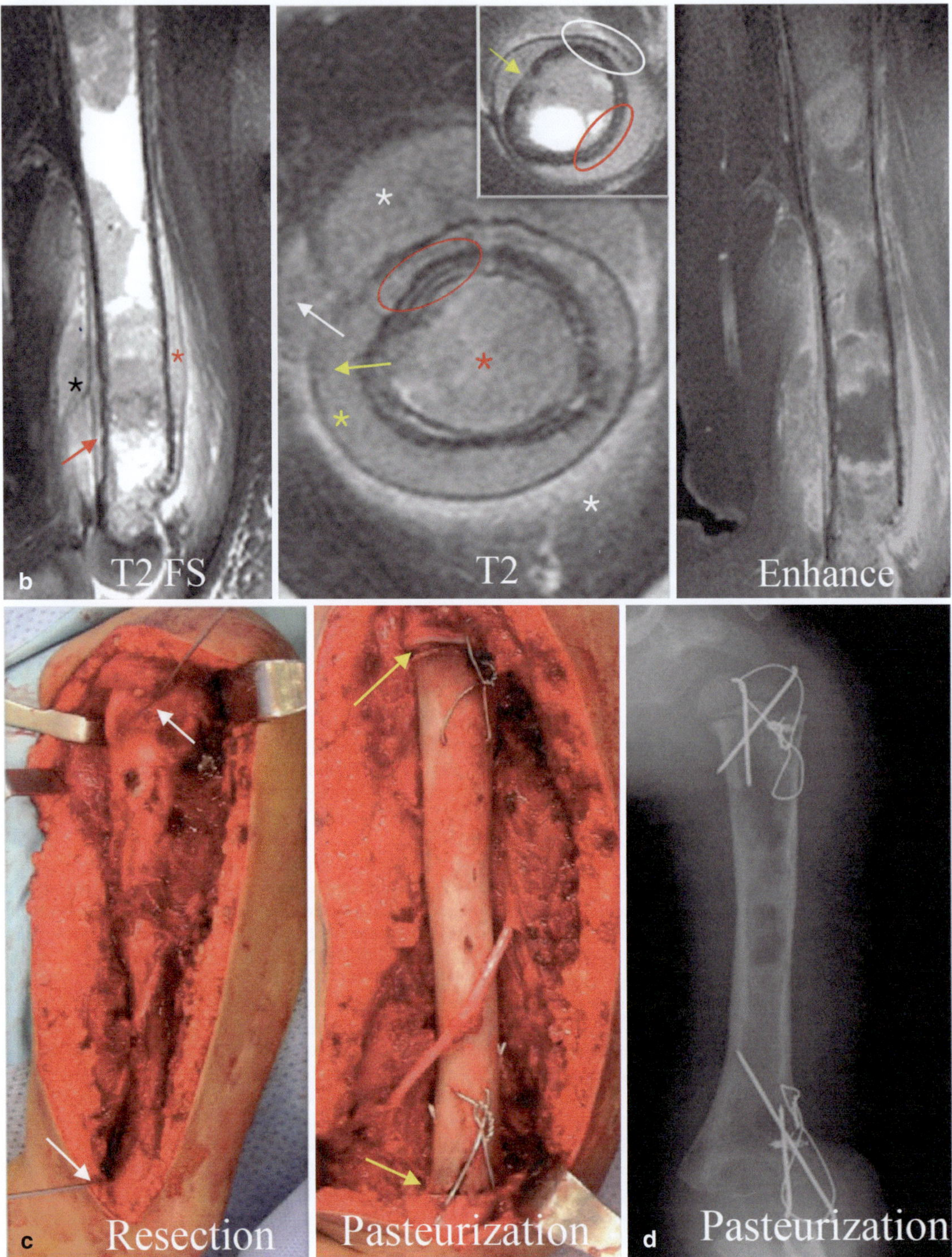

Fig. 25.2 (continued)

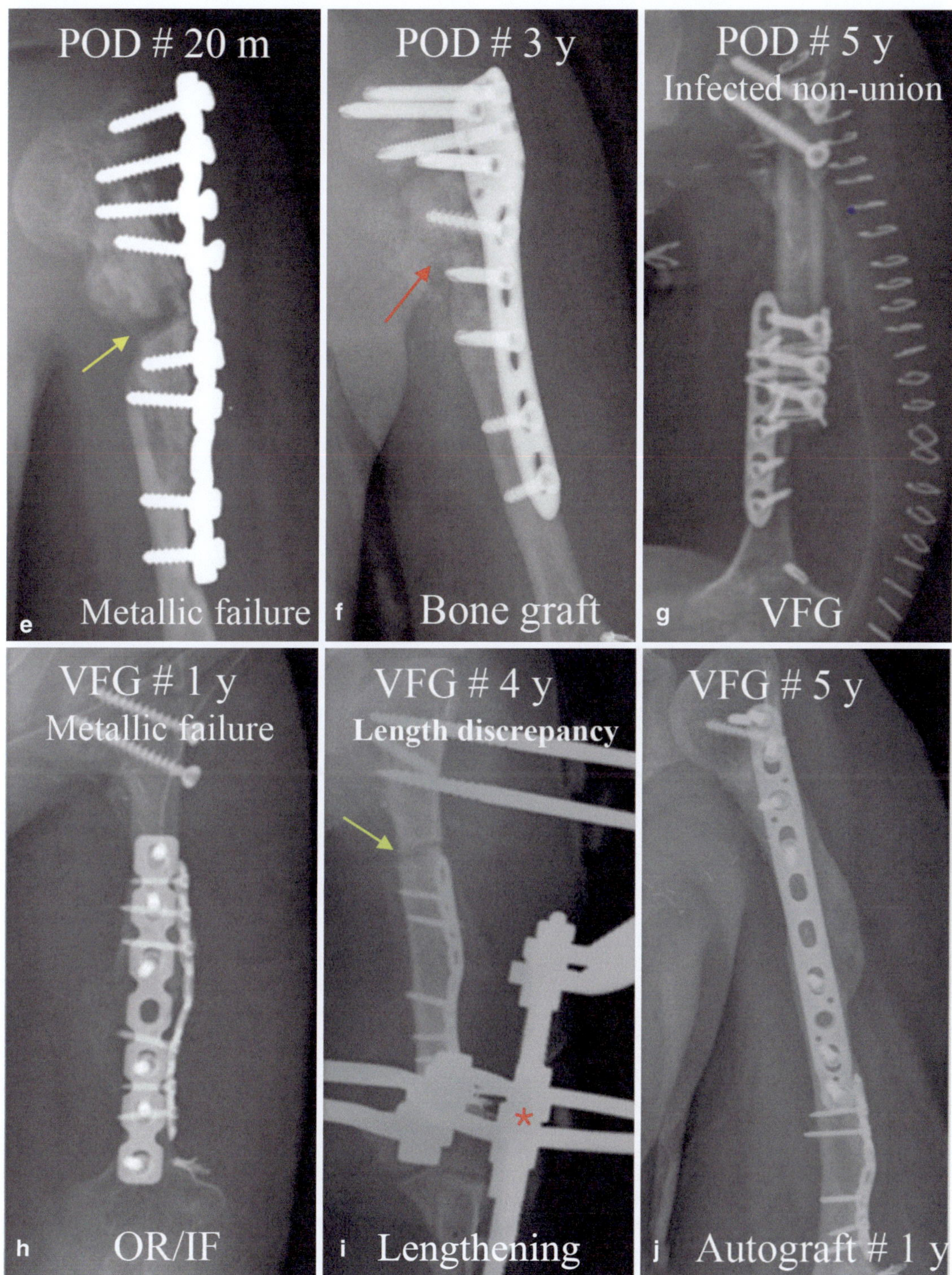

Fig. 25.2 (continued)

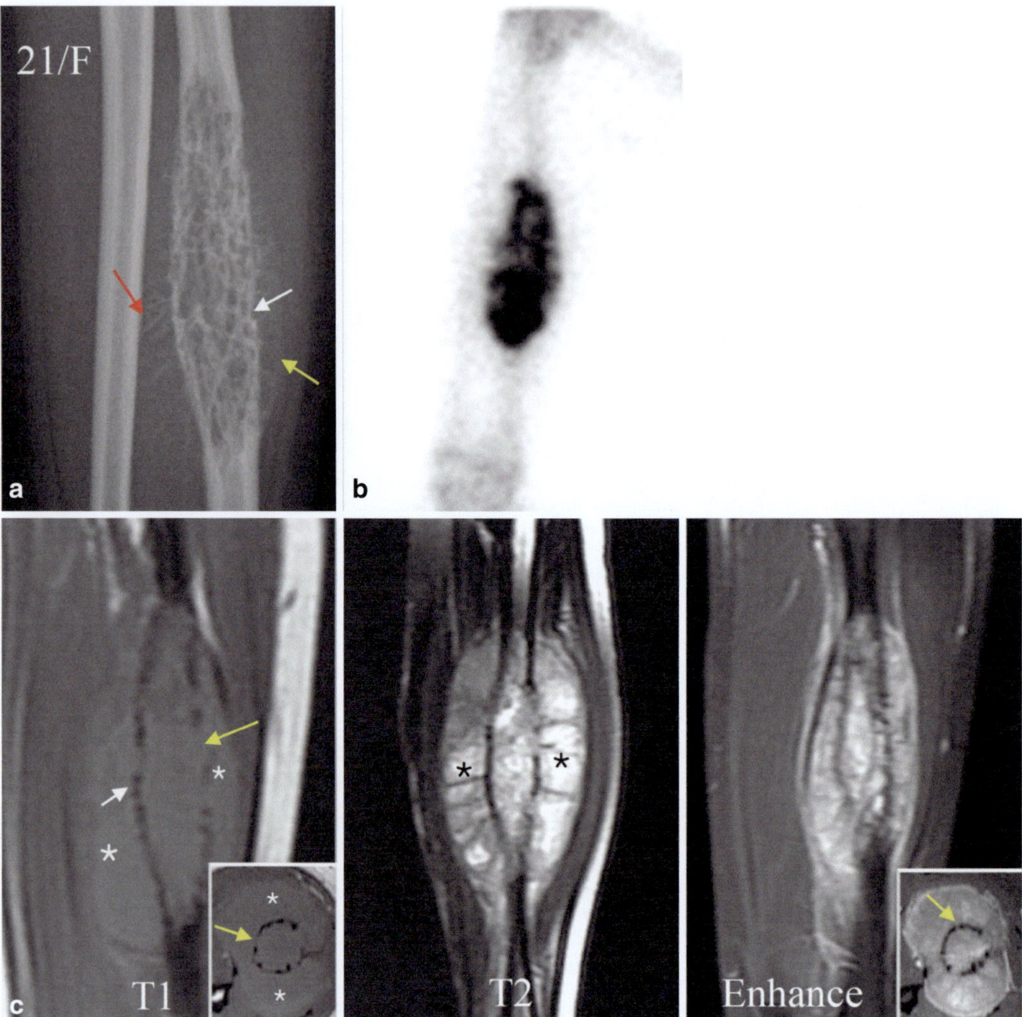

Fig. 25.3 (**a**) Radiograph taken for palpable mass of left forearm of 1-year duration in 21-year-old young lady shows an ill-defined honeycomb-like destructive lesion with a wide zone of transition. Note irregularly thinned with numerous breaches (white arrow) and soft tissue mass surrounded by a thin rim of sclerosis (yellow arrow). The periosteal reaction is a *"sunburst"* type by perpendicular periosteal new bone deposition, which is less common pattern than *"onion-skinning." (red arrow)* (**b**) Bone scan reveals an irregular strong uptake in the medullary lesion and soft tissue mass beyond the cortex but no other bones, suggesting a single lesion. (**c**) MR images demonstrate bone marrow replacement by the lesion with intermediate SI on T1-weighted image and heterogeneous intermediate and high SI on T2-weighted image. Note numerous cortical numerous linear *"penetrating channels"* (white arrow) and small breaches (yellow arrow) with overall preserved cortical architecture, through which a large naked soft tissue mass is produced (asterisks). The mass completely wraps around the ulna, so-called *"wrap-around"* sign (inset). The bone and soft tissue lesion are heterogeneously well enhanced. Note the numerous channels with tumor cells are linearly enhanced (arrow in inset). (**d**) PET/CT scan notes a heterogeneously intense FDG uptake (SUVmax 6.6) only in the lesion but no uptake in the other areas, suggesting no distant metastasis. (**e**) Microscopic examination. (Left) Low-power magnification shows solid densely packed sheets and nests consisting of monotonous undifferentiated small round cells appearing as blue color. (Right) Higher-power magnification reveals biphasic pattern with light and dark cells, which are created by extensive apoptosis of the tumor. The living cells with open chromatin are referred to *"principal light cells"* and those with condensed nuclei by apoptosis to *"secondary dark cells."* The diagnosis of ES was confirmed by positive stains both for CD99 (inset) and FLI-1 as well as positive EWSR1 FISH. (**f**) Wide resection followed by reconstruction with intercalary allograft (between black lines) fixed with locking plate (yellow arrow) was performed after neo-adjuvant chemotherapy. And then, adjuvant chemotherapy was done. (**g**) Follow-up radiograph at 3 years after surgery notes no evidence of local recurrence with complete union of the graft bone (arrows)

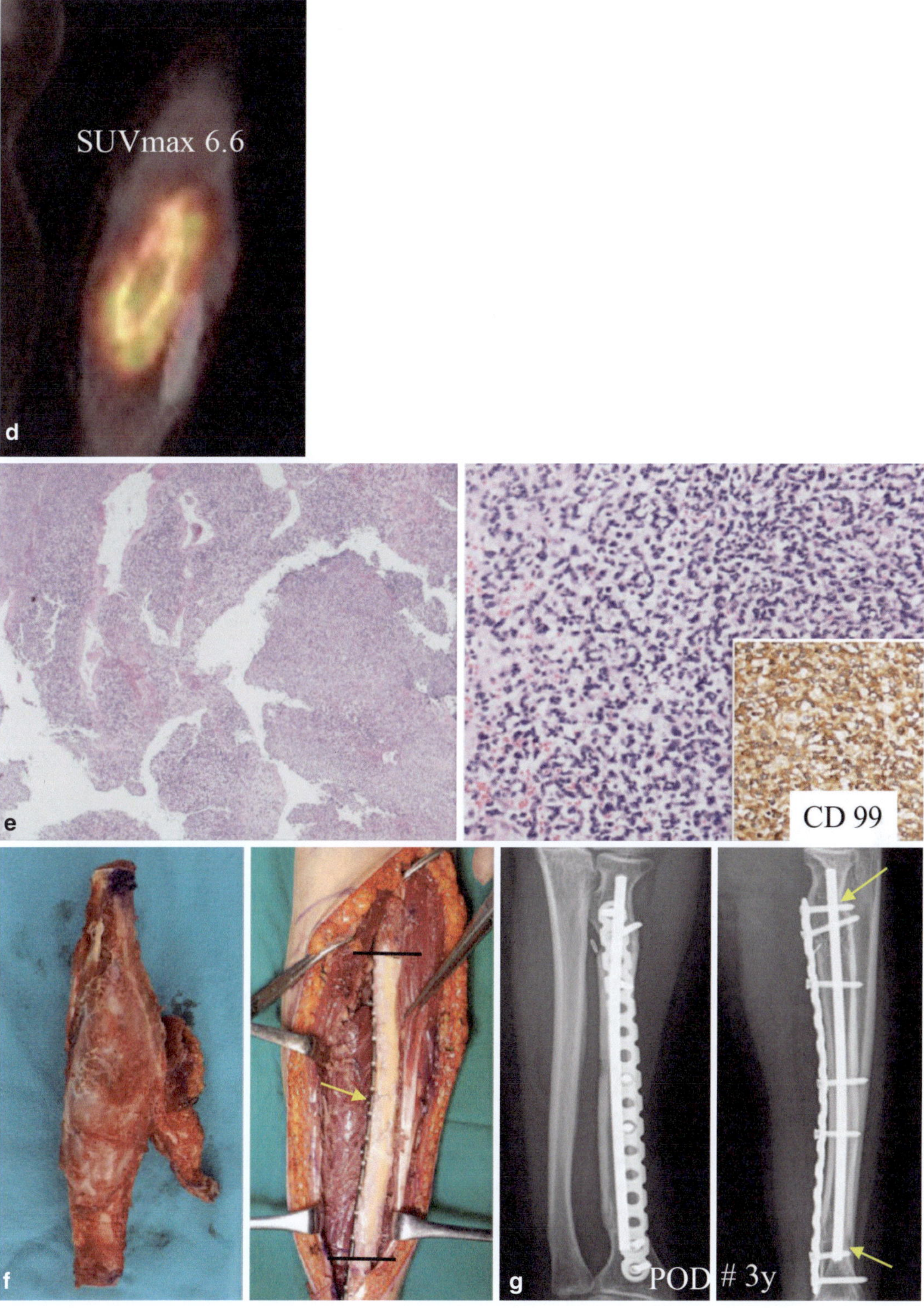

Fig. 25.3 (continued)

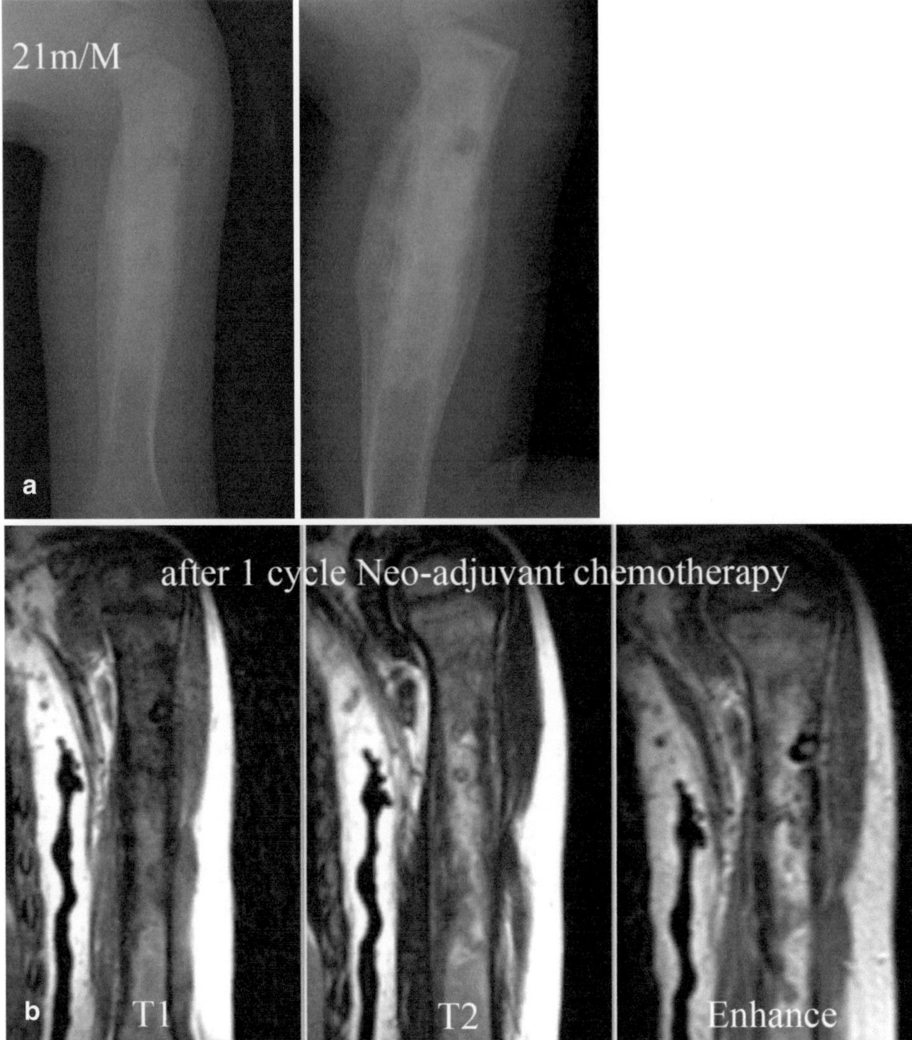

Fig. 25.4 ***The youngest in our series*** (**a**) Radiograph taken for left upper arm pain of 2-month duration in 21-month-old boy toddler shows small multiple radiolucent holes surrounded by significant sclerotic change in the proximal two-thirds of the humerus. Note prominent multiple layers of periosteal reaction, so-called *"onion skinning,"* which becomes solid and extensive leading to a fusiform enlargement of the shaft. (**b**) Initial MR images is not available, but radiologist report described an irregular heterogeneous bone marrow replacement with indistinct focal cortical destruction, prominent soft tissue extension, and multiple lamellate periosteal bone formation in the proximal meta-diaphysis of the humerus. Follow-up MR images after 1 cycle of neo-adjuvant chemotherapy demonstrates decreased tumor volume and periosteal bone formation with subtle increased fibrosis and tumor necrosis. There are remnant tumor nodules in bone marrow and periosteal reaction sites. The lesion is heterogeneously enhanced. (**c**) Bone scan reveals diffuse strong uptake in the meta-diaphysis of humerus with milder uptake in distal portion and periphery of the lesion. (**d**) After completion of neo-adjuvant chemotherapy, wide resection and reconstruction with pasteurized host bone (between yellow lines) augmented by vascularized fibula graft (red asterisk) was performed. And adjuvant chemotherapy was done. (**e**) Follow-up radiograph at 9 months after surgery notes nonunion with significant angulation (yellow arrow) and partial resorption of the pasteurized recycled autobone (white arrow). Open reduction and T-plate fixation with allo-chip bone graft for the nonunion was performed. (**f**) Follow-up radiograph at 18 months after re-operation shows a fracture of the mid-shaft between proximal and distal plate (yellow arrow) due to stress-shielding effect. Open reduction and plate fixation were performed again. (**g**) Last follow-up radiograph at 16 years after initial management when he becomes 18 years old reveals complete healing of the lesion with shortening of the upper arm but evidence of local recurrence. The patient does not want lengthening procedure because he has no pain, functional limitation, and emotional stress despite the severe shortening by 16 cm compared to contralateral upper arm, and the plate is removed (inset)

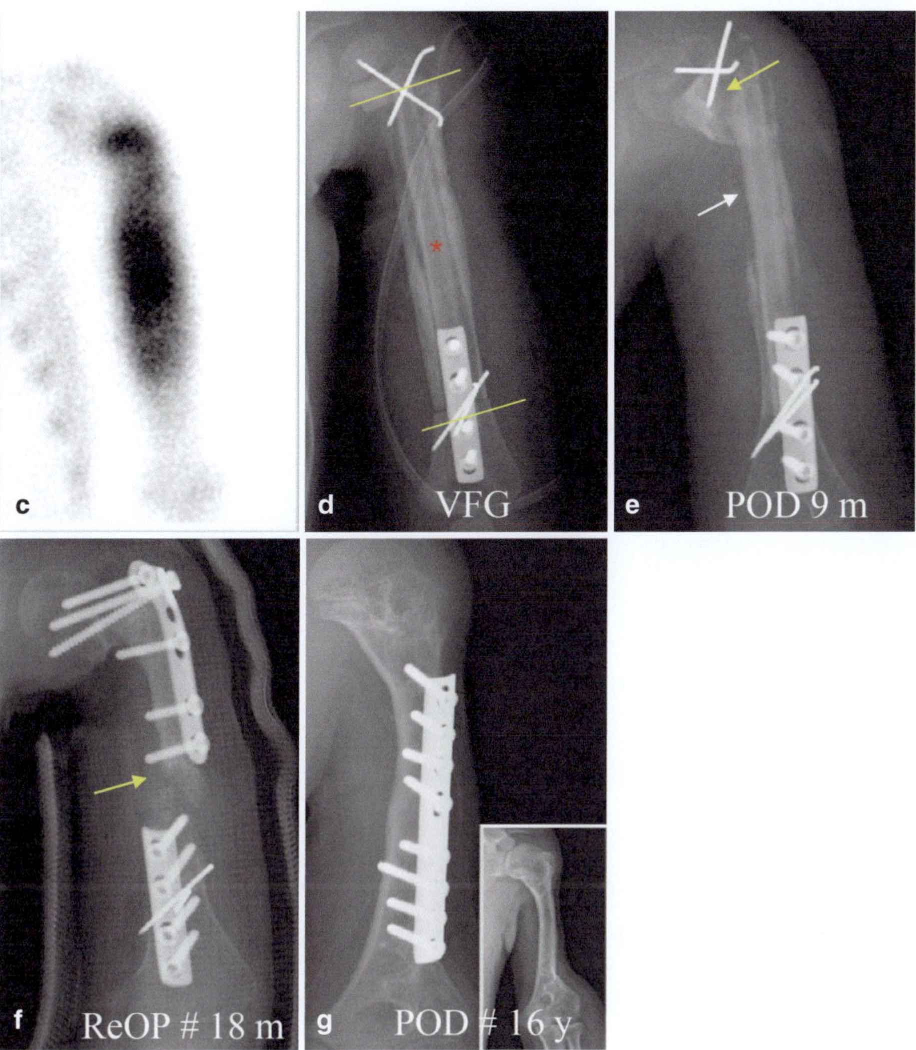

Fig. 25.4 (continued)

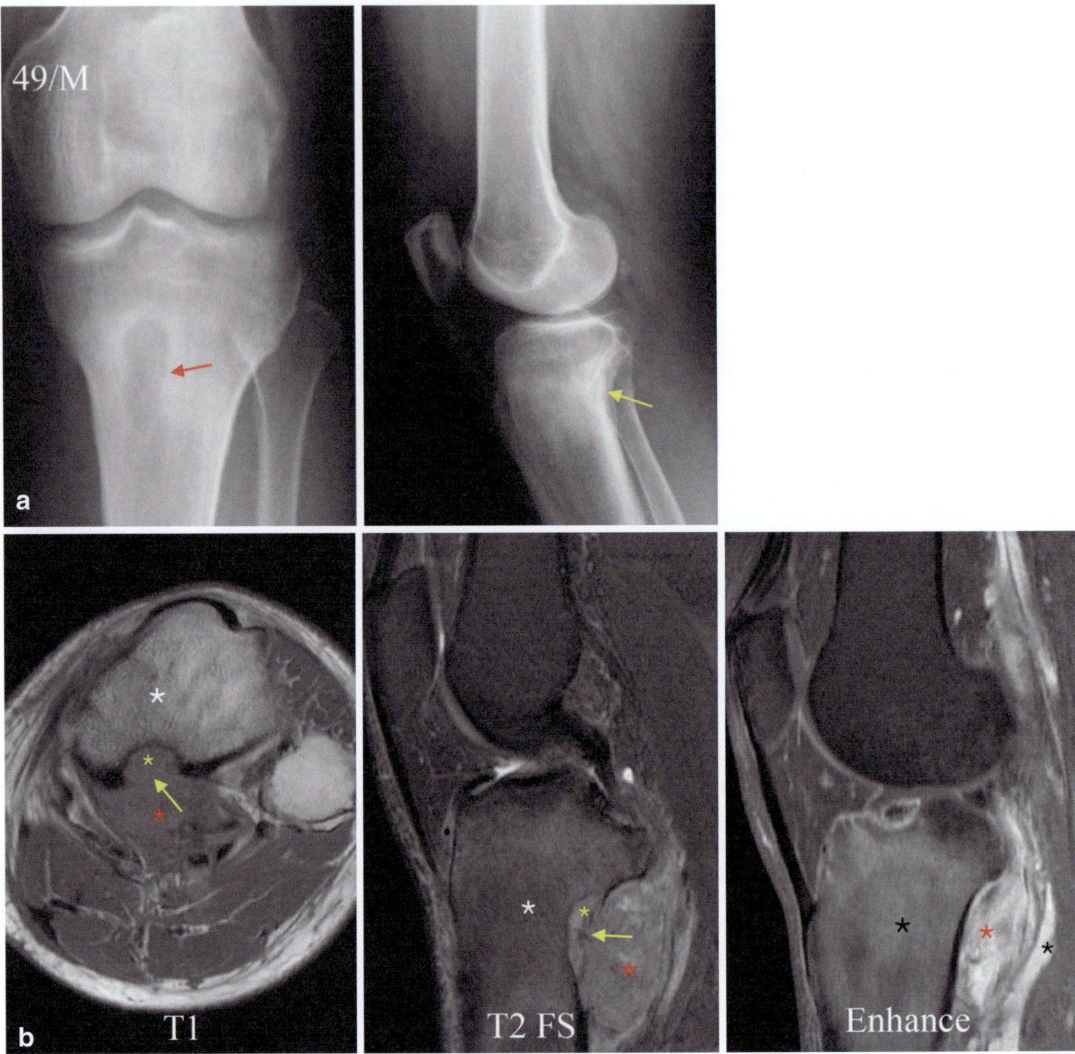

Fig. 25.5 ***Periosteal ES*** (**a**) Anteroposterior radiograph taken for left knee pain of 1-year duration in 49-year-old man shows a well-defined oval radiolucent lesion with a surrounding sclerotic change (red arrow) in the metaphysis of the proximal tibia. However, lateral view reveals an extrinsic erosion with concave cortical defect of the posterior cortex (yellow arrow) probably by a subtle juxtacortical mass, so-called *"saucerization"* with no inequivalent medullary destruction. (**b**) MR images reveal a small periosteal or sub-periosteal mass to produce extrinsic erosion with concave cortical defect of the posterior cortex, so-called *"saucerization"* (yellow asterisks) without no clear medullary involvement (white asterisks). However, the periosteal mass is extending into the adjacent soft tissue through the small cortical breakage (yellow arrows) producing a large naked soft tissue mass (red asterisks). The signal is intermediate on T1-weighted image and heterogeneous intermediate and focal high SI on fat saturated T2-weighted image. The main lesion (red asterisk) as well as bone marrow and soft tissue edema (black asterisks) are heterogeneously well enhanced. (**c**) Bone scan notes a central strong uptake with peripheral weaker uptake. (**d**) PET/CT scan demonstrates a heterogeneously intense FDG uptake (SUVmax 9.1) mostly in the periosteal soft tissue mass (yellow circle) and small area of the cortex invading lesion (red circle). (**e**) Low-power microscopic examination shows multiple solid densely packed nests consisting of monotonous undifferentiated "small round cells" without any matrix formation appearing biphasic pattern created by "light cells" and "dark cells." The nests are focally separated by coarse bands of loose fibrous connective tissue. A diagnosis of *"periosteal ES"* is rendered in consideration of the imaging finding of periosteal location with soft tissue extension. Chemotherapy and radiotherapy were performed, but the patient refused any surgical management. (**f**) Follow-up radiograph after 4 years shows no definite further progression of bone invasion with a surrounding rim of sclerosis (arrow). (**g**) Follow-up MR images also reveal little change of size of the periosteal (yellow asterisk) and soft tissue mass lesion (red asterisk) when compared to the minimal shrinkage on follow-up MR images immediately after chemotherapy and radiotherapy. However, follow-up PET scan notes a possible pulmonary metastasis, and he refused any further study and management

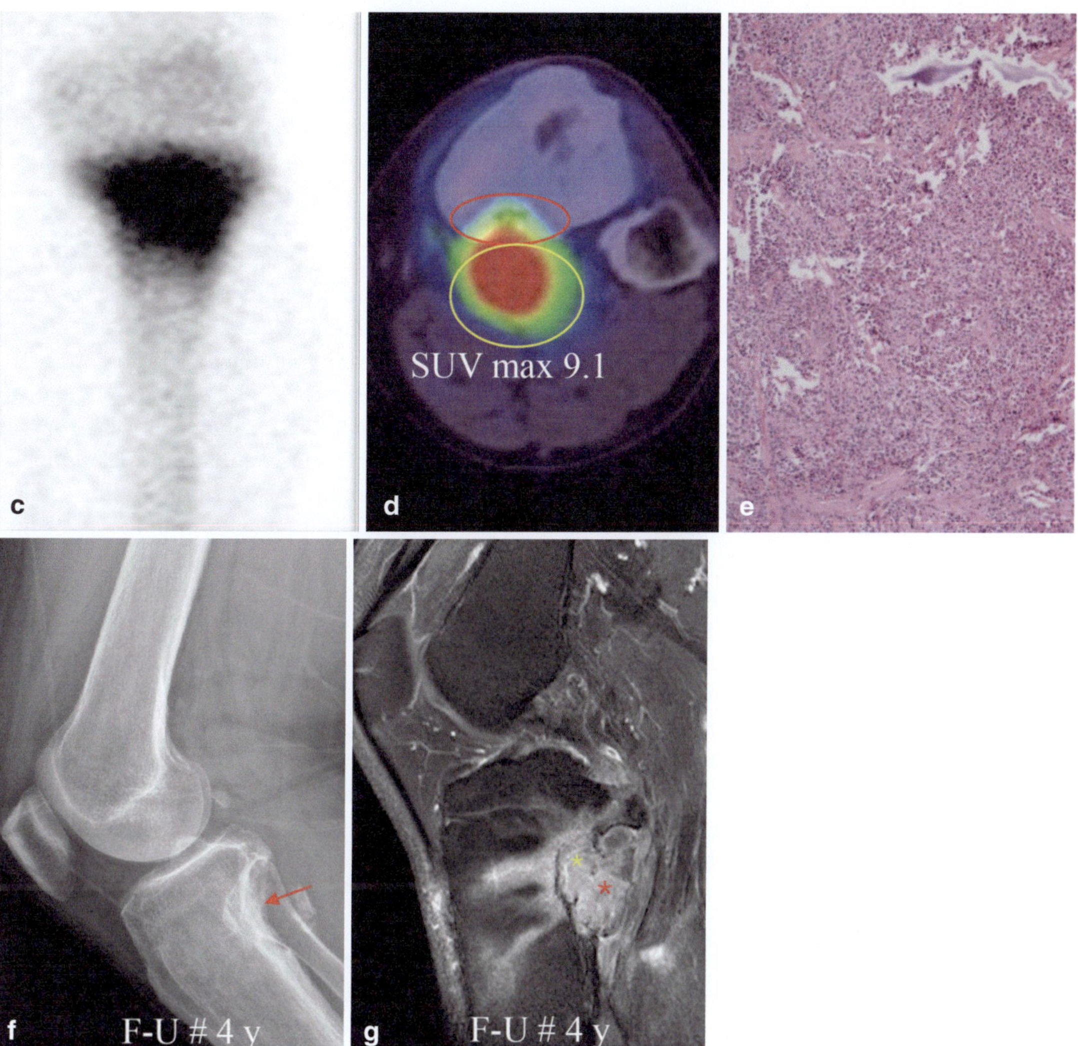

Fig. 25.5 (continued)

replacement with focal cortical breaches or perforation as well as large naked soft tissue masses being more extensive than expected (Figs. 25.1, 25.2, 25.3, 25.4 and 25.5). Rare lesion may only produce a subperiosteal or periosteal mass to cause extrinsic erosion with concave cortical defect of the cortex, so-called *"saucerization,"* without medullary involvement (*"periosteal ES"*) as periosteal osteosarcoma (Fig. 25.5). The SI is low to intermediate on T1-weighted image and heterogeneous high on T2-weighted images. The lesion is usually enhanced by contrast medium either in diffuse or peripheral nodular pattern. A large soft tissue mass through focal cortical breaches with preserved continuity between the medullary and soft-tissue components is highly characteristic. However, there is usually only subtle cortical alteration of numerous linear channels with identical signal to tumor itself and linear enhancement (Figs. 25.1b, 25.2b and 25.3c), but no severe cortical destruction. Through the multiple *"penetrating channels,"* tumor cells extend to the subperiosteal space and adjacent soft tissue from the medullary cavity forming a large soft-tissue mass without extensive cortical destruction (Figs. 25.1, 25.2 and 25.3). This phenomenon is common in in other small round-cell tumors of bone including leukemia and lymphoma. Osseous ES with extensive soft tissue mass or extra-osseous ES shows a large soft tissue mass, which wraps around the adjacent bone best seen on axial image, so-called *"wrap-around"* sign (Figs. 25.1, 25.2 and 25.3).

25.8 Histologic Findings

ES is characterized by solid densely packed sheets or nests consisting of monotonous undifferentiated "small round cells" without any matrix formation appearing on low-power magnification (Fig. 25.6a). The cohesive-sheets of tumor cells are separated by coarse bands of loose fibrous connective tissue making a distinct growth pattern of large lobules or nests. Frequently, a biphasic pattern is created by *"principal light cells"* of living tumor and *"secondary dark cells"* with condensed nuclei representing tumor cells undergoing apoptosis (Fig. 25.6b). The ratio of different cell types varies from tumor to tumor and even in different areas of same tumor. High-power magnification shows the individual cells have centrally located round to oval nucleus with one or more clearly visible nucleoli and high nuclear to cytoplasmic (NC) ratio, which is twice larger and stains less intensely than normal lymphocytes. The cytoplasm is eosinophilic or scanty. It usually contains glycogen in the form of fine droplet to coarse globules, which can be washed out during formalin fixation appearing as cytoplasmic clearing (Fig. 25.6c). The chromatin is finely granular to stipple, and the cytoplasm is usually scarce to pale or vacuolated with an indistinct border. The cells are closely packed in true sarcomatous cohesive sheets rather than spreading as separated cells (not-cohesive). Extensive areas of spontaneous ischemic necrosis with or without hemorrhage are often seen as in other small round cell tumors such as lymphoma. *"Ghost"* outlined cells are often seen in the necrotic area (Fig. 25.6d). The tumor cells are shrunk with decreased amount of glycogen and become individualized in ischemic areas. The shrunk dark cells with dark hyperchromatic nuclei and well-defined cytoplasmic border become abundant and make an interconnecting network of irregular patches, which may simulate lymphocytic lymphoma. With degeneration, a *"rosette-like"* structure may be seen leading to misdiagnosis for neuroblastoma or PNET (Fig. 25.6e). In some cases, tumor cells are arranged in variably sized nests separated by fibrous tissue septa mimicking a pulmonary *"alveolar pattern"* (Fig. 25.6f). Mitotic activity is variable but generally high.

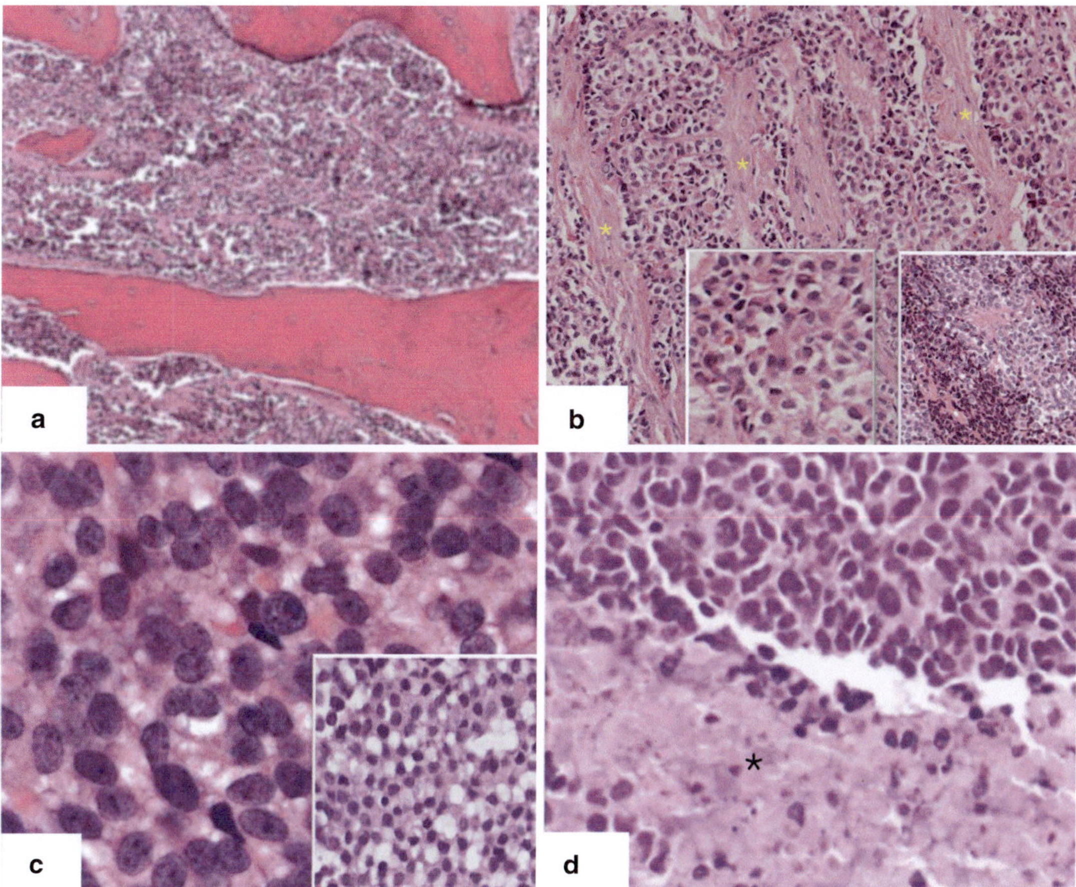

Fig. 25.6 ***Microscopic examination*** (**a**) Scanning-power examination shows a diffuse permeation and replacement of bone marrow by solid densely packed sheets and nests consisting of monotonous small round cells. (**b**) The tumor uniformly consists of cohesive sheets of small round cells without bone or cartilage matrix production, which are separated by coarse bands of loose fibrous connective tissue (asterisks) making a distinct growth pattern of large lobules or nests. Often *principal light cells* with open chromatin (Left inset) and scattered *secondary pyknotic dark cells* with condensed nuclei simulate a biphasic pattern (Right inset). The dark cells with small, condensed nuclei represent tumor cells undergoing apoptosis. The ratio of these different cell types varies from tumor to tumor and even in different areas of same tumor. (**c**) Higher-power magnification shows the neoplastic cells homogeneously growing in cohesive sheets with finely dispersed chromatin, small nucleoli, scarce, pale to lacy, granular or vacuolated cytoplasm with indistinct margin. The nuclei are generally about 1.5 to 2 times larger than normal lymphocytes. The clear vacuolated cytoplasm is caused by intracytoplasmic glycogen, which is not stained or washed out during formalin fixation (inset). (**d**) Areas of spontaneous necrosis is associated with *"ghost"* outlined cells (asterisk). (**e**) Occasionally, degenerated tumor cells forms a *"rosette-like"* structure which are composed of intertwining cytoplasmic processes, simulating neuroblastoma or PNET (asterisks). (**f**) In some cases, tumor cells can be arranged in variably sized nests separated by fibrous tissue septa mimicking a pulmonary *"alveolar pattern."* The cells appear as loosely dispersed and are surrounded by central clear spaces with focal necrosis. (**g**, **h**) Although not pathognomonic, IHC stains both for CD99/MIC2 and FLI-1 are positive in about 90% of cases. The cells show peripheral membranous expression (yellow arrow) of CD99/MIC2 and centered expression (white arrow) in the nucleus of the tumor cells of FLI-1. CD99 is also expressed by many other malignant small round cell tumors such as lymphoma, small cell type osteosarcoma, mesenchymal chondrosarcoma, and small cell carcinoma. However, small cell osteosarcoma and mesenchymal chondrosarcoma are negative for FLI-1

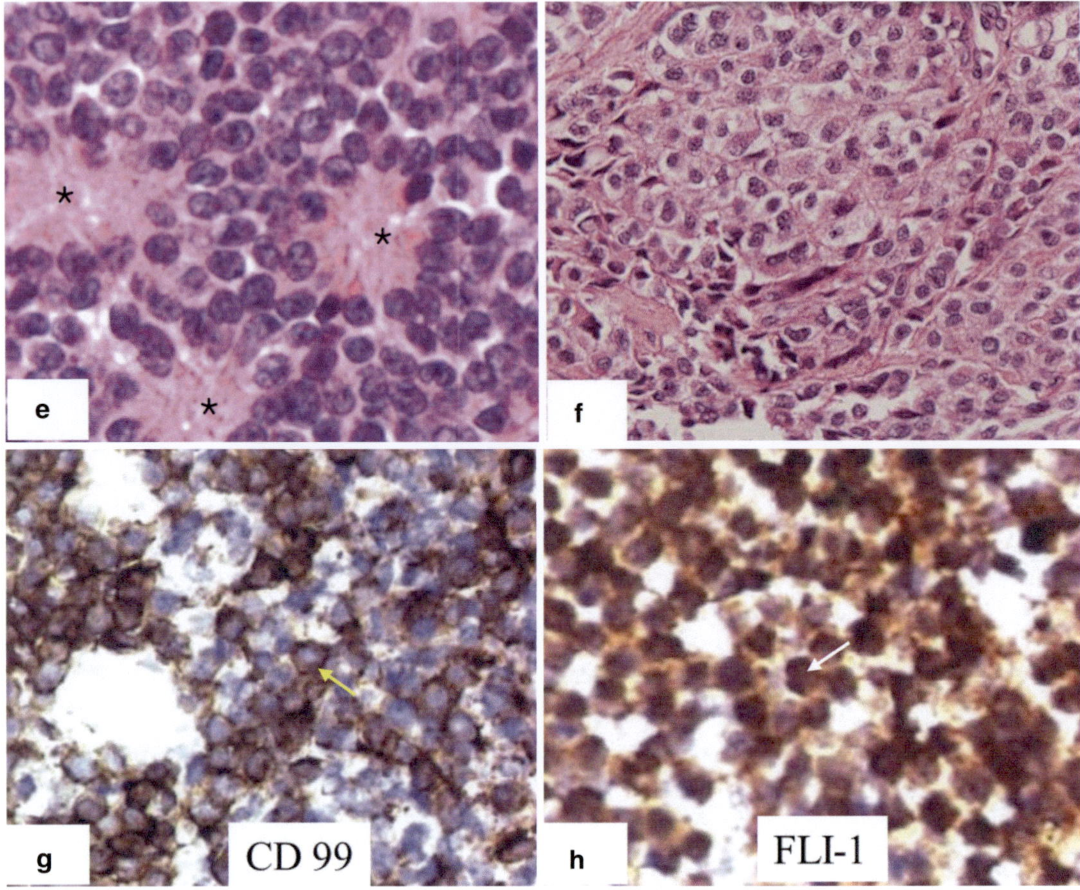

Fig. 25.6 (continued)

25.9 Special Stains

Intracytoplasmic glycogen is clearly detected by periodic acid Schiff (PAS) stain. Immunohistochemical (IHC) stains are mandatory to exclude other types of hematopoietic round cell tumors. IHC stains both for CD99/MIC2 and FLI-1 are positive in most cases (Fig. 25.6g, h). **Molecular genetics** is often required for a diagnostic confirmation of ES. Translocation t(11;22)(q24;q12) is most commonly associated with ESFs in 85% of cases. This fusion of EWS gene on 22q12 with the FLI1 gene on 11q24 results in a chimeric fusion transcript EWS-FLI1 [6].

25.10 Management

Management consists of systemic therapy using neo-adjuvant multidrug chemotherapy and local disease control by wide resection and reconstruction (Figs. 25.1, 25.2, 25.3 and 25.4). Radiotherapy is reserved for tumors located in surgically inaccessible sites, surgical field obtained with inadequate margins, or severely contaminated field. High-dose chemotherapy (HDCT) with autologous stem cell transplantation (ASCT) has been developed to treat patients at high risk of relapse with unpromising result [7, 8]. However, other studies suggested HDCT with ASCT improved survival benefits [7, 9–11].

25.11 Clinical Course and Prognosis

ES is an aggressive malignant tumor with a poor prognosis due to high rate of metastasis at presentation and high incidence of recurrence. Before chemotherapy era, the prognosis was dismal, but the advent of chemotherapy and advanced surgical technique dramatically improve the prognosis. Preoperative chemotherapy allows pathologic assessment of excised specimen for effectiveness of the used drugs. Excised specimens are examined thoroughly mapped into grids to assess the degree of necrosis in the greatest dimension of the tumor. The histological response to chemotherapy is graded quantitatively. Grade 1 is less than 50% of tumor necrosis, grade 2 is more than 50% but less than 90% necrosis, grade 3 is 90–99% necrosis, and grade 4 is 100% necrosis. Patients with a good response to chemotherapy (>90% tumor necrosis, grades 3 and 4) have superior local recurrence-free survival at 5 years than poor responder (86% vs. 51%, $P = 0.015$) [12]. The overall survival of localized disease is improved up to 70–80% at 5 years, but that is still dismal in the patients with initial metastasis at presentation or recurrent disease only with 30–40% survival at 5 years [13–20]. Surveillance, Epidemiology, and End Results (SEER) data analysis by American Cancer Society based on people diagnosed with Ewing tumors between 2012 and 2018 reports 5-year relative survival rates of 82% for localized ES, 71% for reginal ES, 39% for ES with distant metastasis, and 63% for all SEER stages ES [21]. The overall survival rate in infants and toddler was reported to be about 60%, almost identical to the survival rates of the older children [22]. Over 70% of relapses occur within 2 years after completion of chemotherapy and surgery, so-called *"early relapse"* [23–28]. Most local recurrence or relapse (85–90%) occurs within 5 years, and the rest of recurrence (10–15%) occurs after 5 years [18, 25]. The prognosis has been reported to be better in patients with relapse after 2 years than in whom with recurrence within 2 years [18, 25, 29]. *"Periosteal ES"* is very rare and only sporadically reported. Thus, the small number of cases does not allow any conclusion regarding a prognosis. However, the prognosis would be better with long-term survival when compared with its intramedullary counterpart because this type of ES is almost always localized in the juxta-cortical area without involvement of the bone and allow wide local resection easy.

References

1. Czerniak B. Ewing's sarcoma and related tumors. In: Dorfman HD, Czerniak B, editors. Dorfman and Czerniak's bone tumors. 2nd ed. Amsterdam: Elsevier; 2016. p. 760–816.
2. Unni KK, Inwards CY. Ewing's tumor. In: Unni KK, Inwards CY, editors. Dahlin's bone tumors: general aspects and data on 10,165 cases. 6th. ed. Philadelphia, PA: Lippincott William & Wilkins; 2010. p. 211–24.
3. Mirra JM, Picci P. Ewing sarcoma. In: Mirra JM, editor. Bone tumors: clinical, radiologic, and pathologic correlation. 2nd ed. Philadelphia, PA: Lea & Febiger; 1989. p. 1087–117.
4. Goldstein H, McNeil BJ, Zufall E, Treves S. Is there still a place for bone scanning in Ewing's sarcoma? Concise communication. J Nucl Med. 1980;21(1):10–2.
5. Nair N. Bone scanning in Ewing's sarcoma. J Nucl Med. 1985;26(4):349–52.
6. Delattre O, Zucman J, Plougastel B, Desmaze C, Melot T, Peter M, et al. Gene fusion with an ETS DNA-binding domain caused by chromosome translocation in human tumours. Nature. 1992;359(6391):162–5.
7. McTiernan A, Driver D, Michelagnoli M, Kilby A, Whelan J. High dose chemotherapy with bone marrow or peripheral stem cell rescue is an effective treatment option for patients with relapsed or progressive Ewing's sarcoma family of tumours. Ann Oncol. 2006;17(8):1301–5.
8. Meyers PA, Krailo MD, Ladanyi M, Chan K-W, Sailer SL, Dickman PS, et al. High-dose melphalan, etoposide, total-body irradiation, and autologous stem-cell reconstitution as consolidation therapy for high-risk Ewing's sarcoma does not improve prognosis. J Clin Oncol. 2001;19(11):2812–20.
9. Barker LM, Pendergrass TW, Sanders JE, Hawkins DS. Survival after recurrence of Ewing's sarcoma family of tumors. J Clin Oncol. 2005;23(19):4354–62.
10. Burdach S, Jürgens H, Peters C, Nürnberger W, Mauz-Körholz C, Körholz D, et al. Myeloablative

radiochemotherapy and hematopoietic stem-cell rescue in poor-prognosis Ewing's sarcoma. J Clin Oncol. 1993;11(8):1482–8.
11. Tenneti P, Zahid U, Iftikhar A, Yun S, Sohail A, Warraich Z, et al. Role of high-dose chemotherapy and autologous hematopoietic cell transplantation for children and young adults with relapsed Ewing's sarcoma: a systematic review. Sarcoma. 2018;2018:1.
12. Lin PP, Jaffe N, Herzog CE, Costelloe CM, Deavers MT, Kelly JS, et al. Chemotherapy response is an important predictor of local recurrence in Ewing sarcoma. Cancer. 2007;109(3):603–11.
13. Ginsberg JP, Woo SY, Johnson ME, Hicks MJ, Horowitz ME. Ewing's sarcoma family of tumors: Ewing's sarcoma of bone and soft tissue and the peripheral primitive neuroectodermal tumors. In: Pizzo PA, Poplack DG, editors. Principles and practice of pediatric oncology. 4th ed. Philadelphia, PA: Lippincott Williams and Wilkins; 2002. p. 973–1016.
14. Grier HE, Krailo MD, Tarbell NJ, Link MP, Fryer CJ, Pritchard DJ, et al. Addition of ifosfamide and etoposide to standard chemotherapy for Ewing's sarcoma and primitive neuroectodermal tumor of bone. N Engl J Med. 2003;348(8):694–701.
15. Esiashvili N, Goodman M, Marcus RB. Changes in incidence and survival of Ewing sarcoma patients over the past 3 decades: surveillance epidemiology and end results data. J Pediatr Hematol Oncol. 2008;30(6):425–30.
16. Ozaki T, Hillmann A, Hoffmann C, Rübe C, Blasius S, Dunst J, et al. Significance of surgical margin on the prognosis of patients with Ewing's sarcoma: a report from the cooperative Ewing's sarcoma study. Cancer. 1996;78(4):892–900.
17. Dunst J, Schuck A. Role of radiotherapy in Ewing tumors. Pediatr Blood Cancer. 2004;42(5):465–70.
18. Bacci G, Longhi A, Ferrari S, Mercuri M, Versari M, Bertoni F. Prognostic factors in non-metastatic Ewing's sarcoma tumor of bone: an analysis of 579 patients treated at a single institution with adjuvant or neoadjuvant chemotherapy between 1972 and 1998. Acta Oncol. 2006;45(4):469–75.
19. Ahrens S, Hoffmann C, Jabar S, Braun-Munzinger G, Paulussen M, Dunst J, et al. Evaluation of prognostic factors in a tumor volume-adapted treatment strategy for localized Ewing sarcoma of bone: the CESS 86 experience. Med Pediatr Oncol. 1999;32(3):186–95.
20. Rodriguez-Galindo C, Spunt SL, Pappo AS. Treatment of Ewing sarcoma family of tumors: current status and outlook for the future. Med Pediatr Oncol. 2003;40(5):276–87.
21. American Cancer Society. Survival Rates for Ewing Tumors. cancer.org cancer.org | 1.800.227.2345 https://www.cancer.org › detection-diagnosis-staging.
22. Maygarden SJ, Askin FB, Siegal GP, Gilula L, Schoppe J, Foulkes M, et al. Ewing sarcoma of bone in infants and toddlers. A clnicopathologic report from the intergroup Ewing's study. Cancer. 1993;71(6):2109–18.
23. Leavey PJ, Mascarenhas L, Marina N, Chen Z, Krailo M, Miser J, et al. Prognostic factors for patients with Ewing sarcoma (EWS) at first recurrence following multi-modality therapy: a report from the Children's oncology group. Pediatr Blood Cancer. 2008;51(3):334–8.
24. Stahl M, Ranft A, Paulussen M, Bölling T, Vieth V, Bielack S, et al. Risk of recurrence and survival after relapse in patients with Ewing sarcoma. Pediatr Blood Cancer. 2011;57(4):549–53.
25. Bacci G, Longhi A, Ferrari S, Mercuri M, Barbieri E, Bertoni F, et al. Pattern of relapse in 290 patients with nonmetastatic Ewing's sarcoma family tumors treated at a single institution with adjuvant and neoadjuvant chemotherapy between 1972 and 1999. Eur J Surg Oncol. 2006;32(9):974–9.
26. Rodriguez-Galindo C, Billups CA, Kun LE, Rao BN, Pratt CB, Merchant TE, et al. Survival after recurrence of Ewing tumors: the St. Jude Children's Research Hospital experience, 1979–1999. Cancer. 2002;94(2):561–9.
27. Shankar A, Ashley S, Craft A, Pinkerton C. Outcome after relapse in an unselected cohort of children and adolescents with Ewing sarcoma. Med Pediatr Oncol. 2003;40(3):141–7.
28. Ferrari S, Luksch R, Hall KS, Fagioli F, Prete A, Tamburini A, et al. Post-relapse survival in patients with Ewing sarcoma. Pediatr Blood Cancer. 2015;62(6):994–9.
29. Rodriguez-Galindo C, Navid F, Liu T, Billups C, Rao B, Krasin M. Prognostic factors for local and distant control in Ewing sarcoma family of tumors. Ann Oncol. 2008;19(4):814–20.

26 Undifferentiated Pleomorphic Sarcoma

(***undifferentiated*** "anaplastic" + ***pleiōn*** "more, excessive"+ ***morphē*** "form" + ***ōma*** "forming")

26.1 Definition

Intraosseous undifferentiated pleomorphic sarcoma (IUPS), formerly malignant fibrous histiocytoma (MFH), is a rare highly malignant neoplasm of bone typified by a mixture of pleomorphic spindle cells without a specific line of differentiation. Most IUSP (80%) occurs as a primary bone tumor without any underlying conditions, but remained cases (20%) arise secondarily from the pre-existing bone conditions [1–4]. Secondary UPS can be associated with bone infarct, Paget disease, chondrosarcoma, non-ossifying fibroma, fibrous dysplasia, enchondroma, and chronic osteomyelitis, or at the site of irradiation or orthopedic implant [1, 3–8] (Fig. 26.4f).

26.2 Incidence

The incidence may vary depending on the criteria used. UPS is considered one of the most frequent types of soft tissue sarcoma accounting for over 25% of all adult soft tissue sarcomas [9]. However, IUPS is much rarer, only occupying less than 0.6% of primary bone tumors [1, 2] and 1–2% of all primary malignant bone tumors [1, 2, 10]. However, IUPS is the second most malignant bone tumor after chondrosarcoma in adults.

26.3 Age

It can evenly occur in any age groups from a newborn to very old patients. The incidence is gradually increased in older people. The age distribution is wide usually from second to seventh decade of life with a peak incidence in patients older than 50 years of age. The lesion is extremely rare in patients younger than 10 years or older than 80 years. Only 10% of cases are diagnosed in patients younger than age 20 years [2]. Secondary UPS arising from Paget's disease or bone infarct may occur in patients with a more advanced age [4].

26.4 Location

IUPS can involve almost any bones including skull and small tubular bones, but it most commonly occurs around the knee (metaphysis of distal femur and proximal tibia) followed by proximal femur, mid-femur, and proximal humerus [1, 2, 10]. Pelvic bone is the most common site when trunk is involved. Extraordinarily, IUPS can affect multiple bones (Fig. 26.3).

W.-J. Bahk, *Diagnosis and Management of Primary Bone Tumors*,
https://doi.org/10.1007/978-981-99-5498-8_26

26.5 Clinical Features

Pain with or without swelling is the most common symptom usually with short duration of a few months. Pathologic fracture is often complicated particularly when weight bearing part of the long bone is involved. On occasion, vague constitutional symptoms such as fevers, chills, night sweats, and weight loss can be accompanied.

26.6 Radiologic Findings

The lesion exhibits an ill-defined, purely lytic, geographic destruction often with scattered or confluent areas of *"moth-eaten"* to *"permeative"* destruction showing a wide transitional zone, typically in the metaphyseal location of the long bones which may extend into the epiphysis, or pelvic bones (Figs. 26.1a, 26.2a and 26.3a). Pure diaphyseal locations is rarely affected, representing only 10% of cases in the Rizzoli Institute series with 90 cases [11]. Generally, the cortex is destructed extensively and extends into soft tissue to make a mass even in its' early phase. Surrounding rim of reactive sclerosis is not frequent but usually does not completely surround the lesion if presents. Periosteal reaction and new bone formation are not usually seen and minimal if exists. **Bone scan** reveals heterogeneously increased uptake with focal void areas. **PET/CT scan** notes an abnormal FTG uptake indicating hypermetabolic lesion and detects exceedingly rare case of multiple involvement as well (Figs. 26.1c, 26.2c and 26.3c). **CT scan** shows a relatively well-defined medullary lesion with cortical erosion and/or destruction, soft tissue extension with a density typically similar to adjacent muscle, and heterogeneous lower density areas of hemorrhage, necrosis, or myxoid material. **MR images** more clearly reveal a well-defined intramedullary lesion usually with cortical destruction and soft tissue mass formation with low to intermediate SI on T1-weighted image and intermediate to high SI on T2-weighted image. The signal is often heterogeneous if hemorrhage, calcification, necrosis, and myxoid change present. The solid components of the lesion are prominently enhanced (Figs. 26.1, 26.2, 26.3 and 26.4).

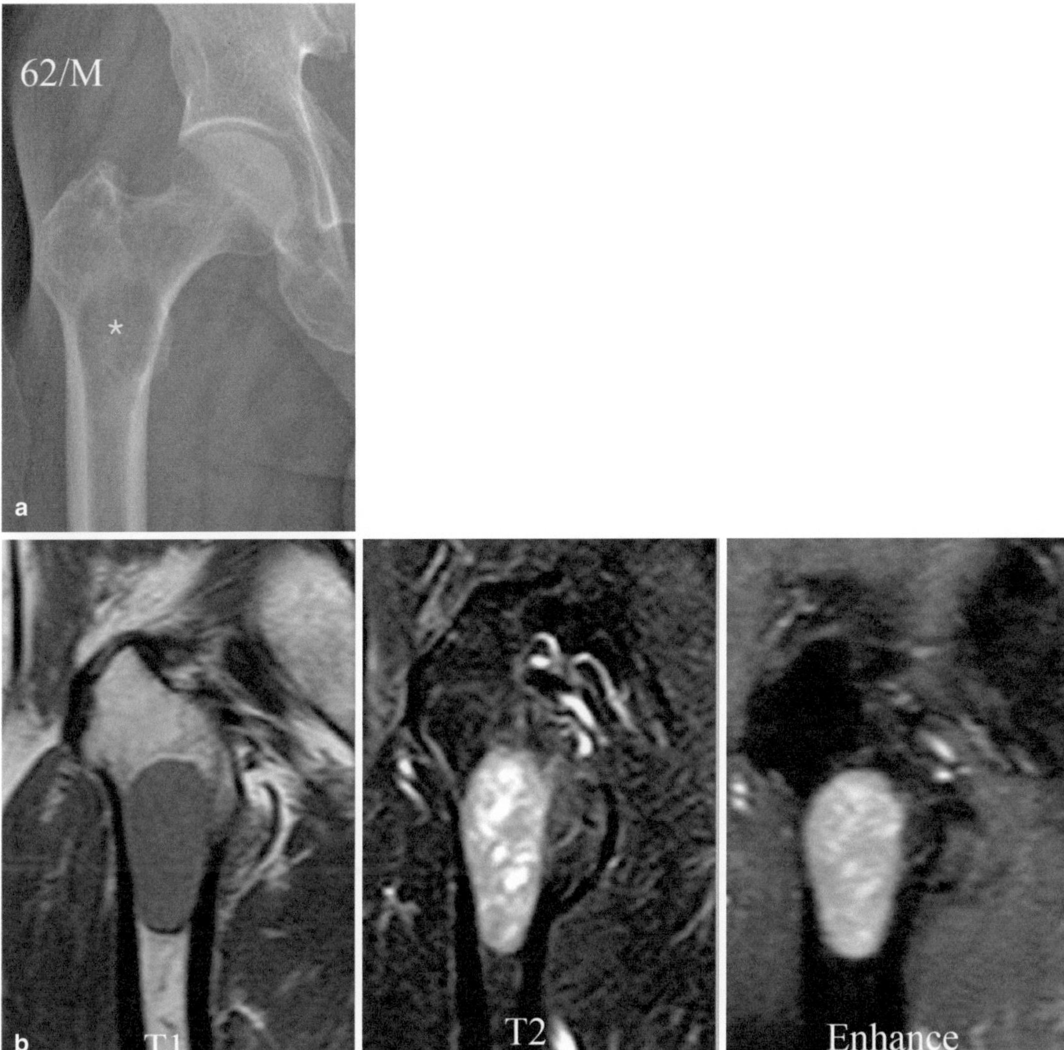

Fig. 26.1 (**a**) Radiograph taken for right hip of 4-month duration in 62-year-old man shows a relatively ill-defined geographic destruction without surrounding rim of sclerosis in the metaphysis of proximal femur (asterisk). (**b**) MR images reveal a well-defined intramedullary large mass-like lesion with low SI on T1-weighted image and heterogeneous intermediate and high SI on T2-weighted image. There is no definite cortical destruction and soft tissue extension. The lesion is focally enhanced. (**c**) PET/CT scan demonstrates increased FDG uptakes in the lesion of right proximal femur as well as in ribs, lungs, and liver, indicating multiple metastases. (**d**) Chest and abdomen CT scan notes a large mass in right upper lung and multiple tiny nodules on both lung fields as well as two large masses in the liver (arrows). (**e**) Microscopic findings of the bone, lung, and liver are identical. (Left) Medium-power magnification reveals proliferation of bland-looking spindle cells in storiform arrangement with larger pleomorphic neoplastic cells. (Middle) There is another area with increased number of multinucleated giant tumor cells with large hyperchromatic nuclei embedded within collagen-rich, even hyalinized stroma as well as hemangiopericytoma-like vascular structure. (Right) Higher–power magnification of more pleomorphic-looking area notes anaplastic large mononuclear spindle or epithelioid cells with abundant granular to foamy cytoplasm, large, bizarre, round to oval, some reniform, or lobulated nucleus in fascicular pattern. IHC stain is strong and even positive only for vimentin but negative to focal weak positive in other stains for mesenchymal tumors and cytokeratin, which supports a diagnosis of UPS of femur, which metastasized to lung and liver. (**f**) Follow-up radiograph at 1 year after minimized surgery of curettage, cementing, and intramedullary nailing for pain control and prevention of pathologic fracture notes no further local progression of the hip lesion. However, his general condition was worsened and transferred to hospice care unit because of progressive lung and liver metastases with hepatic failure

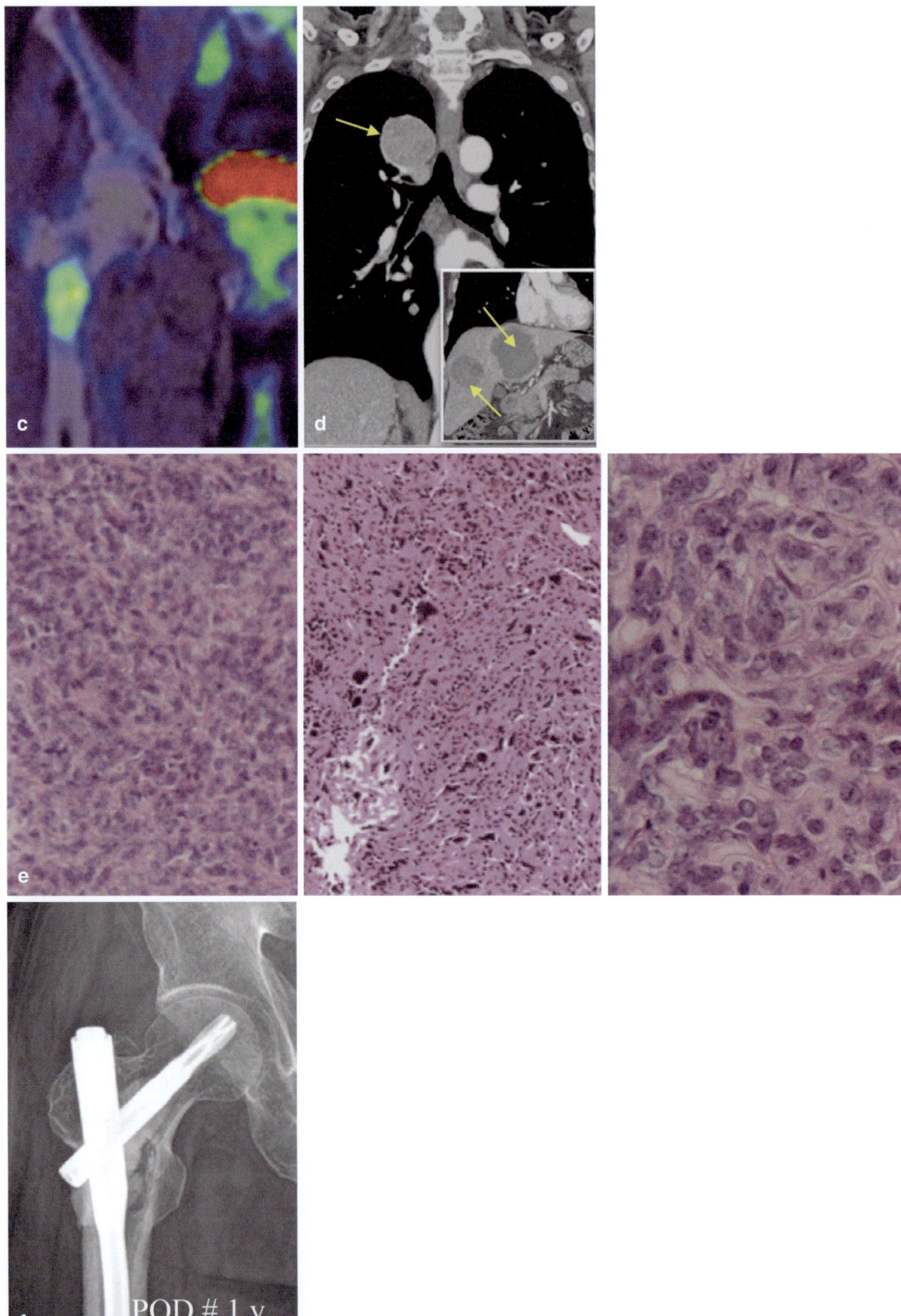

Fig. 26.1 (continued)

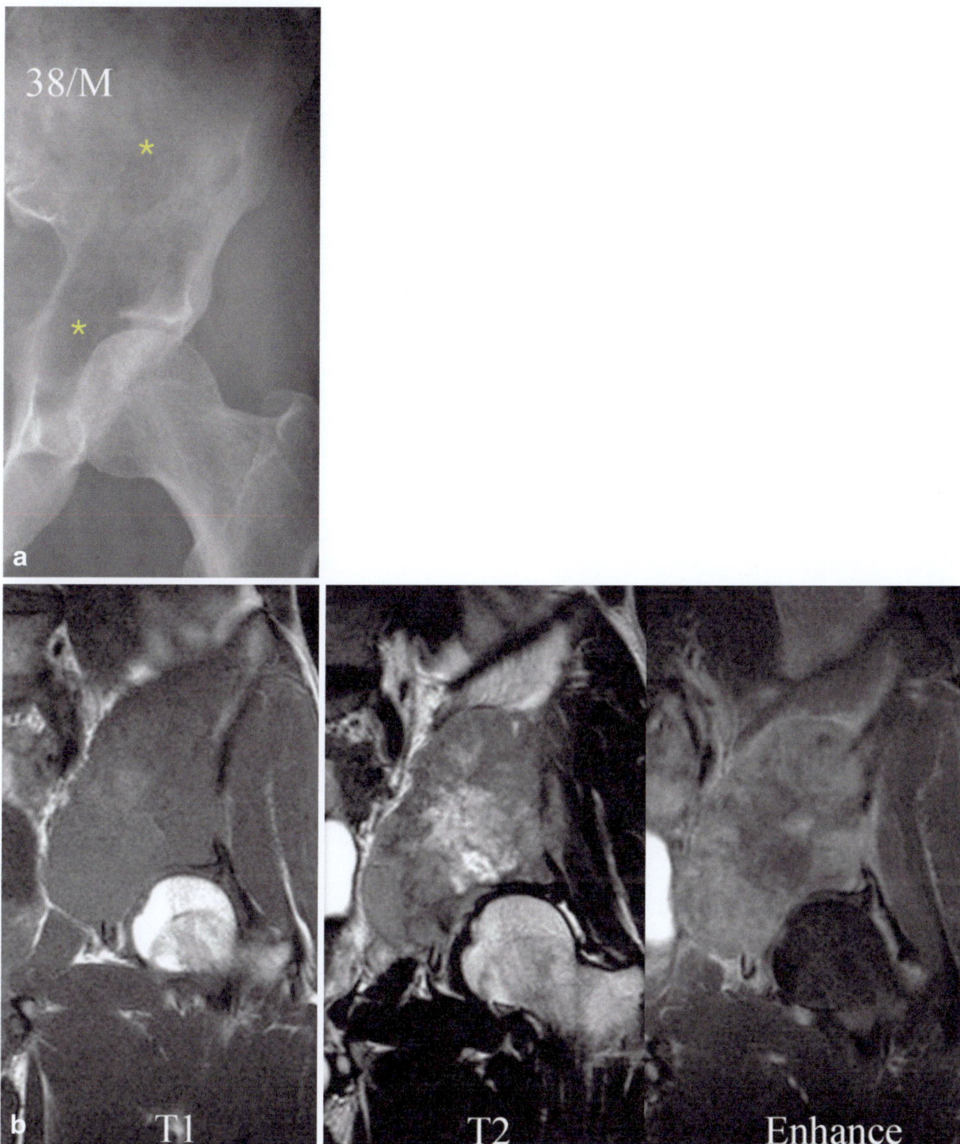

Fig. 26.2 (**a**) Radiograph taken for left hip of 2-month duration in 38-year-old man shows an ill-defined huge radiolucent lesion with a wide transitional margin (asterisks) affecting left acetabulum and iliac wing. (**b**) MR images reveal a huge destructive lesion with an ill-defined margin in the acetabulum, superior pubic ramus, and iliac wing. The lesion totally breaks the inner cortex, extends to surrounding muscles with a huge soft tissue mass, and invades into the hip joint. The SI is low and intermediate on T1-weighted image and heterogeneous intermediate and high SI on T2-weighted image, suggesting hemorrhage and necrosis. The lesion is heterogeneously enhanced. (**c**) PET/CT scan notes a huge hypermetabolic mass in the lesion (SUVmax 13.4). No other abnormal hypermetabolic lesions are observed. (**d**) Microscopic examination. (Left) Lower-power magnification notes a focus of more or less pleomorphic mononuclear cells permeating a host lamellar bone spicule (arrow). (Right) Higher-power magnification shows bizarre pleomorphic mononuclear cells in varying degree of size and shape with an abundant granular to foamy cytoplasm, bizarre, round to oval, some reniform nucleus, and a prominent nucleolus as well as abnormal mitosis (red arrow). Varying size of hemangiopericytoma-like vascular spaces is also seen (asterisks). A diagnosis of UPS affecting left pelvic bones is rendered with exclusion of other sarcomas by strong positive stain for vimentin and negative in all stains for other mesenchymal tumors. (**e**) Follow-up radiograph at 1 year after internal hemi-pelvectomy notes progression of destruction of the remained pelvic bone with significant migration of the resected femur. He died of lung metastasis at 1 year after surgical resection (inset)

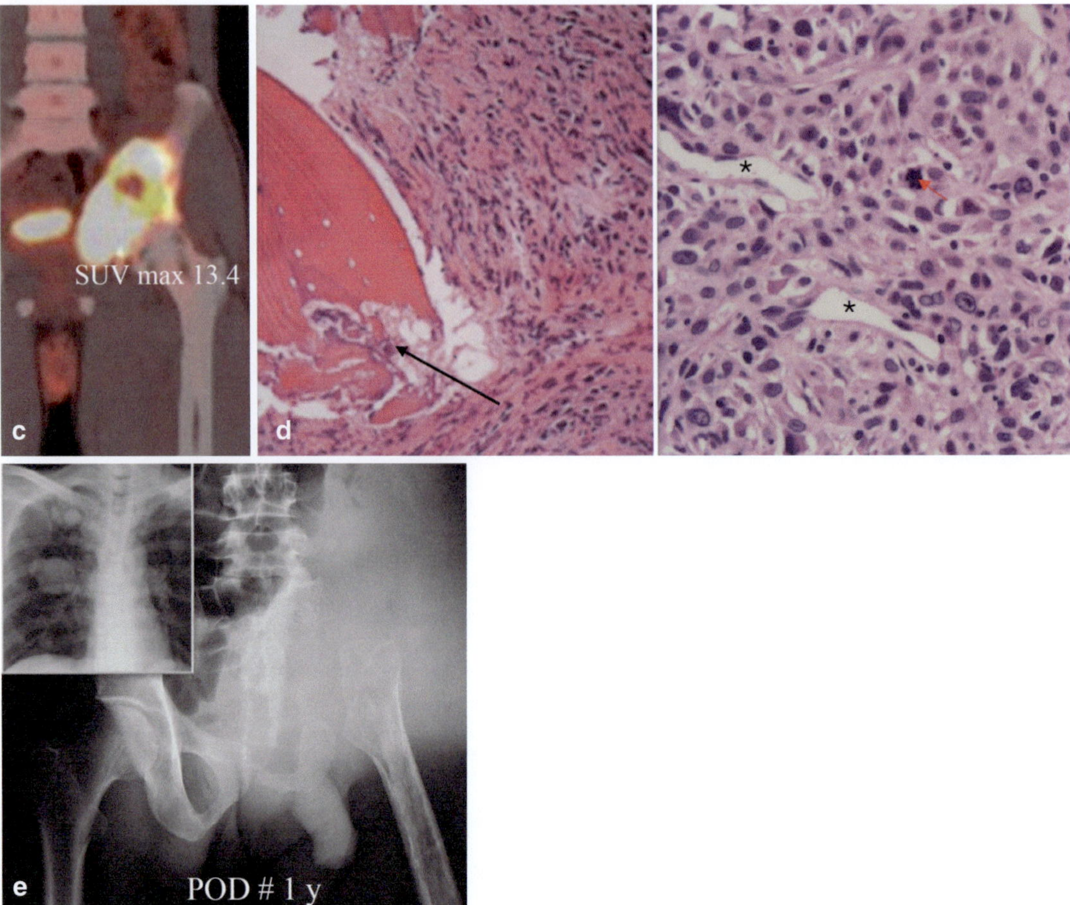

Fig. 26.2 (continued)

Fig. 26.3 ***Multiple IUPSs*** (**a**) Radiograph taken for right pelvic bone pain after fall from 2-m height in 53-year-old man shows an ill-defined huge geographic destruction (yellow asterisk) with compression of the cortex (arrow) in right acetabulum and iliac wing. There is an incidentally observed smaller osteolytic lesion in left acetabulum (white asterisk). (**b**) CT scan reveals a significant bone destruction with a bulging soft tissue density and markedly comminuted fragment as well as cortical breakage (yellow arrow) in right iliac bone and a relatively well-defined osteolytic lesion with a focal cortical disruption (white arrow) in the left iliac bone. (**c**) PET/CT scan notes multiple heterogeneously hypermetabolic lesions (SUVmx 9.8–14.8) in both iliac bones extending to surrounding muscles and left proximal femur, suggesting multiple lesions. (**d**) MR images reveal an ill-defined significant bone destruction and huge soft tissue masses with low to intermediate SI on T1-weighted image and heterogeneous intermediate and high SI on T2-weighted image affecting both acetabuli and iliac bones. There is a relatively well-defined smaller lesion in left intertrochanteric area with similar signal as iliac bone lesions (inset). All of the lesions are heterogeneously enhanced by contrast medium. (**e**) Microscopic examination. (Left) Lower-power magnification shows a mixture of more pleomorphic-looking cells and other blander-looking cells arranged in broad *"storiform"* pattern with abundant collagen production. (Right) Higher-power magnification reveals pleomorphic cells in variable size and shape with bizarre nuclei as well as and frequent abnormal mitoses, which are embedded within collagen-abundant stroma. A final diagnosis of multiple UPSs is confirmed by strong and even positive stain only for vimentin but no other ICH stains. (**f**) Eight months later, follow-up radiograph notes a significant progression of the lesions, and pulmonary metstasis occurs. And then, the patient is lost for follow-up

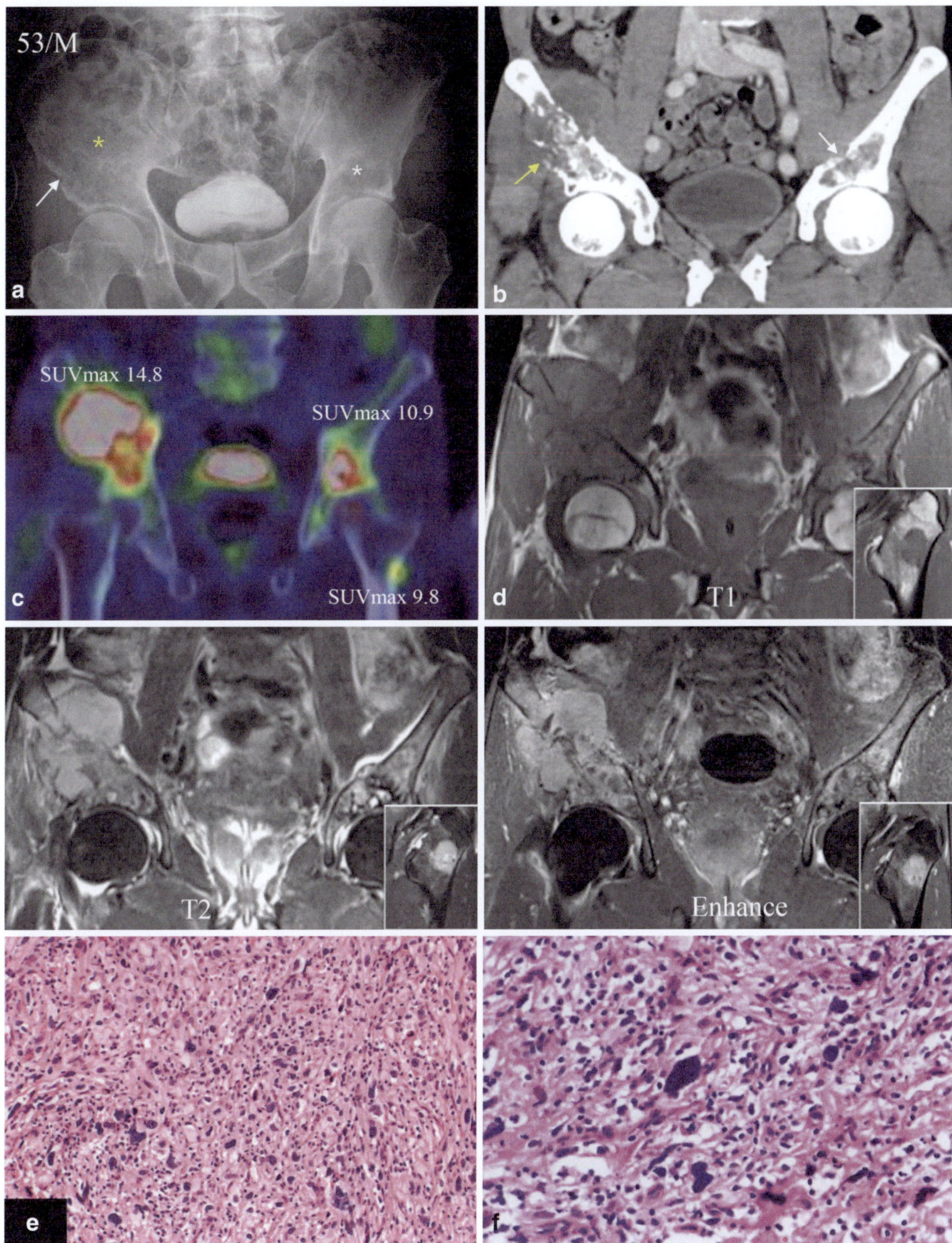
53/M
a
b
SUVmax 14.8
SUVmax 10.9
SUVmax 9.8
c
d
T1
T2
Enhance
e
f

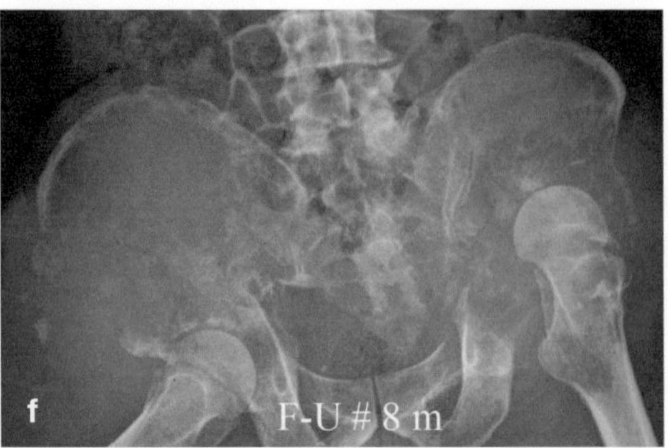

Fig. 26.2 (continued)

Fig. 26.4 ***Rare location of spine*** (**a**) Radiograph taken for back pain of 5-month duration in 48-year-old man shows an ill-defined osteolytic lesion with mild collapse (circle) involving the body of twelfth dorsal spine. (**b**) CT scan reveals an ill-defined osteolytic lesion affecting body and a part of posterior elements with cortical destruction and collapse of the body (circle), which extends into paravertebral space and epidural space on sagittal image (arrow in inset). (**c**) MR images demonstrate irregularly infiltrative medullary lesion extending into paravertebral space and epidural space (yellow arrow in inset) with low SI on T1-weighted image and heterogeneous intermediate and high SI on T2-weighted image, affecting the body and posterior elements of the spine. The body is markedly collapsed with ventral indentation of the spinal cord by the tumor mass (yellow arrows). The lesion is homogeneously well enhanced (inset). There is post-biopsy change around the spinous process and subcutaneous area (yellow asterisk). (**d**) PET/CT scan notes a heterogeneously hypermetabolic lesion mostly localized in the body (SUVmax 6.13) and in a small part of the posterior elements. Otherwise, no other abnormal hypermetabolic lesions are observed. (**e**) Total spondylectomy of D12 and fusion using allogenic strut bone graft fixed by legacy system from D10–11 to L2–3 vertebrae was performed under a histologic diagnosis of UPS after exclusion of other sarcomas by IHC stains. Follow-up radiograph at 1 year after surgery shows good maintenance with no definite evidence of local recurrence. ***Secondary IUPS arsing at the site of total hip replacement*** (**f**) Radiograph taken for left hip of 4-month duration in 60-year-old woman shows peri-prosthetic osteolysis in the femoral trochanteric area (asterisks). She had a past history of radiation therapy for rectal cancer 15 years ago and avascular necrosis of left femur head 13 years ago, which was treated by total hip regalement. (**g**) Pinhole bone scan reveals heterogeneously increased uptake trochanteric area with a focal strong uptake at grater trochanter (red arrow). There is photon defect area (black asterisk) with curvilinear mild uptake at outer part of the replaced prosthetic head (black arrow). Curettage and biopsy showed marked necrosis and fibrosis with no definite malignancy at that time. (**h**) However, follow-up radiograph at 1 year after curettage notes progression of the osteolytic lesion (asterisks). (**i**) PET/CT scan demonstrates a heterogeneous hypermetabolic lesion around the femoral prosthesis stem with a prominent localized uptake at lesser trochanter level (SUVmax 10.1). Biopsy confirmed a diagnosis of UPS of in the peri-stem area of total hip replacement after exclusion of other sarcomas by strong positivity only for vimentin. We are not sure the if this secondary IUPS is associated with irradiation for rectal cancer or just arose at the site of orthopedic implant. (**j**) Wide resection followed by reconstruction with tumor prosthesis was performed and adjuvant chemotherapy was performed. Follow-up radiograph at 9 years after revision surgery reveals no definite evidence of local recurrence. (**k**) Follow-up bone scan notes peri-prosthetic mild uptake particularly in the prosthesis-host bone contact area (black arrow) and distal end of the prosthesis (blue arrow) as well as in the contact acetabular area of prosthetic cup (red arrow). Note photon defect only with a diffuse faint peri-prosthetic uptake in the body of prosthetic stem (asterisk) indicating no local recurrence

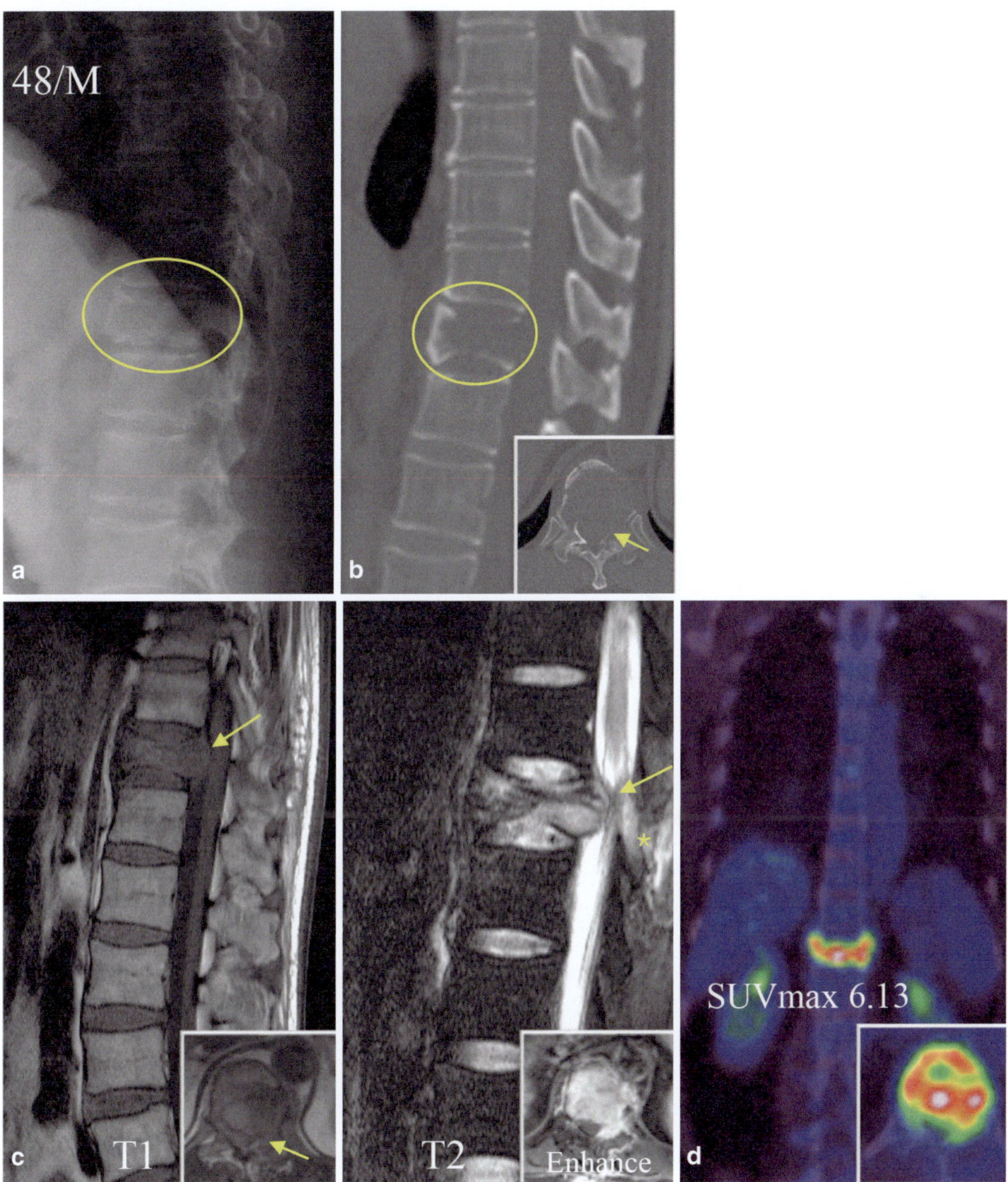
48/M
a
b
T1
c
T2
Enhance
SUVmax 6.13
d

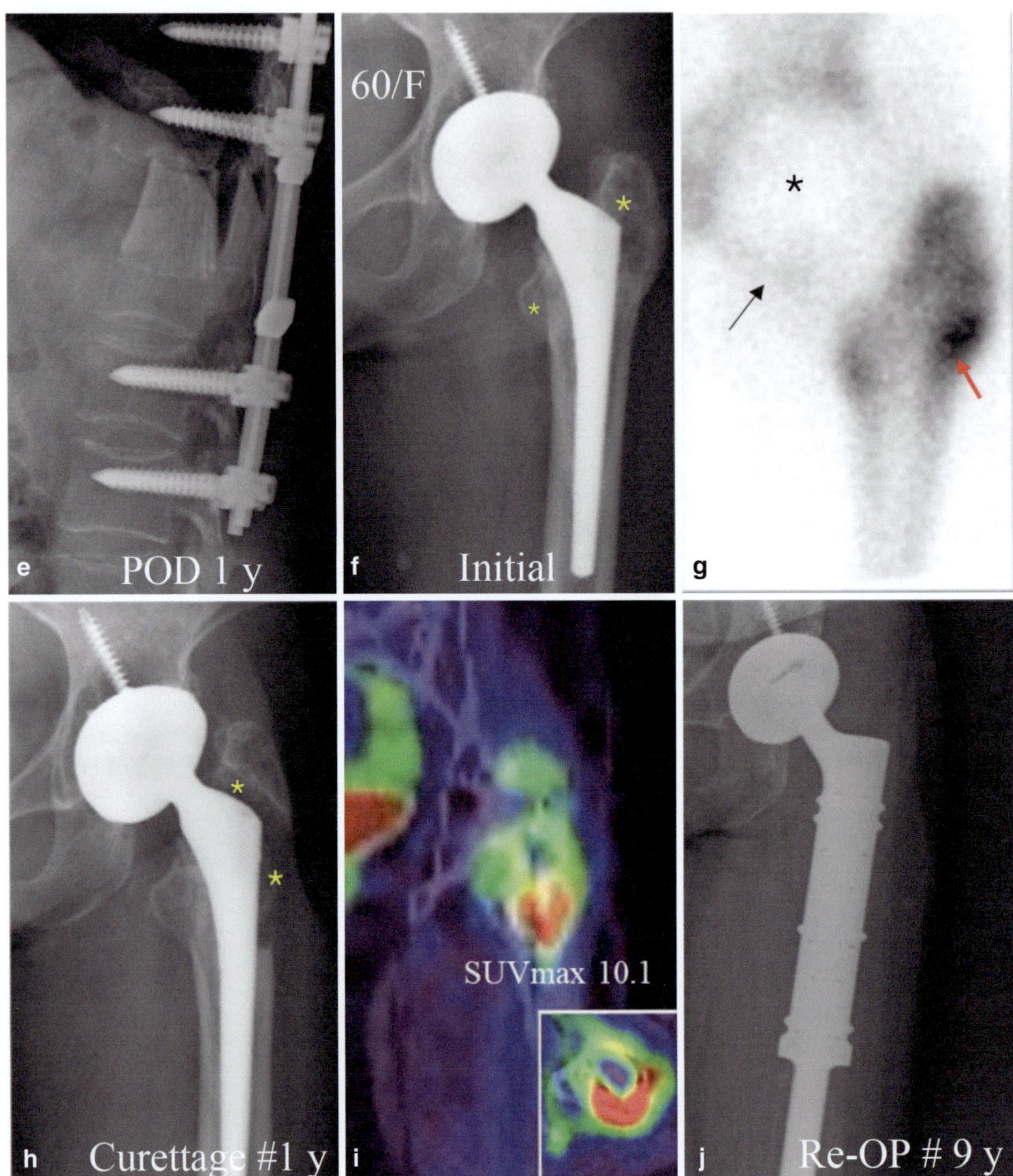

Fig. 26.4 (continued)

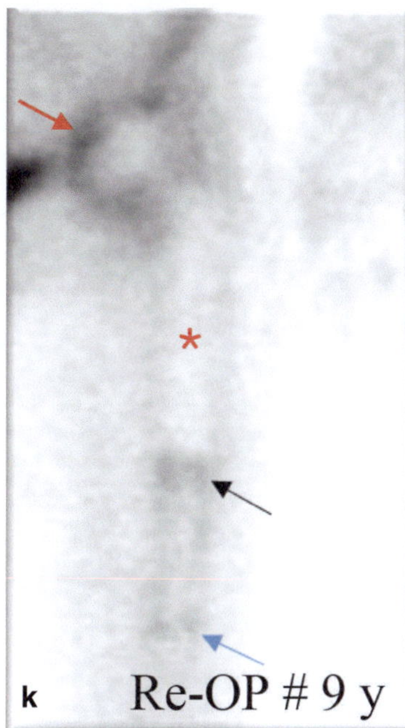

Fig. 26.4 (continued)

26.7 Histologic Findings

Extensive biopsy sample is required for scrutinized examination of presence of even focal deposition of osteoid and/or primitive woven bone to exclude osteosarcoma. The lesion typically consists of a high cellular mixture of more pleomorphic-looking cells and other bland-looking cells of spindle cells with variable amount of collagen production (Fig. 26.5a). The pleomorphic histiocytic cells and bland-looking spindle cells are typically arranged in a *"storiform"* pattern, which is only focally exhibited in most cases and is more evident in areas with prominent collagen production (Fig. 26.5b). In cellular areas where anaplasia is not conspicuous, the cells are more spindle-shaped and smaller, which seem to be similar to normal fibroblasts. Foci of extensive or focal necrosis with scattered foamy histiocytes are often seen. Foci of anaplastic large mononuclear spindle or epithelioid cells with abundant granular to foamy cytoplasm, large, severely bizarre nucleus arranged in haphazard, storiform, or fascicular pattern are an important clue for the diagnosis. In some cases, pleomorphic stromal cells are admixed with diffusely sprinkled prominent multinucleated giant cells, so-called *"giant cell-rich"* variant (Fig. 26.5c). Inflammatory cells including lymphocytes and histiocytes are frequently seen in the collagenous stroma in soft tissue, but distinct inflammatory variant is very rare in IUPS. Bizarre malignant- and benign-looking reactive multinucleated giant cells can be admixed in varying degree. High-power magnification reveals tumor cells with abundant eosinophilic cytoplasm and significant pleomorphism, suggesting high-grade malignant tumor (Fig. 26.5d). Hemangiopericytoma-like vascular structure can be occasionally observed (Fig. 26.5e). Atypical mitoses are usually abundant. UPS of soft tissue has been subclassified into storiform-pleomorphic (the most common type), myxoid, inflammatory, giant cell-rich, and angiomatoid type. All these subtypes can be existed in IUPS [12], but storiform- pleomorphic and giant cell-rich variants are most frequent, but myxoid and inflammatory subtypes have been rarely reported [2].

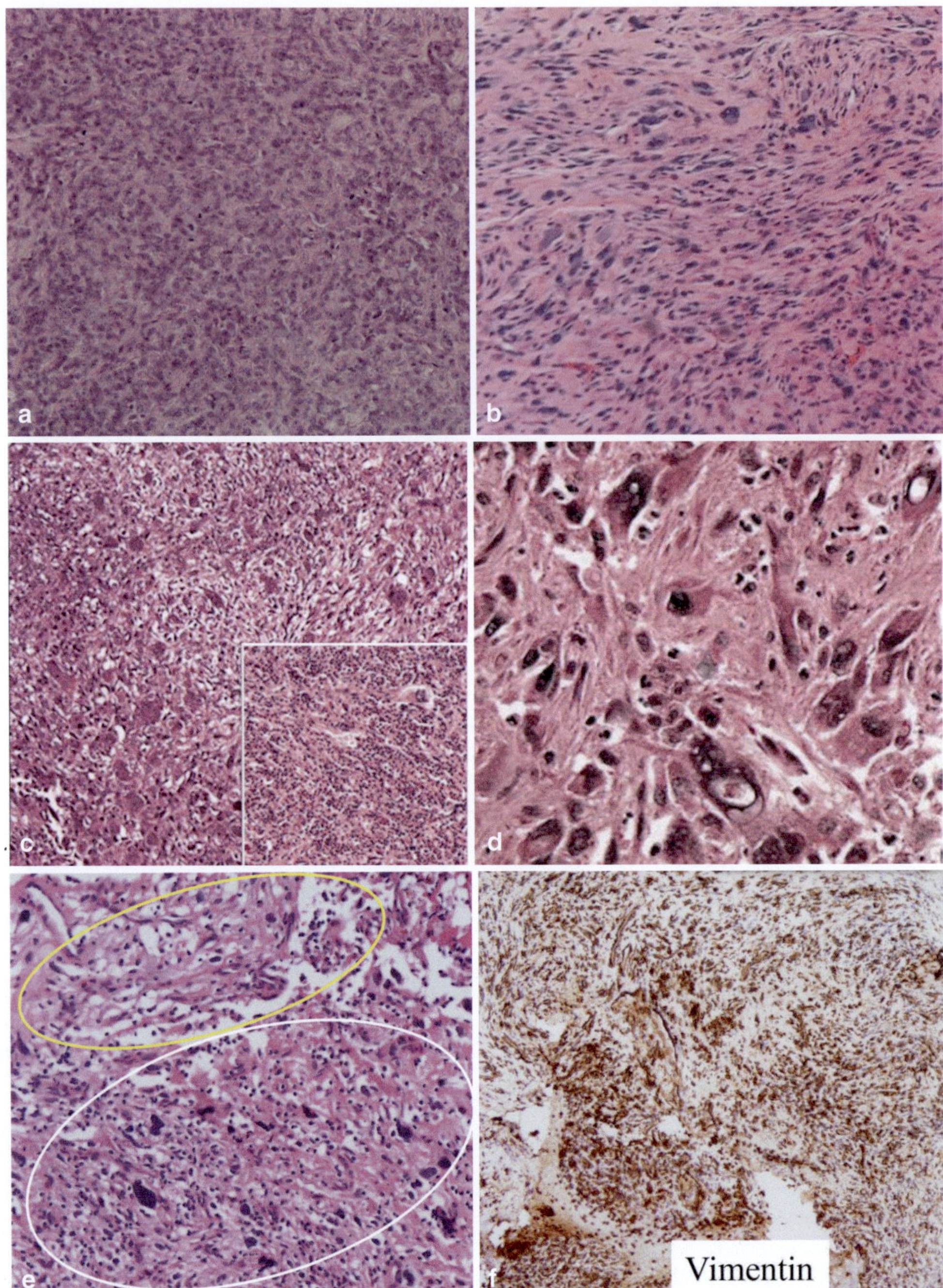

Fig. 26.5 ***Microscopic examination*** (**a**) Low-power magnification shows a mixture consisting of high number of pleomorphic spindle cells interspersed with large anaplastic histiocytic cells and bland-looking spindle cells. (**b**) A *"storiform"* arrangement of pleomorphic and bland-looking spindle cells, a hallmark of IUPS, is more evident in areas with prominent collagen production. (**c**) Some cases reveal pleomorphic stromal cells with profuse scattered multinucleated giant cells (giant cell-rich variant). Inflammatory cells are often focally present (inset), but a distinct inflammatory variant is rare in bone. (**d**) High-power magnification notes tumor cells with abundant eosinophilic cytoplasm and significant pleomorphism showing bizarre nuclei that resembles rhabdomyosarcoma. (**e**) Hemangiopericytoma-like vascular structure is also observed (yellow circle) with abundant collagen production some of which is hyalinized, and there are also significantly pleomorphic cells (white circle). (**f**) ICH stain for fibroblastic marker, vimentin, is strongly and evenly positive, which also shows a characteristic *"storiform arrangement"*

26.8 Special Stains

UPS is a diagnosis of exclusion of other malignant neoplasms by histologic examinations including IHC stains and molecular studies. IHC stain itself gives little role to confirm a diagnosis of UPS, but it is popularly used to exclude other malignant tumors. Stain for vimentin of fibroblastic marker is strongly and evenly positive in UPS (Fig. 26.5f). Stain for smooth muscle actin (SMA) can be weakly and focally positive. However, stains for histiocytic markers such as KP-1 (CD68) are not expressed in the pleomorphic tumor cells. Other stains for keratin, S-100, desmin, myogenin, and MYOD1 can provide an aid to exclude metastatic carcinoma, rhabdomyosarcoma, and melanoma.

26.9 Management

Wide resection with or without reconstruction is the cornerstone of treatment. The role of neo-adjuvant chemotherapy is not entirely clear. However, the amount of tumor necrosis after chemotherapy is one of the most important prognostic factors. Radiation therapy may improve local tumor control by killing residual microscopic disease. It can be given for high-grade, large (>5 cm), deep-seated tumors when adequate margins are not obtained or for unresectable sarcomas.

26.10 Clinical Course and Prognosis

IUPS is a highly malignant and aggressive tumor with a high propensity for distant metastasis, typically to lung (Figs. 26.1, 26.2 and 26.3). Prognostic factors that are known to correlate with survival include tumor grade, location, size, metastatic status, patient's age, and histologic subtype as well as the amount of tumor necrosis by chemotherapy. Favorable prognostic factors include good responder to neo-adjuvant chemotherapy, no metastasis at presentation, younger age less than 40 years old at presentation, and adequate wide surgical margin. A recent review of 408 patients from the National Cancer Database between 2004 and 2016 reported that the overall 5-year and 10-year survival rates were 38.3% and 30.5%, respectively [13].

References

1. Mirra JM, Picci P, Malignant fibrous histiocytoma. Ewing's sarcoma. In: Mirra JM, editor. Bone tumors: clinical, radiologic, and pathologic correlation. 2nd ed. Philadelphia, PA: Lea & Febiger; 1989. p. 766–99.
2. Czerniak B. Fibrous and fibrohistiocytic lesions. In: Dorfman HD, Czerniak B, editors. Dorfman and Czerniak's bone tumors. 2nd ed. Amsterdam: Elsevier; 2016. p. 617–91.
3. Murphey MD, Gross TM, Rosenthal HG. From the archives of the AFIP. Musculoskeletal malignant fibrous histiocytoma: radiologic-pathologic correlation. Radiographics. 1994;14(4):807–26.
4. Nishida J, Sim FH, Wenger DE, Unni KK. Malignant fibrous histiocytoma of bone: a clinicopathologic study of 81 patients. Cancer. 1997;79(3):482–93.
5. Kennedy C, Stoker D. Malignant fibrous histiocytoma complicating chronic osteomyelitis. Clin Radiol. 1990;41(6):435–6.
6. Haag M, Adler C. Malignant fibrous histiocytoma in association with hip replacement. J Bone Joint Surg Br. 1989;71(4):701.
7. Nelson J, Phillips P. Malignant fibrous histiocytoma associated with total hip replacement. A case report. Orthop Rev. 1990;19(12):1078–80.
8. Lindeman G, McKay MJ, Taubman KL, Bilous AM. Malignant fibrous histiocytoma developing in bone 44 years after shrapnel trauma. Cancer. 1990;66(10):2229–32.
9. Enzinger F, Weiss S. Soft tissue tumors. 3rd ed. St Louis, MO: Editorial Mosby; 1995. p. 1067–93.
10. Unni KK, Inwards CY. Malignant fibrous hiticytoma. In: Unni KK, Inwards CY, editors. Dahlin's bone tumors: general aspects and data on 10,165 cases. 6th. ed. Philadelphia, PA: Lippincott William & Wilkins; 2010. p. 184–90.
11. Capanna R, Bertoni F, Bacchini P, Bacci G, Guerra A, Campanacci M. Malignant fibrous histiocytoma of bone the experience at the Rizzoli institute: report of 90 cases. Cancer. 1984;54(1):177–87.
12. McCarthy EF, Matsuno T, Dorfman HD. Malignant fibrous histiocytoma of bone: a study of 35 cases. Hum Pathol. 1979;10(1):57–70.
13. Malik AT, Baek J, Alexander JH, Voskuil RT, Khan SN, Scharschmidt TJ. Malignant fibrous histiocytoma of bone: a survival analysis from the National Cancer Database. J Surg Oncol. 2020;121(7):1097–103.

Leimyosarcoma

27

(***leios*** "smooth" + ***myos*** "muscle" + ***ōma*** "forming")

27.1 Definition

Intraosseous leiomyosarcoma (ILMS) is a very rare aggressive primary malignant mesenchymal tumor involving bone typified by smooth muscle differentiation sharing with identical pathologic characteristics of uterine and soft tissue counterparts.

27.2 Incidence

ILMS is extremely rare to occupy less than 0.1% of biopsy-proven primary bone tumor [1] and less than 1% of all primary malignant bone tumors [2, 3]. Only a small number of studies or case reports are available in the literature.

27.3 Age

The ages of patients are widely varying from first to eighth decades of life with median age of about 45 years [3, 4]. The age distribution is similar to its soft tissue counter part [1].

27.4 Location

The long bone is primarily affected with the most common site being the distal femur followed by proximal tibia around the knee, representing 65–70% of cases [3, 4]. The pelvic and craniofacial bones are next frequently involved. When long tubular bone is affected, ILMS is usually located in the metaphysis rarely extending to the epiphysis (Fig. 27.1) or diaphysis (Fig. 27.2). The pelvic bone is most frequently affected trunk bone.

W.-J. Bahk, *Diagnosis and Management of Primary Bone Tumors*,
https://doi.org/10.1007/978-981-99-5498-8_27

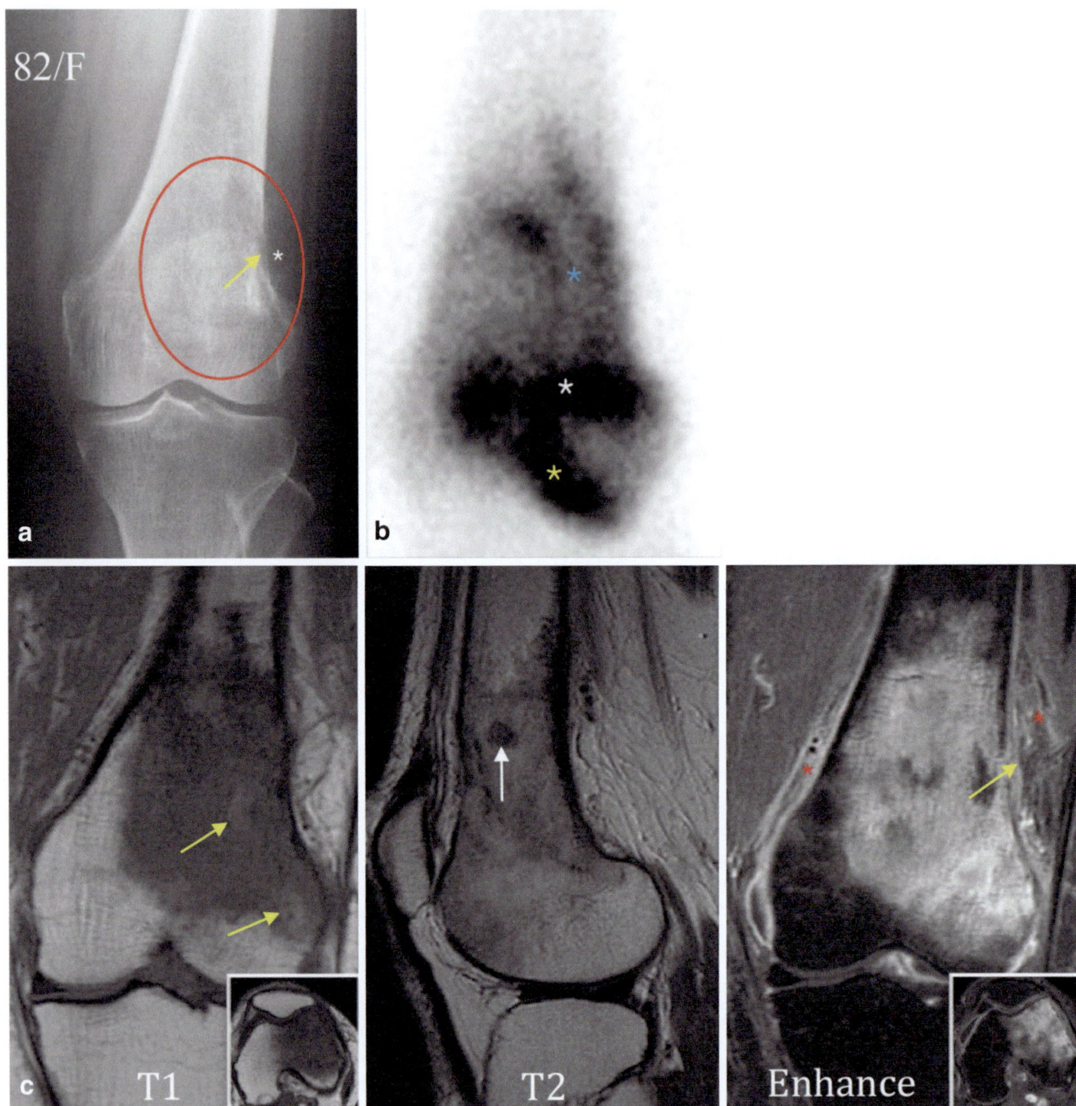

Fig. 27.1 ***The oldest in our series*** (**a**) Radiograph taken for left knee pain of 3-month duration in 82-year-old woman shows an ill-defined, hazy, radiolucent lesion with a wide zone of transition (circle) in the meta-diaphysis of distal femur. The lateral cortex is thinned and focally disrupted (arrow) with a subtle small soft tissue mass formation (asterisk). (**b**) Pinhole bone scan reveals a strong uptake mainly in the metaphysis (white asterisk) and epiphysis (yellow asterisk) as well as heterogeneous milder uptake in the diaphyseal area (blue asterisk) of the distal femur. (**c**) MR images demonstrate an ill-defined intramedullary mass-like lesion with low SI with focal intermediate to high signal of fat (arrows) on T1-weighted image and intermediate to high SI on T2-weighted image, mainly in meta-diaphysis of the distal femur with irregular epiphyseal extension. The lesion contains several small foci with dark signal of calcification (white arrow). The lesion is heterogeneously well enhanced with non-enhancing areas of necrosis and calcification. Note cortical thinning and breaches with focal soft tissue extension (yellow arrow) and adjacent soft tissue edema, which are also heterogeneously enhanced (red asterisks). (**d**) PET/CT scan notes heterogeneous hypermetabolic lesion only in the distal femur (SUVmax 4.2). No other definite hypermetabolic abnormality in the uterus, gastrointestinal, or other soft tissue organs suggesting a primary bone tumor. (**e**) Microscopic examination. (Right) Higher-power magnification notes spindle cells typically with prominent eosinophilic cytoplasm and elongated, "cigar-shaped" nuclei. IHC stain for smooth muscle actin (SMA) shows diffusely and strongly positive. (**f**) Radiograph at 2 years after wide resection and reconstruction using tumor prosthesis shows good maintenance with no evidence of local recurrence

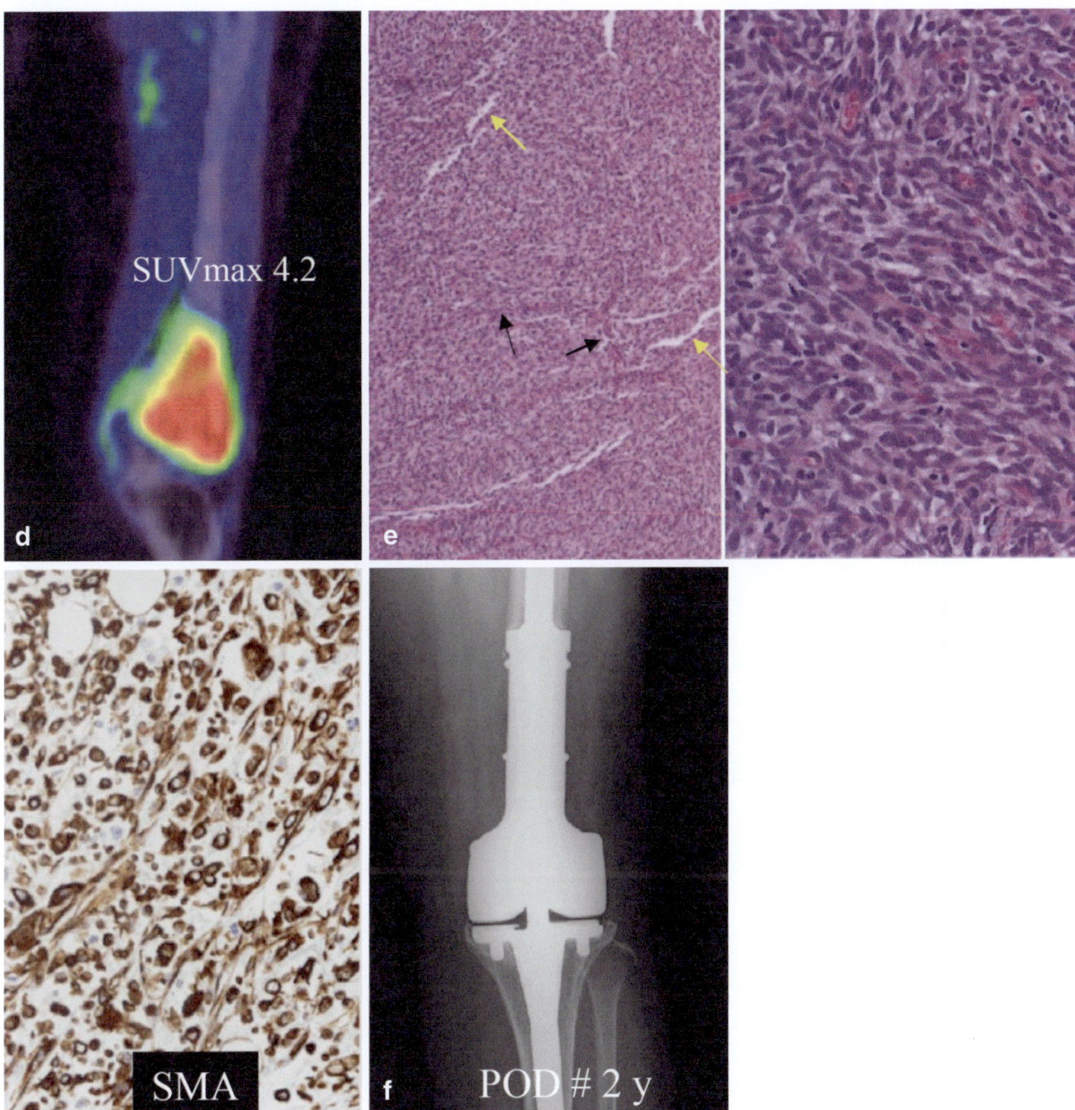

Fig. 27.1 (continued)

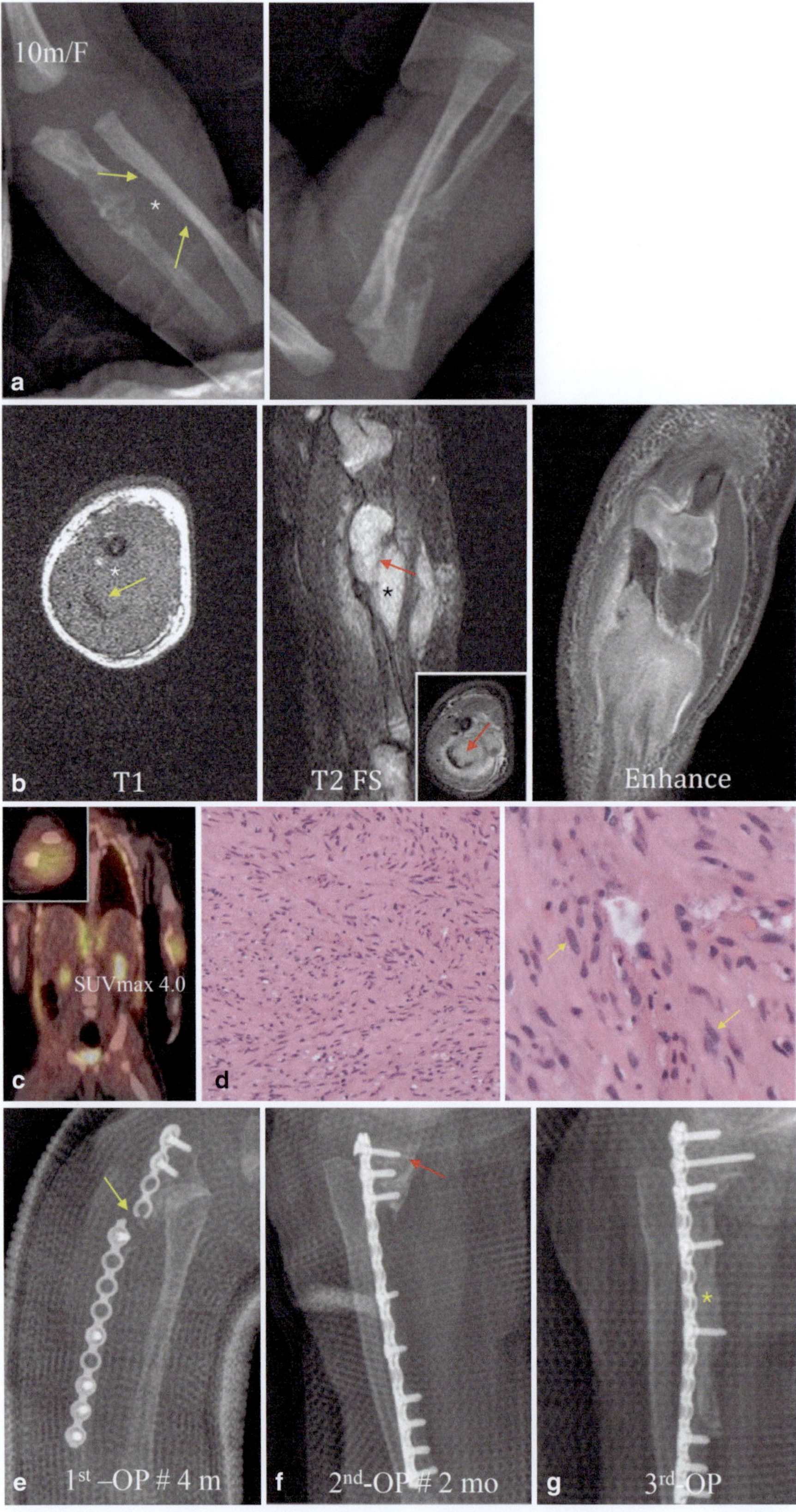
10m/F
a
b
T1
T2 FS
Enhance
SUVmax 4.0
c
d
e
1st –OP # 4 m
f
2nd-OP # 2 mo
g
3rd-OP

Fig. 27.2 ***The youngest in our series*** (**a**) Radiograph taken for palpable mass of left forearm since her birth in 10-month-old infant girl shows an ill-defined aggressive looking mixed geographic and moth-eaten destruction with a wide zone of transition affecting proximal shaft of the ulna. Note marked cortical destruction with a huge soft tissue mass (asterisk) resulting in compression erosion and thinning of the opposite radius shaft (arrows). (**b**) MR images are not adequate in quality because of patient's motion in spite of sedation. MR images reveal of ill-defined medullary mass lesion with marked cortical destruction (arrows) and huge soft tissue mass (asterisks). The SI is iso to surrounding muscle on T1-weighted image and high on fat saturated T2-weight image. The lesion is heterogeneously and peripherally enhanced. (**c**) PET/CT scan demonstrates increased FTG uptake (SUVmax 4.0) in the mid-shaft of ulna and adjacent muscles. No other definite hypermetabolic abnormality in the uterus, gastrointestinal, or other soft tissue organs suggesting a primary bone tumor. (**d**) Microscopic examination. (Left) Low-power magnification notes long thick bundles of prominent spindle cells in *"storiform"* pattern with abundant collagen production. (Right) Higher-power magnification shows spindle cells with prominent eosinophilic cytoplasm with characteristic elongated, *"cigar-shaped"* nuclei (arrows). ICH stains for SMA, MCA, and desmin are strongly and evenly positive. (**e**) Follow-up radiograph at 4 months after wide resection and reconstruction using fibular graft with neo-adjuvant chemotherapy reveals fracture of grafted fibula with metallic failure (arrow). (**f**) Radiograph at 2 months after revision surgery reveals angulation of proximal segment with loosening of screws (arrow). (**g**) Radiograph at 6 months after re-fixation using new osteosynthesis with allomatix (a combination of DBM with cancellous bone) notes good maintenance of the osteosynthesis (asterisk)

27.5 Clinical Features

Most ILMS primarily arises from bone but rarely occurs secondary to prior irradiation. Often, ILMS initially thought to be primary would be proved to be metastatic lesion from the uterus and gastrointestinal LMS. Pain occasionally with swelling or rapidly enlarging mass is the most common presentation. Pathologic fracture can be also associated.

27.6 Radiologic Findings

The radiologic features are nonspecific but typically aggressive-looking with cortical disruption and extension into soft tissue. The lesion is purely osteolytic often with moth-eaten or permeative growth pattern. The lesion usually exhibits a wide zone of transition with indistinct margin indicating malignant lesion. The metaphysis is almost always involved with extension to diaphysis and rarely epiphysis (Figs. 27.1a and 27.2a). In general, sclerosis is usually not accompanied, and periosteal reaction is not visible or subtle to fine if exists. In one series, lesions in long bones are large and typically elongated with the average intraosseous extent measuring 11 cm (7–17 cm) with limited mediolateral expansion and cortical breaching being reminiscent of a pattern associated with lymphoma [5]. Periosteal new bone formation can be found sometimes in the form of Codman's triangle. The cortex is usually thinned and scalloped to focally disrupted with soft tissue extension. But a large soft tissue mass is usually not visible if pathologic fracture is not associated. Pelvic lesion is also purely osteolytic and aggressive-looking often with a large soft tissue mass (Fig. 27.3a). **Bone scan** reveals heterogeneously increased uptake with focal void areas of necrosis (Figs. 27.1b and 27.3e). **PET/CT scan** notes an abnormal FTG uptake indicating hypermetabolic lesion in the bone. It is useful to confirm primary bone tumor by excluding uterine, gastrointestinal, or other soft tissue counterparts which are metastasized to bone (Figs. 27.1, 27.2 and 27.3). **MR images** reveal an ill-defined mass-like infiltrative lesion with low to intermediate (isointense to muscle) SI on T1-weighted image and heterogeneous intermediate and high SI on T2-weighted image. The lesions are mostly sited in the meta-diaphysis but may extend to the epiphysis on occasion (Fig. 27.1c). Soft tissue extension can be frequently observed though subtle alteration or focal breach of the cortex as in small cell tumor of bone such as Ewing's sarcoma, lymphoma, or leukemia (Fig. 27.1c). In addition, elongated, linearly oriented lesion unexpectedly longer on MR images than on radiograph is a striking feature that is not a typical appearance of metastatic cancer but reminiscent of a pattern of lymphoma of bone [5]. Peritumoral edema can be often extensive probably due to inflammatory response to the tumor infiltration through the cortex to adjacent soft tissue. A soft tissue mass is usually small in the long bone (Fig. 27.1c), but pelvic lesions mostly produce a larger extra-osseous mass (Fig. 27.3c). The lesion is heterogeneously well enhanced with non-enhancing area of necrosis.

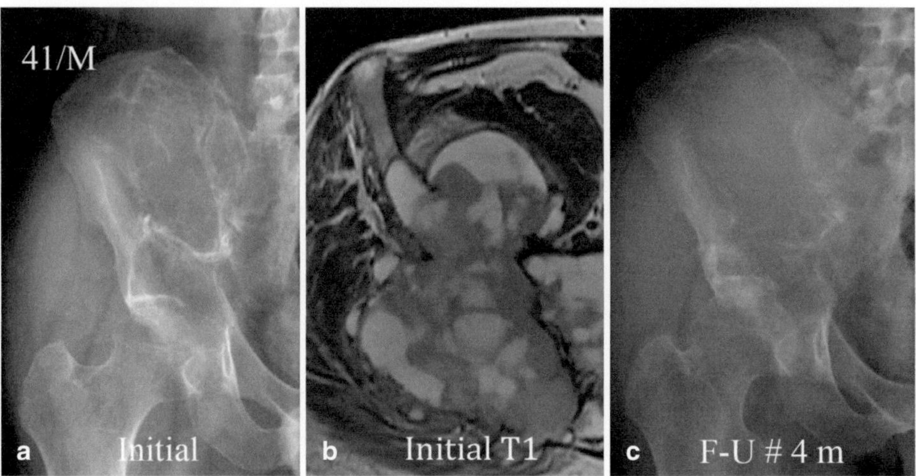

Fig. 27.3 (**a**) Radiograph taken for lower back and right buttock pain of 1-year duration, which is aggravated after slip in 41-year-old man shows a huge multi-septated geographic destruction with a wide zone of transition affecting right pelvic bone. (**b**) MR images reveal a huge multi-lobulated mass-like lesion with heterogeneous low and intermediate SI on T1- weighted image and intermediate and high SI on T2-weighted image (not shown here) involving right sacrum, iliac, and ischial bone, which extensively extends to surround soft tissue and muscles. Histologic diagnosis at another university was rhabdomyosarcoma. (**c**) However, the lesion was significantly progressed during neo-adjuvant chemotherapy and radiotherapy, and he was transferred to our university hospital. Follow-up radiograph at 4 months after initial visit notes that the lesion became enlarged and expansile with loss of the septations indicating a progression of the lesion. (**d**) Follow-up MR images demonstrate that the lesion destructs more severely the bones producing more extensive soft tissue masses with heterogeneous SI on both T1- and T2-weighted images and a prominent enhancement with internal focal non-enhancing areas suggesting a possible necrosis. (**e**) Bone scan notes a strong uptake in the lateral margin of the lesion with central photon defect (asterisk) suggesting a necrosis. (**f**) PET/CT scan demonstrates a heterogeneously increased uptake with central void area in the right iliac bone, acetabulum, right side sacrum, and adjacent muscles. However, there is no hypermetabolic activity in other organs such as uterus and soft tissue counterparts indicating a primary bone tumor. Microscopic examination notes interweaving thick bundles of spindle cells arranged in *"storiform"* pattern with abundant collagen production. Higher-power magnification notes markedly pleomorphic cells and abnormal mitoses indicating grade 4 sarcoma. Stains for SMA and desmin are strong positive. The final diagnosis of ILMS in consideration of no other definite hypermetabolic abnormality in the uterus, gastrointestinal, or other soft tissue on PET/CT scan. (**g**) Preoperative embolization of internal and external iliac arteries was performed. (**h**) Internal hemi-pelvectomy as well as postoperative chemotherapy using Etoposide/Ifosfomide/Cisplatin was performed. At 3 years after, re-operation followed by adjuvant radiotherapy was performed due to local recurrence. (**i**) Follow-up radiograph at 9 years after initial surgery shows progression of the disease with significant upward migration of the femur. He died of local recurrence with multiple metastases to liver, lung, and other bones 3 months later

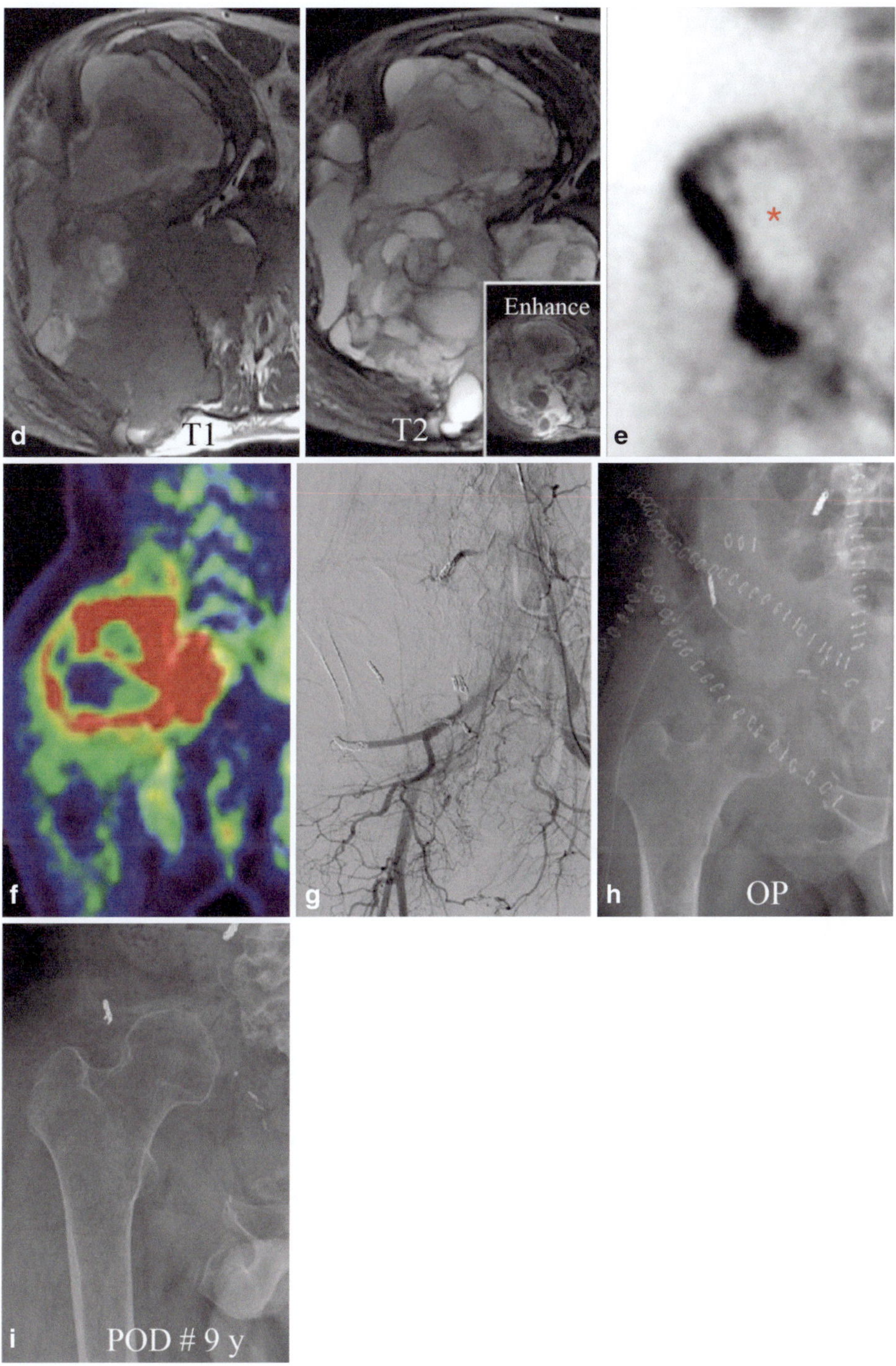

Fig. 27.3 (continued)

27.7 Histologic Findings

Low-power magnification is important to diagnosis and shows interweaving fascicles or thick bundles of spindle cells arranged in *"rolling whorl"* or *"storiform"* pattern with collagen production (Fig. 27.4a). The collagen is variable in amount from case to case and even field to field in same case, and lesion can be focally or diffusely hyalinized. The tumor cells in the fascicles or bundles are arranged in longitudinal orientation and cross each other at wide, sometimes right angle. On higher-power magnification, the spindle cells have prominent eosinophilic cytoplasm

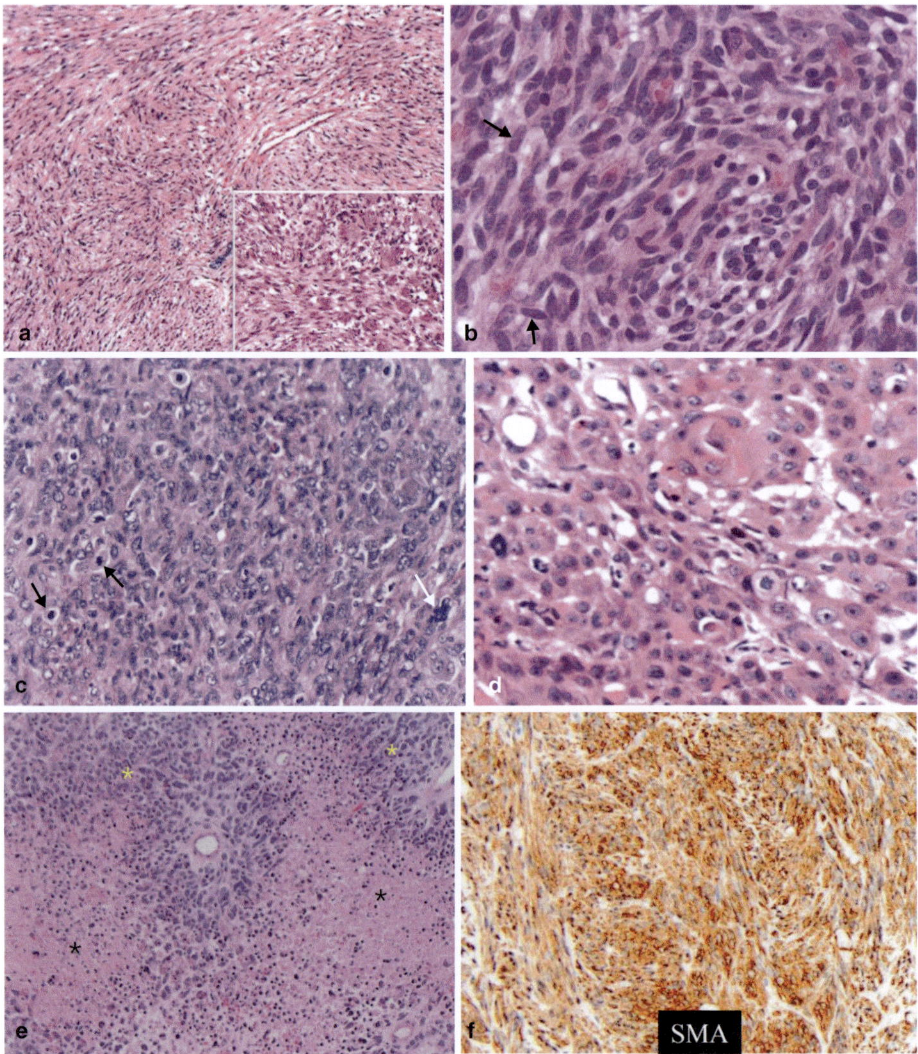

Fig. 27.4 ***Microscopic examination*** (**a**) Low-power magnification shows interweaving fascicles or thick bundles of spindle cells with eosinophilic cytoplasm arranged in *"rolling whorl"* or *"storiform"* pattern and collagen production. The fascicles are arranged in longitudinal orientation and cross each other at wide, often right angle. Variable number of multinucleate giant cells can be frequently scattered throughout the lesion (inset). (**b**) Higher-power magnification reveals the individual spindle cells have prominent eosinophilic cytoplasm with characteristically elongated, blunt end, so-called *"cigar-shaped"* nuclei (arrows), suggesting smooth muscle origin. (**c**) The tumor cells exhibit high degree of pleomorphism with oval to vesicular hyperchromatic nuclei (white arrow), prominent nucleoli, and frequent atypical mitoses (black arrows). (**d**) Some tumor cells are more rounded focally with epithelioid appearance in this field. But more diffuse and prominent epithelioid change is rare in primary ILMS. (**e**) Large geographic areas of spontaneous necrosis (yellow asterisks) are seen in association with areas of marked hyalinization (black asterisks). (**f**) The tumor cells are strongly and diffusely positive for SMA

typically with elongated, *"cigar-shaped"* nuclei with blunt end suggesting smooth muscle origin (Fig. 27.4b). The tumor cells exhibit high degree of pleomorphism with oval to vesicular hyperchromatic nuclei, prominent nucleoli, and frequent atypical mitoses (Fig. 27.4c). Degree of nuclear pleomorphism, mitotic activity, and necrosis correlates with grade of tumor. Pleomorphism and mitotic activity is usually moderate (grade 3) but occasionally prominent (grade 4). The tumor cells may be more rounded with epithelioid appearance. The epithelioid cells can be focally present but are not prominent in most primary ILMSs (Fig. 27.4d). Thus, extensive epithelioid change suggests the lesion would be metastatic from the uterus and other soft tissue LMS rather than primary [6]. Geographic areas of necrosis with or without hyalinization are occasionally present, which can be extensive (Fig. 27.4e). Giant cell reaction is often seen in ILMS.

27.8 Special Stains

The neoplastic cells of LMS express markers indicating a myogenic differentiation. The cells are strongly and diffusely positive for smooth muscle actin (SMA) (Fig. 27.4f), muscle common actin (MCA), and desmin.

27.9 Management

Surgical excision with adequate wide margins with or without reconstruction depending on the location remains the gold standard (Figs. 27.1, 27.2 and 27.3). The role of preoperative chemotherapy remains still debatable with poor response and minimal impact on overall survival benefit [3, 7]. Radiation can be considered for local control particularly in patient with inadequate margin, but its effectiveness is also not promising. Antonescu et al. [4] could not find any difference in survival rates between patients who received surgery alone and patients who received surgery and adjuvant radiation therapy in their series of 33 patients.

27.10 Clinical Course

Data on prognostic factors for ILMS are limited because of its very low prevalence, but clinical outcome reported to be correlated with stage of the diagnosis [3] and histologic grading [4]. The 5-year overall and disease-free survival rates were reported to be 59% to 78%, and 45–82%, respectively, being comparable to that of other skeletal sarcomas [3, 4, 7, 8]. Brewer et al. [3] reported disease-specific survival was 57% at 5 years and 44% at 10 years but for those without metastases was 82% and 60%, respectively. They also concluded high histologic grade and tumor stage with metastasis are predictive of poor outcome as for other bone sarcomas.

References

1. Mirra JM. Primary leiomyosarcomatoma. In: Mirra JM, editor. Bone tumors: clinical, radiologic, and pathologic correlation. 2nd ed. Philadelphia, PA: Lea & Febiger; 1989. p. 874–91.
2. Wirbel RJ, Verelst S, Hanselmann R, Remberger K, Kubale R, Mutschler WE. Primary leiomyosarcoma of bone: clinicopathologic, immunohistochemical, and molecular biologic aspects. Ann Surg Oncol. 1998;5(7):635–41.
3. Brewer P, Sumathi V, Grimer R, Carter S, Tillman R, Abudu A, et al. Primary leiomyosarcoma of bone: analysis of prognosis. Sarcoma. 2012;2012:636849. https://doi.org/10.1155/2012/636849.
4. Antonescu CR, Erlandson RA, Huvos AG. Primary leiomyosarcoma of bone: a clinicopathologic, immunohistochemical, and ultrastructural study of 33 patients and a literature review. Am J Surg Pathol. 1997;21(11):1281–94.
5. Sundaram M, Akduman I, White LM, McDonald DJ, Kandel R, Janney C. Primary leiomyosarcoma of bone. Am J Roentgenol. 1999;172(3):771–6.
6. Czerniak B. Miscellaneous mesenchymal tumors. In: Dorfman HD, Czerniak B, editors. Dorfman and Czerniak's bone tumors. 2nd ed. Amsterdam: Elsevier; 2016. p. 617–91. 1100–1141.
7. Mori T, Nakayama R, Endo M, Hiraga H, Tomita M, Fukase N, et al. Forty-eight cases of leiomyosarcoma of bone in Japan: a multicenter study from the Japanese musculoskeletal oncology group. J Surg Oncol. 2016;114(4):495–500.
8. Adelani MA, Schultenover SJ, Holt GE, Cates JM. Primary leiomyosarcoma of extragnathic bone: clinicopathologic features and reevaluation of prognosis. Arch Pathol Lab Med. 2009;133(9):1448–56.

28 Adamantinoma

(***Adamantine*** "pertaining to the enamel of the teeth"or ***Adamantinos***, "very hard" + ***ōma*** "forming")

28.1 Definition

Adamantinoma (ADA) of long bone is a distinct, rare primary low-grade malignant tumor typically with biphasic histology of epithelial and osteofibrous mesenchymal elements. Early in 1913, Fischer [1] named this tumor "adamantinoma of the tibia" because of its striking histologic resemblance to "adamantinoma" of the jaw bone which is benign but locally aggressive odontogenic tumor originating from the residual epithelium of the tooth germ (ameloblastoma). ADA can be classified into three subtypes: classic, differentiated (osteofibrous dysplasia (OFD)-like), and dedifferentiated ADA.

28.2 Possible Histogenesis

The exact mechanism of development is of ADA of long bone still datable to date. Earlier, Fischer [1] suggested congenital implantation of epithelial cells based on his observation of adamantine epithelium in the tibia as well as in the intraoral enamel during embryonic development. Later, other authors proposed traumatic implantation [2, 3], synovial origin [4, 5], angioblastic [6–9], or dermal inclusion [10]. However, the most widely adopted theory is that of displacement of basal epithelium of skin during embryological development, which is supported by the predominant involvement of anterior tibia where enchondrally formed bone is closest to the skin surface [11]. Many other authors have suggested epithelial origin [12–16].

28.3 Incidence

ADA is very rare, accounting for about 1% of all primary bone tumor [11] and less than 0.5–1% of primary bone tumor [17–21].

28.4 Age

Classic ADA typically affects patients over 20 years with peak incidence between 20 and 40 years. OFD-like ADA usually affects patients younger than 20 years. In Mayor Clinic series, approximately 70% are in their second and third decades of life [20]. The tumor is rarely described in childhood [21].

28.5 Location

ADA exclusively involves diaphysis of tibia and/or fibula. ADA has a strong predilection in the tibia, occupying 80–90% of cases [11,

W.-J. Bahk, *Diagnosis and Management of Primary Bone Tumors*,
https://doi.org/10.1007/978-981-99-5498-8_28

20, 22]. Synchronous involvement of tibia and fibula occurs in about half of the cases [23]. Very rarely, other long bones including humerus, ulna, radius, femur, fibula, and spine, ribs, carpal or metatarsal bones or calcaneum have been reported to be involved [24–31].

28.6 Clinical Features

The initial symptoms are often indolent and nonspecific depending on the extent of the lesion. Generally, The clinical course is, however, prolonged due to its slow growth. A gradual swelling with or without dull aching pain is the main presentation. Anterior bowing of the leg as in OFD is often associated. A palpable mass or pathologic fracture is also presented. A history of previous significant trauma including fracture to the affected site is related in many patients [11, 22].

28.7 Radiologic Findings

In general, classic ADA are radiologically distinct and diagnostic because of their location of predilection and appearance. However, OFD-like differentiated ADA is not distinguishable from OFD on radiographs. Typically, ADA presents eccentric, elongated, single, or multiple variable-sized multilobulated radiolucent lesion and sclerotic foci of interspersed with normal-appearing bone, so-called *"soap-bubble"* appearance, exclusively involving anterior cortex of the shaft of the tibia and/or fibula. Most lesions are mainly confined to the irregularly thickened and sclerotic cortex with scalloping and erosion (intracortical). However, some lesions can extend to medullary space with cortical destruction and soft tissue mass formation. The lesion tends to expand the affected underlying bone due to its slow-growing potential, and each focus is delineated by a ring of the intact cortex to produce *"bubbly"* or *"honeycomb"* appearance (Figs. 28.1a, 28.2a and 28.3a). When involving anterolateral cortex of the tibia, moderate or significant anterior bowing of the leg can be presented as in osteofibrous dysplasia. Periosteal reaction is absent to minimal if exists. When fibula is affected, the eccentricity of the lesion is less evident, and the lesion is centrally located. Expansion of fibular contour is frequent but bowing is not often. **Bone scan** shows (in)homogeneous strong uptake (Fig. 28.1b). In addition, it may find a coexisting fibular involvement. **MR images** are useful to evaluate the extent of intramedullary involvement as well as to depict distant cortical foci and rare cortical destruction with a soft tissue mass, which is essential for the accurate determination of tumor boundaries and the preoperative planning for adequate surgical margin (Figs. 28.1, 28.2 and 28.3). Van der Woude et al. [32] described two morphologic patterns of either a lobulated solitary focus or multiple small nodules in one or more foci interspersed with normal-appearing cortical and/or sponge bone. The authors reported that tumor was confined to the cortical bone without marrow involvement in 40% of ceases, and discrete or more pronounced extension toward the bone marrow was observed in 60%. However, tumor extension into the soft tissues through the cortical breakage was seen in only 10% of patients. The SI is low to intermediate (equal to muscle) on T1-weighted image and high on T2-weighted image. There is usually no periosteal reaction or soft tissue extension through the broken cortex. The lesion tends to be heterogeneously and strongly enhanced suggesting a high vascularity, which was encountered by immunohistochemical (IHC) stain with vascular markers [32].

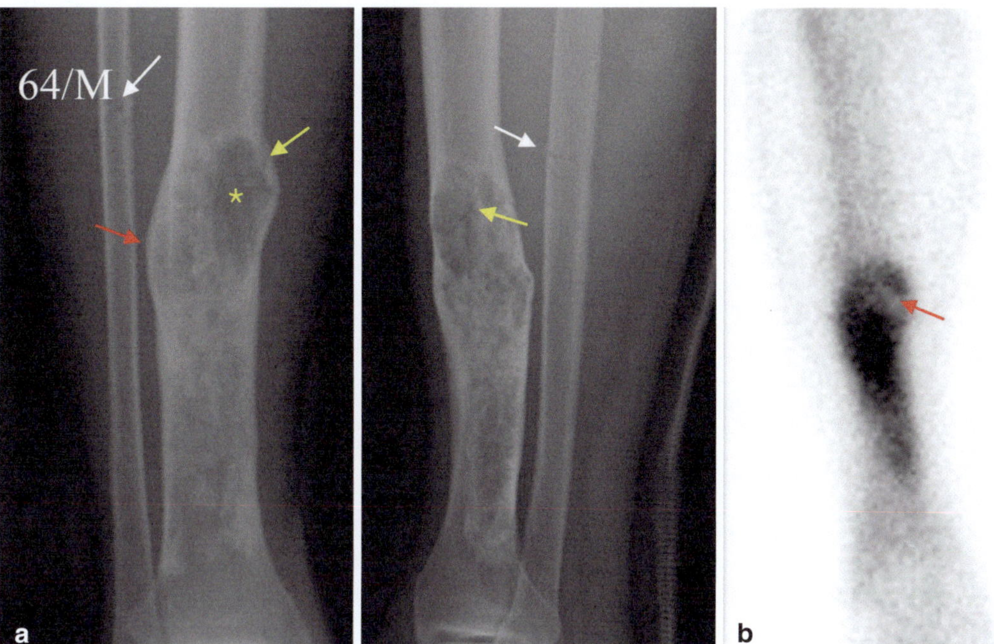

Fig. 28.1 *Classic ADA* (**a**) Radiograph taken for left leg pain with anterior bowing that is aggravated after slip in 64-year-old man shows an elongated large lesion with radiolucent areas (asterisk) and multiple variable sized smaller radiolucent holes with and sclerotic foci of interspersed with normal-appearing bone, so-called *"soap-bubble"* appearance, exclusively involving anterior cortex of the shaft of the tibia. The affected tibia is mildly expanded with mild bowing. The cortex is bulged and markedly thinned without discernible breakage and periosteal reaction (red arrow). There is associated linear fracture line without displacement in the tibia lesion (yellow arrows), suggesting a pathologic fracture as well as in the nonaffected fibular shaft (white arrows). (**b**) Bone scan reveals strong uptake with focal void area (arrow) only in the tibia. (**c**) MR images demonstrate an eccentric expansile intracortical mass-like lesion extending into the medulla cavity (asterisks) with low SI with focal high signals on T1-weighted image and heterogeneous high SI on T2-weighted image. The affected bone is mildly expanded with cortex thinning, endosteal scalloping, and mild bowing but no definite extra-osseous mass formation or periosteal reaction. The lesion is heterogeneously well enhanced by contrast medium. (**d**) Microscopic examination shows scattered conspicuous nests of epithelial-like cells (black arrows) embedded in the bland fibrous stroma with prominent spindle cells arranged in somewhat "*whirling* pattern. There are also variable-sized multiple cyst-like open spaces lined by flattened cells or cuboid cells. The epithelial cells are arranged in combination of mainly basaloid and occasionally tubular pattern, (**e**) IHC stain with cytokeratin reveals keratin-positive cells in solid nests as well as tubular structures. Note prominent anastomosing spaces of vascular channels lined by flattened epithelial cells which are also immunoreactive for keratin. (**f**) Resection specimen shows destructive fleshy tumor lesion (asterisk) with significant cortical erosion and thinning that expands contour of the tibia shaft. There are hemorrhagic areas by linear fracture (arrow). (**g**) Wide resection and reconstruction with allo-strut graft fixed by dual locking plates and auto-chip bone graft around the allo-host bone junction to secure union (yellow arrow) was performed. Fibular osteotomy was simultaneously done for easy position and increased chance of union of allograft by reducing the tension (white arrow). (**h**) Follow-up radiograph at 3 years after surgery shows complete union of host-allograft junction (red arrow) and osteotomized fibula (white arrow) without local recurrence

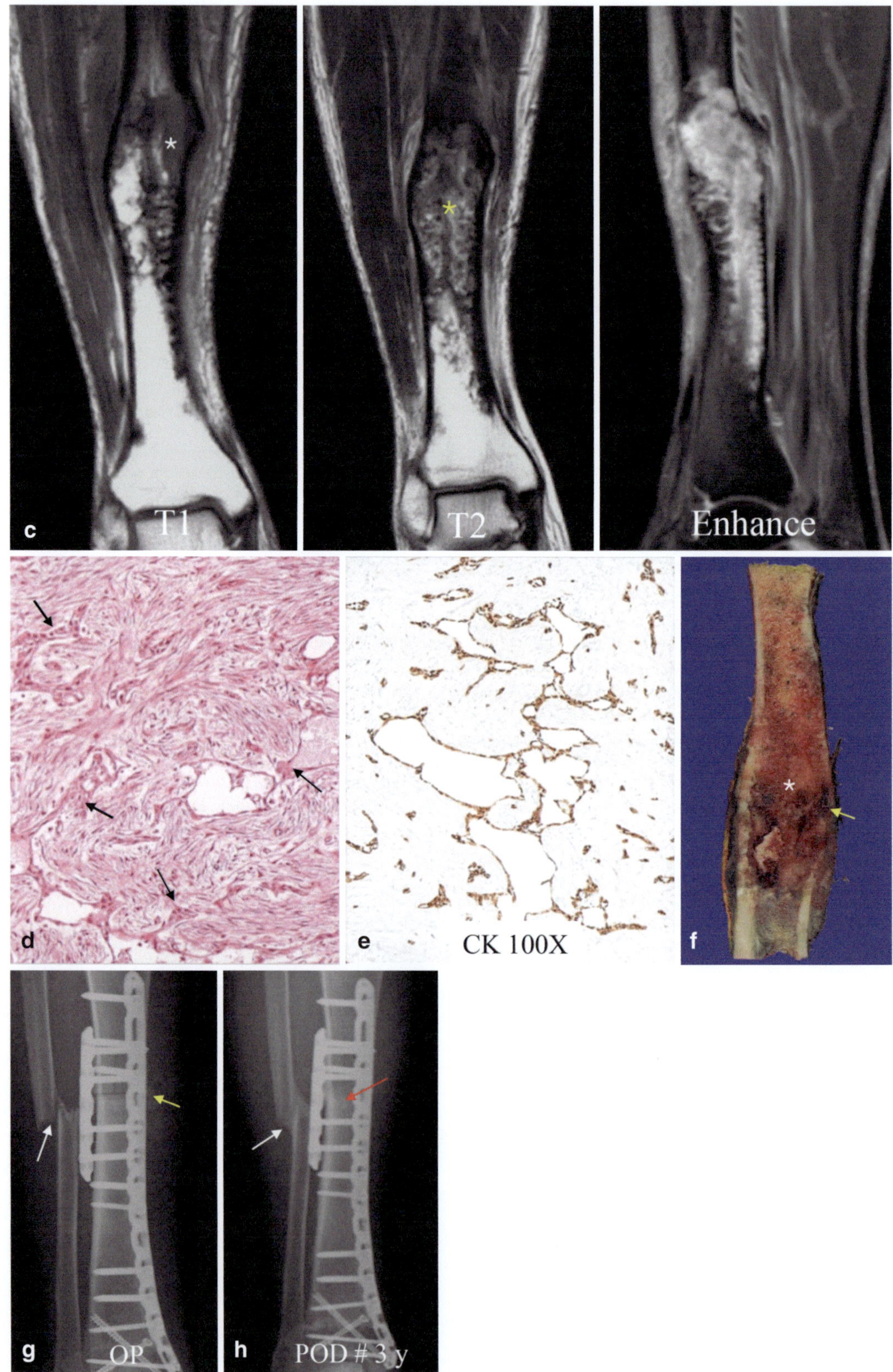

Fig. 28.1 (continued)

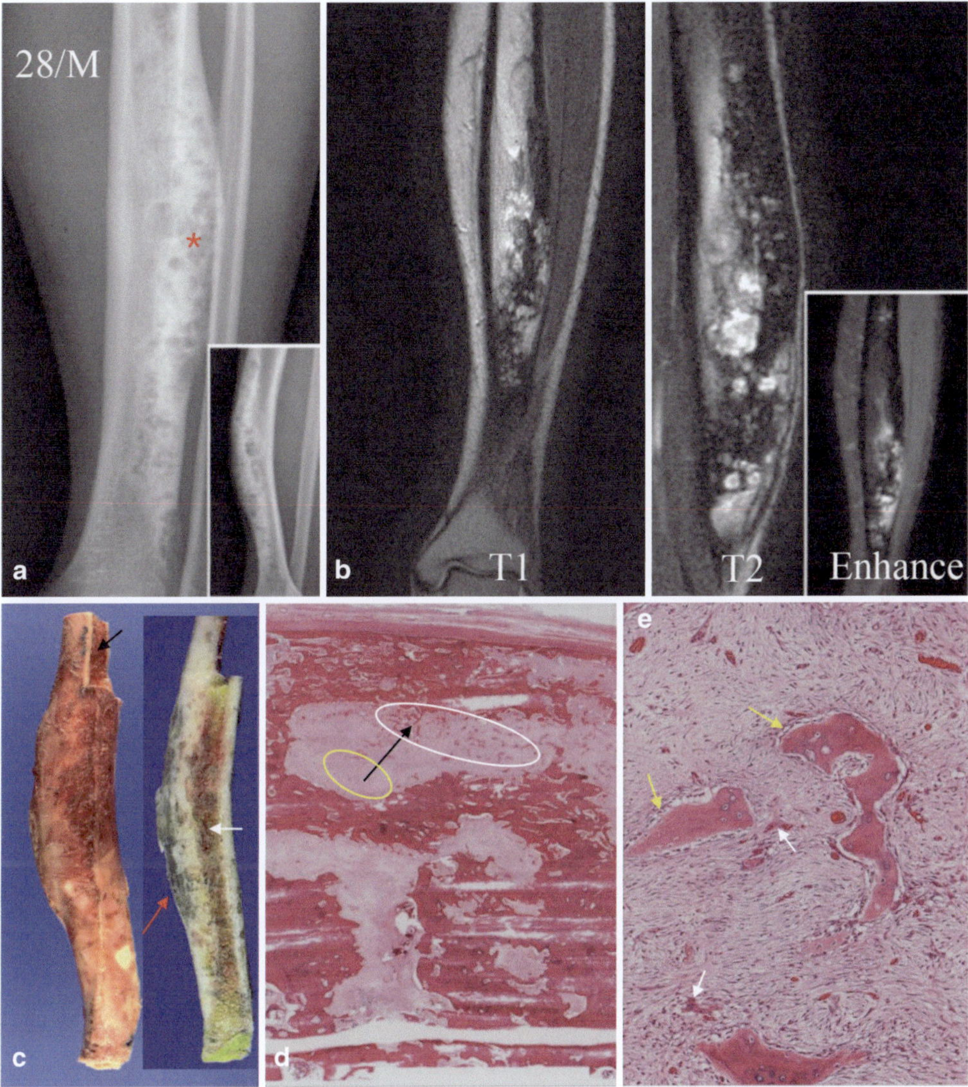

Fig. 28.2 ***OFD-like ADA*** (**a**) Radiograph taken for right leg pain of 5-month duration in 28-year-old man typically shows eccentric, elongated, multiple various sized radiolucent lesions with sclerotic foci, so-called *"soap-bubble" appearance*, mainly in the anterolateral cortex in the distal half of the tibia shaft (asterisk). The involved tibia is laterally expanded with irregularly thickened cortex and sclerotic change but no periosteal reaction. The lesions focally extend into the medullary space. There is marked anterior bowing on lateral view (inset). These findings are indistinguishable from conventional OFD. (**b**) MR images reveal variable-sized multiple lobulated nodules mainly along the anterior cortex of the tibia spreading from the midshaft to the distal metaphysis of the tibia. The SI is heterogeneously mixed low and high on both T1- and T2-weighted images. The intracortical lesion focally extends into the medullary cavity but not into the adjacent soft tissue. The lesion is heterogeneously well enhanced (inset). (**c**) Resection specimen notes destructive fleshy tumor lesion mainly confined to the anterior cortex with significant thickening of the cortex and anterior bowing. There is focal extension of the lesion into the medullary cavity (white arrow) with intact cortex and no evidence of cortical breakage (red arrow). Note proximal step-cut osteotomy (black arrow) to provide a rotation stability of the allograft after fixation. (**d**) Scanning view microscopic examination reveals destructive lesion mostly confined to the cortex. Note a focal area showing a zonal architecture of a central paucity of woven bone trabeculae (yellow circle) with gradual increasing number of progressively matured and mineralized to become lamellar bone toward the periphery (white circle), being reminiscent of de novo OFD (Fig. 8d in OFD chapter in Volume 1). (**e**) Higher-power magnification notes a OFD-like area with woven bone spicules rimmed by osteoblasts (yellow arrows) and inconspicuous small epithelial nests (white arrows), indicating OFD-like ADA. (**f**) IHC stain for keratin shows a few scattered epithelial-like nests (black arrows) in a predominant OFD-like stroma. (**g**) Radiograph at 3 months after wide resection and reconstruction with allograft fixed by dual plates shows good maintenance

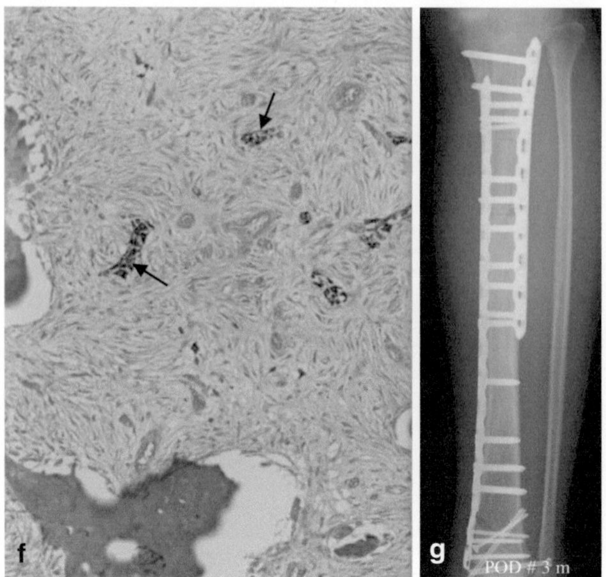

Fig. 28.2 (continued)

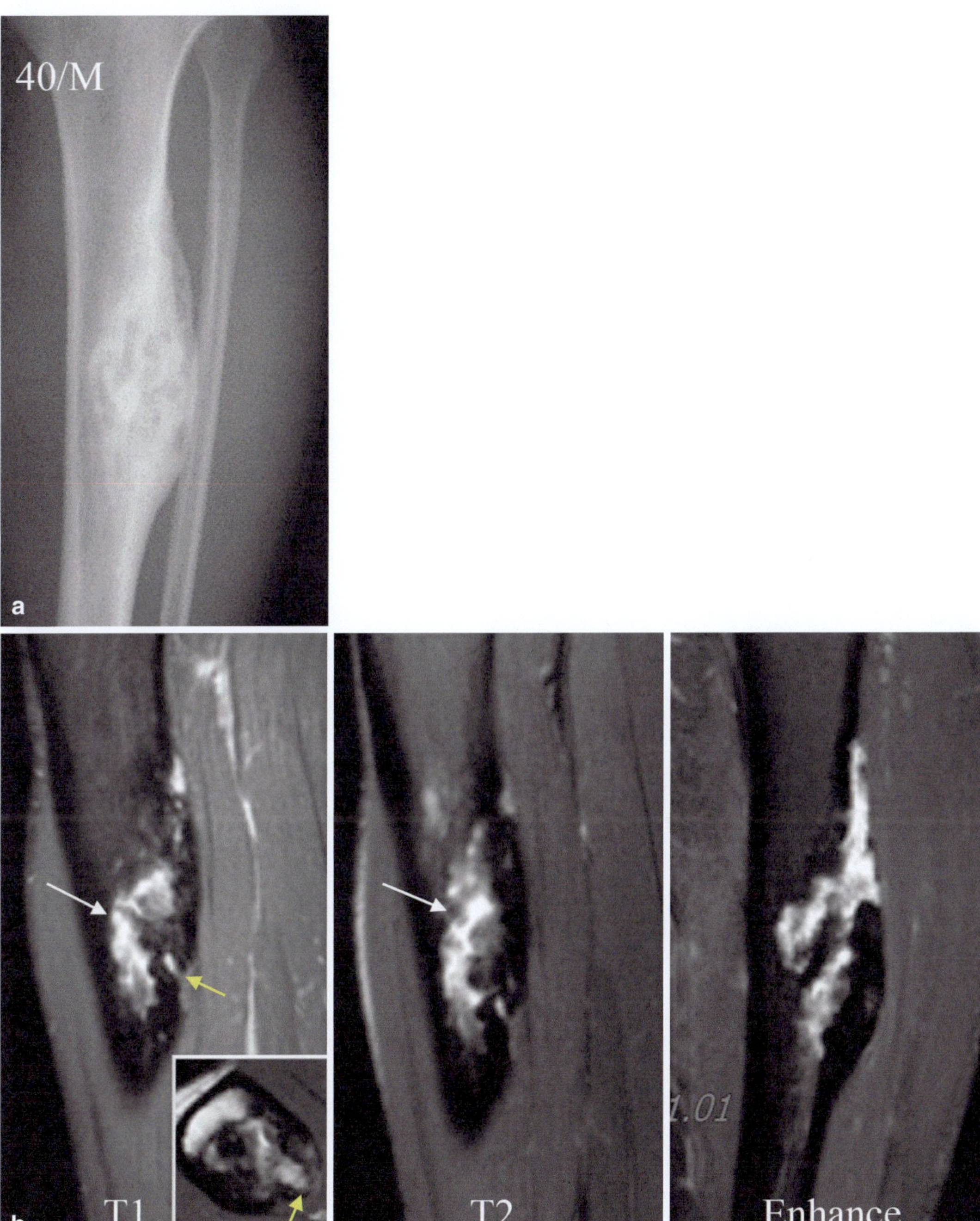

Fig. 28.3 ***OFD-like ADA*** (**a**) Radiograph taken for a hard mass of left leg in 40-year-old man shows cortical-based multiple various sized radiolucent lesions with sclerotic foci mainly confined to the irregularly thickened and sclerotic cortex, which is laterally ballooned and extended into the medullary cavity in the shaft of the proximal tibia. (**b**) MR images demonstrate cortical-based mass lesion significantly extending into the medullary cavity (white arrows) with focal cortical breakage and partial soft tissue extension (yellow arrows). The lesion is homogeneously well enhanced by contrast medium. (**c**) Resection specimen shows that the main cortical lesion (red asterisk) is extending to the medullary space (black asterisk). (**d**) Microscopic examination reveals a predominant OFD-like area of woven bone spicules with osteoblastic rimming (asterisks) as well as a few focal epithelial cell aggregations with inconspicuous to scanty individual epithelial-like cells (arrows). (**e**) The scattered epithelial-like cells are clearly visualized by IHC stain for keratin. (**f**) En-bloc resection and reconstruction using allograft fixed by a plate was performed. (**g**) Follow-up radiograph at 10 years after surgery notes union of the proximal and distal allograft-host junctions (arrows) with no evidence of local recurrence

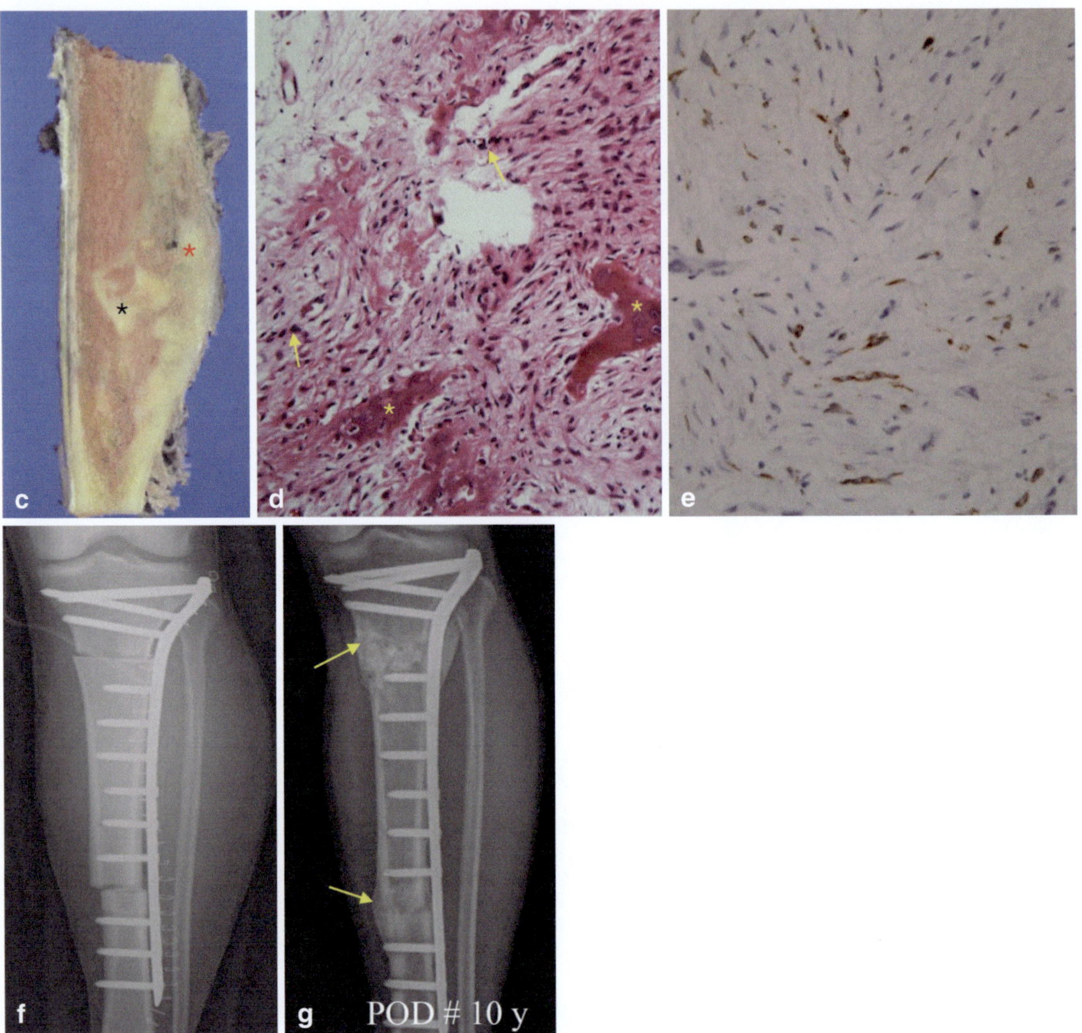

Fig. 28.3 (continued)

28.8 Histologic Findings

ADA is characterized by biphasic histology of *epithelial-like cell aggregation* in various patterns and *bland fibrous or osteofibrous stroma* with various proportions in each case or even each fields of same tumor. The classic ADA is characterized by prominent epithelial-cell component in the center but gradual disappearance toward the smaller peripheral OFD-like areas. The amount of epithelial cells are from prominent (Fig. 28.1d) to inconspicuous tiny to small with dominant fibrous stroma in which cases the epithelial cells are only encountered by careful and scrutinizing search or ICH stains (Fig. 28.2e, f and 28.3d, e). The epithelial nests or islands are variable in size and shape. The stroma cells can be arranged in "*whirling*" pattern with vascular appearing channels. In addition, multinucleated giant cells or foam cells to myxoid change may be occasionally seen. In general, mitotic activity is low. Typically, the principle rounds to oval epithelial-like cells are exhibited with various patterns including *basaloid*, *cord-like or tubular*, *spindle*, *squamous*, and *OFD-like pattern* [11, 22, 23]. (1) The *basaloid pattern* (Fig. 28.1d, 28.4a) is more frequent, and typi-

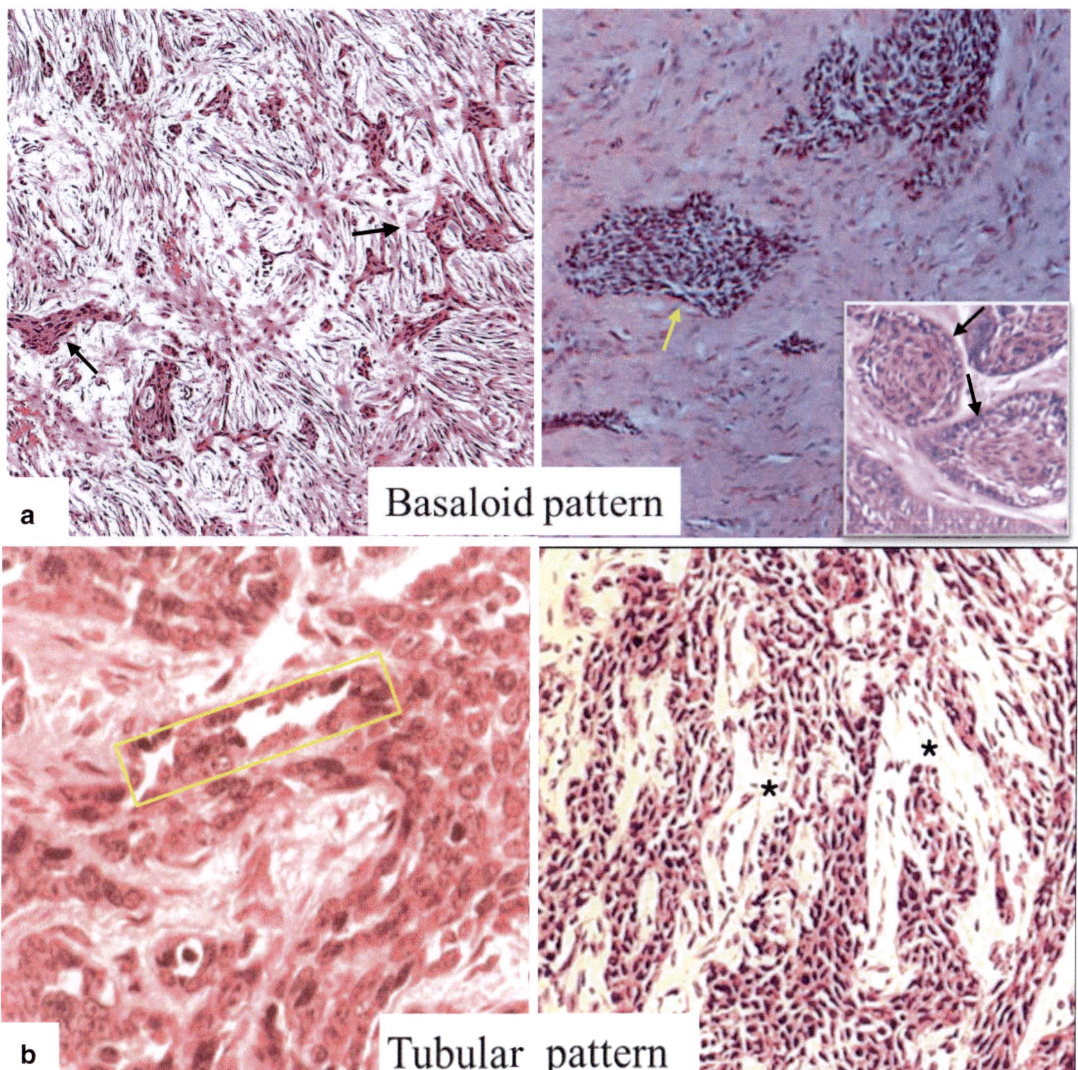

Fig. 28.4 ***Microscopic features*** (**a**) The *Basaloid pattern* is characterized by irregular-shaped nests or island-like aggregation of epithelial cells with peripheral palisading cuboidal basal cells (black arrows) embedded in the bland fibrous stroma, resembling basal cell carcinoma. The stroma cells are arranged in "*whirling*" pattern with prominent cyst-like paces of various size. Higher magnification more clearly shows round to oval epithelial-like cells in the nests (yellow arrow) and the characteristic peripheral palisading arrangement of basaloid epithelial cells (black arrows in inset). (**b**) The *tubular pattern* consists of variable shaped and sized open spaces from small to dilated large size lined by cuboid or flattened cells. Note tubular space lined by cuboid cells in boxcar appearance (yellow box), simulating a metastatic breast carcinoma. You can see also large distended staghorn like tubular spaces (asterisks), resembling hemangioendothelioma. (**c**) The *spindle pattern* mainly consists of bundles of spindle-shaped cells with elongated nuclei arranged in intersecting fascicles "*herringbone*" pattern, resembling a fibrosarcoma. (**d**) The *squamous pattern* demonstrates prickle and keratinized pearls of squamous epithelium focally in the periphery of the tumor nests, resembling a squamous cell carcinoma. (**e**) The *OFD-like pattern* is characterized by predominant OFD-like areas of woven bone spicules with osteoblastic rimming (red arrow) and inconspicuous to scanty epithelial nests (black arrows)

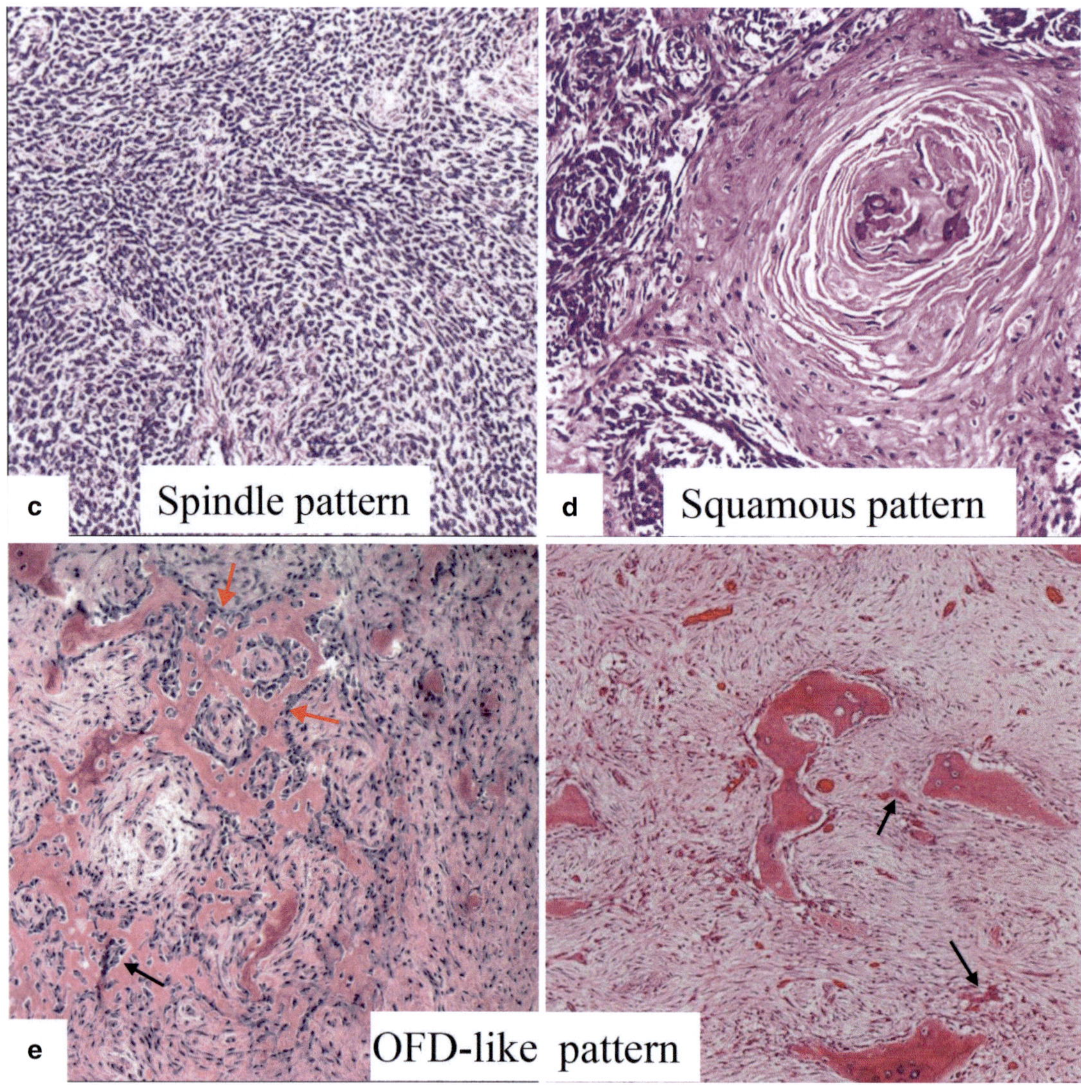

Fig. 28.4 (continued)

cally consists of epithelial nests or islands surrounded by peripheral palisading arrangement of cuboidal basaloid-appearing cells, resembling basal cell carcinoma. There are central micro-cystic structures and stellate-shaped cells reminiscent of the stellate reticulum in ameloblastoma. (2) The *cord-like or tubular pattern* (Fig. 28.4b) is also common and consists of variable-sized gland-like tubular spaces or alveolar cavities lined by cubic or flattened cells arranged in boxcar-like configuration, simulating ductal adenocarcinoma of the breast. Some of the tubular structure may seem to vascular channel mimicking vascular tumor. (3) The *spindle pattern* (Fig. 28.4c) mainly consists of spindle-shaped cells with elongated nuclei arranged in intersecting fascicles or *"storiform"* to "*whirling*" or "*herringbone*" pattern which resembles a fibrosarcoma. (4) The *squamous pattern* (Fig. 28.4d) with prickle and keratinized pearls of squamous epithelium can be focally seen in the periphery of the tumor nests. (5) The *OFD-like pattern* (Figs. 28.2d, e, 28.3d, and 28.4e) is characterized by abundant OFD-like areas of woven bone spicules with predominant osteoblastic rimming but inconspicuous epithelial nests or scattered individual epithelial-like cells which are best visualized by IHC stain for keratin (Figs. 28.2 and 28.3). OFD-like ADA has common feature of OFD with spectrum age in children or young adolescence, slow-growing mass with long history of dull pain and anterior bowing of the tibia, no sign of soft tissue, and intramedullary involvement of the tumor on imaging studies. However, our patients are older adults (Figs. 28.2 and 28.3). The distinction between differentiated (OFD-like) ADA and classic ADA mainly depends on the extent of the epithelial component. A prominent epithelial component with smaller areas of OFD-like woven bone is evident in the classic type. The main feature distinguishing this pattern from OFD-like ADA is the presence of small nests of epithelial cells in the fibroblastic stroma with occasional squamous differentiation. The zonal architecture presenting progressive maturation and increasing numbers of bone trabeculae at the periphery of the lesion can be seen in adequately obtained sample [23]. Over the years, the clinicopathologic spectrum of ADA has been expanded to an extremely rare *dedifferentiated ADA*. Histologically, it is characterized by areas of epithelial differentiation gradually transforming to a diffuse growing pattern of tumor cells with loss of clear epithelial differentiation. The juxtaposed tumor areas consist of highly pleomorphic sarcomatous cells and increased mitotic figures as well as deposition of osteoid or chondroid matrix.

28.9 Management

The standard option for treatment is wide resection and reconstruction using allograft (Figs. 28.1, 28.2 and 28.3) with or without augmented vascularized fibular graft, tumor prosthesis, or distraction osteogenesis. Amputation may be necessary in recurrent lesion or expanded unrespectable lesion.

28.10 Clinical Course

ADA is locally aggressive tumor presenting an indolent clinical course with a potential to spread regional lymph node and metastasizing to lung typically in late during the clinical course. Prognosis is excellent when adequate margin is obtained, but recurrence rate is high after intralesional or marginal excision. Recent study with 92 patients on SEER (the Surveillance, Epidemiology, and End Results) database covering the years between 1975 and 2016 retorted 5- and 10-year survival rates of 98.8% and 91.5%, respectively [33]. The authors also suggested survival time was not related to gender, age group, race, marital status, tumor location, and year of diagnosis. Extremely rarely, ADA may present with sarcomatoid transformation of the epithelial component (*dedifferentiated ADA*), which show more aggressive clinical course [34–36].

References

1. Fisher B. Primary adamantinoma of the tibia. Z Pathol. 1913;12:422–41.
2. Ryrie B. Adamantinoma of the tibia: aetiology and pathogenesis. Br Med J. 1932;2(3752):1000.
3. Dockerty M, Meyerding H. Adamantinoma of the tibia: report of two new cases. JAMA. 1942;119(12):932–7.
4. Lederer H, Sinclair A. Malignant synovioma simulating "adamantinoma of the tibia". J Pathol Bacteriol. 1954;67(1):163–8.
5. Naji A, Murphy J, Stasney R, Neville W, Chrenka P. So-called adamantinoma of long bones: report of a case with massive pulmonary metastasis. J Bone Joint Surg. 1964;46(1):151–8.
6. Changus GW, Speed J, Stewart FW. Malignant angioblastoma of bone. A reappraisal of adamantinoma of long bone. Cancer. 1957;10(3):540–59.
7. Elliott G. Malignant angioblastoma of long bone. J Bone Joint Surg Br. 1962;44(1):25–33.
8. Llombart-Bosch A, Ortuno-Pacheco G. Ultrastructural findings supporting the angioblastic nature of the so-called adamantinoma of the tibia. Histopathology. 1978;2(3):189–200.

9. Reed R. Malignant myxoid angioblastoma of bone. Am J Surg Pathol. 1982;6(2):159–63.
10. Lichtenstein L, editor. Bone tumors. 5th ed. St. Louis, MO: Mosby; 1977. p. 355.
11. Mirra JM. Adamantinoma of long bone. In: Mirra JM, editor. Bone tumors: clinical, radiologic, and pathologic correlation. 2nd ed. Philadelphia, PA: Lea & Febiger; 1989. p. 1204–17.
12. Jaffe HL, editor. Tumors and tumorous conditions of the bones and joints, vol. 34. Phildelphia, PA: Lea & Febiger; 1958. p. 72.
13. Rosai J, Pinkus GS. Immunohistochemical demonstration of epithelial differentiation in adamantinoma of the tibia. Am J Surg Pathol. 1982;6(5):427–34.
14. Ishida T, Iijima T, Kikuchi F, Kitagawa T, Tanida T, Imamura T, et al. A clinicopathological and immunohistochemical study of osteofibrous dysplasia, differentiated adamantinoma, and adamantinoma of long bones. Skeletal Radiol. 1992;21:493–502.
15. Hazelbag HM, Fleuren GJ, Taminiau A, Hogendoorn P. Adamantinoma of the long bones: keratin subclass immunoreactivity pattern with reference to its histogenesis. Am J Surg Pathol. 1993;17(12):1225–33.
16. Jundt G, Remberger K, Roessner A, Schulz A, Bohndorf K. Adamantinoma of long bones: a histopathological and immunohistochemical study of 23 cases. Pathol Res Pract. 1995;191(2):112–20.
17. Moon NF, Mori H. Adamantinoma of the appendicular skeleton--updated. Clin Orthop Relat Res. 1986;(204):215–37. PMID: 3514033.
18. Kitsoulis P, Charchanti A, Paraskevas G, Marini A, Karatzias G. Adamantinoma. Acta Orthop Belg. 2007;73(4):425–31.
19. Puchner S, Varga R, Hobusch G, Kasparek M, Panotopoulos J, Lang S, et al. Long-term outcome following treatment of Adamantinoma and Osteofibrous dysplasia of long bones. Orthop Traumatol Surg Res. 2016;102(7):925–32.
20. Unni KK, Inwards CY. Adamantinoma of long bone. In: Unni KK, Inwards CY, editors. Dahlin's bone tumors: general aspects and data on 10,165 cases. 6th ed. Philadelphia, PA: Lippincott William & Wilkins; 2010. p. 286–94.
21. Van Rijn R, Bras J, Schaap G, Van den Berg H, Maas M. Adamantinoma in childhood: report of six cases and review of the literature. Pediatr Radiol. 2006;36(10):1068–74.
22. Campanacci M. Adamantinoma. In: Campanacci M, editor. Bone and soft tissue tumors. Wien, New York: Springer-Verlag; 1999. p. 721–31.
23. Czerniak B. Adamantinoma of long bone. In: Dorfman HD, Czerniak B, editors. Dorfman and Czerniak's bone tumors. 2nd ed. Amsterdam: Elsevier; 2016. p. 1142–73.
24. Clarke RP, Leonard JR, von Kuster L, Wesseler TA. Adamantinoma of the humerus with early metastases and death: a case report with autopsy findings. Thorofare, NJ: SLACK; 1989. p. 1121–5.
25. Cao K, Susa M, Watanabe I, Nishimoto K, Horiuchi K, Sasaki A, et al. Adamantinoma of the distal femur diagnosed 5 years after initial surgery: a case report. J Med Case Reports. 2016;10(1):1–6.
26. Ulmar B, Delling G, Werner M, Huch K, Reichel H. Classical and atypical location of adamantinomas–presentation of two cases. Oncol Res Treat. 2006;29(6):276–8.
27. Yoshida S, Murakami T, Suzuki K, Itou S, Watanuki M, Hosaka M, et al. Adamantinoma arising in the distal end of the fibula. Rare Tumors. 2017;9(1):14–7.
28. Sherman GM, Damron TA, Yang Y. CD99 positive adamantinoma of the ulna with ipsilateral discrete osteofibrous dysplasia. Clin Orthop Relat Res. 2003;408:256–61.
29. Nerubay J, Chechick A, Horoszowski H, Engelberg S. Adamantinoma of the spine. A case report. J Bone Joint Surg. 1988;70(3):467–9.
30. Chandrasekar C, Mohammed R, Rafalla A, Grimer R. Adamantinoma of the calcaneum—a case report. Foot. 2009;19(1):58–61.
31. Piña-Oviedo S, Del Valle L, Padilla-Longoria R, Mendoza-Ramón H, Ortiz-Hidalgo C. Primary adamantinoma of the rib. Unusual presentation for a bone neoplasm of uncertain origin. Pathol Oncol Res. 2008;14:497–502.
32. Van der Woude HJ, Hazelbag HM, Bloem JL, Taminiau AH, Hogendoorn PC. MRI of adamantinoma of long bones in correlation with histopathology. Am J Roentgenol. 2004;183(6):1737–44.
33. Aytekin MN, Öztürk R, Amer K. Epidemiological study of adamantinoma from US surveillance, epidemiology, and end results program: III retrospective analysis. J Oncol. 2020;2020:1.
34. Hazelbag HM, Laforga JB, Roels HJ, Hogendoorn PC. Dedifferentiated adamantinoma with revertant mesenchymal phenotype. Am J Surg Pathol. 2003;27(12):1530–7.
35. Izquierdo-García FM, Ramos L, Sánchez-Herráez S, Hernández MT, Álava ED. Dedifferentiated classic adamantinoma of the tibia: a report of a case with eventual complete revertant mesenchymal phenotype. Am J Surg Pathol. 2010;34:1388.
36. Nouri H, Jaafoura H, Bouaziz M, Ouertatani M, Abid L, Meherzi M, et al. Dedifferentiated adamantinoma associated with fibrous dysplasia. Orthop Traumatol Surg Res. 2011;97(7):770–5.

MIX
Papier aus verantwortungsvollen Quellen
Paper from responsible sources
FSC® C105338

If you have any concerns about our products,
you can contact us on
ProductSafety@springernature.com

In case Publisher is established outside the EU,
the EU authorized representative is:
Springer Nature Customer Service Center GmbH
Europaplatz 3, 69115 Heidelberg, Germany

Printed by Libri Plureos GmbH
in Hamburg, Germany